Core Topics in Foot and Ankle Surgery

Core Topics in Foot and Ankle Surgery

Edited by

Andrew "Fred" Robinson BSc FRCS (Tr&Orth)
Consultant Orthopaedic Foot and Ankle Surgeon, Cambridge University Hospitals NHS Trust,
Cambridge, UK

James W. Brodsky MD
Clinical Professor of Orthopedic Surgery, University of Texas Southwestern Medical School,
Dallas, TX, USA

John P. Negrine FRACS
Orthopaedic Foot and Ankle Surgeon, Prince of Wales Private Hospital, Sydney, Australia

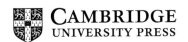

CAMBRIDGE
UNIVERSITY PRESS

CAMBRIDGE
UNIVERSITY PRESS

University Printing House, Cambridge CB2 8BS, United Kingdom

One Liberty Plaza, 20th Floor, New York, NY 10006, USA

477 Williamstown Road, Port Melbourne, VIC 3207, Australia

314–321, 3rd Floor, Plot 3, Splendor Forum, Jasola District Centre, New Delhi – 110025, India

79 Anson Road, #06–04/06, Singapore 079906

Cambridge University Press is part of the University of Cambridge.

It furthers the University's mission by disseminating knowledge in the pursuit of education, learning and research at the highest international levels of excellence.

www.cambridge.org
Information on this title: www.cambridge.org/9781108418935
DOI: 10.1017/9781108292399

First published 2018

Printed in the United Kingdom by Clays, St Ives plc

A catalogue record for this publication is available from the British Library

ISBN 978-1-108-41893-5 Hardback

Cambridge University Press has no responsibility for the persistence or accuracy of URLs for external or third-party internet websites referred to in this publication, and does not guarantee that any content on such websites is, or will remain, accurate or appropriate.

....

Every effort has been made in preparing this book to provide accurate and up-to-date information which is in accord with accepted standards and practice at the time of publication. Although case histories are drawn from actual cases, every effort has been made to disguise the identities of the individuals involved. Nevertheless, the authors, editors and publishers can make no warranties that the information contained herein is totally free from error, not least because clinical standards are constantly changing through research and regulation. The authors, editors and publishers therefore disclaim all liability for direct or consequential damages resulting from the use of material contained in this book. Readers are strongly advised to pay careful attention to information provided by the manufacturer of any drugs or equipment that they plan to use.

Contents

Contributors

Rami J. Abboud PhD HonFRCS(Eng)
Professor and Head of Department of Orthopaedic & Trauma Surgery, Director of Institute of Motion Analysis & Research (IMAR), and Associate Dean for Learning & Teaching, School of Medicine, University of Dundee, Dundee, Scotland, UK

Thomas A. Ball MA MRCP FRCS (Tr&Orth)
Consultant Orthopaedic Surgeon, Torbay Hospital, Torquay, Devon, UK

Cameron R. Barr MD
Department of Orthopaedic Surgery, Scripps Clinic, La Jolla, California, USA

Chris M. Blundell BMedSci MD FRCS (Tr&Orth)
Consultant Orthopaedic Surgeon, Sheffield Teaching Hospitals NHS Foundation Trust, Sheffield, UK

Hilary A. Bosman
Consultant Orthopaedic Surgeon, Broomfield Hospital, Chelmsford, UK

Timothy W. R. Briggs MCh FRCSEd FRCS
Professor of Orthopaedic Surgery, Royal National Orthopaedic Hospital NHS Trust, Brockley Hill Stanmore, Middlesex, UK

James W. Brodsky MD
Clinical Professor of Orthopaedic Surgery, University of Texas Southwestern Medical School, Texas, USA

James Brousil
Fellow in Foot and Ankle Surgery, Cambridge University Hospitals NHS Trust, Cambridge, UK

James D. F. Calder MD FRCS (Tr&Orth) FFSEM
Consultant Orthopaedic Surgeon, The Fortius Clinic, London, UK

Andrew Carne FRCR
Royal Surrey County Hospital, Guildford, UK

Paul H. Cooke ChM FRCS
Consultant Orthopaedic Foot and Ankle Surgeon, Nuffield Orthopaedic Centre, Headington, Oxford, UK

Matthew Costa
Professor of Orthopaedic Trauma, Oxford Trauma, NDORMS, University of Oxford, The Kadoorie Centre, John Radcliffe Hospital, Oxford, UK

Timothy A. Coughlin BMBS BMedSci
Specialist Registrar, Queen's Medical Centre, Nottingham, UK

Nicholas Cullen FRCS (Tr&Orth)
Consultant Orthopaedic Foot and Ankle Surgeon, Royal National Orthopaedic Hospital NHS Trust, Brockley Hill, Stanmore, Middlesex, UK

Mark B. Davies FRCS (Tr&Orth)
Consultant Orthopaedic Surgeon, Sheffield Teaching Hospitals NHS Foundation Trust, Sheffield, UK

Mark S. Davies FRCS (Tr&Orth)
London Foot and Ankle Centre, London, UK

Orla Doody MRCPI FFRRCSI
Consultant Radiologist, Department of Radiology, Tallaght Hospital, Dublin, Ireland

Panagiotis D. Gikas FRCS (Tr&Orth)
Consultant Orthopaedic and Sarcoma Surgeon, Sarcoma Unit, Royal National Orthopaedic Hospital NHS Trust, Brockley Hill, Stanmore, Middlesex, UK

Daniel Z. Goldbloom
Orthopaedic Foot and Ankle Surgeon, The Alfred and Dandenong Hospitals, Melbourne, Australia

Fraser Harrold PhD FRCSEd (Tr&Orth)
Consultant in Foot & Ankle Surgery, Orthopaedic Department, Ninewells Hospital & Medical School, Dundee, Scotland, UK

Melanie A. Hopper MRCS FRCR
Consultant Musculoskeletal Radiologist, Cambridge University Hospitals NHS Trust, Cambridge, UK

Rebecca Kearney
Associate Professor of Trauma and Orthopaedic Rehabilitation (Clinical), University of Warwick, Coventry, UK

Stephen G. B. Kirker FRCP FRCPI
Consultant in Rehabilitation Medicine, Cambridge University Hospitals NHS Trust, Cambridge, UK

Caroline J. Lever FRCS (Tr&Orth)
Fellow in Foot and Ankle Surgery, Cambridge University Hospitals NHS Trust, Cambridge, UK

Ruairi F. MacNiocaill
Consultant Orthopaedic & Foot and Ankle Surgeon, University Hospital Waterford, Waterford, Ireland

John P. Negrine FRACS
Orthopaedic Foot and Ankle Surgeon, Prince of Wales Private Hospital, Sydney, Australia

Paul O'Donnell MA MD FRCP
Consultant Musculoskeletal Radiologist, Royal National Orthopaedic Hospital NHS Trust, Brockley Hill, Stanmore, Middlesex, UK

Ben J. Ollivere MA MRCS
Clinical Associate Professor, Queen's Medical Centre, Nottingham, UK

Jonathan S. Palmer FRCS (Tr&Orth)
Orthopaedic Registrar, Royal National Orthopaedic Hospital NHS Trust, Brockley Hill, Stanmore, Middlesex, UK

Lee Parker FRCS (Tr&Orth)
Consultant Orthopaedic Foot and Ankle Surgeon, St Bartholomew's Health NHS Trust, London, UK

Stephen W. Parsons
Consultant Orthopaedic Foot and Ankle Surgeon, Royal Cornwall Hospital, Truro, Cornwall, UK

Steven M. Raikin MD
Professor of Orthopaedic Surgery and Director of Foot and Ankle Service, Rothman Institute at Thomas Jefferson University Hospital, Philadelphia, USA

Anthony I. Riccio MD
Associate Professor of Orthopaedic Surgery, University of Texas Southwestern Medical Center, Dallas, TX, USA

James F. S. Ritchie FRCS (Tr&Orth)
Consultant Orthopaedic Foot and Ankle Surgeon, The Tunbridge Wells Hospital, Royal Tunbridge Wells, Kent, UK

Andrew "Fred" Robinson BSc FRCS (Tr&Orth)
Consultant Orthopaedic Foot and Ankle Surgeon, Cambridge University Hospitals NHS Trust, Cambridge, UK

Andrew J. Roche MSC FRCS (Tr&Orth)
Consultant Orthopaedic Surgeon, Chelsea and Westminster Hospital, London, UK

Bruce Sangeorzan
Professor, Department of Orthopedics and Sports Medicine, University of Washington, Harborview Medical Center, Seattle, WA, USA

Terence S. Saxby FRCS (Tr&Orth)
Orthopaedic Foot and Ankle Surgeon, Brisbane Private Hospital, Brisbane, Australia

Lew C. Schon MD
Department of Orthopaedic Surgery, The MedStar Union Memorial Hospital, Baltimore, MD, USA

Dishan Singh
Consultant Orthopaedic Surgeon, Royal National Orthopaedic Hospital NHS Trust, Brockley Hill, Stanmore, Middlesex, UK

Matthew C. Solan FRCS (Tr&Orth)
Royal Surrey County Hospital, Guildford, UK

Daniel Thuillier
Assistant Professor of Clinical Orthopaedics,
University of California San Francisco, San Francisco,
CA, USA

Ian G. Winson
Consultant Orthopaedic and Trauma Surgeon
with a Special Interest in Foot and Ankle Surgery,
Brunel Building, Southmead Hospital, Bristol, UK

Brian S. Winters MD
Assistant Professor of Orthopaedic Surgery,
The Rothman Institute, Egg Harbor Township,
NJ, USA

Jacob R. Zide MD
Clinical Assistant Professor of Orthopaedic Surgery,
University of Texas Southwestern Medical School,
Texas, USA

Preface

Editing a book of this nature is a vast amount of work. Is it necessary or worthwhile? This is a question we have asked ourselves repeatedly over the last couple of years – obviously we believe the answer is yes – absolutely yes. In the modern world there is a plethora of information, peer edited, reviewed, appraised, but often not. The aim of this book is to provide expert opinion, a sound rock upon which a new foot and ankle surgeon is able to base his or her practice. While (too) much information is freely available on the internet, the challenge is determining the authority of its source and the authenticity of its content. We have gathered experts to offer "advice" that is reliable, tested, and from true authorities in the field. For those of you who are more experienced, hopefully this distillate will at times confirm your practice, but at other times challenge it, and make you think. We know that in editing we have learned a great deal!

To this end, the assembled group of experts have not only reviewed the literature, but have experience of foot and ankle surgery at the coal face, where they have refined their knowledge to enable them to more effectively and better treat their patients. We hope that this will not only help you to pass exams, if you are not already past that stage, but also better understand foot and ankle pathology and treatment in order to better treat patients. We are grateful to all who have contributed to this book for taking the time to share their experience and wisdom.

We also hope that in turn you are able to hone the principles here outlined, to further improve and develop treatments to improve patient outcomes.

We are all very grateful to Cambridge University Press and, in particular, Jade Scard and Nick Dunton, for their hard work not only in bringing the written word to publication, but also for their encouragement and persistence in what has been a rather longer project than it should have been!

Some individual thanks are of course due:

AHNR: I am very grateful to all who have helped me over the years, not least my two co-editors in this book, and my various fellows and registrars, many of whose names appear in the list of contributors. They have all been unstintingly supportive and, although they may not realise it, they have helped shaped my practice. We all work in a multidisciplinary environment these days, and two very special nurses have been central to me and my patients' welfare: a huge thanks to Jeannette Key and Moira Burgham. Of course, this sort of project is not only undertaken at work. I would like to particularly thank Jane and Alex who have tolerated my "popping off to do a bit of editing" in the evening, in the morning, at weekends, and even on holidays! I am very grateful that they understand, or at least tolerate, the madness that is an orthopedic surgeon.

JWB: Kudos and thanks to Andrew "Fred" Robinson, who conceived of this project, has been the power behind it, and has guided it at every step along the way. Thanks to our co-editor, John Negrine, who is a source of perpetual good sense and wise surgical reasoning. And eternal thanks to Dr. Cynthia Schneidler, a beacon of medical judgment and good advice.

JN: I'd like to thank Andrew "Fred" Robinson for his amazing patience in taking on the important task of writing this book; Jim Brodsky, my mentor, friend, and inspiration in foot and ankle surgery; and my fellows, especially Daniel Goldbloom, for their camaraderie and intellectual stimulation. Special thanks to my wife Dr. JoAnn See and my three boys, Louis, Charles, and Joseph, for their acceptance of an orthopedic father.

Abbreviations

AAOS	American Academy of Orthopaedic Surgeons	**IOL**	interosseous ligament of the ankle syndesmosis
ABC	aneurysmal bone cyst	**IOM**	interosseous membrane of the ankle syndesmosis
ABI	ankle–brachial index		
AFO	ankle foot orthosis	**ITL**	inferior transverse ligament
AITFL	anterior inferior tibiofibular ligament of the ankle syndesmosis	**MMP**	matrix metalloprotease enzyme
		MTPJ	metatarsophalangeal joint
AOFAS	American Orthopaedic Foot and Ankle Society	**NSAID**	non-steroidal anti-inflammatory drug
		ORIF	open reduction and internal fixation
AP	anteroposterior	**PASA**	proximal articular set angle (= DMAA)
ATFL	anterior talofibular ligament	**PB**	peroneus brevis
ATRS	Achilles Tendon Total Rupture Score	**PIPJ**	proximal interphalangeal joint
		P(I)TFL	posterior (inferior) talofibular ligament of the ankle syndesmosis
AVN	avascular necrosis		
CAM	controlled ankle motion	**PL**	peroneus longus
CFL	calcaneofibular ligament	**POPS**	painful os peroneum syndrome
CMT	Charcot–Marie–Tooth	**PQ**	peroneus quartus
COM	center of mass	**PRP**	platelet-rich plasma
CROW	Charcot restraint orthotic walker	**PTFL**	posterior talofibular ligament
CRP	C reactive protein	**PTT**	posterior tibial tendon
CTEV	congenital talipes equinovarus (clubfoot)	**PTTD**	posterior tibial tendon dysfunction
		RA	rheumatoid arthritis
DIPJ	distal interphalangeal joint	**RCT**	randomized controlled trial
DMAA	distal metatarsal articular angle (= PASA)	**RICE**	rest, ice, compression, and elevation
		SACH	solid ankle and cushioned heel
EDB	extensor digitorum brevis	**SPECT-CT**	single-photon emission computed tomography
EDL	extensor digitorum longus		
EHB	extensor hallucis brevis	**SPR**	superior peroneal retinaculum
EHL	extensor hallucis longus	**STIR**	short-tau inversion recovery
ESR	erythrocyte sedimentation rate	**TA**	tendo Achillis (Achilles tendon)
ESWT	extra-corporeal shockwave therapy	**TAA**	total ankle arthroplasty
FDL	flexor digitorum longus	**TGF-β**	transforming growth factor β
FHB	flexor hallucis brevis	**TIMP**	tissue inhibitors of matrix metalloprotease enzymes
FHL	flexor hallucis longus		
GCT	giant cell-rich tumor	**TMTJ**	tarsometatarsal joint
GRS	ground reaction force	**TNJ**	talonavicular joint
GTN	glyceryl trinitrate	**TTA**	trans-tibial amputation
HMSN	hereditary motor and sensory neuropathy	**TTC**	tibiotalocalcaneal
		UCBL	University of California Biomechanics Laboratory (orthosis)
HVA	hallux valgus angle		
IGF-1	insulin like growth factor-1	**USS**	ultrasound scan
IMA	intermetatarsal angle	**WHO**	World Health Organization

Clinical Examination of the Foot and Ankle

Hilary A. Bosman and Andrew "Fred" Robinson

Introduction

Accurate history taking and examination of the foot and ankle are the cornerstones of diagnosis; in turn diagnosis underpins treatment. The complexity of the bony and soft tissue anatomy of the foot and ankle means that modern imaging is no substitute for clinical examination. In some patients pathology is present but not the cause of symptoms; in others, where the imaging technique lacks sensitivity, imaging will miss subtle lesions. For example, in some countries or institutions, ultrasound (US) scanning is preferred over magnetic resonance imaging (MRI) for imaging tendons.

The aim of this chapter is to give you a method that is reliable in clinical practice, as well as under exam conditions. We have divided the examination into "general," which is undertaken on each patient, and "specific," which is aimed at teasing out a specific diagnosis. It is important to bear in mind that foot and ankle pathology is often secondary to systemic disease, for example diabetes mellitus or a hereditary sensorimotor neuropathy. Furthermore the outcome of surgery is closely linked to neurological and vascular pathology. For this reason careful attention and documentation of these systems is mandatory.

If you learn nothing else from this chapter you should remember that knowledge of the surface anatomy is paramount, as diagnosis is related to the precise location of pain and tenderness. Even if the patient has more than one site of tenderness, establishing the region of maximal tenderness will usually yield a differential diagnosis of one or two possibilities, which can be clarified by imaging. We emphasize a simple request to the patient, "point with one finger to where you feel the pain worst." Some patients will wave the hand over an ill-defined broad area of the foot. They should be encouraged to point with a *single finger* to the precise site of the pain – if they are unable to localize their pain precisely this raises the possibility that the pain is "non-surgical,"

for example it may be neurogenic or secondary to a complex regional pain syndrome.

Alternatively the patient may have more than one pathology. In these cases the patient is encouraged to point to the different areas of pain, and quantify the level of pain in the different areas. Thus ask the patient where the most painful area is. The patient is then told that if this area of pain has a severity of ten out of ten, how painful, on the same scale, is the second area? Thus in a patient with two areas of pain at level of ten and eight, both areas should be carefully assessed. Whereas if one area has a severity of ten, and the other of three, it is likely that the lower scoring area is not of such importance, and will settle spontaneously once the primary pathology has been treated.

Descriptive Terms

Understanding descriptive terms is necessary for communication, spot diagnoses, and linking pathologies.

cavus	A hollow or high-arched foot. Associated with varus hindfoot position "cavovarus."
planus	A flat foot – the opposite of cavus. Associated with valgus hindfoot position "planovalgus."
equinus	Flexion of the foot relative to the tibia.
varus	Describes the position of the distal segment, which inclines toward the midline, from proximal to distal.
forefoot varus	Describes a forefoot where the first metatarsal is elevated relative to the fifth metatarsal, i.e., the forefoot is supinated.
adduction	Deviation toward the midline in the horizontal plane. Most commonly used for the mid and forefoot, for example metatarsus adductus.

valgus	Describes the position of the distal segment, being away from the midline relative to the proximal. Most commonly used for the hindfoot.
forefoot valgus	Describes a forefoot where the first metatarsal is lower than the fifth metatarsal, i.e., the forefoot is pronated.
abduction	Similar to valgus, to denote deviation away from the midline in the horizontal plane. Most commonly used for the mid and forefoot.
supination	Complex movement of the foot and ankle composed of inversion, adduction, and plantar flexion. The principal axis is through the talonavicular joint.
pronation	Opposite of supination with eversion, abduction, and dorsiflexion.
plantaris	Plantar flexion of the forefoot, relative to the hindfoot, also called forefoot equinus.
calcaneus	Dorsiflexion of the ankle, the opposite of equinus.

History

The clinical history provides the diagnosis in approximately 75% of general medical patients, there is little to suggest that diagnosis in the foot and ankle is any different. Listen to the patient, "if you only ask questions you will only receive answers in reply[1]." Take a focused history; it will lead to a focused examination.

It is important to take a thorough history, in particular with regards to pain – where is the pain? Is there a history of trauma? How long has the pain been present? Is the pain burning or felt at night? The last is suggestive of neurological pain, which is not an uncommon finding. Early morning and start-up heel pain is characteristic of plantar fasciitis. Instability and giving way should also be noted.

It is important to establish if the patient has a history of arthropathy, psoriasis, skin rashes, vascular disease, neurological disease, or diabetes mellitus.

Smoking cigarettes has been associated with higher non-union and complication rates in foot and ankle surgery, and should be noted.

Enquire what treatments patients have already tried and what the patient is prepared to try. If she

has had physiotherapy, what did the treatment consist of? Exercises? Stretches? "Show me what the physiotherapist taught you," is often a good indicator of their experience.

The use of orthoses and shoe modification should be recorded.

Finding out a patient's expectations is key to being able to meet their expectations. For example, a builder who walks on rough ground and uses ladders extensively is going to have more limitations in his day-to-day activities, following an ankle fusion, than an individual who wishes to walk to the shops and back.

General Examination

Setting and Equipment

The examination should take part in a quiet, well-lit room. There should be available space to observe the patient walking for approximately ten meters. An adjustable examination couch and two chairs should be provided. Examination can usually take place with exposure to the knee, but facility to undertake a full examination should be available. Repetition will lead to a slick technique (Box 1.1).

Special equipment required:

A goniometer.

A hand-held Doppler is useful to assess the vascularity, where pulses cannot be felt.

A 5.07/10 gram Semmes–Weinstein monofilament is a cheap and excellent way of screening for peripheral neuropathy. The monofilament is pressed perpendicular to the skin in five locations until it buckles, it should be held in place each time

---

Box 1.1 Tips for slick examination technique

- Ask the patient to roll up their trousers, not push them up – they will fall down!
- Kneel when observing the patient standing. Ask the patient to turn rather than moving around the patient – it is more efficient.
- Make sure to look at the shoes and orthoses.
- When asking the patient to perform a single-leg heel raise, ask them to stand facing a wall, the vertical surface can be used for balance but not assistance.
- Always examine the patient standing and walking.
- Note any aids.

for about one second and then released. The patient is asked to confirm they can feel the monofilament and the location.

Standing blocks are also essential, both to assess leg length and for undertaking the Coleman block test (see "Special Tests" section).

Tuning fork 128 Hz or biothesiometer. The biothesiometer or neurothesiometer is a simple handheld device that gives semi-quantitative assessment of vibration perception threshold.

Look

The foot can be considered as a tripod. The three legs of the tripod are the calcaneum, the head of the first metatarsal, and the head of the fifth metatarsal. Hindfoot valgus is associated with planus deformity while varus is associated with cavus. The flat foot has a more equal distribution of pressure and therefore is likely to have fewer callosities (areas of thickened skin secondary to high pressure). The cavovarus foot induces higher point pressures and consequently callosities – these will characteristically be under the three "legs" of the tripod – namely the heel, and the first and fifth metatarsal heads. Different kinds of symptoms are seen in cavovarus, compared to planovalgus feet, especially in active or athletic individuals in whom the cavovarus foot is far more symptomatic than the planovalgus. There are a number of common foot pathologies associated with each foot type (Table 1.1).

Examination of Gait, Aids, and Shoes

Observe whether the patient has walking aids and take the opportunity to ask whether they use walking aids during day-to-day life.

Take the insoles out of the shoe and look at them. Have they ever been used or worn just for your benefit? Similarly, has the patient's heel ever contacted the inside of the ankle foot orthosis (AFO)?

What type of shoes does the patient like wearing? Are they the correct fit? Look at the wear pattern on the sole and damage to the upper and any insole as a static imprint of their gait pattern.

Static Inspection

Weight bearing can exacerbate deformity; therefore assessment with the foot in its functional position – standing – is important. Pay attention to the general

Table 1.1 Typical pathologies seen with the principal foot morphologies

Cavovarus foot[2]	Planovalgus foot
ankle instability	hallux valgus
subtalar instability	hallux rigidus
symptomatic os trigonum	tibialis posterior dysfunction
peroneal tendon pathology/tear	spring ligament attenuation/rupture
enlarged peroneal tubercle	midfoot arthritis
painful os peroneum syndrome	peroneal tendon impingement
stress fracture of fourth or fifth metatarsal	ankle instability
sesamoid overload	valgus ankle arthritis
plantar fasciitis	anterior knee pain
vertical stress fracture of medial malleolus	genu valgum
metatarsus adductus	
midfoot arthritis	
varus ankle arthritis	
medial compartment knee arthritis	
iliotibial band friction syndrome	
tibial stress fracture	
exertional compartment syndrome	
tight gastrocnemius	

alignment, rotation, and foot position. Asymmetry and evidence of leg-length discrepancy should be noted.

Look from the side and posteriorly with the patient standing. The hindfoot has a normal valgus of around 5°, in the normal foot this will correct to varus on heel raising (Figure 1.1).

Hindfoot and forefoot positions should be noted independently. One first notes the hindfoot varus or valgus with the patient standing. Then with the patient seated the talonavicular joint is brought into neutral (see below), and the forefoot position is noted. If deformity is present it is important to note whether it is fixed and uncorrectable, or flexible and correctable.

As outlined in the introduction, a thorough understanding of the surface anatomy is key to examination of the foot and ankle. Three-dimensional osteology and surface markings are best appreciated

(a)

(b)

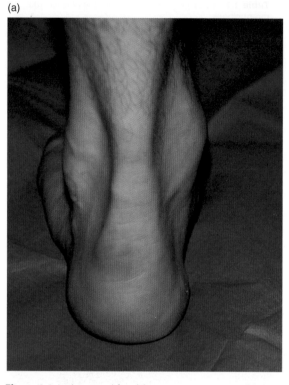
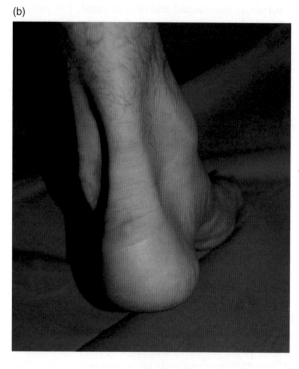

Figure 1.1 In the normal foot **(a)**, on going onto tip toe **(b)** the arch elevates and the heel moves into varus on raising.

by repeated examination comparing the "normal" to "abnormal" (Figure 1.2).

Next, look at the color and quality of the soft tissues. Is the skin woody, hard, or shiny? Is there hair growth? Bare, atrophic skin is a sign of poor vascular supply; coarse hair with shiny skin may be an indicator of a complex regional pain syndrome. Swellings and scars should be recorded.

Look for pressure areas over the dorsum from ill-fitting shoes and callosities of the sole indicating regions of overload.

Finally, check between the toes for soft corns and the condition of the nails.

Gait

While analysis of gait is part of the examination of movement, it is easier to watch the patient before they sit down, as opposed to asking them to stand and walk later. Ask the patient to walk, both in shoes and barefoot. Kneel down to give yourself a level view. Make sure to look from the front, side, and behind.

If the gait type has a specific pattern – describe it (Table 1.2). Otherwise break down the gait cycle to

assess for rhythm, swing and stance phase, overall alignment, and proximal joint movements. Then look specifically at the foot alignment, and point of contact and push off.

Perry[3] described the three "rockers of gait." It helps to consider the subdivisions of the stance phase when observing the patient walk:

Heel rocker: From initial contact of the heel to foot flat, the foot decelerates as a result of eccentric contraction of tibialis anterior and the long toe extensors. The heel rocker may be abnormal in the presence of a tight tendo Achillis (failure of heel strike) or weak tibialis anterior (poor control and a slapping foot).

Ankle rocker: From foot flat to heel rise with controlled forward progression of body weight over the fixed foot. The triceps surae contracts eccentrically while the tibialis anterior is quiet. This rocker is abnormal with ankle pathology and stiffness.

Forefoot rocker: From heel rise to toe off. Gastrocnemius is the prime mover. This rocker is abnormal if the triceps surae is weak or there is forefoot pathology, such as hallux rigidus.

Table 1.2 Abnormal gait patterns

Common gait pattern terminology	Definition
Antalgic gait	Painful gait; asymmetric rhythm with less time spent on the affected, painful limb.
Hemiplegic gait	The patient has a unilateral weakness on the affected side, arm flexed, adducted, and internally rotated. The ipsilateral lower limb is in extension with plantar flexion of the foot and toes (equinus). When walking the patient holds his/her arm to their side and circumducts the foot.
Diplegic gait	Secondary to hypertonicity. The patient walks with an abnormally narrow base, dragging both legs and scraping the toes. The hip adductors may also be tight causing the legs to cross the midline, producing a "scissoring" gait. Fixed flexion at the hip and knee may also be present.
High stepping/foot-drop gait	Active dorsiflexion of the foot is weak. The foot may drag or is lifted clear of the floor through the swing phase with additional hip and knee flexion. Causes include proximal (spinal) and distal neurology with deep peroneal nerve dysfunction.

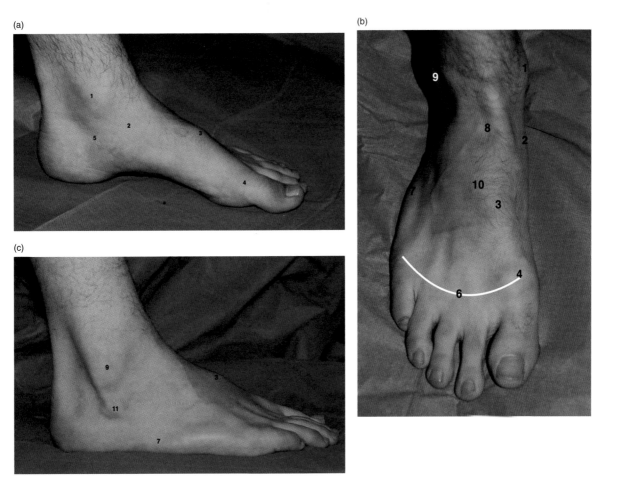

Figure 1.2 The bony landmarks of the foot and ankle. (1) medial malleolus; (2) navicular tuberosity; (3) first tarsometatarsal joint; (4) first metatarsophalangeal joint; (5) sustentaculum tali; (6) metatarsophalangeal joint parabola; (7) base of fifth metatarsal; (8) talonavicular joint; (9) lateral malleolus; (10) second tarsometatarsal joint; (11) peroneal tubercle.

Table 1.3 Gage's prerequisites for normal gait cycle: (4) and (5) relate to the foot

1	Energy conservation
2	Adequate step length
3	Sufficient foot clearance
4	Appropriate pre-positioning of the foot in swing phase
5	Stability in stance

An adequately functioning foot and ankle are essential for two of Gage's five prerequisites for a normal gait cycle (Table 1.3)[4].

The midtarsal and subtalar joints are inter-related and influence one another. When the talonavicular and calcaneocuboid joints are in a valgus position they are parallel, and the midfoot is supple; when they are in a varus position they are divergent and, consequently, the foot is stiff. These interactions in the hindfoot allow two foot morphologies. Firstly, from heel rocker through ankle rocker, with the subtalar joint everted and the transverse talar joints parallel, the foot is supple for shock absorption and to allow for irregularity in the ground. Secondly, from heel rise in forefoot rocker, the subtalar joint is inverted, the transverse talar joints are not parallel, and the hindfoot is locked, facilitating the propulsion by creating a rigid segment between the tendo Achillis and the forefoot.

As shock absorption and energy conservation are dependent on hindfoot version and transverse tarsal position, errors in the positioning of any element of the kinetic chain from pelvis to toes will have a detrimental effect on gait efficiency.

At heel strike the subtalar joint starts to evert making the foot suppler. Foot pronation provides flexibility to adapt to uneven surfaces. A stable platform is provided throughout the stance phase. Hindfoot valgus (or subtalar joint eversion) then moves to inversion (or hindfoot varus) through the stance phase, and on heel raise the heel inverts providing a stiff lever for propulsion. This can be observed in a simple heel raise with the normal valgus position changing to varus as the heel is elevated.

Feel

This is best done with the patient seated on a high couch, with the examiner seated opposite.

With focused and systematic palpation for areas of bony or soft tissue thickening, focal lesions, and tenderness, the differential diagnosis can often be narrowed. History and the patient pointing to the area of maximal pain gives a good indication of the site of maximal tenderness. Careful palpation, combined with knowledge of the deep and surface anatomy, allows the affected structure or structures to be identified. This is illustrated in the regional "feel maps" later in the text. Where areas of tenderness are found, try to define the exact limits of the tenderness, and how they are related to, or changed by, motion of the joints and tendons.

Move

While the patient remains seated, this is an excellent position to assess the movements of the foot and ankle. Start from the ankle and hindfoot and move distally. It is also important to establish the relationship between the hind and forefoot.

When examining the foot and ankle it is important to understand the basic biomechanics. The ankle joint is not a simple hinge. Stiehl suggested that the articular surface of the talus was an approximation of a frustum (a section of a cone)[5], the apex of which is directed medially. The axis of rotation is just distal to the intermalleolar axis, which is easily located by palpation. The obliquity of the axis of rotation results in a change in foot position with pure ankle movements, with internal rotation of the foot in plantar flexion and external rotation in dorsiflexion. The normal arc of movement of the ankle is 50 to 60°. Ankle movements can be separated from dorsiflexion and plantar flexion of the midtarsal and tarsometatarsal joint (TMTJ) by grasping the heel with the foot rested along the forearm (Figure 1.3). Ankle dorsiflexion should be recorded with the knee flexed and extended by performing Silferskiöld's test. This is also a good time to assess the ankle ligaments – see "Special Tests" later in the chapter.

The range of motion in the subtalar joint is most accurately assessed prone with the knee flexed; however, the inconvenience to the patient is rarely necessary and examination can usually be undertaken with the patient sitting. It is usually sufficient to compare the two sides, expressing the range of movement as a percentage of the normal side. The patient remains seated and the calcaneus is aligned with the tibia. The

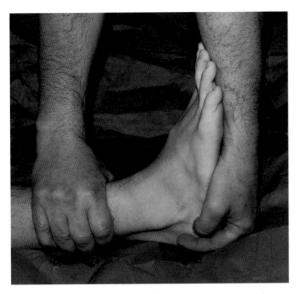

Figure 1.3 When examining the ankle it is useful to place the forearm along the sole of the foot to isolate the ankle movement from the midfoot.

heel is then moved from inversion to eversion. The normal subtalar joint range of movement is about 20 to 60°, with twice as much inversion as eversion.

The range of first TMTJ motion is difficult to test accurately, nevertheless it is more important to assess stability than range. The foot is taken in two hands, one hand taking the first ray in isolation, the other hand taking the lateral four rays. The two hands are then moved dorsally and plantarwards. If the inferior aspect of the first metatarsal does not reach that of the lesser rays the first ray is considered stiff, whereas if it dorsiflexes above the dorsal aspect of the lesser rays, the first ray is considered hypermobile.

The metatarsophalangeal joints (MTPJs) are assessed individually. Pain at the limits of movement of the first MTPJ is assessed. Midrange pain of the first MTPJ is recorded, as this helps determine if a patient is suitable for a cheilectomy to treat hallux rigidus.

The Relationship Between the Hindfoot and Forefoot

The ability of the midfoot to compensate for hindfoot position is core to understanding foot and ankle pathology, as well as the establishment of a plantigrade foot with varying hindfoot morphologies.

Imagine a theoretical solid foot, where no movement, or compensation, were possible. If the heel is placed in varus, the forefoot will twist so that the first ray is elevated (*forefoot varus*). In such a foot weight bearing will lead to pressure and symptoms under the entire lateral border of the foot, often with a callus under the fifth metatarsal base and head. Thus compensation for the forefoot varus is necessary. This compensation occurs through rotation in the midfoot, thus *forefoot valgus* compensates for *hindfoot varus*. On the other hand, a *valgus hindfoot* requires a compensatory *forefoot varus* to elevate the first ray. These compensatory rotations of the forefoot occur in the coronal plane, and are fundamental to maintain a plantigrade foot.

Clinically establishing the position of the hind- and forefoot is achieved by placing the subtalar joint in neutral. The talonavicular joint forms a ball and socket in the midfoot – the "acetabulum pedis." Subtalar neutral is established by centering the navicular on the talus. This is achieved by placing a finger on either side of the talar neck. There is usually a deeper recess palpable laterally than medially. As the heel, through the subtalar joint, is brought into varus, the depth of the soft tissues equalizes on both sides of the talar neck. When the soft tissues are equal, the talonavicular joint is said to be in neutral.

Thus the hindfoot position is established with the patient standing, then in the seated patient the heel is held and moved to "subtalar neutral." The position of the forefoot is then noted. If the forefoot lies in varus or valgus, use your second hand to establish if this deformity is correctable, or flexible.

The importance of this in surgical practice is in establishing the surgery required to correct a deformity. For example, a patient with a significant hindfoot valgus may well have compensatory forefoot varus (supination). If this forefoot deformity is fixed, surgical correction will require a bony procedure, often a fusion, through the midtarsal joint to produce a plantigrade foot. If the forefoot is flexible, or correctable, simply addressing the hindfoot should be acceptable. The Coleman block test is a weightbearing variation of these principles (see below).

The importance of this examination has been magnified in recent years, by the advent of total ankle arthroplasty, because coronal plane deformity of the foot has been shown to be the major driver of failure, due to transmission of coronal plane forces to the ankle replacement.

(a) 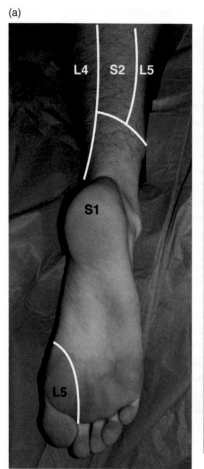 (b)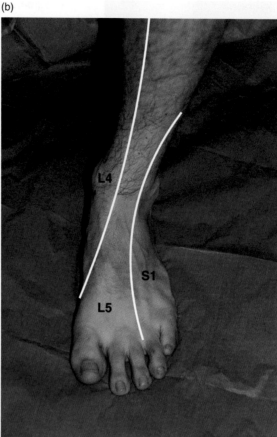

Figure 1.4
Dermatomes of the foot.

Extras

- The need for complete examination of the spine, hip, and knee is determined by the patient's history. Be sure to check the spine and any cutaneous manifestations of neuromuscular disease, such as café au lait spots, if the history is suggestive.

Neurology

Test light touch in the dermatome regions. Sensibility with a 5.07/10 g Semmes–Weinstein monofilament is probably easiest. A 128 Hz tuning fork and a monofilament have similar specificity for detecting diabetic neuropathy, but the monofilament is more practical[6]. Neurological pain is not uncommon in the foot and ankle, and the dermatomes and peripheral nerve distributions are important (Figures 1.4 and 1.5).

Power and muscle balance should be assessed and compared to the contralateral side. Relate muscle weakness to the myotome where a proximal nerve cause has been identified, or with the peripheral supply if local causes are suspected (Table 1.4). Documentation of the Medical Research Council (MRC) grade should be noted (Table 1.5).

Vascular

Look for general signs of venous and arterial insufficiency. Visible varicosities, edema, and hemosiderin pigmentation should be noted. Skin color, warmth, and soft-tissue quality should be assessed. Are there any signs of active or healed ulceration?

Check the presence and quality of the dorsalis pedis pulse, just lateral to the extensor hallucis longus (EHL) tendon at the midfoot, and the posterior tibial

Table 1.4 The actions and innervation of the principal long muscles of the foot and ankle

Muscle	Test	Myotome	Peripheral nerve
Gastrocnemius–soleus complex	Resisted plantar flexion in neutral	S1, S2	Tibial nerve
Tibialis posterior	Resisted inversion in plantar flexion Ability to invert across midline of limb	L5, S1, S2	Tibial nerve
Tibialis anterior	Resisted inversion in dorsiflexion	L4, L5, S1	Peroneal nerve
Peroneus brevis/longus	Resisted eversion	L4, L5, S1	Peroneal nerve
Extensor hallucis longus	Resisted great toe extension	L5	Deep peroneal nerve

(a)

(b)

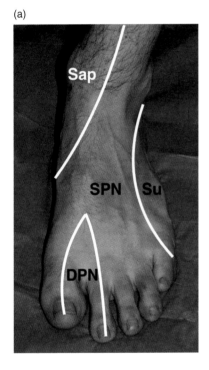
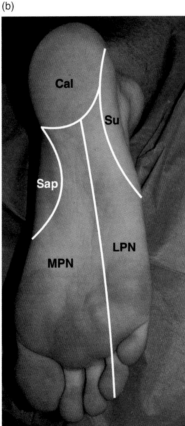

Figure 1.5 Sensory innervation of the foot. Sap: saphenous nerve; Su: sural nerve; SPN: superficial peroneal nerve; DPN: deep peroneal nerve; Cal: calcaneal branches of posterior tibial nerve; MPN: medial plantar nerve; LPN: lateral plantar nerve.

pulse, posterior to the medial malleolus. It is worth bearing in mind that the presence of pulses and absence of symptoms gives a 96% accuracy in excluding vascular disease.

If pulses are not easily palpable, use the handheld Doppler to measure the pressure. The blood pressure cuff is inflated until the pulse disappears. The blood pressure cuff is then slowly deflated and when the pulse is redetected through the Doppler probe the pressure in the cuff at that moment indicates the systolic pressure of that artery. Measure the ankle brachial pressure index (ABPI). The ABPI is obtained by dividing the ankle systolic pressure by the higher of the two brachial systolic pressures. An ABPI of >0.9

Table 1.5 The Medical Research Council (MRC) grading of muscle strength. Grade 4 is sometimes divided into 4–, 4, and 4+

MRC Grade	
0	No muscle contraction
1	Flicker of contraction but no movement
2	Active joint movement with gravity eliminated
3	Active movement against gravity, but not resistance from examiner
4	Movement against resistance, but reduced power
5	Full and normal power against resistance

Table 1.6 The components of the Beighton score for hypermobility

	Score
Passive extension of the little finger >90°	1 each side
Passive apposition of thumb to flexor aspect of forearm	1 each side
Hyperextension at the elbow	1 each side
Hyperextension at the knee	1 each side
Ability to touch hands flat on floor from standing with knees extended	1
Total score	**9 (>4 "hypermobility")**

is normal, <0.8 is associated with claudication, and <0.4 is commonly associated with ischemic rest pain and tissue necrosis. Note that the lower extremity measurements may be spuriously elevated in advanced diabetes due to calcification of the vessels.

Hypermobility

There are several hypermobility scores. The Beighton score (Table 1.6) remains the most widely used and the one on which exam knowledge is expected[7,8]. Test the upper limbs first; if a zero score is achieved there is no need to assess the lower limbs.

Systemic hypermobility is important in many aspects of foot and ankle disease, maybe most notably hallux valgus/first ray instability and lateral ankle ligament instability. It should also be borne in mind that patients with Ehlers–Danlos syndrome have more foot and ankle problems than the normal population, and hallux valgus, generalized foot pain, pes planus, or ankle instability may be their presenting complaint. Most hypermobility is mild, benign, and idiopathic and is not part of the Ehlers–Danlos spectrum, which is associated with many serious organ (e.g., cardiac) abnormalities.

Specific Examination

The patient is asked to put his or her finger on the point of maximal tenderness. The location of pain gives rise to a differential diagnosis. Many of the eponymous tests are described in the "Special Tests" section.

Hindfoot

See Figure 1.6 – the numbers in the text relate to the figures.

Central/Calcaneal Tuberosity

Differentials: Insertional tendinopathy of the tendo Achillis (1), retrocalcaneal bursitis (2), Haglund's deformity (2), and Achilles enthesophytes (3).

Features: Tenderness at the tendo Achillis insertion, tenderness and swelling of the retrocalcaneal bursa, pain and limitation on dorsiflexion.

Central/Midtendon

Differentials: Non-insertional tendinopathy (4), tendo Achillis rupture (4).

Features: Tendinopathy – tenderness and nodule of the tendon, crepitus (paratendinopathy). Positive Silfverskiöld's test. Palpate medially to assess for plantaris involvement[9].

Rupture: Perform (Simmonds'/Thompson's) calf-squeeze test. If it produces passive ankle plantar flexion, equal to the contralateral limb, the triceps surae and tendo Achillis are intact. Acutely feel for a palpable gap in the tendon. If the rupture is chronic there will be excess ankle dorsiflexion, a gait with a weak push off, and recruitment of the long toe flexors.

Posteromedial

Differentials: Posterior ankle impingement by an os trigonum (5), fracture of posterior process of

(a)

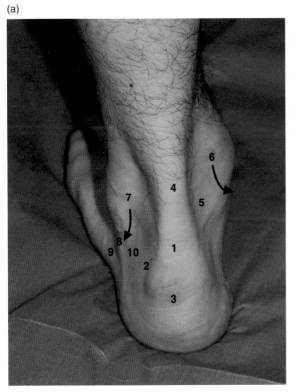

(b)

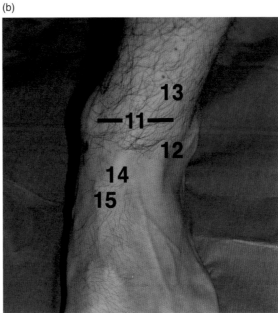

(c)

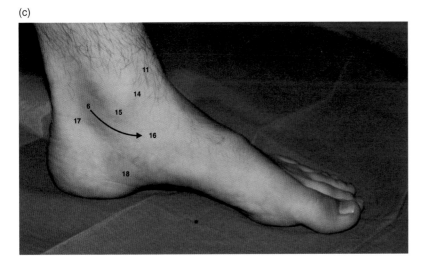

Figure 1.6 Hindfoot feel map (see text for numbering).

talus or symptomatic long posterolateral process of talus (Stieda's process) (5), FHL entrapment/tenosynovitis (5), tibialis posterior dysfunction (6).

Features: Tibialis posterior dysfunction specific examination is covered in "Exam Pearls."

Posterior ankle impingement: Presents with ankle pain in maximum plantar flexion, which is provoked by rapid hyperplantarflexion of the ankle.

Diffuse intrinsic wasting is most often associated with longstanding peripheral neuropathy, and most easily observed in the abductor hallucis muscle along the plantar-medial foot. Tarsal tunnel syndrome is rarely associated with intrinsic muscle wasting. Test for Tinel's sign and sensory dysfunction in the nerve distribution in the sole of the foot. A provocation test with the ankle in dorsiflexion and eversion may be helpful[10,11].

Posterolateral

Differentials: Peroneal tendon tear/tendinopathy (7), peroneal tendon (7) subluxation.

Features: Pain and swelling along the course of the tendon with overlying synovitis. Pain and weakness in resisted eversion. Palpate for snapping or flicking of the tendon in circumduction – the patient may be able to demonstrate tendon subluxation.

Lateral Calcaneum

Differentials: Peroneal tendon pain around a hypertrophied peroneal tubercle (8), painful os peroneum syndrome (POPS) (9), subtalar joint degeneration (10).

Features: Carefully examine the exact location of pain. Pain around the peroneal tubercle may indicate pathology. Peroneal tendon pain may be exacerbated with resisted eversion. With POPS, the patient is tender over the peroneus longus as it passes under the lateral border of the foot. With subtalar pain hindfoot movements may be reduced.

Anterolateral Ankle

Differentials: Synovitis (11), meniscoid lesion (12), impingement due to Bassett's ligament (12) (a hypertrophied inferior portion of the anterior tibiofibular ligament), syndesmosis injury of the ankle (13), lateral ankle ligament injury (12).

Features: Palpable thickening in the lateral gutter and/or a joint effusion. Meniscoid lesions can be provoked by passive dorsiflexion of the ankle with thumb pressure in the lateral gutter[12]. Palpate directly over the syndesmosis to assess for syndesmotic injury. In the "squeeze" test for syndesmosis injury the fibula is squeezed against the tibia by grasping the leg just above the ankle. This test is positive if the squeeze provokes pain. Local syndesmosis tenderness and pain with forced external rotation of the foot are the most sensitive tests[13] for a syndesmotic injury.

Anterior Ankle

Differentials: Anterior tibial osteophyte or footballer's ankle (11), talonavicular joint osteoarthritis (14), navicular stress fracture (15).

Features: Anterior ankle osteophytes and dorsal osteophytes of the talonavicular joint may be palpable. Examine range of movement, in particular impingement pain on full ankle dorsiflexion. Navicular stress fracture may be associated with swelling, although there are usually few clinical signs.

Medial Ankle

Differentials: Medial gutter osteophytes of the ankle (14), deltoid ligament injury (15), tibialis posterior tendinopathy (6), symptomatic accessory navicular (16).

Features: Check the range of movement of the ankle and associated impingement. Tenderness over the medial ligament complex and excessive valgus on forced eversion should be compared to the contralateral side. Look for signs of tibialis posterior tendinopathy and dysfunction (see "Common Case Scenarios").

Heel Pain

Differentials: Tarsal tunnel syndrome (17), entrapment of Baxter's nerve (17) (first branch of the lateral plantar nerve to abduct or digiti quiniti minimi), plantar fasciitis (18), calcaneal stress fracture (18).

Features: Tenderness primarily at the plantar fascia insertion extending into the medial arch. Examine also for Achilles tightness, which is commonly associated. Check for altered sensation in the tibial nerve distribution, in particular the medial and lateral plantar nerves. A calcaneal stress fracture typically is tender with compression of the calcaneal tubercle between the heels of the examiner's two hands.

Midfoot

See Figure 1.7.

Medial Border

Differentials: Tibialis posterior (1), accessory navicular (2), spring ligament rupture (1), first TMTJ instability and degeneration (3), midsubstance plantar fasciitis (4).

(a)

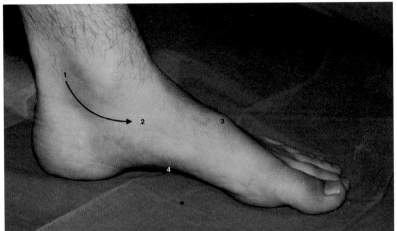

Figure 1.7 Midfoot feel map (see text for numbering).

(b)

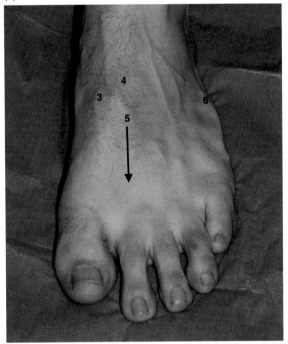

Features: Palpate for prominent bony landmarks. A large accessory navicular will usually be visible, and tender if it is symptomatic. Look for signs of tibialis posterior tendinopathy and dysfunction (see "Common Case Scenarios"). Osteophytes at the TMTJs may be focally tender. Stress the first TMTJ for pain and move the first ray relative to the lesser to assess for instability.

Dorsal Midfoot

Differentials: Second and lesser TMTJ degeneration (4), Lisfranc injury (4), proximal second metatarsal stress fracture (5), osteophyte impingement on deep peroneal nerve (4).

Features: Palpate and localize the region of maximal tenderness. The metatarsal head of each

Table 1.7 A classification of the causes of metatarsalgia, after Espinosa[14]

Primary	First ray insufficiency	Hallux valgus, hallux rigidus, first ray instability
	Abnormal metatarsal parabola	Congenitally long/short metatarsals, malunited fracture
	Prominent metatarsal head	Plantar flexed ray (isolated or as part of plantaris), large metatarsal head
	Equinus	
Secondary	Inflammatory arthritis	Rheumatoid arthritis, etc.
	Gout	
	Osteoarthritis	
	Trauma	Plantar plate injury, intra-articular fracture
	Neurological disease	Morton's neuroma
	Freiberg's disease	
Iatrogenic	Failed first metatarsal surgery	First ray shortened/elevated
	Excision of first MTPJ	Including failed first MTPJ replacement
	Unbalanced length or flexion of lesser rays	

ray is taken between the fingers of one hand, the head is moved up and down to stress the more proximal TMTJ, and if the joint is painful, or tender to palpation, this is indicative of joint disease, which is usually degenerative. Check for a Tinel sign over, and sensation in, the deep peroneal nerve territory, in the first web space, as impingement on the nerve by an osteophyte is not uncommon.

Lateral

Differentials: Base of fifth metatarsal fracture (6), peroneus brevis insertional tendinopathy (6).

Features: Note any swelling and tenderness consistent with acute injury. Test power in eversion and discomfort in passive inversion.

Forefoot

Medial Forefoot

Differentials: Hallux valgus/rigidus

Features: Note the overall foot position. Is there evidence of pressure over the bunion? Pronation of the great toe is important, relevant to severity and likely progression. Comment on associated lesser toe deformity. Measure the passive range of motion at the MTPJ. Is there mid-range pain or impingement pain only?

Lesser Metatarsals ("Metatarsalgia")

Differentials: Lesser MTPJ synovitis, lesser toe deformity, Morton's/interdigital neuroma.

Table 1.8 The positions of the joints of the toes in lesser toe deformity. There is great variability in the literature regarding the position of the joints

Description	Definition
Mallet	MTPJ neutral
	PIPJ neutral
	DIPJ flexion
Hammer	MTPJ neutral
	PIPJ flexion
	DIPJ extension or neutral
Claw toe	MTPJ extension
	PIPJ flexion
	DIPJ flexion

Features: Metatarsalgia is a symptom – metatarsal pain – and it is important to determine the underlying cause (Table 1.7). Note the principal ray affected and, if there is toe deformity, whether the deformity is fixed or correctable. The nomenclature for toe deformity can be confusing and varies between texts[15] (Table 1.8).

The location of pain is important, and needs careful examination. Sequentially squeeze the metatarsal heads and spaces between the thumb and index finger, working across the foot. There are two principal locations of pain:

- Interspace tenderness from a Morton's neuroma[16], with a "Mulder's click," (see "Special Tests"). Check for sensation on the medial and lateral side of each toe, carefully comparing. There is often a subtle difference, with both hypo- and hyperalgesia being a reliable sign of a neuroma.

- Tenderness in the joint. This is often associated with synovitis of the MTPJ. The synovitis may be from systemic disease, such as inflammatory arthritis, or local pathology. The commonest scenario is an insufficient first ray, with overload of the second ray, such that the second MTPJ becomes synovitic, and eventually dislocates (see forefoot case scenario below).

MTPJ synovitis and a neuroma often coexist. Nevertheless, accurate diagnosis is important and there is often confusion between the two diagnoses; the most useful distinguishing finding is loss of sensation in the distribution of the common digital nerve with a neuroma.

Plantar Forefoot Pain

Differentials: Sesamoiditis, sesamoid bursa, plantar fibromata, transfer lesion.

Features: Look carefully at the soles of the feet for areas of high pressure loading, indicated by callosities. Plantar callosities build up in areas of high pressure, for example under the metatarsal head of a dislocated MTPJ. Painful callosities under metatarsal heads are often called "transfer lesions."

Medial and lateral sesamoids should be individually palpated – with careful examination it is usually possible to determine which sesamoid is symptomatic.

An idiopathic plantar keratosis – an "IPK" – is a plantar callosity, usually under the fourth or fifth metatarsal head, which is associated with prominence of the metatarsal head condyles.

Plantar fibromas may be obvious and are commonly found in the medial arch. These are associated with Dupuytren's disease of the hands in 10 to 50% of cases.

Nails

Toenail pathology is common. Presentation of nail problems may provide a clue to systemic pathology, genetic abnormality, or even a malignant process. Simple classification systems (Table 1.9) will aid diagnosis, but often a spot diagnosis approach is required.

Common nail abnormalities include:

(i) Onychocryptosis

Ingrowing toenail most often occurs due to errors in nail trimming or tight-fitting shoes, with

Table 1.9 Classification systems for nail disease

Pardo–Castello and Pardo classification[17]	Nzuzi classification[18]
<ul><li>dermatologic and systemic disorders</li><li>congenital and nail bed disorders</li><li>common nail abnormalities and onychodystrophies</li></ul>	<ul><li>nail plate disorders</li><li>nail bed disorders</li><li>nail fold disorders</li><li>nail matrix disorders</li></ul>

a nail spike progressively growing into the nail fold. A secondary infection or paronychia is the usual reason for presentation.

(ii) Onychauxis and onychogryphosis

Onychauxis, or hypertrophied nail, is very common in the elderly and may be related to trauma, minor infection, systemic disease, or peripheral vascular disease. Usually affecting the hallux, there is uniform thickening of the nail often with brownish or yellow discoloration. With onychogryposis there is severe nail thickening with deformity, the appearance is likened to a ram's horn.

(iii) Onchomycosis

Nails are prone to fungal infection, dermatophytes utilize the keratin as a food source. Nails will appear thickened and discolored. Established infection can prove difficult to eradicate.

(iv) Psoriatic nail changes

80% of patients with psoriatic arthopathy have associated nail changes. Nail plate changes, pitting, onycholysis, and subungual keratosis are common findings. Inflammation of the nail and adjacent distal interphalangeal joint can mimic infection.

(v) Glomus tumor

Commonly presenting with exquisite tenderness and purple subungual discoloration. Glomus tumor is a benign vascular lesion (angioleiomyoma) that may be only a few millimeters in size, it may be treated by excision biopsy.

(vi) Subungual exostosis

The exostosis usually causes pain and lifting of the nail plate. Histologically these are osteochondromas, and reconstruction of the overlying nailbed is a surgical challenge.

(vii) Subungual melanoma

Usually painless; may be visible as a pigmented spot or band beneath the nail. Look for spread to periungual soft tissues. Prognosis is poor with five-year survival rates below 50%. Differential diagnosis is subungual hematoma from shoes or trauma. Nail removal may be required to make the diagnosis.

Special Tests

Simmonds'/Thompson's Test

Described by Simmonds in 1957 and Thompson in 1962[19–20]. Do not declare whether the test is "positive" or "negative," but rather if it indicates a rupture or not. The patient is asked to kneel on a chair, facing away from the examiner. The feet are left free. The unaffected calf is squeezed and the presence or absence of passive plantar flexion of the foot noted. This is repeated on the injured side. The absence of plantar flexion indicates complete rupture of the tendo Achillis.

Mulder's Click

Described by Dutch surgeon Mulder in 1951[16]. The forefoot is grasped across the metatarsal heads with one hand. The thumb of the second hand is used to push the neuroma between the metatarsal heads. The metatarsal heads are then compressed from side to side by squeezing the foot and this causes the neuroma to escape with a characteristic Mulder's click, and often pain. The absence of a Mulder's click does not exclude the presence of a neuroma – and vice versa.

Silfverskiöld's Test

Nils Silfverskiöld was an orthopedic surgeon, Swedish aristocrat, bon vivant, Olympic gymnast, left wing intellectual, and anti-Nazi[21]; he described his test in relation to isolated gastrocnemius contracture.

The Silfverskiöld test assesses gastrocnemius tightness. With the patient positioned supine, with the knee extended and the talonavicular joint in neutral, the ankle is passively dorsiflexed. It is important to place the talonavicular joint in inversion to lock the subtalar joint. This prevents eversion of the subtalar joint, which is important because dorsiflexion is a component of eversion. The test is repeated with the knee flexed to 90°. Knee flexion relaxes the

gastrocnemius, which crosses the knee joint, but leaves the soleus, which does not cross the knee joint, unaffected. An increment in dorsiflexion with the knee flexed implies isolated gastrocnemius tightness. Normal ankle dorsiflexion with the knee in extension is 5 to 10°.

Anterior Draw of the Ankle

The equivalent of the anterior draw/Lachman test for the knee. The anterior talofibular ligament (ATFL) is the primary restraint to anterior subluxation.

With the patient seated and the knee slightly flexed, firmly stabilize the lower calf just above the ankle. Allow the foot to drop into plantar flexion and grasp it around the heel, attempt to sublux the ankle anteriorly. Compare anterior translation to the contralateral side. In marked instability the lateral skin is sucked into the joint – the "sulcus" sign.

Squeeze Test

Combined with tenderness over the anterior inferior tibiofibular ligament (AITFL) and provocation on the external rotation test, the squeeze test is an important indicator of syndesmosis injury.

The "squeeze" test is where the fibula is squeezed against the tibia by grasping the leg just above the ankle. This test is positive if the squeeze provokes pain in the syndesmosis.

Peek-a-Boo Heel Sign

First described by Manoli in 1993, the "peek-a-boo" heel sign is seen in subtle hindfoot varus, it is the reverse of the "too many toes" sign seen in the flat foot.

The medial aspect of the heel is visible on the medial side when viewing the patient from the front with the feet in neutral rotation (Figure 1.8).

Coleman Block Test

The patient is asked to stand with the fourth and fifth metatarsals on a wooden block. The hallux is allowed to hang free. This neutralizes the plantar flexion of the first ray. The test is positive if the heel moves to a more valgus position. Correction of the heel varus with the block in place confirms both that the subtalar joint is mobile and that the plantarflexed first ray is driving the hindfoot varus (Figure 1.9). The same can be shown simply by

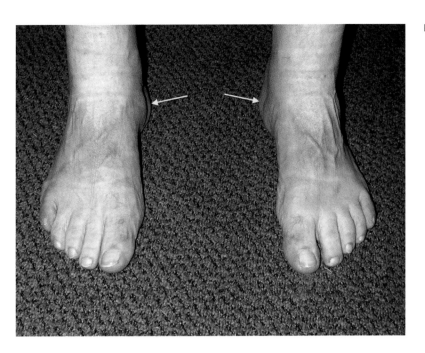

Figure 1.8 "Peek-a-boo" heel sign.

(a)

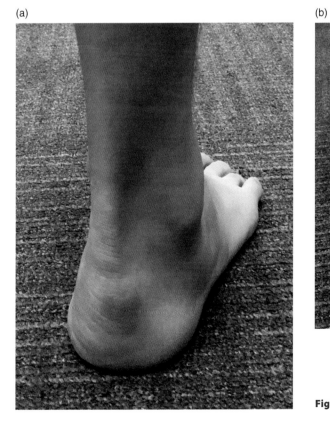

(b)

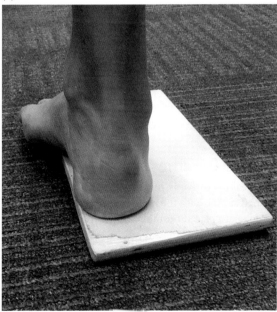

Figure 1.9 Coleman block test.

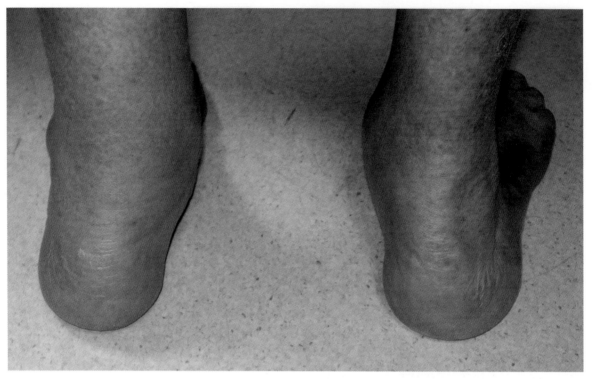

Figure 1.10 "Too many toes" sign. Note the heel valgus and three toes visible on the right, when compared to the left foot.

demonstrating that the heel passively moves in to valgus when the patient is sitting.

Described in 1977, this "simple test" is key to the surgical management of cavovarus[22], as if positive it implies that a dorsiflexion osteotomy of the first metatarsal should correct the heel varus.

Peroneal Overdrive

Peroneal overdrive is measured with the patient positioned supine with the knee extended. The examiner's thumbs are placed on the plantar aspect of the foot at the level of the metatarsal heads, one thumb medially under the first metatarsal and the other under the lesser metatarsals. With the ankle in neutral, the patient is asked to plantar flex the foot against the examiner's resisting thumbs. A positive test is when the examiner's thumbs are pushed away with more force by the first metatarsal than the lateral forefoot. The foot plantar flexes into a pronated position.

The significance of peroneal overdrive is in the patient with mild cavovarus, which is forefoot driven. In this condition it is considered that the primary deformity is plantar flexion of the first ray driven by

an overactive peroneus longus, which inserts to the base of the first metatarsal.

Too Many Toes Sign

Described by Johnson in 1989, now a widely taught method of recognizing tibialis posterior deficiency. Beware of false positives, as too many toes will also be seen in other causes for flat foot, most notably abduction through the tarsometatarsal joints due to arthritis, or a previous Lisfranc dislocation, and in more proximal external rotation deformity (Figure 1.10).

"Too many toes" is a sign of forefoot abduction. View the standing patient from behind. If more than two toes are visible lateral to the leg, when compared to the contralateral side, this confirms the "too many toes" sign. Hindfoot valgus is also liable to be present.

Common Case Scenarios

Cavovarus Foot

These patients may well have an underlying neurological condition, and full neurological evaluation is important. Note calf and intrinsic muscle wasting. Assess sensation. The hands, lower back, and lower limbs should also be examined for signs of hereditary sensorimotor neuropathy (HSMN). Champagne bottle, or stork-like, calf shape is associated with a high stepping gait and a foot drop in HSMN.

Look: Shoe wear pattern should be noted, increased wear under the lateral border and damaged uppers may occur. Check for the presence and nature of any orthoses.

Stand the patient barefoot. Foot alignment and arch height should be recorded from the front and behind. Toe clawing is often associated with extensor recruitment and intrinsic weakness.

The heel alignment should be observed, paying particular attention to subtle varus, including the peek-a-boo heel sign. A normal hindfoot lies in slight valgus. Proximal malalignment should also be excluded, whether varus/valgus or rotational.

Feel: Tenderness around the lateral ankle and the peroneal tendons should be assessed. There may be callosities under a plantar flexed first ray of the fifth metatarsal head. In severe cases there may be a callus along the lateral border of the foot, with the fifth metatarsal head being tender.

Move: Check muscular strength of all groups, but in particular look for weakness of dorsiflexion and the peroneal tendons (HSMN). Establish if the hindfoot varus is correctable, and if there is compensatory forefoot valgus. Achilles tightness should be established using Silfverskiöld's test.

A Coleman block test is important. The gait pattern should be noted.

Lateral Ankle Ligament Instability

The history should be indicative of instability, but pain may be the primary presenting complaint. Detail any precipitating injury, the exact mechanism may lead to the diagnosis. Ask about sport and leisure activities, past and present, any treatments and outcome.

Examine the foot position and alignment; a subtle cavus can often lead to instability[2]. Is the hindfoot in varus? Does the patient have peek-a-boo heels?

It is important to check for tenderness, as anterolateral synovitis is common, as are peroneal tendon tears, which lead to pain and clicking behind the

fibula. Examine for laxity of the lateral ligaments and also the strength of the peroneal tendons. The tibiofibular syndesmosis should also be evaluated by direct palpation for tenderness, a calf squeeze, and an external rotation test.

Tibialis Posterior Dysfunction

Classically seen in a middle-aged, overweight, female patient, whose foot shape has flattened. Often the patient is hypermobile.

Look: View the patient standing from in front and behind, look at arch height and medial swelling. Severe dysfunction will be accompanied by forefoot abduction and hindfoot valgus. Look for the "too many toes" sign. Lateral ankle pain from impingement, secondary to valgus, may also be present. Carefully note the presence of a hallux valgus and TMTJ arthritis. First-ray insufficiency may predispose to posterior tibial tendon insufficiency. TMTJ arthritis and collapse can present a similar clinical picture, with a painful flat foot.

Feel: Palpate carefully over the tibialis posterior tendon. There may also be lateral tenderness and impingement.

Move: There are two ways of undertaking the single heel raise. Both have advantages.

1. Ask the patient to stand close to and facing a wall, they may rest their fingertips on the wall for balance; "cheating" is lessened with minimal ability to use the wall to assist upward movement.

2. The alternative is to ask the patient to face you and place the palms of their hands on the examiner's. This allows the examiner to watch the patient as well as feeling through the palms of their hands if the patient is weak.

Whichever technique is used, in early dysfunction a heel raise may still be possible, but the patient fatigues on repeated heel raises. The single heel raise should be repeated to establish weakness. A positive test is indicated not just by diminished height of heel raise, but especially by the failure of the heel to move from valgus to varus, as the patient goes up on her toes.

With the patient now seated, the strength of the tibialis posterior is tested with the foot plantar flexed and abducted to neutralize the power of tibialis anterior.

Check for ankle and hindfoot flexibility, as secondary changes will result from end-stage tendinopathy making the deformity not correctable. Thus the heel valgus is corrected and the presence and correctability of forefoot varus is recorded. The presence of a secondary Achilles contracture should also be noted with a Silfverskiöld's test.

Johnson and Strom (1989) proposed a staging system, which is in general use in the orthopedic foot and ankle community. They recognized three basic stages:

- stage 1: no deformity
- stage 2: a flexible planovalgus foot
- stage 3: fixed planovalgus deformity

Myerson added stage 4, where there is valgus tilting of the talus in the ankle mortise.

Forefoot

Look: Simple observation of the standing foot is very informative in forefoot diagnosis. Ask the patient to stand barefoot. Note the overall foot alignment and arch height. Pes planus with hindfoot valgus is often associated with hallux valgus. Describe the position of the hallux and any lesser toe deformities. Is the forefoot abducted? Is the great toe pronated? Does the patient have a pure medial bunion or a dorsomedial bunion, the later implying degenerative change. The latter is associated with hallux rigidus.

Feel: Feel for osteophytes and tenderness around the first MTPJ. Note sensibility over the dorsum of the great toe; it is often reduced.

Hallux pathology is often associated with lesser toe problems. This may be because of first-ray insufficiency, leading to transfer lesions and lesser toe deformity. The earliest stages of this manifest with tender thickening of the MTPJ from synovitis.

When examining the lesser rays, note plantar callosities and their position. These will be under areas of high pressure, whether it be the fifth ray from a varus heel or the second metatarsal head from a dislocated second MTPJ.

Metatarsalgia is a symptom, not a diagnosis. For treatment, the causes of metatarsalgia need to be defined. It is important to identify areas of tenderness by careful palpation. Morton's neuromas with interspace tenderness and a Mulder's click may also be present.

Examine the stability of the first TMTJ as well as noting systemic hypermobility.

Move: Note the active and passive range of motion of the MTPJ. If there is hallux valgus does it correct? Check for midrange pain if there is degenerative change of the first MTPJ. The latter will be more responsive to dorsal cheilectomy.

Examine the lesser rays; assess whether tenderness is related to a metatarsal head, often due to synovitis or plantar plate injury, or in the interspace, which is usually due to a Morton's neuroma. Is there a "Mulder's click," or any altered sensibility in the appropriate toes? This is best detected by lightly touching the medial and lateral borders of the toes and asking about difference in sensation. The toe may be hyper- or hypoesthetic.

Where there are lesser toe deformities, differentiate between fixed or correctable deformity at the MTPJs and interphalangeal joints. Check between the toes, in particular between the fourth and fifth, for a soft corn.

Rheumatoid Foot

A common exam case, but the incidence is reducing in clinical practice. Subdivide observations into general rheumatoid, forefoot, and hindfoot.

General rheumatoid features include poor skin quality and nodules. The hip and knee should also be examined. Multilevel changes can make gait description complex.

Deformity can be severe. Common patterns include pes planus with a valgus hindfoot, abduction at the TMTJ, and hallux valgus with lesser toe deformity. Often the lesser toes are dislocated with callosities under the metatarsal heads. Detail each component systematically. Note the circulation, as there may be a vasculitic component.

References

1. Hope RA, Longmore JM, McManus SK, Wood-Allum CA. *Oxford Handbook of Clinical Medicine*, 4th edn (Oxford: Oxford University Press, 1998).

2. Manoli A, Graham B. The subtle cavus foot, "the underpronator," a review. *Foot Ankle Int.* 2005; 26: 256–63.

3. Perry J. Kinesiology of lower extremity bracing *Clin Orthop.* 1974; 102: 18–31.

4. Gage JR, Deluca PA, Renshaw TS. Gait analysis: principles and

applications. *J Bone Joint Surg Am*. 1995; 77: 1607–23.

5. Stiehl JB. *Inman's Joints of the Ankle*, 2nd edn (Baltimore: Williams & Wilkins, 1991), p. 155.

6. Al-Geffari M. Comparison of different screening tests for diagnosis of diabetic peripheral neuropathy in Primary Health Care setting. *Int J Health Sci*. 2012; 6(2): 127–134.

7. Beighton P, Solomon L, Soskolne CL. Articular mobility in an African population. *Ann Rheum Dis*. 1973; 32: 413–18.

8. Beighton P, Horan F. Orthopaedic aspects of the Ehlers-Danlos syndrome. *J Bone Joint Surg Br*. 1969; 51: 444–53.

9. Alfredson H. Midportion Achilles tendinosis and the plantaris tendon. *Br J Sports Med*. 2011; 45: 1023–5.

10. Ahmad M, Tsang K, Mackenney PJ, Adedapo AO. Tarsal tunnel syndrome: a literature review *Foot Ankle Surg*. 2012; 18: 149–52.

11. Kinoshita M, Okunda R, Morikawa J, Jotoku T, Abe M. The dorsiflexion-eversion test for diagnosis of tarsal tunnel syndrome. *J Bone Joint Surg Am*. 2001; 83-A: 1835–9.

12. Molloy S, Solan MC, Bendall SP. Synovial impingement in the ankle: a new physical sign. *J Bone Joint Surg Br*. 2003; 85: 330–3.

13. Sman AD, Hiller CE, Refshauge KM. Diagnostic accuracy of clinical tests for diagnosis of ankle syndesmosis injury: a systematic review. *Br J Sports Med*. 2013; 47: 620–8.

14. Espinosa N, Myerson MS. Current concepts review: metatarsalgia. *Foot Ankle Int*. 2008; 8: 871–9.

15. Schrier JC, Verheyen CC, Louwerens JW. Definitions of hammer toe and claw toe: an evaluation of the literature. *J Am Podiatr Med Assoc*. 2009; 99: 194–7.

16. Mulder, JD. The causative mechanism in Morton's metatarsalgia. *J Bone Joint Surg*. 1951; 33B: 94–5.

17. Pardo-Castello V, Pardo OA. *Diseases of the Nails*, 3rd edn. (Springfield, Ilinois: Charles C Thomas, 1960).

18. Nzuzi SM. Common nail disorders. *Clin Podiatr Med Surg*. 1989; 6: 273–94.

19. Simmonds FA. The diagnosis of the ruptured Achilles tendon. *Practitioner*. 1957; 179: 56–8.

20. Thompson TC. A test for rupture of the tendo Achillis. *Acta Orthop Scand*. 1962; 32: 461–5.

21. Singh D. Nils Silfverskiöld (1888–1957) and gastrocnemius contracture. *Foot Ankle Surg*. 2013; 19: 135–8.

22. Coleman SS, Chesnut WJ. A simple test for hindfoot flexibility in the cavovarus foot. *Clin Orthop* 1977; 123: 60.

21

Chapter 2

Biomechanics of the Foot and Ankle

Fraser Harrold and Rami J. Abboud

Introduction

Biomechanics is the study of engineering mechanics, specifically Newton's laws, as applied to the musculoskeletal system. An understanding of the biomechanics of the foot and ankle enables appreciation of the intricate function of individual components, their inter-relationships, and aids in an understanding of pathology and the potential impact of surgical intervention. Although the focus of this chapter is on foot and ankle biomechanics, the foot and ankle should not be considered in isolation, but as an open chain. Foot and ankle biomechanics are intimately related to the knee, hip, and spine. The principles are outlined with clinical correlates.

Function

The foot has evolved for bipedal locomotion, providing a mechanism for the absorption and transfer of energy during propulsion, and stability during stance. Additionally, the foot is important for balance and provides an interface with the environment.

Energy Absorption and Transfer

The foot has a unique ability to change from a flexible, compliant structure to a rigid lever. To absorb and transfer energy efficiently it must be able to conform to even and uneven surfaces and make good contact with almost any supporting surface, while also forming a rigid platform that does not collapse under body weight. The forces transmitted through the foot during walking and running are between one and three times body weight[1] and up to 16 times in jumping[2]. Energy is either dissipated or absorbed by the foot, protecting the skeletal structures more proximally. The specialized cells of the plantar skin, subcutaneous fat pads under the heel and metatarsal heads, plantar aponeurosis, ligaments, and the intrinsic and extrinsic musculature all absorb the forces and store the potential energy. The plantar aponeurosis and musculature release the energy during propulsive activity.

Stability

A combination of dynamic and static stabilizers created by the relatively stiff medial longitudinal arch, bony congruence, the close packing of individual bones in certain foot positions, the plantar soft tissue structures, and traversing musculature maintain foot stability during standing, walking, or running.

Proprioceptive nerve endings within the intrinsic musculature, ligaments, and joint capsules feed back to allow the intrinsic and extrinsic musculature to maintain the center of gravity in a 4 cm^2 area just anterior to the ankle joint[3]. In the resting state, soleus, tibialis posterior, and peroneus brevis control anteroposterior oscillations[4]. In patients who have been immobilized in cast, the proprioceptive mechanism becomes dormant, making balance difficult when standing and walking unsteady.

Sensory

The skin in contact with the ground can be over 5 mm thick in unshod individuals[5]. It responds to increases in pressure by creating callosities to reduce soft tissue trauma. The specialized skin covering the surface of the foot is also densely populated with nociceptive fibers, which sense pain and temperature, enabling subtle and constant changes in pressure by constantly adjusting the center of gravity. Neuropathic individuals, for example diabetics, lose the ability to sense increases in pressure or trauma to the foot, resulting in ulceration. Neuropathy also affects proprioception and thus balance.

Evolution of the Foot

A detailed treatise on the evolution of the foot is beyond the scope of this chapter but, for the

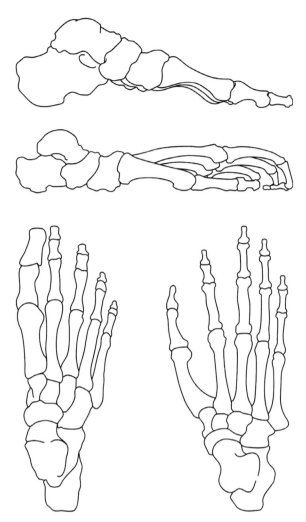

Figure 2.1 The major evolutionary changes in foot morphology including a broader and straighter first ray, longer calcaneus, and higher medial arch. The human left foot (top and left), and simian left foot (lower) and right foot (right). (From Schultz 1963[9])

foot once used for grasping, many other features reflect its adaption for weight bearing. The human calcaneus is larger than its primate origins, resulting in a longer moment arm for the tendo Achillis to improve propulsion. The plantar surface is also larger, reducing point loading by increasing the contact area. The subtalar facet joints are less obliquely oriented relative to the ground, reducing the shear stresses through the joint in bipedal locomotion.

The bony architecture of the midfoot has also changed. The cuboid and cuneiforms have evolved to become wedge shaped, apex plantarwards, in the formation of the transverse arch. This has been further strengthened by the relative hypertrophy of the plantar ligaments. The overall effect is to make the midfoot more rigid, with the ability to absorb and store energy during standing and locomotion.

The first ray is broader and straighter than the other four rays with less transverse and sagittal plane motion, and is almost parallel with the second ray. Stability is also conferred by slightly flatter first metatarsocuneiform joint and the surrounding intrinsic musculature and deep transverse metatarsal ligament, which is unique to humans.

A recent study by Wang et al. (2014)[10] compared foot structure in humans and apes, examining the influence of foot proportions on force, torque, and work in the foot joints during simulated bipedal walking. The authors concluded that the geometric proportions of the feet in humans and apes exert a discernible effect on these variables. Their results showed that during simulated human-like bipedal walking: (1) the human and ape feet experience similar joint forces, although the distributions of the forces differ; (2) the ape foot incurs larger torque across the joint than the human foot. The human foot has higher torque in the first tarsometatarsal and metatarsophalangeal joints, whereas the ape foot incurs higher torque in the lateral digits; (3) total work in the metatarsophalangeal joints is lower in the human foot than in the ape foot.

Thus the proportions of the human foot are more advantageous for bipedal walking than the ape's. The authors have also shown that short toes play an important role in human walking. These subtle changes have improved the propulsive potential of the foot as well as its stability, and created an important evolutionary step, freeing the upper limb to develop fine motor skills with parallel brain development.

interested reader, Olson and Seidel (1983)[6] published an in-depth review. There are a number of key developments worth highlighting. The origins of the foot are from tree-dwelling apes in which the "foot" functioned as a grasping appendage (Figure 2.1). Although the foot has been evolving for over 2 million years, the anatomical variation found within the human population suggests that the foot remains a work in progress[7]. The foot is evolving to improve its function in balance, propulsion, and upright stance[8].

While the lateral torsion in the first ray and slight medial torsion in the lateral four rays are features of a

(a)

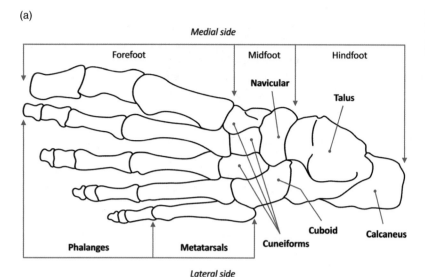

(b)

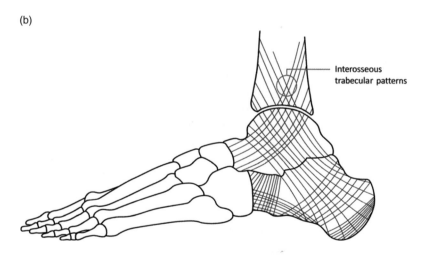

Figure 2.2 (a) The 26 bones of the foot and their division into hindfoot, midfoot, and forefoot. (b) Interosseous trabecular patterns of the ankle and foot.

Anatomy

The soft tissue structures are built around and on a constrained bony anatomy comprising 26 bones, which, for practical purposes, are grouped into the hindfoot, midfoot, and forefoot (Figure 2.2a).

The hindfoot comprises the talus and calcaneus, which are the first and second bones to ossify, respectively. The three parts of the talus (body, neck, and head) are oriented to transmit reactive forces from the foot through the ankle to the leg. Lying between the calcaneus and tibia, the talus communicates thrust from one to the other. The calcaneus is the largest and most posterior bone in the foot and provides a lever arm for the insertion of the tendo Achillis and associated triceps surae, which imparts plantar flexion forces to the foot. The calcaneus' height, width, and structure enable it to withstand high tensile, bending and compressive forces. Trabecular lines, formed according to Wolff's law, run through the hindfoot. They are contiguous with the trabecular patterns from the tibia and extend into the midfoot and forefoot, crossing joints. The anterior trabecular system in the tibia curves posteriorly into the talus and posterior calcaneus. The posterior trabecular system in the tibia curves anteriorly extending into the medial column. A plantar-based system joins the posterior and anterior systems and is accompanied by a number of smaller systems within each of the bones of the foot (Figure 2.2b).

The midfoot comprises the navicular, cuboid, and the three cuneiforms – medial, intermediate, and lateral. The navicular is boat shaped, as its name suggests, and articulates with the head of the talus proximally and the three cuneiforms distally. The navicular forms the keystone at the apex of the medial longitudinal arch. It is the last bone to ossify in the foot. These features may be why it is vulnerable to osteochondrosis (Köhler's disease) in childhood and vulnerable to the development of avascular necrosis[11]. The cuboid articulates with the calcaneus proximally, the lateral cuneiform medially, and the fourth and fifth metatarsals distally. In a small proportion of the population, there is an articulation between the navicular and the cuboid, and occasionally the two are joined as a coalition[12]. The three cuneiforms are trapezoidal, with a broad dorsal aspect and narrower plantar surface. They form an intrinsically stable transverse arch. The medial, intermediate, and lateral cuneiforms articulate individually with the first, second, and third metatarsals in turn.

The forefoot comprises the metatarsals and phalanges. There are five metatarsals in the forefoot. These are all tapered distally and articulate with the proximal phalanges. The first metatarsal is the shortest and widest. The head of the first metatarsal also articulates with two sesamoids, the tibial and fibular sesamoids, which are situated within the flexor hallucis brevis tendon on the plantar articular surface. The second metatarsal is recessed proximally between the medial and lateral cuneiforms, and articulates with the intermediate cuneiform. This results in the second metatarsal being "locked" in place. The third, fourth, and fifth metatarsals are broad at the base and narrow in the shaft. The fifth has a prominent styloid, laterally and proximally at its base, to which the peroneus brevis tendon and plantar fascia are attached. The phalanges represent the digits. The big toe (hallux) consists of two phalanges and the remaining four toes typically have three phalanges (Figures 2.2a). The heads of the proximal and middle phalanges tend to be trochlear shaped, creating good stability.

Joint Motion

By convention, motion occurs around three axes: X, Y, and Z (Figure 2.3). Plantar flexion and dorsi-flexion describe sagittal plane motion (Y–Z plane), inversion and eversion describe coronal plane motion (X–Y), and adduction and abduction describe transverse plane motion (Z–X).

The foot needs to remain flat on the ground and must accommodate the rotational moments that are transmitted from the pelvis and lower limb to enable efficient forward propulsion during gait. This is accomplished through composite motion created by the variable axes of each of the joints of the foot and ankle. There is a marked degree of variability in the range of motion of each joint within the normal population. This variability can result in variation of foot posture, which, in turn, defines an individual's gait.

Pronation and supination are composite triplanar motions of the foot: pronation describes abduction in the transverse plane, dorsiflexion in the sagittal plane, and eversion in the coronal plane; supination is the opposite, i.e., adduction, plantar flexion, and inversion.

The next section covers each of the major joints in turn. For several reasons, considering a joint axis as a simple hinge joint is an oversimplification. Firstly, arbitrarily selecting sagittal, coronal, and transverse planes for reference means that out-of-plane joints will, by definition, produce multiplanar motion. Secondly, the varying topography and congruency between articular surfaces results in an instantaneously changing center of rotation during motion. The result is motion around a series of helical axes, exemplified at the ankle and subtalar joints[12].

Ankle Joint

Inman describes the ankle joint as uniaxial, with its axis a few millimeters distal to the tips of the malleoli and a few millimeters anterior to the lateral malleolus[13]. The result is a downward and laterally oriented axis with a range in the coronal plane from 74 to 94° (Figure 2.4).

There is great variability in the ankle joint range of motion described in the literature. This probably reflects the differences in methodology. For example, Sammarco et al. (1973)[14] reported 23 ± 7° of ankle dorsiflexion and 23 ± 8° of plantar flexion under weightbearing conditions. However, only 10° of dorsiflexion and 20° of plantar flexion are deemed necessary for normal locomotion[15].

Additionally, there is variation in the curvature of the lateral and medial components of the talar dome, which results in differing axes of rotation in plantar

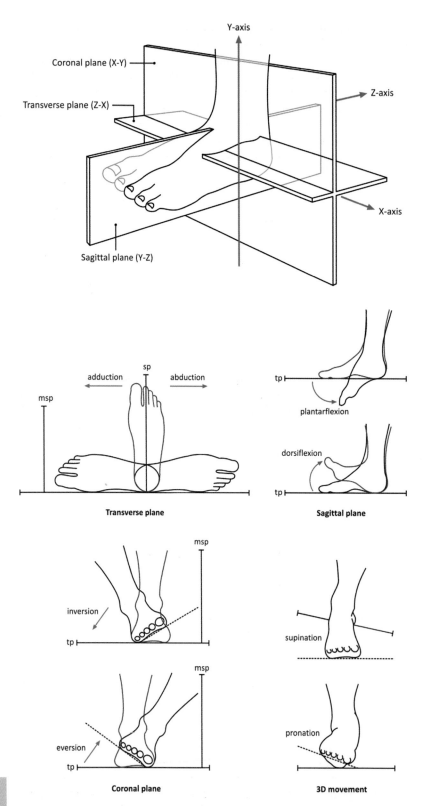

Figure 2.3 Convention for the axes around the foot and the associated motion around each axis.

flexion and dorsiflexion[16]; this accounts for the foot being 1° internally rotated in plantar flexion and 9° externally rotated in dorsiflexion[17] (Figure 2.5).

There is also tibial rotation during the normal gait cycle. During the early stance phase, with forward progression of the tibia and ankle dorsiflexion, there is internal tibial rotation. In contrast, in late stance phase, with the ankle plantar flexing, there is external tibial rotation[13].

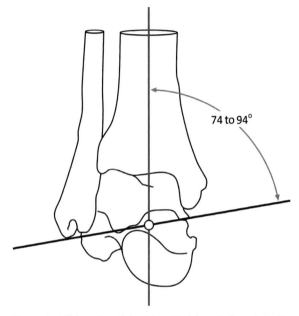

Figure 2.4 Orientation of the right ankle joint axis (frontal view).

74 to 94°

The position of arthrodesis of the ankle joint in all three planes is critical to the function of the joints above and below the ankle. Fusion in plantar flexion results in an increase in leg length, with a back-knee thrust and increased stress across the midfoot. By contrast, fusion of the ankle in dorsiflexion results in excessive loading of the heel. Fusion with the ankle in internal rotation results in increased stresses at the knee and subtalar joint, and external rotation may increase loading at the first MTPJ and can lead to the development of hallux valgus. Finally, varus positioning of the talus can lead to lateral column loading as well as increased stress through the midfoot, if subtalar joint motion is limited[18].

The ankle is stabilized by the congruent articular surfaces, the ligaments, and the muscles traversing joint. The congruency of the bony structures is particularly important during weight bearing and is dependent upon the position of the talus within the mortise, being less stable in extreme plantar flexion.

The ligamentous structures around the ankle joint are critical in the unloaded ankle, with each ligament providing variable contributions depending on the position of the foot and ankle. Serial sectioning reveals the relative contributions of each ligament and their primary mode of failure[19]: the anterior talofibular ligament (ATFL) is the most commonly injured ligament and primarily prevents anterior translation of the talus, resists internal rotation of the talus in the ankle mortise, and resists adduction when the foot is plantar flexed; the calcaneofibular

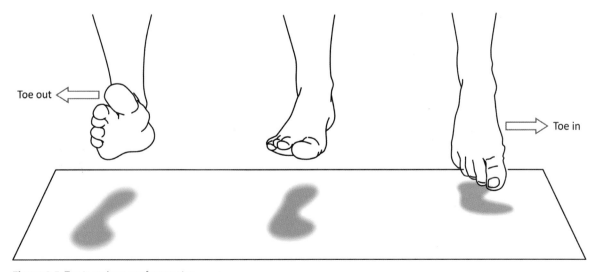

Toe out

Toe in

Figure 2.5 Toe-in and toe-out foot motion.

ligament (CFL) also resists adduction but its primary role is with the foot in neutral or dorsiflexed; the posterior talofibular ligament (PTFL) and deep deltoid resist external rotation of the dorsiflexed ankle. Finally, extreme dorsiflexion is resisted by the posterior tibiotalar ligament.

Peroneus longus and peroneus brevis muscle activity further protects against lateral ankle ligament injury when subjected to external forces[20-21]. Additionally, tibialis anterior, extensor digitorum longus, extensor digitorum brevis, and peroneus tertius play a role through eccentric contraction – resisting forced supination of the hindfoot and protecting the lateral ligament structures.

The Subtalar Joint

The subtalar joint is the articulation between the talus and calcaneus, which has three facets – posterior, middle, and anterior. Like the ankle joint, it is a single axis joint, which is angled 16° medial to the longitudinal axis of the foot and slopes 42° inferolaterally compared to the transverse plane (Figure 2.6)[22]. Nevertheless, there is a wide degree of variation.

There are two functional components: the posterior talocalcaneal facet, and the talocalcaneonavicular joint or "acetabulum pedis." The acetabulum pedis is a deep socket that accommodates the head of the talus. It is made up of the navicular, the anterior and middle facets of the calcaneus, and the spring ligament complex (superomedial and inferior calcaneonavicular ligaments) (Figure 2.7).

The oval shape of the articular surfaces and oblique orientation of the subtalar joint axis means that the subtalar joint allows the coupled movements of supination and pronation; it also enables the joint to act as a shock absorber and torque converter, converting rotation around a vertical axis to rotation around a horizontal axis, while minimizing shear through adjacent joints as energy is transferred; the ankle and subtalar joints, considered together, accommodate 19° of transverse plane rotation of the tibia, 8° through the subtalar joint and 11° through the ankle. As described above, in early stance phase, as the tibia shifts forward over the dorsiflexing ankle it rotates internally and, at the same time, the calcaneus everts. In contrast, during late stance phase, as the ankle plantar flexes, the tibia externally rotates and

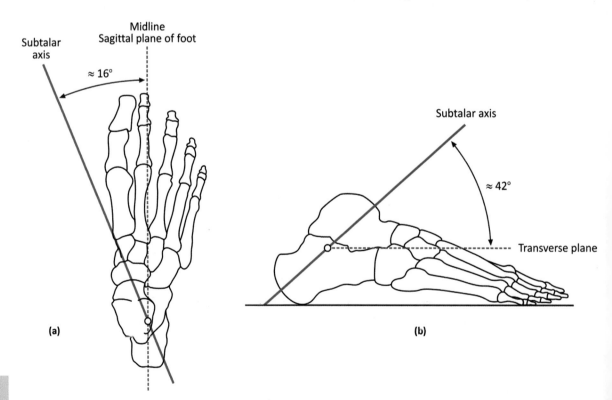

Figure 2.6 The orientation of the subtalar joint axis in (**a**) the sagittal plane; (**b**) the transverse plane.

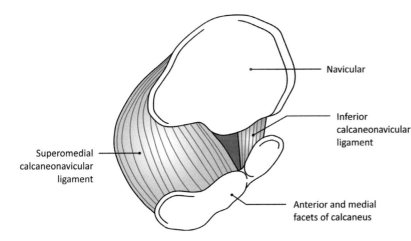

Figure 2.7 Components of the acetabulum pedis. View with the talar head removed.

Navicular

Inferior calcaneonavicular ligament

Superomedial calcaneonavicular ligament

Anterior and medial facets of calcaneus

the calcaneus inverts. These small movements are vital for the foot to accommodate uneven surfaces.

Tarsal coalition is a congenital anomaly, which can cause a painful flat foot. Calcaneonavicular or talocalcaneal coalition reduces subtalar movement and increases stress across the proximal and distal joints. The loss of the torque converter function of the subtalar joint may be taken up by the ankle joint, which, in the developing skeleton, can result in the development of a ball-and-socket ankle joint. Furthermore, the gliding motion is also restricted and the joints act as a hinge, with periosteal damage and the talar beaking that is a radiographic feature of this condition[23].

The subtalar joint is stabilized by components of the deltoid and lateral collateral ligaments, the interosseous ligaments of the sinus tarsi, and by its lateral capsule[12]. The ligaments of the sinus tarsi separate the posterior facet from the anterior and middle facets of the subtalar joint. The interosseous talocalcaneal ligament within the tarsal canal is the most important as it limits eversion. It consists of two thick short bands, which act as the center of rotation for the subtalar joint. Additionally, there are four weaker ligaments, which contribute to overall stability: the anterior talocalcaneal ligament; posterior talocalcaneal ligament; lateral talocalcaneal ligament; and calcaneofibular ligament. The tibialis posterior, flexor hallucis longus, and flexor digitorum longus provide dynamic stability to the hindfoot in general.

Transverse Tarsal Joint (Chopart's Joint)

The rotation that occurs at the subtalar joint would translate along the whole of the forefoot, everting and inverting it with tibial rotation during gait. However, the transverse tarsal joint, or Chopart's joint, allows movement and acts as a pivot in the midfoot. It consists of the talocalcaneonavicular and calcaneocuboid joints and is the key to enabling transition from a flexible to a rigid structure. The talocalcaneonavicular joint functions as a ball-and-socket joint in a similar way to the hip joint – hence the acetabulum pedis. The calcaneocuboid is saddle shaped. The convex and concave surfaces are perpendicular to each other; the convex surface is horizontal and the concave surface is vertical. The degree of congruency between the two surfaces means that motion is essentially limited to rotation.

The calcaneocuboid and talonavicular joints work together; they are parallel when the calcaneus is everted (Figure 2.8a) and non-parallel when the calcaneus is inverted (Figure 2.8b). Thus as the foot makes contact with the ground, the heel is everted, the joints are parallel, and hence the foot is flexible, accommodating any unevenness and absorbing the impact. As the calcaneus inverts, the joints diverge, converting the foot into a rigid lever upon which the tendo Achillis can act to push off[24]. In the parallel configuration, joint motion occurs around two axes: the longitudinal axis slopes medially and upward enabling inversion and eversion; the second oblique axis allows dorsiflexion/abduction and plantar flexion/adduction[16]. The composite motion (pronation/supination) results in a plantigrade foot with varus and valgus hindfoot motion.

The importance of the talonavicular joint is reflected in the effect of fusion on the remaining hindfoot mechanics. Astion et al. (1997)[25] found that

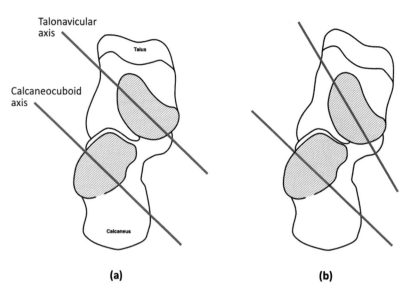

Figure 2.8 Relative change in orientation of the calcaneocuboid and talonavicular joints converting the foot from a compliant to a stiff structure. A view of the midfoot, navicular and cuboid removed. Talar head and anterior calcaneus shaded. As the heel goes into varus (**b**) the joints diverge.

fusion of the talonavicular joint, either alone or in combination with either the subtalar joint or calcaneocuboid joint, limited the motion of the remaining joints to 2°, effectively "locking" the triple complex.

The main support of the transverse tarsal joints is ligamentous. The four ligaments connecting the calcaneus and cuboid are the medial, dorsolateral, long, and short plantar ligaments. The medial calcaneocuboid ligament forms part of the bifurcate ligament, with the calcaneonavicular ligament, or ligament of Chopart. The anterior talonavicular capsule is defective, anteriorly, and is reinforced by the talonavicular ligament and the lateral calcaneonavicular ligament. Inferomedially the capsule is strengthened by the inferior calcaneonavicular ligament (the spring ligament)[12]. Further stability in subtalar inversion is provided by the two joints diverging, as described above.

Intertarsal Joints

The naviculocuboid, naviculocuneiform, and intercuneiform joints that form the arch of the midfoot are, individually, relatively rigid. However, their cumulative motion enables the transverse arch to flatten and rise with hindfoot pronation and supination, respectively. Stability is conferred by the bony congruence, and dorsal and plantar ligaments. The plantar ligaments are the strongest.

Tarsometatarsal Joints (Lisfranc)

The TMTJ consists of the three cuneiforms and their articulation with the first, second, and third metatarsals, as well as the cuboid articulation with the fourth and fifth metatarsals. In the coronal plane the tarsal bones are trapezoidal in shape, creating a "Roman arch." The configuration is stable in compression. Stability of the medial column is partially bony, with the long second metatarsal locked between the bases of the first and third metatarsals and the three cuneiforms. The articular surfaces are relatively flat, limiting overall motion. There are also strong dorsal, plantar, and intermetatarsal ligaments, which stabilize the TMTJ. The relatively stronger plantar ligaments resist flattening of the arch during stance. However, the largest and strongest interosseous ligament is the Lisfranc ligament, which arises from the lateral surface of the medial cuneiform and inserts onto the medial aspect of the second metatarsal base near the plantar surface. The integrity of the Lisfranc ligament is considered crucial to the integrity of the TMTJ complex[12]. The first metatarsal base is anchored to the medial cuneiform by plantar and dorsal longitudinal ligaments. The peroneus longus attachment to the lateral base of the first metatarsal provides dynamic resistance to first metatarsal varus and supination of the forefoot during toe off. The tibialis anterior also stabilizes the first TMTJ. Longitudinal and oblique ligaments stabilize the remainder of the metatarsals to the cuneiforms and cuboid on the dorsal and plantar surfaces. The first to third TMTJs have little motion, with the second TMTJ being the stiffest of all.

By contrast, the fourth and fifth TMTJs are mobile with approximately twice the range of motion of the medial three rays. This relative difference reflects the functional demands, with the stiffer medial column allowing a more efficient transfer of energy and creating a more effective moment arm for the tendo Achillis. The flexible lateral column enables the foot to accommodate variation in terrain with shock absorption and equitable distribution of force through the midfoot.

The importance of lateral column mobility makes the management of symptomatic degenerative change of the fourth and fifth TMTJs challenging. Thus surgery for degenerative change of the TMTJs is focused on fusion of the first, second, and third TMTJs, with retention of mobility of the fourth and fifth TMTJs. The outcome for lateral column fusion is generally poor[26], consequently replacement and interposition arthroplasty with tendon have been tried.

Forefoot

The forefoot comprises the metatarsals and phalanges with their associated joints. The metatarsophalangeal joints (MTPJs) form an arch in the transverse plane.

Two distinctive foot types have been recognized in both science and in art: one with a long first ray, the "Greek" or "Roman" foot, and the other with a relatively long second ray, the "Egyptian" foot. The long first ray was recognized in Assyrian and Greek art and is later reflected in work by Versalius and Leonardo da Vinci after its adoption by the Romans. This contrasts with Egyptian, Mexican, and Nigerian art, which depicts the second ray as longer. Morton (1927)[27] described a congenitally short first metatarsal as part of a triad, along with a hypermobile first ray and calluses under the second and third metatarsal heads, calling it metatarsus atavicus, implying atavism, or an evolutionary throwback.

The long second toe is thought to affect less than 10% of the population and is clinically more relevant in shod societies where the second toe can impinge on the toe box of the shoe. The relevance of relative toe length also relates to gait and the initial phase of push off, which occurs through an oblique axis, which passes through the second to fifth metatarsal heads – the oblique metatarsophalangeal break line (Figure 2.9). The angle of the break line varies between 50 and 70° in the transverse plane[28], and

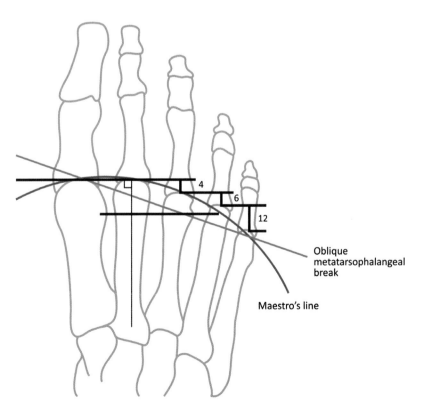

Figure 2.9 The MTPJ break line and Maestro's line. The first and second rays, in this idealized model, are the same length with a progressive shortening of 4, 6, and 12 mm of the lesser metatarsals – a Fibonacci sequence.

4

6

12

Oblique metatarsophalangeal break

Maestro's line

enables the tibial axis to remain vertical at toe off with the majority of force transmitted through the medial column of the first three rays.

Maestro et al. (2003)[29] described an arc from first to fifth metatarsal heads as a parabola with a sequential step approximating a Fibonacci sequence (Figure 2.9).

The first ray is the main load-bearing structure in the forefoot and has a key role in maintaining the medial arch. The sesamoids enhance the load-bearing capacity of the first ray. The effective shortening of the hallux either through the pathology (primary metatarsalgia) or following corrective surgery (iatrogenic metatarsalgia) may result in overloading of the lateral rays[30–31], and subsequent metatarsalgia. Hallux valgus is another predisposing factor for the development of metatarsalgia in the lateral rays. As the toe drifts into valgus it becomes unstable, defunctioning the load-bearing capacity of the first ray, placing increasing demand on the lesser toes. Pedobarography is a useful tool in the assessment process of the forefoot[32].

The metatarsophalangeal and interphalangeal joints are hinge joints, which allow flexion and extension in the sagittal plane enabling the toes to grip the ground for stability and provide proprioceptive feedback. The angle of the MTPJs in neutral is influenced by the angle of the metatarsal to the ground in the sagittal plane. The first metatarsal subtends the highest angle of between 18 to 25°. There is a progressive reduction, or flattening, of the metatarsal to the ground, to approximately 5° for the fifth metatarsal. An awareness of this cascade is important in avoiding metatarsalgia in forefoot surgery, for example following Weil osteotomy.

Foot Stability

The foot is stabilized by a combination of dynamic and static stabilizers; intrinsic and extrinsic musculotendinous structures around the foot provide dynamic stability and the congruence of the bony architecture, ligaments, and plantar fascia provides static stability.

Arches of the Foot

The foot is traditionally described with a transverse, and medial and lateral longitudinal arches. However, an arcuate structure can behave as an arch, a truss, or a curved beam.

- An arch is a segmented curved structure, normally with a keystone at the apex and the two curved limbs being supported by two columns. The lateral longitudinal arch of the foot is an example of such an arch, with the cuboid acting as a keystone between the calcaneus and fourth and fifth metatarsals.
- A truss is a variant of an arch with a tie rod holding in the two ends. In the foot the arch has two joists, one with a long arm, including the metatarsals, and one with a short arm, including the os calcis. This arch is prevented from splaying by the plantar fascia acting as a truss.
- A curved beam is unsegmented and relies on tension on the convex side and compression on the concave side to resist bending. These properties are used along the first metatarsal as part of the medial longitudinal arch.

Thus the bony anatomy of the foot forms an arcuate structure, with a plantar vault composed of longitudinal and transverse arches (Figure 2.10). In a plantar vault, all tensile and compressive forces are dissipated via the summit – in this case the ankle – to three equidistant points – in this case the heel and first and fifth metatarsal heads.

The medial arch is made up of the calcaneus, talus, navicular, the three cuneiforms and their three metatarsals. The foundations of the arch are formed by the tuberosity of the calcaneus, proximally, and the heads of the three metatarsals, distally. The lateral arch consists of the calcaneus, the cuboid, and the lateral two metatarsals. The medial and lateral arches are relatively rigid during standing but become more compliant during walking as a result of Hicks' windlass mechanism (see below). The middle three metatarsals are relatively rigid providing the main anchor and stability at push off, with the second and third metatarsals absorbing the highest pressures under the ball of the foot[33–34].

There is a transverse arch through the TMTJ. The wedge shape of the cuneiforms and metatarsal bases stabilizes the transverse arch. Furthermore the second metatarsal is recessed, which stabilizes both the medial longitudinal and transverse arches. There is also a transverse tarsometatarsal arch at the level of the metatarsal heads, which is flatter than the arch at the level of the TMTJ.

The plantar fascia acts as a truss. It is a broad, dense band of longitudinally arranged collagen fibers,

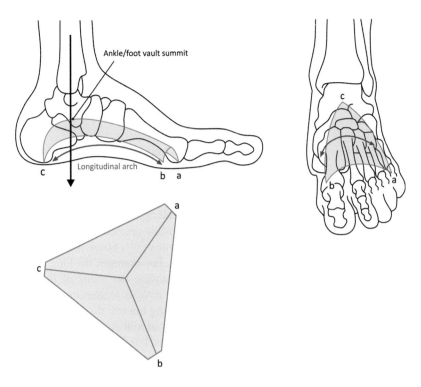

Figure 2.10 Biomechanical structure of the foot as a plantar vault. The main loading points are the first and fifth metatarsal heads and the heel (**a**, **b**, and **c**). The forces are transmitted through the vault summit, the ankle, and then proximally through the tibia.

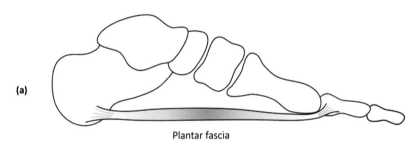

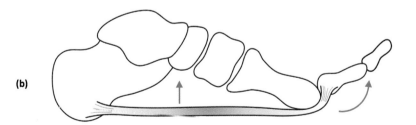

Figure 2.11 (**a**) The plantar fascia proximal and distal attachments. (**b**) Note as the toe extends the plantar fascia tightens around the metatarsal head elevating the arch – Hicks' windlass mechanism.

which originate predominantly from the medial calcaneal tuberosity. Distally the fascia inserts into the plantar aspects of the proximal phalanges of all five toes[35–36]. Hicks (1954)[37] described the windlass mechanism of the foot. He referred to the plantar fascia as a "tie rod" with collagen fibers resisting the tensile forces created by loading of the bony arch above it. The plantar fascia functions as a windlass mechanism (Figure 2.11); as the MTPJs dorsiflex, the metatarsal head acts as a drum, or windlass, around which the plantar aponeurosis tightens, stiffening and elevating the longitudinal arch. The medial insertion of the plantar fascia into the calcaneus also creates an inversion moment through the subtalar joint and the heel moves into varus, which locks Chopart's joint and further stiffens the midfoot. The extrinsic and intrinsic musculature contribute to the overall effect, pre-tensioning the aponeurosis[6]. This mechanism stiffens the foot and optimizes the propulsive effect of the tendo Achillis at toe off.

Ligaments

The plantar ligaments, including the spring ligament, provide approximately 20% of the resistance to the tensile forces created in the arch during vertical loading. They are stronger than the dorsal ligaments and this reflects the functional demands placed upon them. Expanding on the twisted-plate theory described by MacConaill (1945)[38], as the weight progresses through the medial column, the plate untwists with pronation of the heel and supination of the midfoot and forefoot. The plantar ligaments, particularly the spring ligament, are under tension and hold the talonavicular joint, in particular, in a close-packed configuration. The calcaneocuboid ligaments are also under tension, contributing to locking of the midfoot. Similarly, with eversion of the heel and pronation of the midfoot, the tension in the ligaments relaxes, increasing the overall compliance of the foot.

Metatarsophalangeal joint stability is provided by the collateral ligaments and intermetatarsal ligaments.

The plantar plates, which are connected to the plantar fascia and the deep transverse metatarsal ligament, help prevent longitudinal and transverse splaying of the foot.

The Dynamic Stabilizers and Ankle Foot Motors

Intrinsic and extrinsic muscles of the foot function both as dynamic stabilizers during balance and as the motors involved in propulsion. The flexor/extensor and everter/inverter groups work as force couples around the foot, controlling and stabilizing the foot during gait and stance while providing power for gait and protection from injury[20-21]. Some muscles have more than one function. For example, the long extensors of the toes first stabilize the joints of the toes during propulsion, then serve as accelerators in ankle joint dorsiflexion following toe off, then finally assist as decelerators of the foot at foot strike. The gait cycle is discussed in detail below, but Table 2.1 summarizes the involvement of the foot motors during the gait cycle. The plantar flexors of the ankle are the strongest muscle group and are able to generate four times more work (force × distance) than the dorsiflexors. The triceps surae generates 90% of the posterior muscle group's power. The flexor hallucis longus, flexor digitorum longus, tibialis posterior, peroneus longus, and peroneus brevis contribute the remaining 10% of ankle plantar flexion power. The dorsiflexors of

Table 2.1 Muscle function during gait cycle (adapted from Mayich et al. 2014)[39]

Phase of gait	Period	Muscles	Contraction type	Function
Stance	First rocker	Anterior muscle group[a]	Eccentric	Control of foot plantar flexion
	Second rocker	Intrinsic muscles of the foot	Eccentric	Intrinsic muscles of the foot plus tibialis posterior maintain the longitudinal arch throughout second rocker
		Peroneus longus Posterior muscle group[b]		Posterior muscle groups control forward motion of the tibia over the ankle
	Third rocker	Posterior muscle group[b]	Concentric	Locks Chopart's joint, permitting the heel to rise, rotating about the MTPJs Provides a small propulsive force
Swing	N/A	Peroneus brevis plus anterior muscle group[a]	Concentric	Dorsiflexion of the foot at the ankle for foot clearance and preparation for heel strike

[a] Anterior muscle group: tibialis anterior, extensor hallucis longus, extensor digitorum longus muscles.
[b] Posterior muscle group: tibialis posterior, flexor hallucis longus, flexor digitorum longus, gastrocnemius, and soleus muscles.

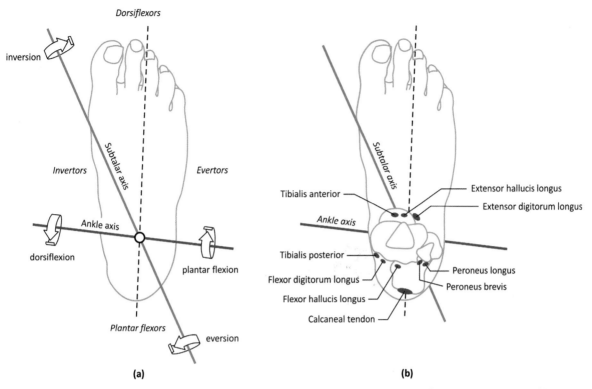

Figure 2.12 Position of the muscles around the foot relative to the ankle and subtalar joint axes: (**a**) foot motion around the ankle and the subtalar axes; (**b**) relative positions of the foot motor tendons.

the ankle joint are tibialis anterior, extensor digitorum longus, extensor hallucis longus, and peroneus tertius.

The oblique nature of the subtalar joint enables the muscle group medial to the subtalar joint's axis, i.e., the tibialis posterior, tibialis anterior, flexor digitorum longus, and flexor hallucis longus muscles, to act as inverters of the foot. Peroneus longus and brevis, extensor digitorum longus, peroneus tertius, and extensor hallucis longus on the lateral side of the subtalar joint axis act as everters. Figure 2.12 depicts the relative position of the extrinsic muscle motors in relationship to the subtalar joint. Further joint stability is achieved with the long flexors of the foot acting from their distal insertions as ankle plantar flexors and foot inverters. The long extensors act as ankle extensors and foot everters.

Gait

Normal gait describes forward propulsion of the body in which the center of mass (COM) of the body is constantly moving, constantly losing and recovering its balance. During the gait cycle, the joints of the foot and ankle transition from a flexible, compliant structure to a stable, rigid lever enabling forward propulsion of the body in a smooth, energy-efficient manner. The degree of stability or flexibility of each joint depends on the phase of the gait cycle and the joint's role in that particular phase.

An understanding of the gait cycle and its component parts is important in the diagnosis and management of foot and ankle pathology. Analysis of gait is complex and is aided by breaking the gait cycle into discrete components and analyzing the ground reaction force's (GRF) line of action and magnitude (Figure 2.13b, white arrow). At each point of the cycle, the GRF creates a moment around each joint of the lower limb. This moment acts to flex or extend the foot, ankle, knee, and hip joints to allow the body to progress forward.

The normal gait cycle is divided into two phases (Figure 2.13). Stance phase constitutes approximately 62% of the gait cycle and swing phase involves the remaining 38%. Both phases are further subdivided:

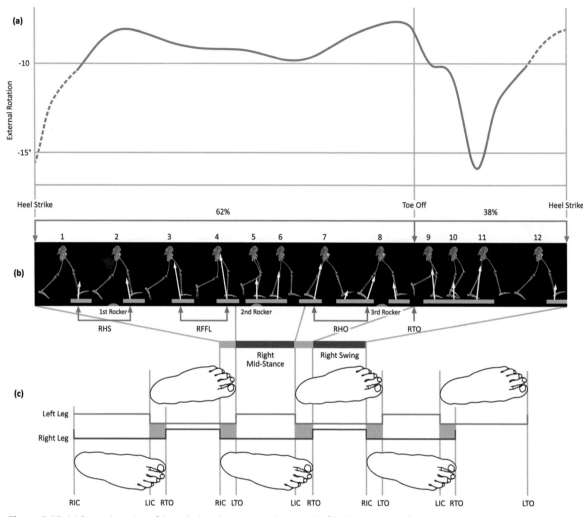

Figure 2.13 (a) External rotation of the right leg during a typical gait cycle; (b) 3D annotation of the gait cycle describing the line of action and magnitude of the ground reaction force vector; (c) reciprocating gait cycle. RIC = right initial contact; LIC = left initial contact; RTO = right toe off; LTO = left toe off; RHS = right heel strike; RFFL = right forefoot loading; RHO = right heel off; RTO = right toe off.

Stance phase is divided into single- and double-limb support in walking. In running there is no double-limb support phase.

Swing phase is divided into initial swing (point 9); mid swing (points 10–11); and terminal swing (points 11–12).

Within the gait cycle, there are a number of important events: foot strike (points 1–2 and point 12; RHS); opposite toe off (points 1 and 12); opposite foot strike (point 7); toe off (point 8, RTO); foot clearance (swing phase); tibia vertical (points 3–4); midstance (points 4–6); and second foot strike (point 12). All of these points are associated with a ground reaction

vector that changes in direction and magnitude accordingly[15] (Figure 2.13b, white arrow).

The traditional terminology describes a normal gait cycle and was developed after World War II with the development of lower extremity prosthetics. Gait is broken down into discrete events, such as heel strike, heel rise, and toe off. This traditional terminology has largely been replaced by that developed at Rancho Los Amigos, which can also be used to describe pathological gait. The Rancho Los Amigos terminology describes gait in terms of processes or segments of time. For example, initial contact, which in most cases will be heel strike, refers to the instant when the limb contacts the ground (Figure 2.13b:

points 1 and 2). In some pathological gaits (for example clubfoot and cerebral palsy) heel strike is not the initial contact with the ground, which is the advantage of the Rancho system.

Point 1 is known as *heel transient* and it plays an important part in stabilizing the foot at heel strike. The second rocker starts at point 5. In biomechanical terms, the GRF changes from being anterior to both the ankle and knee joints at point 1 to posterior, with an increase in magnitude, until the end of the second rocker at points 5 to 6.

At point 1, the moment around the ankle is a dorsiflexor and helps keep the foot dorsiflexed. At point 2, the GRF is posterior to the ankle and creates a plantar flexor moment, which triggers the tibialis anterior muscle and extensor hallucis longus to contract eccentrically. This eccentric contraction decelerates the forefoot as it approaches the ground (points 3 and 4), and stops the foot "slapping" on the ground[32].

Between points 2 and 6 the left foot is in the swing phase and only makes contact with the ground at point 7, which is heel transient of the left side. Heel transient of the left leg coincides with the start of heel rise of the right foot. This is the double-support phase, when both feet are in contact with the ground

(points 7 to 8). The third rocker of the right foot commences, ending between points 8 and 9 with right toe off (RTO), when the right foot moves into swing phase.

Determinants of Gait

Saunders et al. (1953)[40] identified six key determinants of gait to allow a smooth transition of the COM of the body during gait: pelvic rotation; pelvic obliquity; knee flexion in stance; foot and ankle motion; lateral displacements of the pelvis; and axial rotation of the lower limbs.

The COM displaces, on average, 4 cm in the vertical plane and 5 cm in the transverse plane in a smooth double sinusoid. The third component is forward displacement and occurs as a series of controlled "falls," in the way a horizontally thrown ball falls under the influence of gravity (Figure 2.14). The fall is broken by the swing forward of the non-weightbearing limb, which makes contact with the ground just at the moment the COM reaches maximum vertical displacement. The point of maximum inferior displacement occurs during double-limb stance phase, and the highest point is at single mid-stance phase. The maximum lateral displacement

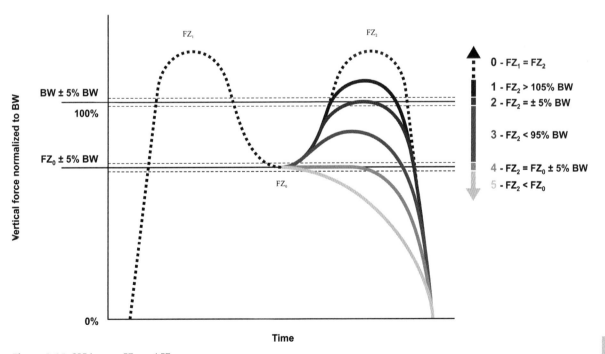

Figure 2.14 GRF humps, FZ_1, and FZ_2.
(Adapted from Williams et al. 2011[41])

also occurs at midstance phase. Any pathology that interferes with two or more of the determinants of gait will impact on the vertical and horizontal displacement as well as the sagittal plane velocity and overall loss of efficiency.

Gait Analysis

There are five main components of gait analysis: (1) temporal-spatial; (2) kinematic; (3) kinetic; (4) integrated biomechanics; and (5) electromyography[39].

Temporal-Spatial

This is the simplest and most clinically practical description. It has been referred to as the "vital signs of gait"[42] and includes: gait velocity, step length, stride length, cadence, single- and double-leg support time, and stance duration. Gait velocity can be quantified in centimeters per second, meters per minute, or by the product of cadence (the number of steps per minute) and step length. Step length is defined as the distance between one foot strike and the next on the contralateral foot. Stride length describes the distance covered between two sequential foot strikes of the ipsilateral limb. The duration of stance phase is prolonged when there is intrinsic weakness resulting, but shortened when there is pain – an antalgic gait.

The "vital signs" correlate with an individual's level of function and degree of disability. However, the patient's age and gender, concomitant pathology (cardiovascular or respiratory), the environment in which the data are collected, and footwear may influence the results. These factors make comparison between patient groups challenging but temporospatial analysis is a reliable form of assessment when assessing a patient before and after a surgical intervention.

Kinetics of Gait

Kinetics is the study of the forces acting on a moving body and is measured in Newton meters. Forces are determined using force plate analysis. Force-plate data can be used to measure vertical force, medial and lateral shear forces, and fore and aft shear forces, as well as rotational forces (torque).

At foot strike there is a spike in the vertical force component, which exceeds body weight, before dropping to approximately 80% of body weight during midstance. A further peak occurs toward toe off

and, again, exceeds body weight. At toe off the vertical force rapidly declines to zero. The body decelerates on contact with the ground and then accelerates again as the COM passes over the extended, planted limb. Deceleration and acceleration account for GRFs that exceed body weight.

In the AP direction, there are two fore and aft shear force peaks of approximately 10% of body weight. The first is at heel strike where heel contact exerts a horizontal forward shear force. The second peak occurs just prior to toe off, with a posteriorly directed shear force. A similar pattern is seen with the medial/lateral forces and both peak at 10% body weight at foot strike and just prior to toe off. Rotational forces are generated by tibial rotation. Maximum internal rotation is at foot strike, at approximately 15% of the gait cycle, and maximum external rotation is at 50% of the cycle, prior to toe off[12]. This changes when dealing with pathological gait, where FZ_2 (the second force hump/peak in a traditional GRF graph) is significantly reduced when compared to normal subjects' gait graphs and this mainly occurs in cerebral palsy patients and those with artificial limbs (Figure 2.14)[40].

The use of force-plate analysis in isolation has not been found to be a robust tool in the clinical setting. Some abnormalities of the foot and ankle have been found to produce characteristic force–time profiles that differ from the normal population, such as ankle arthritis or following arthrodesis[43].

Kinematics

Kinematics is the study of movement without considering the forces involved. The easiest way to remember the difference between "kinetic" and "kinematic" is to remember that "MA" appears in "kineMAtics" and "Movement Analysis."

Out-of-plane motion is difficult to assess by observation alone. Three-dimensional (3D) motion analysis using reflective markers and an array of cameras to acquire data on body segment motion allows more detailed analysis (Figure 2.15). Data coupled from two or more cameras are used to reconstruct a 3D view of motion, including translation, rotation, distance, velocity, and acceleration (Figure 2.15). Translation describes linear displacement while rotation describes movement around a fixed axis and is always perpendicular to that axis. As a result, motion can be assessed in three planes and around three axes.

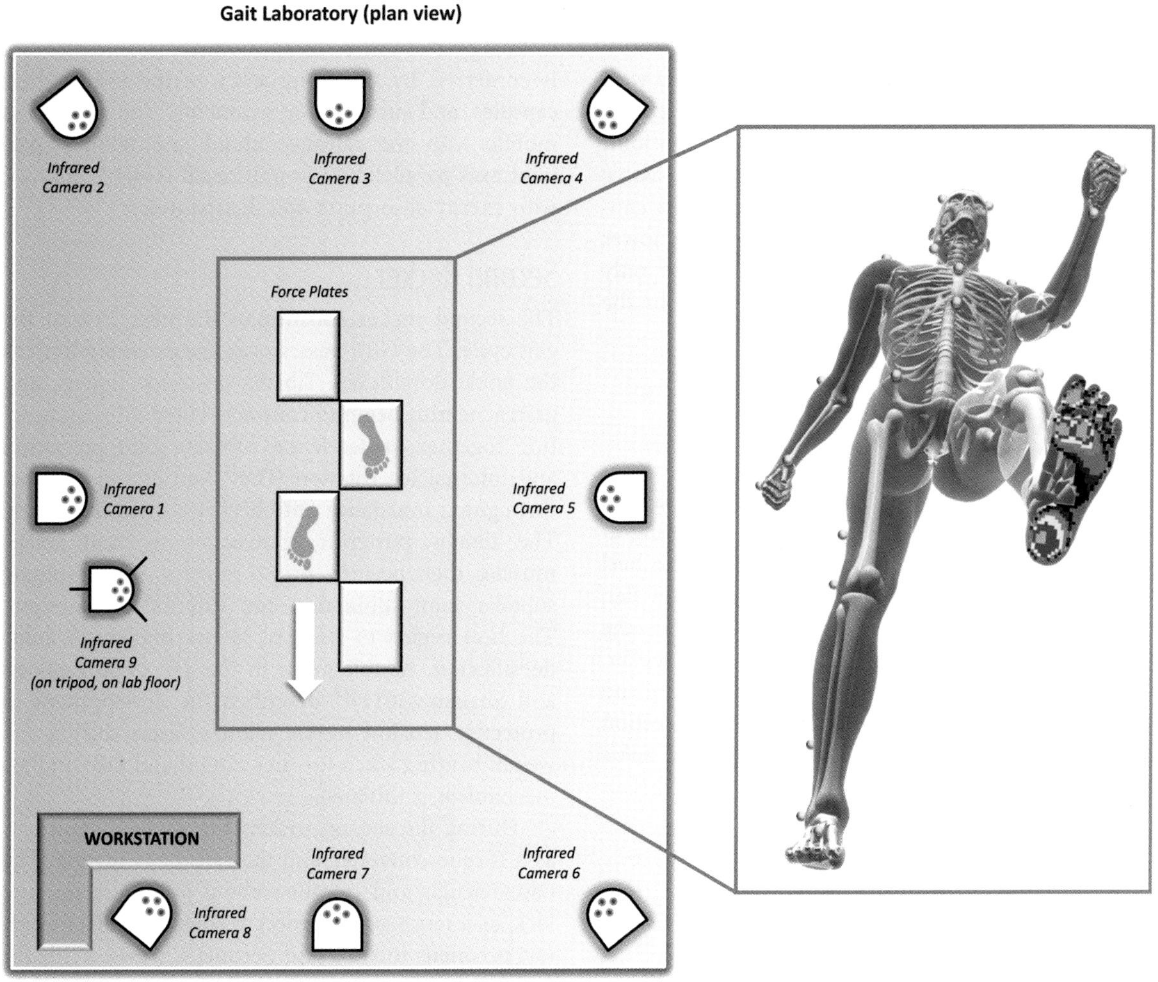

Gait Laboratory (plan view)

Figure 2.15 Annotation of the Institute of Motion Analysis and Research 3D Gait Laboratory depicting the central calibrated volume to produce accurate 3D kinematic and kinetic data.

A complex inter-relationship exists between the 26 bones of the foot and the associated joints. Each joint contributes to triplanar motion. Current technology is insufficiently sensitive to discriminate between the different bones and joints of the foot. Initial model simulations treated the foot as a single unit, grossly oversimplifying analysis. However, technological development has now enabled segmental analysis, assessing the hindfoot, midfoot, and forefoot separately. The impact of underlying pathology, such as ankle arthritis, on kinematics can be assessed[39].

Electromyography

Electromyography (EMG) measures the electrical activity of individual muscles. EMG analysis can provide information on muscle activity and the level of motor recruitment in terms of frequency (temporal summation) and quantity of motor units involved (spatial summation). This can provide an indication of the overall activity of the neuromuscular units being studied. EMG cannot be used to calculate dynamic muscle forces or assess whether the muscle is contracting eccentrically or concentrically.

Integrated Biomechanics

When kinetic, kinematic, EMG, and anthropomorphic data (mass of a body segment, position of center of gravity) are combined, joint moments and power can be calculated. These forces can either be within the joint (internal moments) or acting on the joint

39

(external moments) and are determined mathematically using a technique called inverse dynamics.

For example, it has been found that patients with ankle arthritis have reduced strength in muscle contraction in those muscle groups traversing the joint (dynamic stabilizers) and rely more on the passive restraints from the congruency of the joint, the capsule, and surrounding ligaments. The result is lower moments across the joint. However, one can only speculate whether this is a conscious process or the result of pain inhibition.

Summary of the Foot and Ankle During Gait

Perry (1992)[44] divided the gait cycle in the sagittal plane into the three discrete rotations, occurring at three different points: the first rocker at the heel lasting from initial contact to the time of foot flat; the second rocker, at the ankle, lasting from the time of foot flat to heel rise; and the third rocker, at the forefoot, lasting from heel rise until the end of stance (Figure 2.13b). The following section summarizes the three rockers of the foot and ankle during gait.

First Rocker

The first rocker of gait is approximately 15% of the gait cycle. The GRF starts anterior to both the ankle and knee joints and passes posterior to both. In the initial phase, at heel strike, the tibialis anterior and extensor hallucis longus contract eccentrically, producing an external dorsiflexion moment, which decelerates the rate of ankle joint plantar flexion. The synergistic action of these two muscle groups allows the foot to passively plantar flex in a smooth, regulated manner such that ankle joint plantar flexion is virtually stopped as the forefoot makes contact with the ground. The intrinsic muscles of the foot and posterior compartment of the calf muscles play no part in this phase. In diabetic patients there is evidence of asynchronous activity of the tibialis anterior muscle resulting in delay in activation and alteration to the normal modulating role of the muscle in lowering the foot to the ground after heel strike, leading to forefoot slap and higher plantar pressures[32]. Clinically a rupture of the tibialis anterior often also presents with a slapping-foot gait. At foot strike the heel moves into valgus and the medial longitudinal arch flattens as the body's weight passes directly over it. Energy is absorbed by the soft tissues and stability is conferred by the congruency of the joints, their capsules, and surrounding ligaments. The midfoot is mobile with the calcaneocuboid and talonavicular joint axes parallel. The overall result is stable contact, with energy absorption and dissipation.

Second Rocker

The second rocker constitiutes the next 25% of the gait cycle. The GRF passes over the extended limb as the ankle dorsiflexes. Tibialis posterior, soleus, and gastrocnemius begin to contract. These muscles function together to decelerate subtalar joint pronation and internal leg rotation. They continue to contract throughout midstance until heel rise when they relax. The tibialis posterior, gastrocnemius, and soleus muscles then become prime movers, which initiate subtalar joint supination and external leg rotation. The heel begins to rise just before maximum ankle dorsiflexion. At this point in the gait cycle Kelikian and Shahan (2011)[12] described the development of protective tension in the plantar fascia during full weight bearing when the toes extend and the windlass mechanism is initiated.

During the second rocker, the subtalar joint acts as a torque converter and the calcaneus inverts. The talonavicular and calcaneocuboid joints diverge and lock, as a result of the action of soleus, tibialis posterior, peroneus longus, and peroneus brevis. With the midtarsal joint complex locked, the peroneus longus can function, pulling the first ray, while the tibialis posterior pulls medially. Thus the opposing actions of peroneus longus and tibialis posterior compress the tarsus and improve medial/lateral stability.

Third Rocker

The third rocker lasts from heel lift to toe off. It starts 40% of the way through the gait cycle and finishes at toe off, 62% through the gait cycle. The body accelerates forward over the foot as the gastrocnemius–soleus complex contracts with a rapid increase in the GRF. Simultaneously, the vertical GRF generated exceeds that of body weight. The ball of the foot is subjected to high torque and shear forces.

Heel rise is a result of momentum of the body, deceleration of the tibia, and passive knee flexion. The body moves forward over the foot, with forward trunk momentum carrying the thigh and leg with it.

Immediately prior to heel rise the knee begins to flex. Thereafter the tibia continues to move forward while the heel rises. Shortly after heel rise, the lateral side of the foot lifts from the ground. Weight is transferred to the medial side of the forefoot where it is normally concentrated through the great toe during the final stages of toe off. The two muscles primarily producing this propulsive event are peroneus longus and brevis[45]. The lesser toes are stabilized against the ground and each toe is extended at both the proximal and distal interphalangeal joints. The long and short plantar flexors of the lesser digits stabilize the toes against the ground with the extensors helping to make the toes into rigid beams.

The major function of the intrinsic muscles during gait is to provide the tensile forces necessary to stabilize the bones of the midfoot and forefoot. When the foot is abnormally pronated, such as in a planovalgus foot, the intrinsic musculature functions more strongly and for a longer period during midstance. Conversely, less intrinsic muscle function is required during the midstance and propulsive periods in a supinated foot.

Key Points

- The foot has evolved for bipedal motion with the ability to adapt and conform to the surfaces it encounters, changing from a compliant shock absorber to a rigid lever for propulsion.
- Joint motion occurs around three axis (X, Y, and Z) and in three planes (sagittal, coronal, and transverse).
- There are two important functional components to the subtalar joint: the posterior talocalcaneal facet joint and the acetabulum pedis enabling the joint to act as a torque converter.

- The midtarsal or Chopart's joint has an important role in altering the relative compliance of the foot from a flexible shock absorber in initial foot contact to a rigid lever for propulsion at toe off.
- The stability of the Lisfranc joint is conferred partly by the bony anatomy as the second metatarsal is recessed in between the first metatarsal, third metatarsal, and the three cuneiforms, and partly by the soft tissues, including the dorsal, intermetatarsal, and plantar (strongest) ligaments, as well as the peroneus longus and tibialis anterior.
- The foot forms a plantar vault comprising a series of longitudinal and transverse arches, with the first metatarsal, fifth metatarsal, and heel forming the stable base.
- The plantar aponeurosis attaches to the medial calcaneal tuberosity and the plantar aspect of all five proximal phalanges. When the toes are extended, the plantar fascia acts as a windlass mechanism, stiffening and raising the longitudinal arch.
- There are five main components of gait analysis: temporo-spatial; kinematic; kinetic; integrated biomechanics; and electromyography.
- The gait cycle can be divided into stance phase (62% of gait cycle) and swing phase (38%). Each can be further divided: stance phase into heel strike, midstance, and toe off; and swing phase into initial swing, midswing, and terminal swing.
- There are three rockers of gait during stance phase: (1) heel strike, (2) foot flat, (3) heel raise.

Acknowledgement: The authors would like to thank Mr. Ian Christie for his editorial support and for the illustration of the figures used in this chapter.

References

1. Cavanagh PR, Lafortune MA. Ground reaction forces in distance running. *J Biomech*. 1980; 13:5, 397–406.

2. Hay JG. Citius, altius, longius (faster, higher, longer): the biomechanics of jumping for distance. *J Biomech*. 1993; 26: Suppl 1, 7–21.

3. Saltzman CL, Nawoczenski DA. Complexities of foot architecture as a base of support. *J Orthop Sports Phys Ther*. 1995; 21:6, 354–60.

4. Houtz SJ, Walsh FP. Electromyographic analysis of the function of the muscles acting on the ankle during weight-bearing with special reference to the triceps surae. *J Bone Joint Surg Am*. 1959; 41, 1469–81.

5. Myerson MS. *Foot and Ankle Disorders* (Philadelphia: W.B. Saunders Company, 2000).

6. Olson TR, Seidel MR. The evolutionary basis of some clinical disorders of the human foot: a comparative survey of the living primates. *Foot Ankle*. 1983; 3:6, 322–41.

7. Crelin ES. The development of the human foot as a resume of its evolution. *Foot Ankle*. 1983; 3:6, 305–21.

8. Conroy GC, Rose MD. The evolution of the primate foot from the earliest primates to the

Miocene hominoids. *Foot Ankle.* 1983; 3:6, 342–64.

9. Schultz AH. The relative lengths of the foot skeleton and its main parts in primates. *Symp Zool Soc Lond.* 1963; 1, 199–206.

10. Wang W, Abboud RJ, Günther MM, Crompton RH. Analysis of joint force and torque for the human and non-human ape foot during bipedal walking with implications for the evolution of the foot. *Journal of Anatomy.* 2014; 225:2, 152–66.

11. Maceira E, Rochera R. Muller–Weiss disease: clinical and biomechanical features. *Foot Ankle Clin.* 2004; 9:1, 105–25.

12. Kelikian ASS, Shahan K. *Sarrafian's Anatomy of the Foot and Ankle: Descriptive, Topographic, Functional* (Lippincott Williams & Wilkins, 2011).

13. Inman VT. *The Joints of the Ankle* (Baltimore: Williams & Wilkins, 1976).

14. Sammarco GJ, Burstein AH, Frankel VH. Biomechanics of the ankle: a kinematic study. *Orthop Clin North Am.* 1973; 4:1, 75–96.

15. Abboud RJ. Relevant foot biomechanics. *Current Orthopaedics.* 2002; 16, 165–79.

16. Hicks JH. The mechanics of the foot. I. The joints. *J Anat.* 1953; 87:4, 345–57.

17. Lundberg AI, Goldie I, Kalin B, Selvik G. Kinematics of the ankle/foot complex: plantarflexion and dorsiflexion. *Foot Ankle.* 1989; 9:4, 194–200.

18. Coughlin MJ, Mann RA, Saltzman CL. *Surgery of the Foot and Ankle* (St Louis, USA: Elsevier, 2006), Chapter 1.

19. Rasmussen O. Stability of the ankle joint: analysis of the function and traumatology of the ankle ligaments. *Acta Orthop Scand Suppl.* 1985; 211, 1–75.

20. Kerr R, Arnold GP, Drew TS, Cochrane LA, Abboud RJ. Shoes influence lower limb muscle activity and may predispose the wearer to lateral ankle ligament injury. *J Orthop Res.* 2009; 27:3, 318–24.

21. Ramanathan AK, Wallace DT, Arnold GP, Drew TS, Wang W, Abboud RJ. The effect of varying footwear configurations on the peroneus longus muscle function following inversion. *Foot (Edinb.)* 2011; 21:1, 31–6.

22. Close JR, Inman VT, Poor PM, Todd FN. The function of the subtalar joint. *Clin Orthop Relat Res.* 1967; 50: 159–79.

23. Vincent KA. Tarsal coalition and painful flatfoot. *J Am Acad Orthop Surg.* 1998; 6:5, 274–81.

24. Elftman H. The transverse tarsal joint and its control. *Clin Orthop.* 1960; 16, 41–6.

25. Astion DJ, Deland JT, Otis JC, Kenneally S. Motion of the hindfoot after simulated arthrodesis. *J Bone Joint Surg Am.* 1997; 79:2, 241–6.

26. Russell DF, Ferdinand RD. Review of the evidence: surgical management of 4th and 5th tarsometatarsal joint osteoarthritis. *Foot Ankle Surg.* 2013; 19:4, 207–11.

27. Morton DJ. Metatarsus atavicus: the identification of a distinct type of foot disorder. *J Bone and Joint Surg.* 1927; 9, 531–44.

28. Isman RE, Inman VT. Athropometric studies of the human foot. *Bulletin of Prosthetics Research.* 1969; Spring edition.

29. Maestro M, Besse JL, Ragusa M, Berthonnaud E. Forefoot morphotype study and planning method for forefoot osteotomy. *Foot Ankle Clin.* 2003; 8:4, 695–710.

30. Espinosa N, Maceira E, Myerson MS. Current concept review: metatarsalgia. *Foot Ankle Int.* 2008; 29:8, 871–9.

31. Espinosa N, Brodsky JW, Maceira E. Metatarsalgia. *J Am Acad Orthop Surg.* 2010; 18:8, 474–85.

32. Abboud RJ, Rowley DI, Newton R. Lower limb muscle dysfunction may contribute to foot ulceration in diabetic patients. *Clin Biomech (Bristol, Avon)* 2000; 15:1, 37–45.

33. Putti AB, Arnold GP, Cochrane L, Abboud RJ. The Pedar® in-shoe pressure system: repeatability and normal pressure values. *Gait Posture.* 2007; 25, 401–5.

34. Putti AB, Arnold GP, Cochrane L, Abboud RJ. Normal pressure values and the repeatability of the Emed® system. *Gait Posture.* 2008; 27:3, 501–5.

35. Huang CK, Kitaoka HB, An KN, Chao EY. Biomechanical evaluation of longitudinal arch stability. *Foot Ankle.* 1993; 14:6, 353–7.

36. Iaquinto JM, Wayne JS. Computational model of the lower leg and foot/ankle complex: application to arch stability. *J Biomech Eng.* 2010; 132:2, 021009.

37. Hicks JH. The mechanics of the foot. II. The plantar aponeurosis and the arch. *J Anat.* 1954; 88:1, 25–30.

38. MacConaill MA. *The Postural Mechanism of the Human Foot*? Proceedings of the Royal Irish Academy. Section B: Biological, Geological, and Chemical Science, Royal Irish Academy. 1945; 50: 265–78.

39. Mayich DJ, Novak A, Vena D, Daniels TR, Brodsky JW. Gait analysis in orthopedic foot and ankle surgery – Topical review, Part 1: Principles and uses of gait analysis. *Foot Ankle Int.* 2014; 35:1, 80–90.

40. Saunders JB, Inman VT, Eberhart HD. The major determinants in normal and pathological gait. *J Bone Joint Surg Am.* 1953: 35-A:3, 543–58.

41. Williams SE, Gibbs S, Meadows B, Abboud RJ. Classification of the reduced vertical component of the ground reaction force in late stance in cerebral palsy gait. *Gait Posture*. 2011; 34:3, 370–3.

42. Kirtley C. *Clinical Gait Analysis: Theory and Practice* (New York, NY: Elsevier, 2006).

43. Flavin R, Coleman SC, Tenenbaum S, Brodsky JW. Comparison of gait after total ankle arthroplasty and ankle arthrodesis. *Foot Ankle Int*. 2013; 34:10, 1340–8.

44. Perry J. *Gait Analysis: Normal and Pathological Function* (Thorofare, New Jersey: Slack Incorporated, 1992).

45. Schwartz RP, Heath AL, Morgan DW, Towns RC. A quantitative analysis of recorded variables in the walking pattern of normal adults. *J Bone Joint Surg*. 1964; 46A, 324–34.

Radiology of the Foot and Ankle

Orla Doody and Melanie A. Hopper

Introduction

There are a number of imaging modalities available to the clinician to assist in the evaluation of foot and ankle pathology. An understanding of each technique and its limitations is crucial in providing a rational approach to radiological investigation. The variety of techniques will be described, highlighting the particular advantages and shortcomings of each. Recent advances and variations relating to the individual modalities are discussed together with the normal imaging appearance of ankle and foot structures. The imaging findings for a range of common and important abnormalities are used to emphasize how imaging can be best utilized.

Radiography

The initial evaluation of many conditions of the foot and ankle is with plain radiographs. A radiograph is produced through variations in the absorption of ionizing radiation by the body's tissues, resulting in excellent spatial resolution between soft tissues and bone, due to their relative attenuation values. Excepting acute trauma, radiographs should be performed weight bearing, if tolerated by the patient. This provides standardization of views and allows review of subtle malalignments, giving important biomechanical information.

In the ankle and hindfoot, routine radiographs include a lateral, an anteroposterior (AP), and mortise view. The mortise view is acquired with 15 to 20° of internal rotation to allow unobstructed assessment of the talar dome. Variations of the standard radiographs can be used to answer specific queries; this is particularly helpful in the ankle and foot where complex anatomy can obscure important findings. For example, the Harris–Beath view provides an axial assessment of the calcaneum including the sustentaculum tali and is particularly informative in suspected fracture assessment and in imaging suspected coalition. The Harris–Beath view is taken from behind with the patient standing with the sole of the foot on the radiographic plate, and the ankle flexed, a position similar to that adopted for skiing. The X-ray beam is angled 45° downward, toward the midline of the heel.

In the foot the standard views include an AP view and a lateral view. The addition of an external oblique radiograph is essential for fracture assessment and optimizes visualization of the lateral midfoot, it is also useful in diagnosis of calcaneonavicular coalition[1] (Figure 3.1).

Advantages

Radiographs are widely available and relatively inexpensive. Many institutions are now "filmless" allowing radiographs to be acquired, viewed, and stored digitally. The Picture Archive and Communication System (PACS) facilitates rapid comparison with previous imaging studies. Plain radiographs are particularly useful in the diagnosis of bony abnormalities. The presence of a joint effusion or soft tissue swelling can help in cases of radiographically occult injuries[2] (Figure 3.2). Soft tissue calcification can point to underlying connective tissue disease, arthropathy, or even tumor (Figure 3.3).

Disadvantages

The acquisition of plain radiographs involves ionizing radiation and while the dose to the extremity is minimal, the potential hazards of radiation should not be ignored. A detailed assessment of the soft tissues is not possible on radiographs as a result of the narrow range of attenuation values of the various soft tissues, even when injured. It is important that the clinician interprets the result of any radiographic examination in the context of the clinical scenario, and that additional imaging is performed if concern persists.

(a)

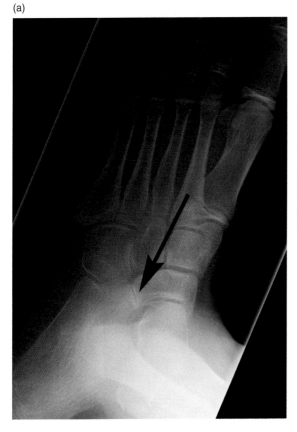

(b)

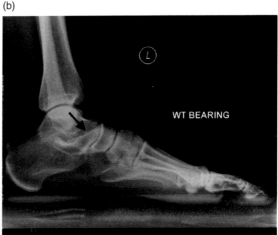

Figure 3.1 **(a)** Oblique radiograph showing fibrous calcaneonavicular coalition. **(b)** The lateral view showing a prolonged anterior process of the calcaneum, said to resemble an anteater's nose.

Variations

Stress Views

Active or passive stress views may demonstrate indirect evidence of an associated ligamentous injury. The combination of the additional applied force and an underlying ligamentous disruption results in widening of the joint space. In the ankle, stress views can evaluate for disruption of the lateral ligament complex, the medial ligament complex, and the tibiofibular syndesmosis.

Fluoroscopy

Fluoroscopic techniques are typically used in orthopedic surgery and across radiological services to guide fracture reduction or aid interventional procedures. Similar to standard radiography this modality utilizes a related x-ray source but produces real-time dynamic assessment.

Arthrography

Arthrography involves the injection of a radio-opaque contrast agent into a joint. This is typically under fluoroscopic guidance, although ultrasound (US) guidance is also used. Indirect information pertaining to the soft tissues can be deduced from the pattern of distribution of the injected contrast medium. Both diagnostic and therapeutic joint injections are frequently undertaken with arthrographic control to ensure that the agent has been injected into the correct joint. Arthrography also establishes with which joints the injected joint communicates, this is important if the injection is diagnostic.

In current practice, arthrography is often performed in conjunction with MRI scanning and less frequently with CT (Figure 3.4). In the ankle joint both direct and indirect MR arthrography have a role in the evaluation of ligamentous injuries, impingement syndromes, cartilage lesions, loose bodies, osteochondral lesions of the talus, and synovial joint disorders[3].

Tomosynthesis

Conventional radiography can be modified to acquire numerous low-dose images of a specific

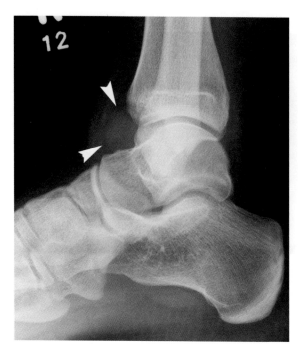

Figure 3.2 Lateral radiograph demonstrates an ankle joint effusion (arrowheads) but no fracture, following trauma.

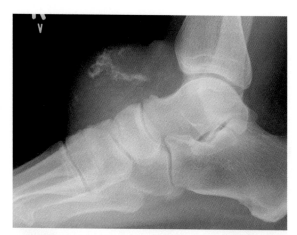

Figure 3.3 Lateral radiograph shows a synovial sarcoma anterior to the ankle joint with coarse intrinsic calcification.

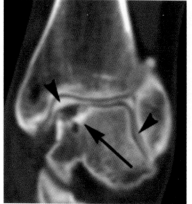

Figure 3.4 Computed tomography (CT) arthrogram, coronal reformatted image showing an established osteochondral defect (arrow). Iodinated contrast is seen within the ankle joint (arrowheads) but not within the talar dome defect.

body part resulting in the acquisition of digital tomosynthesis images. This modality was established both for breast imaging and in the evaluation of pulmonary nodules, but has been extended into musculoskeletal imaging[4]. The radiation dose is greater than for conventional radiography but lower than in CT. Tomosynthesis shows promise in the evaluation of postoperative patients as it can reduce streak artifact. Streak artifact is the dark and bright streaks from metalwork that distorts CT images. Studies have demonstrated the value of tomosynthesis in relation to wrist fractures, but it also has the potential to evaluate the foot and ankle for occult bony injury, where complex anatomy limits evaluation by plain radiography[5] (Figure 3.5).

Ultrasound

Ultrasound plays a key role in the diagnosis and management of musculoskeletal abnormality. High-frequency sound waves produced by the probe reverberate back from internal structures and the resultant echoes received by the probe are converted into the displayed image. For the evaluation of superficial musculoskeletal structures a high-frequency probe is necessary, typically a linear array probe of at least 7 MHz and ideally 10 MHz or greater. These higher frequency probes offer better spatial resolution, but reduced depth penetration. A small footprint probe is a useful adjunct in the foot and ankle. While intrinsic evaluation of bone is not possible with US, the periosteum is well visualized and occult stress fractures of the ankle or metatarsals can be detected.

Advantages

Ultrasound is a high-resolution, rapid real-time examination and involves no radiation. Compared to other imaging modalities it offers the advantage of dynamic review with structures being evaluated during active and passive movement. Due to the superficial location of the ankle and foot tendons,

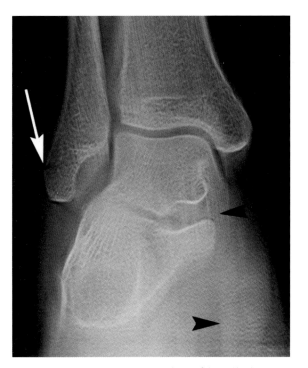

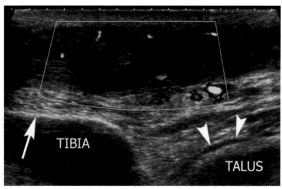

Figure 3.6 Longitudinal USS of the anterior ankle with severe tendinosis within tibialis anterior including abnormal vascularity on power Doppler. Note normal smooth bony cortex and periosteum of the anterior tibia (arrow) and normal hypoechoic articular cartilage covering the anterior aspect of the talar dome (arrowheads).

Figure 3.5 Anteroposterior tomosynthesis of the ankle showing a minimally displaced fracture of the lateral malleolus, which was not evident on conventional radiographs. Note the blurring of structures that are not at the same focal depth (arrowheads) unlike standard radiography.

US is an ideal tool to evaluate these structures. In the ankle, dynamic US is routinely used to assess for subluxation or dislocation of the peroneal tendons.

Doppler evaluation of vascularity is used in the imaging of joints for synovitis, tendons for neovascularity (Figure 3.6), and assessing blood flow within soft tissue masses. As the US wave is reflected from the moving blood there is a change in the frequency of the wave that is received by the US probe. Power Doppler uses signal amplification to increase sensitivity so that even small, low-flow vessels are recognized. Traditional color Doppler is less sensitive, but can be used to determine the speed and direction of blood flow; important, for example, in deep vein thrombosis imaging. Although both Doppler techniques can be used in musculoskeletal assessment, power Doppler is generally preferred as it is more sensitive to blood flow and the directional information provided by color Doppler is not required.

Ultrasound is widely used for image-guided musculoskeletal procedures and allows excellent visualization of the needle tip during injection, aspiration, or biopsy.

Disadvantages

Ultrasound is operator dependent and there are a number of intrinsic artifacts that can influence image quality. The most frequently encountered in musculoskeletal US is anisotropy. Anisotropy is an artifact that occurs in muscles and tendons during musculoskeletal US as a result of the linear arrangement of the structures being assessed. When the US beam is perpendicular to a tendon, the normal tendon has a characteristic hyperechoic, fibrillar appearance. If the beam is at an angle to the structure, the tendon becomes hypoechoic, simulating tendon pathology such as tendinosis. Anisotropy may lead to an incorrect diagnosis of tendinosis or tendon tear. This is an important potential pitfall in the imaging of tendons, ligaments, and muscle[6].

Variations
Beam Steering

When beam steering is applied to the transducer array the beam can be electronically tilted by 30 to 40°. This technique, either alone or in conjunction with manual angulation of the probe, allows the operator to acquire images from varying angles and helps reduce, or even eliminate, anisotropic artifact.

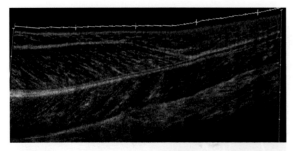

Figure 3.7 An extended field of view (EFOV) sonogram of the calf demonstrates normal medial gastrocnemius and soleus. Note the organized linear appearance of the muscle fascicles running obliquely.

Extended Field of View (EFOV) Imaging

Panoramic scanning or EFOV US can be used to demonstrate an abnormality that is greater than the width of the US probe by reconstructing several images to form a composite view of the structure under review (Figure 3.7). While the diagnostic quality of the US is not improved, this technique produces a continuous image, which can be a useful overview for the referring clinician.

Contrast Enhanced US (CEUS)

Standard sonography can be combined with the intravenous administration of specific microbubble contrast agents. These are markedly echogenic and can be used to assess microcirculation. At present, for musculoskeletal pathologies, these techniques lie firmly within the research forum, but CEUS is emerging as a promising adjunct in musculoskeletal US imaging, particularly in rheumatological conditions[7].

Ultrasound Elastography

Traditional or B-mode US relies on morphological changes within a structure to denote an underlying pathological process. Modification of the technique and equipment with elastography can provide a measure of tissue stiffness by gentle manual compression of the tissues under evaluation. The benefit of sonoelastography over conventional techniques in musculoskeletal US has not yet been fully evaluated[8]. Nevertheless, tissue softening has been identified as an early indicator of several pathological processes, including tendon degeneration. Thus elastography can be used as an adjunct to B-mode US in, for example, evaluation of the tendo Achillis (Figure 3.8).

Computerized Tomography (CT)

Multiple parallel images are produced through an array of x-ray detectors that move circumferentially around a patient, while the patient is moved through the CT scanner. The spatial resolution of calcified structures on CT renders it an ideal modality to evaluate bone and soft tissue mineralization. While acquired axially, images can subsequently be reconstructed in multiple planes, typically coronal and sagittal. For surgical planning a 3D surface rendered image can be generated from the 2D data.

Intravenous contrast is not routinely utilized in musculoskeletal CT, although it may be administered to evaluate peripheral vascularity in cases of trauma with suspected vascular compromise or in the further evaluation of a soft tissue mass.

Advantages

The process of acquiring a CT takes seconds and is well tolerated by patients. Cross-sectional imaging with CT can help detect loose bodies, osseous coalitions, and help in the preoperative planning of complex fracture fixation.

Disadvantages

As with conventional radiography, CT involves ionizing radiation – but at a higher dose. The soft tissue structures have similar attenuation values, consequently the predominant limitation of musculoskeletal CT is poor soft tissue evaluation. Even when abnormal the soft tissues cannot be differentiated from the adjacent normal soft tissues. While much more problematic with MRI, metallic artifact from a surgical prosthesis can obscure diagnostic detail on CT.

Advances
Dual-Energy CT

In dual-energy CT two x-ray tubes at different kilovoltages simultaneously acquire two data sets of the desired region. A comparison between different materials' attenuation values at these two acquisitions allows differentiation between uric acid and calcium, and allows imaging of uric acid crystals in tophaceous gout (Figure 3.9)[9]. Dual-energy CT also has potential in the evaluation of traumatic bony injuries and detecting acute bone marrow edema. It may provide an alternative assessment technique for bone bruise

(a)

(b)

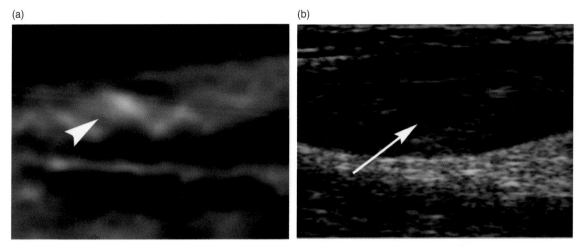

Figure 3.8 **(a)** Elastogram and **(b)** B-mode USS of Achilles tendinosis. Focal softening (arrowhead in **(a)**), corresponds to a partial thickness tear (arrow in **(b)**).

and stress response in the foot and ankle. Dose-reduction techniques both in standard and dual-energy CT are being utilized without compromising the diagnostic ability of the study[10-11].

Magnetic Resonance Imaging (MRI)

Magnetic resonance imaging has revolutionized musculoskeletal imaging and offers excellent spatial and contrast resolution. Magnetic resonance images are produced by the effect of a strong homogeneous magnetic field on the body's hydrogen nuclei in water molecules, hence avoiding ionizing radiation and its associated risks.

Magnetic resonance technology is rapidly advancing, in particular functional MRI techniques. The complexity of MRI is not helped by the vast variety of sequences available, with inconsistency in the terminology between different manufacturers for similar sequences.

In routine musculoskeletal imaging, three general groups of MR sequences are commonly used, although there are many variations.

In T1-weighted images, fat returns a high signal and appears bright; water returns a low signal and appears dark. T1 is particularly useful in anatomical evaluation.

Fat and fluid both return a high signal in T2–weighted sequences, and to increase fluid conspicuity sequences are often performed with fat suppression to reduce the fat signal. These sequences are denoted as T2fs. A frequently used alternative to fat saturation is the short tau inversion recovery (STIR) sequence.

For simplicity, proton density (PD) sequences can be considered fluid-sensitive intermediate-weighted sequences, particularly useful for hyaline cartilage assessment. Proton density sequences are often combined with fat suppression, denoted PDfs.

Advantages

Magnetic resonance imaging provides excellent spatial and contrast resolution of the ankle and foot without any associated ionizing radiation. Consequently it is widely utilized in the evaluation of bony and soft tissue abnormalities of the foot and ankle.

Disadvantages

As a result of the strong magnetic field, patients with many implantable devices, including pacemakers, are currently unsuitable for MRI, although this is an area of rapid advancement. The development of wide, short-bore MRI scanners has increased compliance in claustrophobic patients, and some centers use open-bore scanners to further help in scanning the claustrophobic patient[12]. Each sequence of a diagnostic study requires the patient to remain completely still, as even minor movement during image acquisition can cause significant artifact and loss of diagnostic detail. This can be problematic as sequences take several minutes to acquire with a much longer overall scanning time compared to CT. Although there are

(a)

(b)

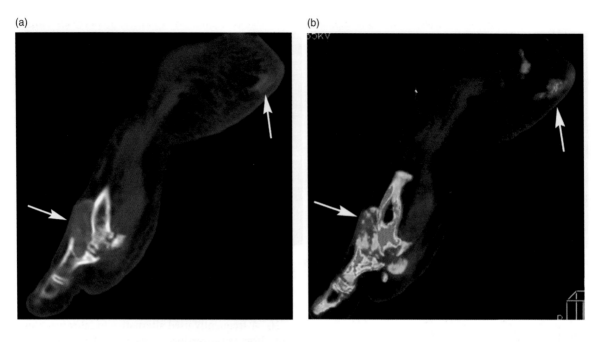

(c)

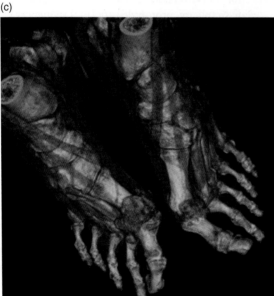

Figure 3.9 Dual-energy CT images of a patient with severe gout. **(a)** Sagittal reformatted CT; **(b)** corresponding color-coded dual-energy image, **(c)** volume rendered, color-coded two-material image. The images show extensive erosions of the first MTPJ and uric acid tophaceous deposits at the MTPJ and plantar soft tissues (arrows).

exceptions, the majority of routinely used sequences can only be viewed in the form in which they are obtained, as it is not possible to manipulate images into alternative planes, in contrast to CT.

Ferrous materials create artifacts, which impact on image quality as a result of image distortion and signal voids. The newer generation orthopedic titanium and non-ferrous prostheses are less of a problem; however, imaging of prostheses is an ongoing challenge with development of metal artifact reduction sequences (MARS) to maximize the diagnostic information achievable in these patients[13].

While MRI is highly sensitive, it is not always specific and study findings must be interpreted in the context of the clinical scenario and the appearance on other imaging modalities. For example, an MRI examination will detect increased fluid or edema, but cannot always differentiate between the various etiologies, which include trauma, infection, or malignancy.

Advances

Magnetic Resonance Arthrography

Magnetic resonance arthrography is widely used in the evaluation of the labrum of the hip and gleno-humeral joints. Both direct and indirect arthrography have a role in the evaluation of a variety of ankle joint pathologies, including ligamentous injuries, evaluation of loose bodies, and osteochondral lesions[14]; however, with the advent of more advanced MR sequences and higher Tesla scanners, many units no longer routinely use arthrography.

Cartilage Imaging

Magnetic resonance imaging provides an excellent non-invasive evaluation of articular cartilage, which as the treatment of chondral damage evolves has led to an increased focus on the development of accurate cartilage-specific sequences. These sequences focus both on the biochemical alterations and on the morphological changes including fissuring, thinning, and cartilage loss. Morphological changes are excellently evaluated with fluid-sensitive fast-spin echo and 3D T1 weighted spoiled gradient recalled echo sequences. Alterations in the water or sodium content of cartilage, or in the proteoglycan composition or distribution, can predict cartilage damage. Evaluation with T2 mapping or sequences such as delayed gadolinium-enhanced MR imaging cartilage (dGEMRIC) can identify an irregularity of chondral make-up, which precedes any morphological abnormality[15-16].

Nuclear Medicine

A standard bone scintigram is the most common nuclear medicine technique used for the evaluation of musculoskeletal disorders and is particularly useful in the evaluation of acute stress fractures of the metatarsals. A radioactive substance, typically technetium-99m labeled methylene diphosphonate (99mTcMDP), is injected into the patient. As this

undergoes radioactive decay gamma rays are emitted and detected by a gamma camera, with a resolution of 5 to 8 mm. Three-phase imaging to include an arterial phase, blood pool phase, and bone scan image can be performed to improve differentiation between bone and soft tissue. The tracer detects increased osteoblastic activity and hence areas of increased bone turnover.

Advantages

Bone scintigraphy is widely available and allows evaluation of bone metabolism of the entire skeleton in a single study. It is highly sensitive for a range of osseous conditions that result in increased bone turnover.

Disadvantages

While bone scintigraphy is highly sensitive, it has a low specificity. A wide range of bone disorders including trauma, degeneration, malignancy, and infection result in increased bone turnover. Processes without associated osteoblastic activity, such as multiple myeloma or lytic metastases, may be occult on scintigraphy. The spatial resolution is inferior to other imaging modalities and as a result the evaluation of complex anatomical areas can be limited. The radiation dose involved is greater than standard radiography.

Variations

Multiplanar data can be acquired using single photon emission computed tomography (SPECT-CT) utilizing similar radiopharmaceuticals to traditional scintigraphy (Figure 3.10). Multiplanar SPECT-CT combines both SPECT and CT imaging, resulting in greater anatomical evaluation of many musculoskeletal conditions[17].

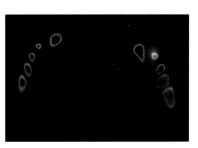

Figure 3.10
SPECT-CT showing increased radiotracer uptake due to a second metatarsal stress fracture.

Normal Imaging Appearances

Radiographs

Bones

Radiographs offer an excellent primary evaluation of bone and joint conditions. In the setting of trauma most fractures or dislocations are readily identifiable. In cases of symptomatic joints or bones, bony changes or underlying osseous lesions can be detected. The cortex is dense, well defined, and of varying thickness with a distinct cortico-medullary junction. The medulla has a trabecular structure, which can be evaluated on plain radiographs. The ratio of cortex to medulla varies depending on the bone and can impact on the appearance of certain pathologies.

Soft Tissues

Radiographs have poor sensitivity in evaluating soft tissue disorders, but the presence of a large joint effusion or marked soft tissue swelling can be an indication of underlying soft tissue injury (Figure 3.2).

Ultrasound

Bone and Joints

Internal bone structure cannot be evaluated by US. Conversely, periosteal reaction can be detected. In skeletally immature patients the normal growth plate should not be mistaken for a fracture, it is a distinct hypoechoic interruption to the contrasting hyperechoic cortex.

Ultrasound is increasingly being used to evaluate joint disease in rheumatological practice. In the evaluation of a joint the synovium, its vascularity, and the presence of fluid can all be readily demonstrated. Simple joint fluid, which is hypoechoic and compressible, can be differentiated from complex effusions with internal echoes. These echoes may be secondary to debris, an underlying crystal arthropathy, proteinaceous fluid, or loose bodies. Normal synovium is not visible, whereas abnormal synovium has a range of appearances from hyperechoic to anechoic. The bony cortex is a well-defined continuous hyperechoic structure (Figure 3.6). When imaging close to the articular surface it is important not to misdiagnose normal cortical grooves as erosions.

Soft Tissues

The subcutaneous fat is a well-defined layer, deep to the dermal tissues, and is predominately hypoechoic with linear, hyperechoic connective tissue septae traversing the fat.

Skeletal muscle is less echogenic in appearance than the subcutaneous fat and is a highly organized structure (Figure 3.7). The degree of echogenicity depends on muscle contraction, with relaxed muscle appearing more echogenic. When imaging muscles care is needed to avoid anisotropy, as a result of their frequently oblique course.

Given the superficial nature of the tendons surrounding the ankle and foot, these structures are suitable for USS evaluation. Each tendon is composed of a fibrillar array of echogenic fascicles, which are orientated parallel to the long axis of a tendon. The tendon sheath, or paratenon, is identified as a thin, highly echogenic line. Ideally, tendons should be evaluated both under tension and in their relaxed state. Under tension a tendon is taut, reducing anisotropy, which allows internal hypoechoic foci to be more readily demonstrated and also allows more confidence in assessing tendon integrity. Tension will, however, compress small vessels, thus the assessment of neovascularity should be in the relaxed state.

Ligaments are composed of Type 1 collagen, the fibers of which are arranged in a fibrillar pattern, with an echogenic US appearance. Normal ligaments vary in size, and comparison with a normal contralateral side is useful. When injured the normal linear structure is lost and hypoechoic foci are identified within the normally homogeneously echogenic ligament. Ideally ligaments should be evaluated under tension.

Ultrasound clearly demonstrates the fascicular arrangement of nerves with the hypoechoic fascicles surrounded by the echogenic perineurium. On longitudinal evaluation the parallel fascicular arrangement is shown (Figure 3.11).

Computed Tomography

Bone

Cortical bone is a dense high-attenuation layer, which in long bones thins at the metaphyses. On CT scan the trabeculae within the medullary cavity can be appreciated.

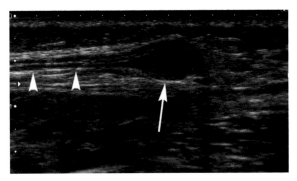

Figure 3.11 Sonogram of the sural nerve shows a terminal neuroma (arrow) due to previous nerve graft harvest. Arrowheads denote the normal longitudinal appearance of the more proximal sural nerve with normal neural fascicular bundles.

Soft Tissues

Evaluation of soft tissue structures is limited on CT, and while fat and skeletal muscle can be differentiated as structures, a detailed assessment is not possible.

Magnetic Resonance Imaging

Bone

Through its ability to differentiate hematopoietic and fatty marrow, MRI offers an invaluable method for the assessment of bone marrow. The composition and distribution of bone marrow follows well-recognized, age-dependent patterns, but this is not normally a consideration in the foot and ankle.

Joints

Unlike the other imaging modalities, MRI is unique in its ability to directly evaluate internal joint structure. The accurate evaluation of cartilage is increasingly important with advances in the treatment of chondral injuries. Hyaline cartilage is routinely evaluated on PD sequences as a discrete intermediate signal layer, distinguishable from high-signal fluid and low-signal bony cortex (Figure 3.12). Chondromalacia, fissuring, irregularity, and full thickness loss can be appreciated, although it is more challenging to detect in the smaller joints of the ankle and foot, as opposed to larger joints such as the knee.

Soft Tissues

Normal fat has a high signal on T1 and fast spin echo (FSE) T2 weighted sequences. Normal

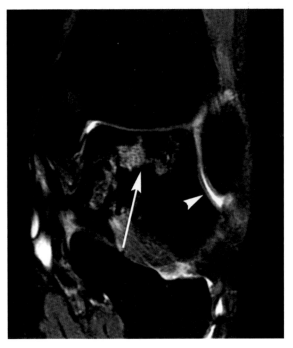

Figure 3.12 Coronal PDfs MR image showing the geographic area of abnormal bone marrow signal within the talus as a result of avascular necrosis (arrow). Normal intermediate signal cartilage within the lateral aspect of the ankle joint (arrowhead).

fat also has internal connective tissue septae, and should completely saturate with fat suppression sequences, such as STIR. The deep fascia is a defined low-signal band, which separates the subcutaneous fat from the underlying muscle compartments.

Abnormalities within the muscle can be broadly divided into masses, anatomical variations, atrophy, and conditions resulting in muscular edema. To fully evaluate for these, the correct combination of sequences is essential and will typically include T1 and T2 fat saturated or STIR sequences. On T1 weighted sequences the normal skeletal muscle signal is much lower than fat and slightly higher than water. On T2 weighted images the signal of skeletal muscle is higher than fat and lower than fluid. On STIR and fat suppressed T2 weighted imaging, normal muscle returns a higher signal than fat and a lower signal than fluid (Figure 3.13).

Tendons and ligaments are mainly composed of Type 1 collagen, and are similar in their MR appearance, returning a low signal on all conventional sequences, when normal.

(a)

(b)

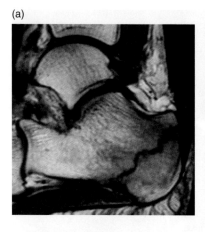
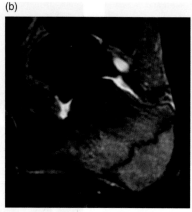

Figure 3.13 Stress fracture of the calcaneum with low-signal fracture line surrounded by bone marrow edema on MRI. **(a)** Sagittal T1 weighted; **(b)** sagittal T2fs. Note the normal signal within the adjacent skeletal muscle.

Specific Clinical Scenarios

The following clinical scenarios, while not exhaustive, highlight important imaging principles.

Fractures

Stress Fractures

While the majority of fractures will be diagnosed on standard radiography, more involved imaging modalities play an important role in the diagnosis of stress fractures, pathological fractures, and in the detection of clinically suspected, but radiographically occult, fractures in the setting of trauma. In the ankle and foot stress fractures are common, frequently involving the second metatarsal, calcaneus, and less commonly the talus or navicular. A fracture line on MR is depicted as a very low signal intensity line with associated changes in the adjacent bone consistent with edema and hemorrhage (Figure 3.13). A bone bruise is radiographically occult but on MRI is depicted as an ill-defined area of low signal on T1 and high signal on T2 or STIR, which is confined to the medullary cavity. Stress fractures in nuclear medicine studies are revealed as focal areas of increased radiotracer uptake (Figure 3.10).

Osteochondral Fractures

In the ankle osteochondral fractures typically involve the middle third of the lateral talar dome and the posterior third of the medial talar dome[18]. An osteochondral fragment partially or completely detaches as a result of single or multiple traumatic insults. The staging of these lesions is based on the condition of the subchondral bone and the integrity of the articular cartilage. Both plain radiographs and CT can detect these lesions (Figure 3.4); however, MRI provides important information as to the condition of the articular cartilage, the viability and stability of the bone fragment, and the extent of any healing[19]. As with injuries elsewhere, there are several classification systems used to describe talar dome lesions. Berndt and Hardy is the most widely used and is based on plain radiographic findings. Subsequent grading systems have been developed for CT and MR imaging. Given the variability of the classification systems many radiologists avoid using them and rely instead on a descriptive report to avoid confusion or misinterpretation.

Lisfranc Injury

Conventional radiographs can indicate a fracture or malalignment in the case of Lisfranc injury, but changes can be subtle and may be missed. The important radiographic signs of a Lisfranc injury are:

- Alignment of the lateral border of the base of the first metatarsal with the lateral border of the medial cuneiform on the AP view.
- Alignment of the medial border of the second metatarsal with the medial border of the intermediate cuneiform on the AP view.
- The medial and lateral borders of the lateral cuneiform should align with medial and lateral borders of third metatarsal on the oblique view.
- Alignment of the medial border of the fourth metatarsal with the medial border of the cuboid on the oblique view.
- The presence of a bone fragment related to the Lisfranc ligament – the "fleck sign."

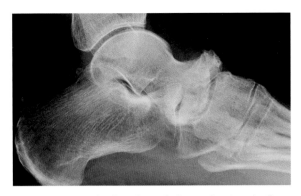

Figure 3.14 Lateral ankle radiograph shows sclerosis and collapse of the navicular in longstanding AVN.

It has to be recognized, however, that conventional radiographs miss 30% of Lisfranc injuries[20]. Thus CT and MRI scanning have a role in both diagnosis and preoperative planning.

Avascular Necrosis (AVN)

In the foot and ankle AVN typically involves the talus, metatarsal heads (Freiberg's disease), or the navicular (Kohler's disease). More generalized AVN is also seen, for example secondary to high-dose steroids. Whatever the underlying etiology, the findings on imaging are similar. Radiographs initially can be normal, even with extensive involvement. Early changes include lucency followed by sclerosis and bony collapse (Figure 3.14).

The talus is particularly prone to AVN following fracture, as its blood supply traverses the talar neck from distal to proximal. The plain film finding of subchondral lucency within the talar dome developing after fracture is known as Hawkin's sign. The sign is reassuring as the radiolucency is the result of bone hyperemia, and indicates that the blood supply is preserved. Thus AVN is highly unlikely to arise. On MRI, AVN gives the classical finding of a geographic bone marrow signal (Figure 3.12). This can be followed over time to demonstrate the recovery from the AVN, as the normal marrow fat signal re-establishes.

Tendon Dysfunction

The tendons of the foot and ankle are particularly prone to acute and chronic injury. Acute tenosynovitis initially presents with increased fluid in the tendon sheath with a normal appearing tendon. In chronic tenosynovitis, the tendon may appear nodular or diffusely thickened. Tendinosis, depending on its severity, will cause mild to severe thickening and heterogeneity of the tendon and can make assessment for a partial tear more difficult[21].

MRI and US are widely used in the evaluation of the tendo Achillis. Both modalities readily detect all aspects of tendo Achillis disease (Figures 3.8b and 3.15). The greater resolution of US also allows confident assessment of alternative causes of calf pain, including the presence of plantaris, which is a possible cause of Achilles tendinosis. Insertional Achilles tendinosis may be associated with a Haglund's deformity, or retrocalcaneal bursitis and edema within Kager's fat pad. Intrasubstance calcification is more readily assessed using USS or plain films. On MRI, calcaneal marrow edema and increased signal within the distal tendon may be demonstrated (Figure 3.15b)[21].

Tendons are particularly vulnerable to injury at specific anatomical sites, and these areas need to be carefully assessed. The features on imaging are the same no matter what the location of involvement. For example, the flexor hallucis longus (FHL) tendon is prone to injury within its fibro-osseous tunnel posterior to the talus and also more distally at the knot of Henry (Figure 3.16).

Partial tendon tears can be more difficult to assess, especially in the context of underlying degeneration or inflammation, an exception is the tendon of peroneus brevis, which develops a distinctive inverted V shape on MRI, enveloping the adjacent peroneus longus (Figure 3.17). Ultrasound scanning is particularly helpful in evaluating intermittent peroneal tendon subluxation, as it is dynamic, a particular advantage over a static MRI study[22].

Ligament Injury

In the acute setting, injuries to the lateral and medial ankle ligament complexes are well demonstrated on MRI[23]. Early diagnosis of significant ligament injury is important to prevent secondary osteoarthritis, impingement syndromes, or chronic instability[22]. Normal ligaments are crisply defined, linear, low-signal structures. Ligament injury on MRI is diagnosed by morphological and signal intensity alterations including discontinuity, detachment,

(a)

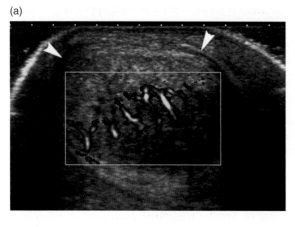

(c)

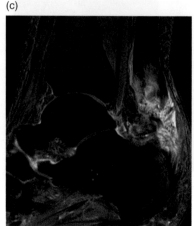

(b)

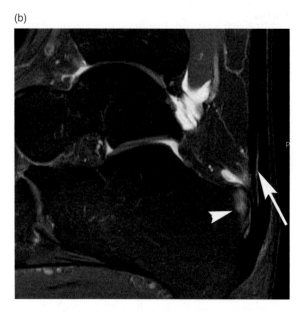

Figure 3.15 Tendo Achillis disease in different patients.
(a) Transverse sonogram of the Achilles showing severe tendinosis with abnormal vascularity and thickening of the paratenon (arrowheads). **(b)** Sagittal PDfs MRI of the ankle showing bone marrow edema in a Haglund's deformity (arrowhead) with excess fluid in the retrocalcaneal bursa. The arrow denotes insertional Achilles tendinosis with a partial thickness tear. **(c)** Sagittal PDfs of the ankle shows complete rupture of the distal tendo Achillis with edema and discontinuity of fibers.

thinning, thickening, or irregularity of the ligament (Figure 3.18). Coexistent bony edema, soft tissue edema, and extravasation of joint fluid may be present. In a chronic tear the affected ligament may appear thinned, thickened, wavy, elongated, or irregular in contour with adjacent scarring or synovial proliferation[21].

Contusional injuries, in particular of the medial deltoid ligament complex of the ankle, have a high association with inversion sprains[24]. These contusions result in loss of the normal striations within the deltoid, with the ligament demonstrating homogeneous intermediate signal intensity (Figure 3.18b).

Coalition

Tarsal coalitions can be radiologically assessed with plain film, CT, and MRI. Even when there is a complete bony synostosis, the radiographic features can be subtle but classic findings are described in the more common types of coalition (Figures 3.1 and 3.19a). The anteater sign describes the prolongation of the anterior process of the calcaneus seen with a calcaneonavicular coalition on the lateral view. It is said to look like an anteater's nose (Figure 3.1b). A talocalcaneal coalition classically has talar beaking and a C-sign on the lateral standing radiograph (Figure 3.19a). Fibrous and cartilaginous coalition

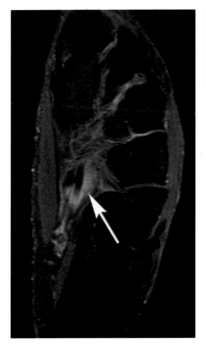

Figure 3.16 Axial PDfs MRI shows tendon sheath fluid and adjacent edema (arrow) from tenosynovitis at the knot of Henry.

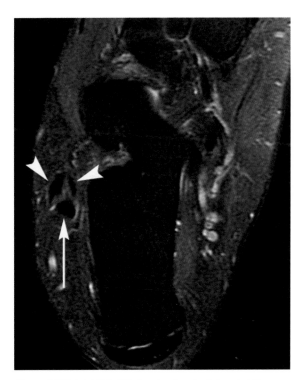

Figure 3.17 Axial PDfs MRI showing the classic inverted V (arrowheads) of a longitudinal tear in the peroneus brevis tendon enveloping the peroneus longus (arrow).

causes cortical irregularity and theses are often associated with osseous edema (Figure 3.19b).

Infection

While established bone destruction can be detected on serial plain radiographs, MRI is frequently used in the evaluation of osteomyelitis to diagnose abscess formation, to differentiate soft tissue infection from osteomyelitis, and to establish the extent of involvement (Figure 3.20a). Small locules of gas can be difficult to appreciate on MRI, but are evident both on plain film and CT (Figure 3.20b). Bone scanning is also helpful. Indium-labeled white cell scans are time consuming and have largely been supplanted by MRI scanning. The anatomic localization is also poor, although this can be got around to some degree by superimposing the scan on traditional modalities, such as CT scanning (Figure 3.20c).

The Neuropathic Foot

Diabetes mellitus is the leading causes of Charcot neuroarthropathy in the foot and ankle in modern society; however, the imaging appearances are identical to other causes of Charcot neuroarthropathy, such as spina bifida, syringomyelia, leprosy, syphilis, and spinal trauma. The chronic stage of neuroarthropathy is easily recognized on plain films with sclerosis, dislocation, debris, bony destruction, and deformity. The early stages are often radiographically occult. In these cases MRI and scintigraphy are useful to identify neuropathy before the destruction and deformity occur. MRI also helps differentiate neuroarthropathy from infection. In diabetes and other causes of neuropathy, infection is almost always contiguous with a soft tissue ulcer, reinforcing the importance of clinical examination in this patient group[25]. The presence of an ulcer and the secondary signs of infection, such as an abscess, can help differentiate infection from neuroarthropathy. Bone marrow changes on MRI scanning and increased radiotracer uptake in scintigraphy tend to be periarticular and subchondral in neuroarthropathy. Nevertheless, imaging the diabetic foot can be particularly challenging as infection, neuroarthropathy, and post-surgical changes have similar appearances and frequently coexist. An indium-labeled white cell scan can be valuable in diagnosing infection (Figure 3.20c).

(a) (b)

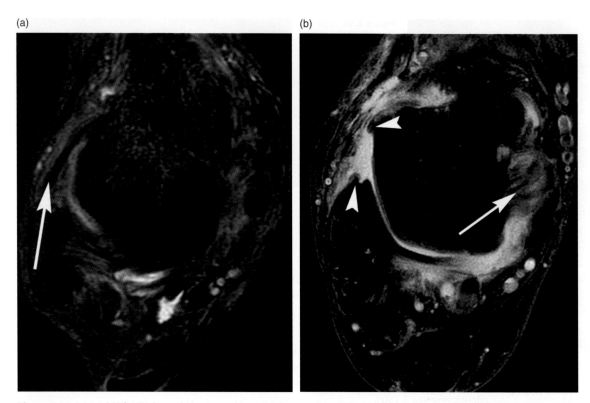

Figure 3.18 **(a)** Axial PDfs MRI shows thickening and loss of definition of the ATFL due to a recent sprain (arrow). **(b)** Axial T2fs in a different patient showing complete ATFL rupture. Arrowheads denote stumps of the ligament. There is a concomittent injury to the deltoid ligament complex, which is thickened and edematous (arrow).

(a) (b)

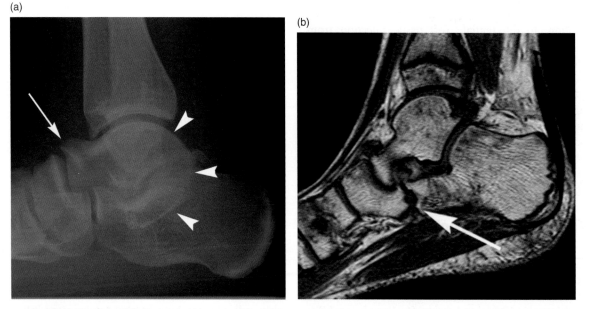

Figure 3.19 **(a)** Lateral weightbearing radiograph showing classical features of talocalcaneal coalition with talar beaking (arrow) and the C-sign (arrowheads). **(b)** Sagittal T1 of a different patient with a fibrous calcaneonavicular coalition (arrow).

(a)

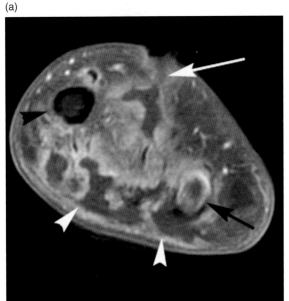

(b)

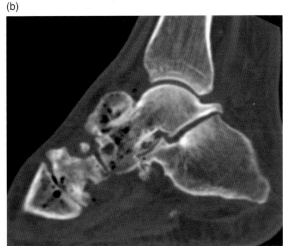

(c)

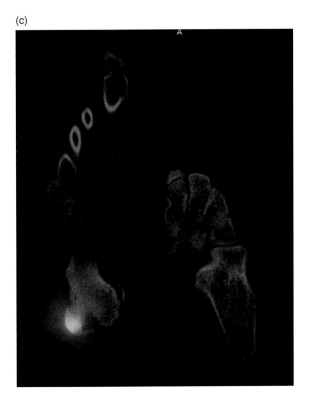

Figure 3.20 (a) Axial T2fs MRI following gadolinium contrast showing a large plantar abscess (white arrowheads) tracking to a dorsal sinus (white arrow). There has been previous surgical amputation of the second, third, and fourth digits. Note osteomyelitis within the fifth metatarsal (black arrow) compared to the normal signal of the great toe (black arrowhead). (b) Reformatted sagittal CT image of a different patient showing multiple locules of air due to extensive joint, bony, and soft tissue infection. The patient was unable to tolerate MRI. (c) CT and coregistered indium-labeled white cell scan showing focal radiotracer uptake as a result of calcaneal osteomyelitis in a patient with established Charcot neuroarthropathy and an equivocal MR examination (not shown).

Meta-analysis shows that at the current time MRI is still considered the investigation of choice for imaging infection in the diabetic foot. It has a sensitivity of about 90% and specificity of approximately 85%. Triple-phase bone scans are sensitive (80–90%) but are limited by low specificity (30–45%), while radio-labeled white cell scanning demonstrates sensitivity and specificity of about 80%[26].

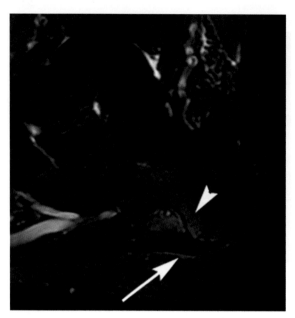

Figure 3.21 Sagittal PDfs MRI shows plantar fasciitis with thickening and edema of the origin (arrow). There is bone edema in the adjacent calcaneum (arrowhead).

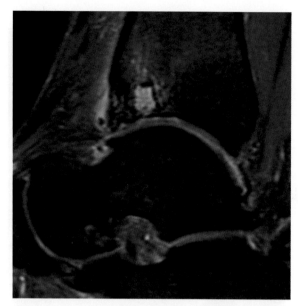

Figure 3.22 Sagittal PDfs of the ankle shows features of anterior impingement in a footballer. There is synovitis and edema with anterior cartilage loss and secondary degenerative changes within the anterior aspect of the tibia.

Plantar Fascia

The plantar fascia is readily evaluated with both USS and MRI. The normal plantar fascia is a thin, fibrous band measuring up to 4 mm in thickness at its origin with low signal intensity on all MR sequences[27]. The plantar fascia has a uniform fibrillar structure on US.

Plantar fasciitis is either the result of repetitive microtrauma, or it can be associated with a seronegative spondyloarthropathy. It has characteristic MRI findings with thickening and edema, typically at the origin of the medial band[27]. Edema may be present within the adjacent calcaneum (Figure 3.21) and heel fat pad. On US scanning plantar fasciitis appears as hypoechoic thickening. US can be used to guide injection or dry needling as part of treatment.

The fibrous proliferation of plantar fibromatosis can be demonstrated as single or multiple hypoechoic or isoechoic fusiform nodules within the plantar fascia on US. On MRI scanning the fibromata are of intermediate signal intensity on T1 and T2. Larger nodules may be heterogeneous and locally aggressive involving the plantar musculature on MRI[28].

Impingement Syndromes

Painful limitation of ankle movement can occur as a result of both anterior and posterior ankle impingement. The typical anterior impingement of footballer's ankle is between the anterior tibial spurs and the neck of the talus. This is often adequately imaged with plain radiographs, although oblique views and CT scanning can be helpful in demonstrating the anatomy.

A meniscoid lesion of the ankle is a soft tissue lesion, usually anterolaterally, in which both MRI and US can demonstrate excess joint fluid and synovitis, which can be targeted with US for diagnostic and therapeutic injection[29]. MRI can provide additional information regarding bone and cartilage injury (Figure 3.22).

Posterior ankle impingement may be caused by bony impingement from an os trigonum or a long posterior talar process (Stieda's process). In other cases the FHL tendon becomes entrapped, and can become tenosynovititc. MRI is probably the most useful imaging technique for posterior ankle pain, as it helps differentiate the osseous and soft tissue components. However, USS-guided injections can be helpful in diagnosis.

Soft Tissue Mass Lesions

In imaging soft tissue lesions, US readily differentiates between cystic and solid masses. The increased

(a)

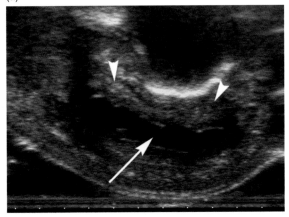
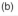

(b)

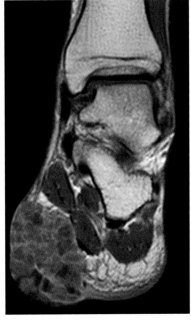

Figure 3.23 (a) Sonogram of an adventitial bursa of the plantar aspect of the first metatarsal head. Centrally hypoechogenicity (arrow) with posterior acoustic enhancement (arrowheads). (b) Coronal T1 post-gadolinium contrast image shows an extraskeletal Ewing's sarcoma as a partially enhancing solid mass, abutting the fascia but without deep invasion.

transmission of the US waves through the fluid contrasts with the solid tissue lying deep to the cyst, which causes posterior acoustic enhancement (Figure 3.23a). As previously discussed, US is extremely sensitive to blood flow. The presence or absence of flow within a lesion is an important diagnostic aid. It is only possible to confirm the cystic nature of a lesion on MRI by demonstrating lack of enhancement following gadolinium contrast administration. Consequently US is preferred by many in the initial assessment of likely cystic lesions, such as ganglia or bursae. The greater resolution of US, when compared to MRI, is of particular benefit for smaller lesions.

For deep lesions, or when more sinister pathology is suspected, MRI is invaluable in the provision of detailed information regarding involvement of the adjacent structures, including bone. MRI is also helpful for surgical planning, as the images are available to the surgeon and detail the anatomical abnormalities and their extent (Figure 3.23b).

Key Points

- The basis of foot and ankle imaging, for the majority of patients, is weightbearing radiographs.
- Ultrasound, CT, and MRI scanning have helped enormously in the refinement of foot and ankle diagnosis over the last 20 years.
- While MRI scanning evaluates all structures, often the dynamic nature of US scanning is more helpful in evaluating tendon disease.
- Modern techniques can be used to limit artifacts from metalwork in MRI and CT.
- The poor anatomical information with bone scans is overcome with newer nuclear medicine techniques such as SPECT-CT.
- Clinical correlation is crucial as there is overlap in the imaging appearances of some pathologies, in particular neuroarthropathy and infection.

References

1. Crim J. Imaging of tarsal coalition. *Radiologic Clinics of North America*. 2008; 46:6, 1017–26.

2. Clark TW, Janzen DL, Ho K, Grunfeld A, Connell DG. Detection of radiographically occult ankle fractures following acute trauma: positive predictive value of an ankle effusion. *AJR. American Journal of Roentgenology*, 1995; 164:5, 1185–9.

3. Chandnani VP, Harper MT, Ficke JR, et al. Chronic ankle instability:

evaluation with MR arthrography, MR imaging, and stress radiography. *Radiology*. 1994; 192:1, 189–94.

4. Dobbins JT 3rd. Tomosynthesis imaging: at a translational crossroads. *Medical Physics*. 2009; 36:6, 1956–67.

5. Ottenin MA, Jacquot A, Grospretre O, et al. Evaluation of the diagnostic performance of tomosynthesis in fractures of the wrist. *AJR. American Journal of Roentgenology*. 2012; 198:1, 180–6.

6. Crass, JR, van de Vegte GL, Harkavy LA. Tendon echogenicity: ex vivo study. *Radiology*. 1988; 167:2, 499–501.

7. McNally EG. The development and clinical applications of musculoskeletal ultrasound. *Skeletal Radiology*. 2011; 40:9, 1223–31.

8. Drakonaki EE, Allen GM, Wilson DJ. Real-time ultrasound elastography of the normal Achilles tendon: reproducibility and pattern description. *Clinical Radiology*. 2009; 64:12, 1196–202.

9. Nicolaou S, Yong-Hing CJ, Galea-Soler S, et al. Dual-energy CT as a potential new diagnostic tool in the management of gout in the acute setting. *AJR. American Journal of Roentgenology*. 2010; 194:4, 1072–8.

10. Guggenberger R, Gnannt R, Hodler J, et al. Diagnostic performance of dual-energy CT for the detection of traumatic bone marrow lesions in the ankle: comparison with MR imaging. *Radiology*. 2012; 264:1, 164–73.

11. Pache G, Bulla S, Baumann T, et al. Dose reduction does not affect detection of bone marrow lesions with dual-energy CT virtual noncalcium technique. *Academic Radiology*. 2012; 19:12, 1539–45.

12. Hunt CH, Wood CP, Lane JI, Bolster BD, Bernstein MA, Witte RJ. Wide, short bore magnetic resonance at 1.5 T: reducing the failure rate in claustrophobic patients. *Clinical Neuroradiology*. 2011; 21:3, 141–4.

13. Olsen RV, Munk PL, Lee MJ, et al. Metal artifact reduction sequence: early clinical applications. *Radiographics: A Review Publication of the Radiological Society of North America, Inc.* 2000; 20:3, 699–712.

14. Cerezal L, Llopis E, Canga A, et al. MR arthrography of the ankle: indications and technique. *Radiologic Clinics of North America*. 2008; 46:6, 973–94.

15. Roemer FW, Crema MD, Trattnig S, Guermazi A. Advances in imaging of osteoarthritis and cartilage. *Radiology*. 2011; 260:2, 332–54.

16. Gold GE, Chen CA, Koo S, Hargreaves BA, Bangerter NK. Recent advances in MRI of articular cartilage. *AJR. American Journal of Roentgenology*. 2009; 193:3, 628–38.

17. Even-Sapir E, Flusser G, Lerman H, Lievshitz G, Metser U. SPECT/ multislice low-dose CT: a clinically relevant constituent in the imaging algorithm of nononcologic patients referred for bone scintigraphy. *Journal of Nuclear Medicine: Official Publication, Society of Nuclear Medicine*. 2007: 48:2, 319–24.

18. Flick AB, Gould N. Osteochondritis dissecans of the talus (transchondral fractures of the talus): review of the literature and new surgical approach for medial dome lesions. *Foot Ankle*. 1985; 5:4, 165–85.

19. De Smet AA, Fisher DR, Burnstein MI, Graf BK, Lange RH. Value of MR imaging in staging osteochondral lesions of the talus (osteochondritis dissecans): results in 14 patients. *AJR. American Journal of Roentgenology*. 1990; 154:3, 555–8.

20. Rankine JJ, Nicholas CM, Wells G, Barron DA. The diagnostic accuracy of radiographs in Lisfranc injury and the potential value of a craniocaudal projection. *AJR. American Journal of Roentgenology*. 2012; 198:4, W365–9.

21. Rosenberg ZS, Beltran J, Bencardino JT. From the RSNA Refresher Courses. Radiological Society of North America. MR imaging of the ankle and foot. *Radiographics*. 2000; 20, S153–79.

22. Neustadter J, Raikin SM, Nazarian LN. Dynamic sonographic evaluation of peroneal tendon subluxation. *AJR. American Journal of Roentgenology*. 2004; 183:4, 985–8.

23. Perrich KD Goodwin DW, Hecht PJ, Cheung Y. Ankle ligaments on MRI: appearance of normal and injured ligaments. *AJR. American Journal of Roentgenology*. 2009; 193:3, 687–95.

24. Klein MA. MR imaging of the ankle: normal and abnormal findings in the medial collateral ligament. *AJR. American Journal of Roentgenology*. 1994; 162:2, 377–83.

25. Lipsky BA, Pecoraro RE, Wheat LJ. The diabetic foot. Soft tissue and bone infection. *Infectious Disease Clinics of North America*. 1990; 4:3, 409–32.

26. Lipsky BA, Aragón-Sánchez J, Diggle M, et al. IWGDF guidance on the diagnosis and management of foot infections in persons with diabetes. *Diabetes Metab Res Rev.* 2016; 32:Suppl 1, 45–74.

27. Berkowitz JF, Kier R, Rudicel S. Plantar fasciitis: MR imaging. *Radiology*. 1991; 179:3, 665–7.

28. Morrison WB, Schweitzer ME, Wapner KL, Lackman RD. Plantar fibromatosis: a benign aggressive neoplasm with a characteristic appearance on MR images. *Radiology*. 1994; 193:3, 841–5.

29. Hopper MA, Robinson P. Ankle impingement syndromes. *Radiologic Clinics of North America*. 2008; 46:6, 957–71.

Orthoses for the Foot and Ankle

James Brousil and Andrew "Fred" Robinson

Introduction

The treatment of the foot and ankle differs from many other areas of orthopedic practice, in that a large proportion of patients are treated non-operatively, many with orthoses. An *orthosis* is defined as "an externally applied device used to modify the structural and functional characteristics of the neuromuscular and skeletal systems."

The reason for using an orthosis will fall into one or more of the following categories:

- pain relief
- deformity management
- restriction or promotion of movement through a joint
- to correct the imbalance of neuromuscular structures
- to compensate for abnormalities of body-segment shape or volume
- to protect tissues during healing.

In prescribing an orthosis the diagnosis and goal of treatment must be clear. Specific considerations should be documented in the prescription, such as weightbearing limitations, recommended movement restrictions, and neurovascular pathology. The prescription for an orthosis needs tailoring to the patient and their practical needs, to ensure an appropriate, wearable device is produced. Detailed prescription will help ensure that the orthosis is acceptable to the patient, corrects the abnormality, and fits the limb to which it is applied.

The orthotist will evaluate the patient, specify the device, and make the orthosis. The orthotist should also educate the patient and, if necessary, fit or adjust the device.

Terminology

The terminology for orthoses is defined by the International Organisation for Standardisation (ISO),

based in Geneva. ISO-8549 defines the vocabulary for prostheses and orthoses, these definitions facilitate communication and limit the use of eponyms, which can introduce error and variability.

Orthoses are described by the part of the body they pertain to. Relevant devices to the scope of this chapter are: foot orthosis (FO), ankle–foot orthosis (AFO), knee–ankle–foot orthosis (KAFO), and hip–knee–ankle–foot orthosis (HKAFO).

Materials

The materials used in the manufacture of an orthosis determine its properties and function. The materials may be classified in many ways. Rigid (for example metal or plastic) or soft (for example leather, cork, or cellular plastics) is one way. In the end soft and hard materials are often combined to produce a supportive appliance (hard), which is comfortable (soft).

Rigid Materials
Metals

Steel struts were the basis for the first generation of orthoses. Steel is rigid and may be used in combination with leather strapping to correct deformity. Steel can be contoured to the shape of the limb, and joints can be fashioned to allow movement. The struts are linked to the shoe and the addition of springs and movement stops can be used to address motor deficits and instability. Nevertheless steel's stiffness risks damaging the soft tissues and it is therefore used with a soft interface, such as leather.

Plastics and Composites

Two main families of plastics are in common use in the fabrication of orthoses: thermosetting and thermoforming. The two groups behave differently with heat and their method of manufacture differs.

Thermosetting Plastics and Composites

Thermosetting plastics are formed from syrup-like resins composed of long chain, synthetic organic polymers. The two in most common use are polyester (cheap) and epoxy (expensive). Thermosetting plastics are worked in their liquid phase. They may be poured into molds to form complex shapes or laminated to form rigid structures. The result is a tough plastic, which has a high strain modulus, but which is relatively brittle and will fatigue and crack under extreme deformation.

Depending on the plastic and the desired properties of the finished product, thermosetting plastics may be cured at room temperature or using heat and pressure. In the case of epoxy, a nitrile hardener is added to cross-link it and form a rigid structure. Once curing is complete, strong, permanent bonds form between the linear-chain polymers. Once these strong covalent bonds are formed, they cannot be undone by heat. Instead the plastic will be destroyed if its glass transition temperature is exceeded. An appropriate analogy is with that of boiling an egg. Once the albumin protein is denatured by heat a solid structure is formed, and this process cannot be reversed.

The properties of these plastics may be enhanced significantly by the addition of glass, carbon, or aramid fibers to the resin base. The fibers can either be added as sheets or mixed into the liquid plastic prior to setting. The addition of glass increases tensile strength by up to 90%. Carbon fibers are lighter, improve the stiffness to weight ratio, but are more expensive. Aramid fibers added to a thermosetting plastic form Kevlar®. All of these composite materials are brittle and lack yield capacity. This may result in dramatic failure when stressed to failure, for instance during impact loading.

Epoxy and polyester are the dominant materials used in fashioning rigid orthoses:

- Polyester is quick setting but unpleasant to work with as a result of its odor. It can be toxic in confined spaces. It is versatile and may be manipulated to alter its flexibility. This is usually achieved by the addition of styrene to the mix, which increases its elastic deformation. A ratio of 60:40 of polyester:styrene is used for most foot orthoses. The resultant plastic is more flexible than epoxy, but will flex and fail upon excessive loading. It is permeable to moisture.

- Epoxy is more expensive but produces a better performing plastic when cured. Its bonding strength is four times that of polyester and it is less prone to cracking and fatigue. It is also impervious to moisture. Epoxy is used in most high-pressure lamination plastics; it may also be formed by vacuum or direct pressure molding.

Thermoforming Plastics and Composites

Thermoforming plastics are long-chain polymers, resembling strands of spaghetti. They are formed by an addition polymerization reaction. This requires heat, pressure, and a catalyst. There are no discrete bonds between the strands. They are held in apposition by temperature-sensitive, weak electrostatic attraction. These bonds become weaker with heating and form again upon cooling. Prolonged application of force to these plastics causes the molecules to slide over each other, a deformation process known as "creep."

The macroscopic organization of these long-chain polymers has an effect upon the properties of the plastic. Organization of the plastic may be amorphous (loosely packed) or crystalline (tightly packed). Molecules that have few side chains will lie in close apposition to each other, resulting in stronger intermolecular forces. Polymer strands held apart by side chains form weaker intermolecular bonds, leading to loosely associated amorphous zones within the plastic.

Composite plastics, which contain both crystalline and amorphous elements, are in common use. As with the thermosetting plastics, the addition of glass, carbon, or aramid fibers greatly improves the performance of the finished composite.

- Amorphous plastics include acrylonitrile butadine styrene (ABS), polystyrene, polycarbonate, polyethermide, and acrylic. Amorphous plastics tend to be heat moldable over a broad range of temperatures making them easy to thermoform. When cured, the polymer chains of amorphous plastics are held together by weak electric bonds, heating allows these long-chain molecules to slide over each other during the molding process. There is a window when the material is pliable and heat moldable, after this it melts. If the plastic melts, the long-chain polymers will break and the plastic degrades. Amorphous plastics tend to set clear and can be bonded to other plastics using solvents or adhesives. They are prone to creep and stress fatigue. Their main application is in the structural components of orthoses in which bending and shear stress are not involved, for example in the base layer of an in-shoe orthosis.

- Common crystalline plastics include polyethylene, polypropylene, polyether ether ketone (PEEK), and nylon. These plastics have much sharper melting points, making heat molding more difficult. They tend to be opaque when set and are difficult to bond to other plastics. They display excellent resistance to fatigue and cracking. They are used for structural orthoses that are required to resist bending and shear forces. Polyethylene and polypropylene are commonly used in AFOs. Polyethylene is available in two formats: ortholene and subortholene. Subortholene is more extensively used in sports bracing as it is more flexible, but also prone to plastic fatigue. Polypropylene is more rigid and durable than polyethylene and is more commonly used for corrective AFOs. Its thermoformable properties allow adjustment of the orthosis post manufacture.

Soft Materials

Leather

Soft materials dissipate force and accommodate deformity. Leather is still widely used, and should not be forgotten. It is soft, comfortable, breathable, readily available, and can be easily worked.

Cork

Cork is flexible and moldable. It is often used as the base layer of in-shoe orthoses. It is also used for posting and wedging hindfoot orthoses. Cork is impervious to moisture, and rigid enough to be corrective when added to an orthosis. It is used in the welting process of shoe production to fill the void between the upper and sole. Cork is commercially available in heat moldable forms, which are utilized in custom foot orthoses.

Synthetics

Soft deformable plastics are divided into open- and closed-cell foams. Open-cell foams dissipate heat and are less resistant to deformation than closed-cell materials. They allow moisture evaporation and are more durable. Polyurethane is an open-celled plastic used in the middle and base layers of cushioning insoles and training shoes. It has excellent deformation memory but poor shear resistance, and consequently is not used as an interface layer. Its most commonly available commercial form is Poron®.

Closed-cell foams are characterized by discrete, non-communicating cells. Closed-cell foams are prone to "compression settling" under load. This property is harnessed to accommodate bony prominences, for example when fitting a total contact insole in a neuropathic foot.

The most common closed-cell foam in use is a cross-linked polyethylene compound, commercially available as Plastazote®. The foam consists of nitrogen bubbles in a polyethylene base. It is both soft and deformable and is commonly used in total contact orthoses. Three densities are produced and color coded accordingly – in order of increasing density – pink, white, and black. Plastazote® is heat moldable and will adhere to other plastics if heated above its yield temperature. Aliplast®, Pelite®, and ethylene vinyl acetate (EVA) are similar polyethylene foams, all of which are available in differing grades of stiffness. These foams are used in prosthetic socket fabrication and may be formed to the shape of the limb by direct molding. Ethylene vinyl acetate is the most commonly used cushioning component used in athletic shoes, as a result of its combination of shock absorption and support.

Viscoelastic materials, such as Sorbothane®, are unique among the soft materials in that they display rate-dependent resistance to compression. This shock-absorbing property is utilized in custom foot orthoses. Sorbothane® cannot be heat formed or molded to accommodate or correct foot shape but can be shaped, or contoured, by sublayering it with harder materials.

Neoprene is a polymer of chloroprene and has a wide range of applications. It forms an ideal top layer for foot orthoses. It is impervious to moisture and resists shear stress. Neoprene is available as an open-cell variant, which has superior heat-dissipation properties, but at the expense of its cushioning ability.

Manufacture

Fabrication techniques have changed to reflect changes in material technology. The first generation of orthoses were made of leather straps and steel struts. These have now largely been replaced by moldable, bespoke devices constructed from lightweight thermoplastic materials, often reinforced with carbon fiber. Nevertheless, the techniques required to fit modern devices continue to rely on the original principles of fitting, established by "brace makers."

Orthoses may be prefabricated or custom made. Prefabricated orthoses include most of the simple in-shoe devices such as heel cups, metatarsal bars, and semi-rigid contoured orthoses. These can often be bought over the counter and are less expensive.

Custom made orthoses are molded to the limb to which they are applied. The first step in custom orthosis manufacture is the creation of a positive model of the limb to be braced. Two techniques are in common use to form this model: casting and foam-block molding.

Casting

The mold for the positive model is usually made from a complete below-knee plaster of Paris or synthetic cast. The steps are:

1. Apply a single layer of stockingette around the limb, with a length of tubing down the anterior portion of the limb to allow cast removal without damaging the skin beneath.
2. Mark joint axis and bony prominences on the stockingette. These marks transfer to the plaster.
3. Apply a layer of plaster.
4. Remove the cast with shears and then reseal it to form a negative mold of the limb.

The mold is then filled with liquid plaster, creating a positive model of the limb. The positive model can be used as a template around which a heat formable plastic can be applied.

Foam-Block Molding

The creation of a model of the foot is undertaken in a block of low-density polyurethane. The patient's weight is used to create an impression of the foot (Figure 4.1). This negative space is in turn filled with liquid plaster, to create a model of the foot. This technique is commonly used in the production of total contact insoles, which are used for patients with deformed feet, for example diabetics with Charcot neuroarthropathy. It is less reliable when fitting a corrective orthosis, as an impression of the foot in neutral alignment is not usually achieved. This is because the foot is usually partially loaded during acquisition of the impression.

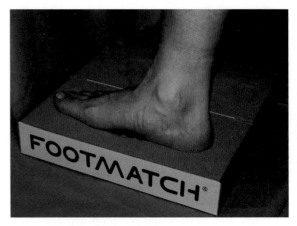

Figure 4.1 Creating a foot impression in foam. The foot is placed onto a preformed polyurethane block to create a negative impression of the foot.

Lamination and Vacuum Molding

If the orthosis is to be predominantly made of plastic, vacuum and lamination molding are usually the techniques of choice. Both techniques require a positive model of the limb and will result in a custom-made device, bespoke to accommodate the foot, or limb, shape.

Vacuum Molding

Thermoplastic sheeting may be vacuum formed to a shape using negative pressure to draw a heated, moldable sheet against the contours of a model. Reinforcements may be incorporated to provide extra rigidity in key areas. Corrugating the thermoplastic sheet can also reinforce the orthosis. Extra layers may be added to improve durability, for example on the sole of an AFO. These layers are usually added during molding of the initial shell layer. Once the orthosis has been formed, it is finished with the removal of prominent surfaces or ridges.

Lamination Molding

Lamination is a production method by which beneficial properties may be imparted into a finished plastic by layering the plastic with additional or "base" materials. Commonly used bases include nylon, Dacron® fibers, glassfiber, boron, and aramid.

The lamination process uses a polymer (thermosetting or thermoplastic) in its workable state, and a base material applied in alternate layers over a positive mold. The layers adhere to each other during production, as they are added while the polymers are still in a workable state. For example, if epoxy is used, the base material is draped over a positive mold and saturated in resin prior to the application of a further layer. Resin can be layered one on top of the other.

Lamination requires the application of pressure. Three variants are in common use:

- High-pressure lamination

This method uses a thermosetting plastic applied over a positive mold using a press capable of exerting between 7 and 14 MPa to the material. A highly durable plastic is produced. Specialized machinery is required, usually in a factory setting.

- Low-pressure lamination

This technique uses a vacuum to exert pressure on the laminated plastic and can be performed in the

hospital workshop. Local production speeds up the production process.

- Contact-pressure lamination

This technique is used to fashion multiple bespoke sections of an orthosis or to adjust an existing device by creating an addition. Pressures of approximately 1 MPa are used to manually apply layers over a positive model.

Recent advances in technology now allow models to be produced from CT/MRI data without the need for a molding visit to the orthotist. It is possible to use 3D printing to produce positive models of a limb. The printed model of the limb is then used in construction of the orthosis.

In building a metallic orthosis, which is rare for the foot and ankle, the positive model is used to ensure the contours and hinges are at the correct level.

Table 4.1 A summary of common conditions and recommended orthotic prescriptions

Disease	Goals of treatment	Prescribed device
Hallux rigidus/turf toe	Reduce the moment through the first MTPJ	Morton's extension Rocker bottom shoe
Metatarsalgia	Redistribution of plantar pressures	Metatarsal dome or bar
Midfoot arthritis	Reduce bending moment across midfoot joint	Arch support and rocker-sole shoe
Acquired flat foot – correctable	Pain relief, offloading eccentric force across medial hindfoot	Plaster or walker boot (acute phase) Rigid correcting through shoe orthosis Arizona brace
Acquired flat foot – stiff	Pain relief, realignment of ankle, redistribution of plantar pressures	Custom-molded through-shoe accommodative orthosis
Cavovarus foot	Relief of high-pressure areas under the first MTPJ and base of fifth metatarsal	Through-shoe semi-rigid accommodating orthosis
Ankle arthritis	Pain relief, restriction of sagittal plane movement across ankle	Lace-up leather or neoprene brace extending to the mid-calf
Heel-pad pain	Cushioning at heel strike, pain relief	Cushioned heel cups
Plantar fasciitis	Cushioning of heel pad	Cushioned heel cups
Insertional Achilles tendonopathy	Cushioning the heel and reducing the working length of the Achilles	Semi-rigid heel cups
Ligamentous ankle instability	Preventing extraphysiological varus across the ankle	Neoprene stirrup with added metal or plastic inserts
Flaccid instability across ankle due to paralysis (polio, nerve injury, etc.)	Holding ankle alignment through each phase of gait	Ankle–foot orthosis
Neuropathic foot with deformity	Redistribute plantar pressures	Total-contact insole

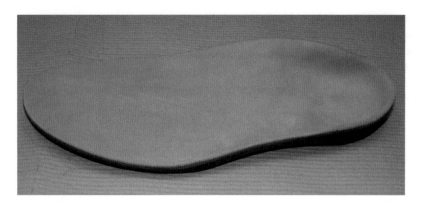

Figure 4.2 A total-contact insole, composed of three layers.

Orthoses

Virtually all diseases of the foot are treatable using an orthosis. These devices may be either in-shoe orthoses or ankle–foot orthoses, the indications for which differ depending upon the disease being treated.

Both foot orthoses and AFOs can be utilized in correcting flexible deformities within the foot. Foot orthoses are small, and more cosmetically acceptable, but achieve less correction than an AFO.

Foot Orthoses

The foot orthosis provides, and may modify, the interface between the foot and the floor. Both corrective and accommodative foot orthoses have been shown to be clinically beneficial[1-2].

In-shoe orthoses are commonly manufactured in three layers:

1. Top layer – compressible open- or closed-cell, e.g., Poron®
2. Middle layer – often compressible polyurethane
3. Base layer – firm non-compressible layer made of cork, dense foam, or thin plastic.

Assessment and Evaluation

While the measurement of pressures under the foot is possible, careful examination of the foot, weight bearing and non-weightbearing, gives the majority of the information. The deformity, its correctability, and assessment of the range of movement in each of the major motion segments of the foot should be recorded. Callosity develops under the sole of the foot in areas of high pressure. It is the callused areas that will need offloading by the orthosis. It is also important to confirm that the foot is sensate – hard insoles under an insensate foot may well lead to ulceration.

Following assessment the orthosis is prescribed. Foot orthoses can either be soft, semi-rigid, or rigid. Soft, accommodative insoles are designed to support and cushion the foot, without correction of deformity. An example is the total-contact insole, which is often used in diabetics with insensate feet and is made of three layers (Figure 4.2). The cushioning upper layer is usually made from a closed-cell polyethylene. This rests upon shock-absorbing polyurethane, which in turn sits upon a tough ethylene vinyl acetate layer that is placed in the shoe. Cut-outs are contraindicated in the neuropathic foot as pressure is generated around the cut-out, with the risk of ulceration. Similarly, patients with degenerative disease will find corrective, hard insoles painful and also need soft, accommodative insoles.

On the other hand, sportsmen usually need corrective insoles, for example to correct a flat foot. Such insoles will need to be more rigid and will consequently be harder.

Foot orthoses are also classified by their length – hindfoot, full-length, three-quarter, and forefoot.

Hindfoot Orthoses

Simple heel orthoses can usually be bought off the shelf. Their commonest indication is plantar fasciitis, where soft inserts are used to cushion heel strike. Simple prefabricated off-the-shelf heel inserts, for example made of silicon rubber, associated with an Achilles stretching program, have been shown to be more effective than a customized polypropylene insole in the treatment of plantar fasciitis[3].

A simple in-shoe heel raise can also be used to treat insertional Achilles tendinopathy by reducing the motion segment[4-6]. A heel raise can also be used to address leg length discrepancies of up to 1.5 cm, raises greater than this need to be built into the shoe.

More complex, corrective insoles can be divided into two principal groups: cavovarus and planovalgus. The cavovarus foot is stiff with reduced shock absorption, and increased pressure under the heel and first and fifth metatarsal heads. Manoli described successful management of 92% of patients with mild cavovarus feet with an orthosis with a small heel raise, to accommodate tightness of the calf, a recess under the first ray, and a laterally based forefoot wedge to correct the hindfoot varus[7]. The medial arch of this orthosis is low.

At the opposite end of the spectrum is the physiological flat foot, which is supple and more evenly distributes the pressure. In later life, flat foot may develop, or worsen, as a result of tibialis posterior tendon insufficiency, or degenerative change in the tarsometatarsal joint. In asymptomatic patients with physiological pes planus, orthoses are not indicated[8]. There is no objective evidence that orthoses alter the shape of the foot, in the short or long term. The beneficial effect seen in patients with flexible deformities is thought to result from a favorable alteration in kinetics, by modifying the position of the joints of the foot and the shoe–orthosis interface[9–10].

The correctable, *painful* flat foot can often be successfully treated with orthoses[11–12]. The orthosis has a medial hindfoot post to correct the valgus and an arch support to raise and support the midfoot. The most powerful example of this device is the University of California Biomechanics Laboratory (UCBL) insert (Figure 4.3). This is a corrective,

in-shoe device, fashioned from injection-molded polypropylene. It has a molded heel cup, which controls the subtalar joint. The UCBL insert has fallen out of favor recently, as they are bulky and difficult to fit into shoes and can be uncomfortable.

Forefoot Orthoses

Forefoot orthoses are mostly used in the treatment of metatarsalgia. Metatarsalgia is a symptom, with a number of etiologies. Not all metatarsalgia, for example the synovitis of inflammatory arthropathy, will be helped by insoles. In other cases, for example a Morton's neuroma, an orthosis can be used to offload the forefoot. Offloading can be achieved by using a metatarsal dome for a single ray, or a metatarsal bar across the width of the forefoot to offload multiple metatarsals (Figure 4.4). The bar, or dome, is placed just proximal to the pathology and redistributes the pressure.

Other devices used in the forefoot include toe spacers, caps (Figure 4.5), and sleeves to prevent the formation of soft corns between the toes and callosities over the tips of the toes. Toe props are cushioned fillers, placed in the concavity under a lesser toe to prevent pressure and calluses under the tips of the toes.

Braces to correct hallux valgus have their advocates, although, once again, there is no objective evidence that they have any impact on the natural history of the disease.

Hallux rigidus can be managed non-operatively with a full-length orthosis with a rigid forefoot extension (a Morton's extension) under the first ray. The

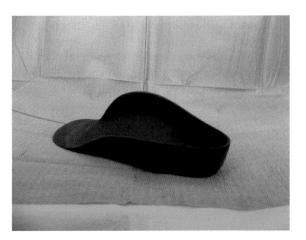

Figure 4.3 The University of California Biomechanics Laboratory (UCBL) insole is used to correct flexible deformities. Note the raised flange around the heel and sides of the device, which control the foot position, but add bulk.

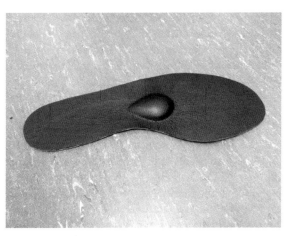

Figure 4.4 A metatarsal dome within a basic insole.

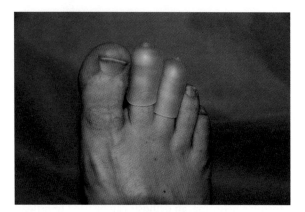

Figure 4.5 Gel toecaps to protect the sides and ends of the toes.

extension reduces movement of a painful first MTPJ. This can be used in combination with a rocker-bottom on the shoe.

Ankle–Foot Orthoses (AFOs)

An AFO is fitted from below the knee, across the ankle, and extends along the foot to provide control of the foot and ankle in the coronal and sagittal planes. An AFO can be used to:

- limit and control movement (ankle arthritis)
- correct deformity (tibialis posterior tendon insufficiency)
- compensate for weakness (foot-drop splint)
- increase the efficiency of walking (cerebral palsy).

Traditional AFOs were made of steel uprights, with an attachment to the shoe and a calf band (Figure 4.6). The metal uprights key into horizontal slots in the heel of the shoe. The uprights can be disarticulated from the shoe to help in taking it on and off. The shape of the metal interface with the shoe can be used to control ankle movement. Round pegs in round holes allow ankle movement, whereas rectangular articulations will immobilize the ankle. The problem with the hinge being at the heel, and not the ankle, level is that the device pistons up and down during gait. For this reason the round pegs in round holes design is rarely used when sagittal movement of the ankle is wanted. An adjustable hinge is accommodated in the uprights at the level of the ankle to allow movement. The hinge itself can be modified, with a lock to prevent movement, or an assist mechanism to promote motion. Most metal/leather AFOs have bilateral upright struts but variations with single-sided support do exist. These AFOs are lower profile

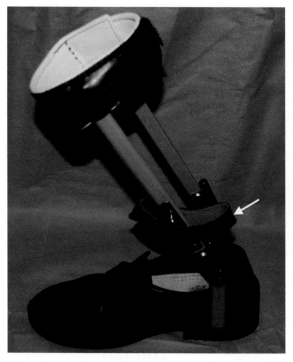

Figure 4.6 A metal and leather AFO with a strap (white arrow) to correct hindfoot varus. Note the hinges at the center of rotation of the ankle, which allow movement.

and less noticeable under a trouser, but are subject to twice the deforming force.

The metal/leather AFO may be further adapted to correct deformity. The principle of three-point fixation will be familiar to the reader from its role in deformity correction when applying a plaster. An AFO can be used in a similar way. A strap, at the apex of the deformity, pulls the deformity to the upright in the concavity.

Modern AFOs are more usually made of plastic, as it is light, easy to clean, simple to manufacture, and is easily modified. They consist of a calf shell, a foot plate, and a securing strap. The securing strap is usually Velcro®. Pressure areas can be protected with Plastazote® cushioning. Customized plastic AFOs are manufactured by molding over a plaster model. The flex of the "ankle" can be altered by trimming the plastic around the ankle – the "trim lines." The more plastic that is cut away the greater the flex.

There are numerous variants of the AFO; we will consider a few that illustrate the main design and functional principles.

The solid ankle AFO (Figure 4.7) has trim lines anterior to the malleoli. This creates a rigid construct

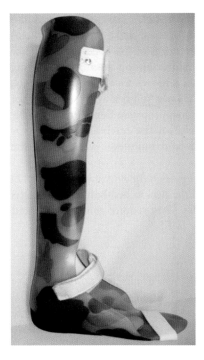

Figure 4.7 A solid ankle AFO. Note the trim lines at the level of the ankle, which sit anterior to the malleoli. This results in greater rigidity in both the sagittal and coronal planes.

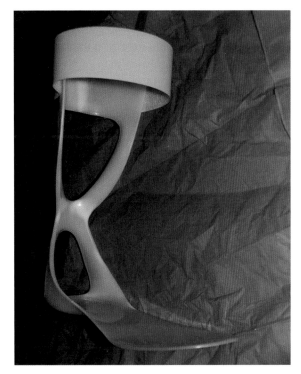

Figure 4.8 A posterior leaf-spring AFO.

and effectively abolishes both sagittal and coronal movement of the hindfoot. This is useful in the hypertonic and flaccid limb. The AFO may also prevent knee hyperextension in the stance phase by preventing equinus. Heel strike is firm and may necessitate a cushioned heel. The addition of a rocker sole also helps to normalize gait.

The posterior leaf-spring AFO is indicated for patients with a foot drop or weak ankle dorsiflexion, for example following tibialis anterior tendon rupture. The AFO controls plantar flexion at heel strike and maintains dorsiflexion during swing phase. The trim lines run behind the malleoli and allow some flexibility during gait. This flexibility is important as it allows some plantar flexion to reduce pressure in the hindfoot at heel strike. The AFO must be worn in combination with a sock or protective sleeve as it will piston slightly during gait, as the centers of rotation of the ankle and AFO are at different levels. Models with a cut-out posteriorly are available to prevent friction over the tendo Achillis (Figure 4.8).

An alternative to the posterior leaf-spring AFO is the foot-up splint (Figure 4.9). This consists of an ankle strap, which attaches to the laces of the shoe. It allows dorsiflexion, but prevents plantar flexion. It is lightweight and well tolerated, but offers no varus/valgus support.

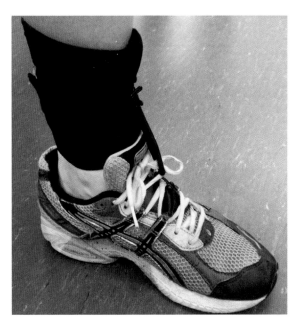

Figure 4.9 A foot-up splint.

A hinged AFO (Figure 4.10) allows movement at the ankle joint through a metal or plastic hinge; plastic is lighter but less durable and is commonly used in children. Hinged AFOs control the subtalar

71

joint and coronal plane stability and can be used in the treatment of tibialis posterior tendon insufficiency. A relative contraindication to the hinged AFO is spasticity of the limb, which may result in painful clonus, causing uncontrolled movement across the ankle.

The ground reaction AFO (or GRAFO) (Figure 4.11) is dynamic and includes a rigid band across the anterior tibia, which forces the knee into extension during stance. Prerequisites for GRAFO usage are a knee that

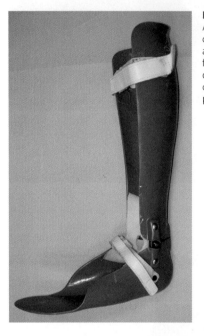

Figure 4.10
A hinged AFO. The constrained device allows plantar flexion and dorsiflexion, while controlling coronal plane movement.

has full extension and an ankle that can be moved into neutral dorsiflexion. At heel strike the GRAFO helps to prevent hyperextension of the knee. In midstance both knee flexion and extension are held, stabilizing the joints as the body moves forward. At toe off the GRAFO extends the knee, improving the efficiency of gait by preventing inappropriate flexion of the knee. It is especially useful in the cerebral palsy patients with a crouch gait and multilevel weakness of the knee and ankle.

Pressure-relieving AFOs (or PRAFOs) (Figure 4.12) are used to offload the heel in bed-bound neuropaths at risk of heel ulcers. They require good eyesight and patient compliance to fit.

Shoes

Shoes are a basic element of modern clothing and are subject to the vagaries of fashion and the commercial mores of modern society. Function and comfort are often a secondary consideration. Modern fashionable shoes are narrow with a shallow profile, often with a high heel. In patients with deformity or reduced sensation, accommodation of the foot and function may have to override fashion. Explaining this to patients can be challenging. A useful trick is to ask the individual to stand on a piece of paper. The outline of the foot is traced (Figure 4.13). The shoe can then be placed on the paper and the mismatch between the foot and the shoe becomes apparent. The overlap of many toes on the outline is illustrative that simple correction of a bunion, for example, may not allow

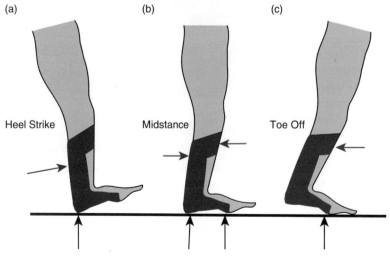

(a)   (b)   (c)

Heel Strike   Midstance   Toe Off

Points of Ground Reaction Force During Gait

Figure 4.11 A ground reaction force orthotic and the biomechanical forces exerted during wear. The three rockers of gait are shown; at each phase the force exerted by the GRAFO is shown by the red arrows.

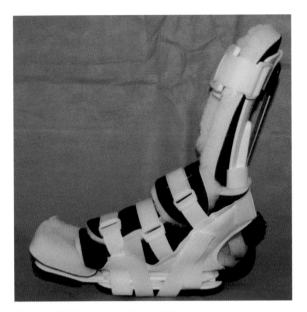

Figure 4.12 A pressure-relieving AFO.

the wearing of fashionable shoes. With middle age, and reduced soft tissue compliance, compromise may need to be learned!

It is useful to consider the characteristics of the upper and the sole separately.

The Upper

Shoe uppers are usually made from leather, as it is hard wearing and can easily be worked, stretched, and sewn into the desired shape. The main exceptions are sports shoes, which are made of canvas or nylon to give strength, breathability, and to allow drying.

The upper is divided into (Figure 4.14):

- the toe box – the material that covers the toes
- the vamp – which covers the foot, between the toe box in front and the quarter posteriorly
- the quarter – this is the section of the upper anterior to the heel
- the tongue – a section of upper that covers the dorsum of the foot
- the throat – the opening of the shoe, which admits the foot.

The throat of a shoe may be of a Balmoral, Blucher, or U-throat design (Figure 4.15). A Balmoral throat is seen in the majority of formal men's shoes, with the sides of the lace stays coming together before the toe box. This allows the laces to draw together and control the foot, preventing it moving around in the shoe.

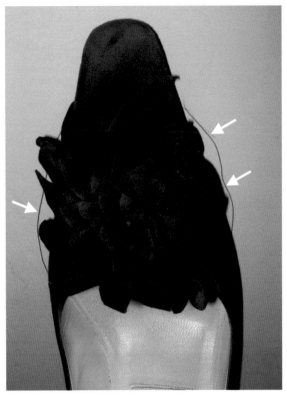

Figure 4.13 A fashionable shoe with a narrow toe box. Note the outline of the patient's weightbearing foot, showing the mismatch between shoe and foot.

The Balmoral style is not used in orthopedic shoe manufacture as it renders the quarter inflexible to expand and accommodate midfoot deformities. With the Blucher design the lace stays do not meet, and are separated by the tongue. The U-throat is an extension of the Blucher design, with the lace stays being extended to the toe box. The Blucher and U-throat designs expand to accommodate the midfoot and allow greater adjustment for feet requiring more depth – for example in the cavus foot.

The Sole

The sole of the shoe is the point of contact with the ground. It is extremely important that it provides support, grip, flexibility, and protection. The sole of the shoe is subdivided into:

- an insole or "foot orthosis," as discussed above
- the midsole – this is an optional layer, which sits directly beneath the insole and may add further support or rigidity

73

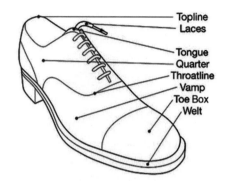

Topline
Laces
Tongue
Quarter
Throatline
Vamp
Toe Box
Welt

Figure 4.14 The anatomy of the modern shoe.

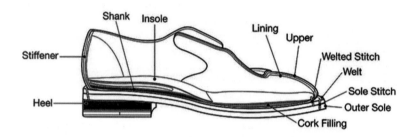

Shank   Insole
Stiffener
Heel
Lining
Upper
Welted Stitch
Welt
Sole Stitch
Outer Sole
Cork Filling

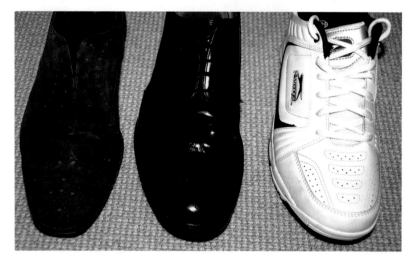

Figure 4.15 Throat designs of shoes. (From left to right) Balmoral, Blucher, and U-throat.

- the outsole – the outermost layer of the shoe, which contacts the floor
- the shank, which is the portion of the sole between the ball of the foot and the heel – this may be reinforced with steel or carbon fiber to increase rigidity.

The outsole can be manufactured from a number of materials including the following.

Leather. This traditional material has poor traction or grip, especially in wet conditions. It also wears relatively quickly.

Rubber. This is heavy and durable and does not lose grip in the wet. It can be easily molded during manufacture to improve grip. It is easily worked, for example to accept the recess for a calliper or stirrup.

Vibram® soles. These are made of dense lightweight rubber with lugs to improve grip. Vibram® soles are the choice for safety shoes, where traction is essential.

Crepe soles. These are made of naturally occurring latex rubber. They are lighter than Vibram® soles, as a result of the microscopic honeycomb structure, but have good grip and working properties.

Ethylene vinyl acetate (EVA). This has become ubiquitous in shoe production within the last 20 years. It is rubber-like, lightweight, flexible, and easily worked. It is typically used as a shock absorber in the soles of sports shoes, but is also used in insoles.

Lasting

In "lasting" the shoe upper is stretched over a last, or model of the foot. The outsole is then bonded into place in a process called bottoming. The shoe is then "de-lasted." There are several variations of lasting.

Board lasting. A fiber board is attached to the edges of the leather as it is stretched over the last. This piece of board is attached to the outsole of the shoe.

Slip lasting. This method is often used in the manufacture of lightweight sports shoes and involves stitching the upper to the insole. The last is then inserted and the upper is heat shrunk onto the last while the sole is bonded to the upper.

Injection molding. This method involves heat-sealing a thermoplastic outsole to the upper. It is a common method of mass shoe manufacture, but widths are limited by the number of "forms" or molds available. The construct makes modifications to the shoe difficult.

The Goodyear welt (Figure 4.16). This involves chain-stitching a flat piece of leather – the "welt" – to both the upper and insole. The welt is then sewn to the sole of the shoe. The void between the insole and the sole is filled, usually with cork, which is flexible and cushioning. The shoe tends to be stiffer as a result of this.

The Littleway and McKay method involves stitching the upper to the insole of the shoe. The outsole layer is then attached with a continuous stitch. This creates a pliable shoe and is the primary method seen in moccasin manufacture.

Shoe Fitting and Dimensions

Three standard measurements should be considered when determining the dimensions of a foot.

1. Overall foot length. This is determined using a Ritz stick or a Brannock device.
2. The arch length. This is the distance from the heel to the metatarsal heads.
3. Foot width, measured across the widest part of the foot.

These measurements should be taken while weight bearing for both feet. The feet are rarely identical. The shoe should be approximately 15 mm longer than the foot to allow for movement. The fit should be assessed during weight bearing. The upper should not be stretched tight over the forefoot while weight bearing and should have some "give" within it. When assessing fit, the widest part of the foot and shoe should correspond during stance phase. The depth of the shoe should be appropriate and accommodate the instep. Extra-depth shoes may be required for patients with claw toes or a cavus deformity, and to accommodate insoles.

There are seven broad categories of shoe. These are:

- The boot – this refers to any footwear that extends above the ankle.
- The clog – a backless shoe, usually fashioned from wood, which allows the wearer to slip them on with ease.

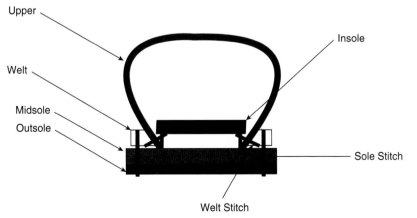

Figure 4.16 The Goodyear welt. Welted shoes may include a midsole and outsole, which makes adaptation with flares and wedges easier.

Upper

Welt

Midsole

Outsole

Insole

Sole Stitch

Welt Stitch

- The Oxford – a shoe with a low-cut top line fastened with laces.
- The moccasin – this is usually made of a single piece of fabric or leather forming both the sole and sides of the shoe. The leather is continuous under the foot, and is then brought around the last and sewn across the top of the shoe.
- The mule – a backless fabric shoe with a flat heel.
- The sandal – a shoe in which the upper consists of strapping only.
- The pump or court shoe – a thin-soled slip-on shoe, worn predominantly by women, often with a heel.

Only the boot and Oxford shoe have significant relevance for orthotic adaptation. The Oxford shoe is the basic design from which most others are derived. Oxford shoes have a low top-line passing below the ankle and an enclosed toe box with a standard securing mechanism, such as laces or Velcro. As well as Blucher, Balmoral, and U-shaped throat adaptations mentioned above, Oxford shoes may be altered to include lace-to-toe shoes to accommodate complex midfoot deformities.

Outsole Modifications

Shoe modifications are a cost-effective, practical method of adapting off-the-shelf shoes. The techniques used include:

1. Stiffening with a shank.

    The original sole of the shoe is removed. A midsole is then attached under the upper, into which a carbon fiber or steel shank is incorporated. This stiffens the shoe and reduces the bending forces across the mid- and forefoot. The original sole is then reattached to restore the functional tread. Stiffening can be used for degenerative disease of the mid- and forefoot, as well as with a rocker sole.

2. Applying a rocker sole.

    A rocker sole enhances forward movement during stance phase and can compensate to some degree for stiffness in one portion of the kinetic chain. There are two principal types each with different indications.

    - The mild rocker sole has small rockers at the level of the heel and the MTPJs. It is useful with early degeneration of the ankle and forefoot.

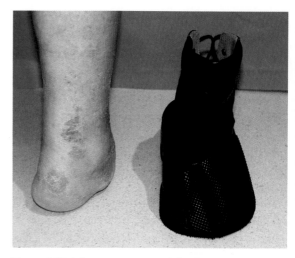

Figure 4.17 A flare to correct varus deformity.

- The heel–toe rocker consists of a single arc extending the length of the sole of the shoe and is indicated in patients with midfoot degeneration or postsurgical fusion. It is also helpful in patients fitted with a stiff AFO. The stance phase is shortened during ambulation so caution should be used when recommending these shoes to patients with poor balance.

3. Heel wedges and flares (Figure 4.17).

    Wedges are occasionally added to the heel of a shoe to correct varus or valgus. A medially based wedge is used for valgus and a laterally based wedge for varus. However, a Manoli insole, as described above, is usually preferred for the cavovarus foot. A flare is more powerful, extending up to the shoe upper. It is less cosmetically acceptable, but is more stable. A flare is useful where, for example, the peroneal tendons are non-functional.

4. Leg-length inequality.

    Up to 1.5 cm of correction can usually be achieved with an in-shoe heel raise. For greater corrections the heel starts to escape from the heel cup of the shoe, making the shoe impractical. Thus larger raises are applied to the sole of the shoe. Heel only build-ups should not exceed 2 cm to avoid an equinus contracture. Therefore larger build-ups require full-length additions to the sole, with extra width of the sole, to increase stability.

Special Considerations

Two conditions illustrate many of the principles of treatment with orthoses – the sensory neuropathy of diabetes mellitus and the paralysis of poliomyelitis.

Diabetes Mellitus

The primary aim of orthoses and shoes in the neuropathic limb is to accommodate deformity, and prevent ulceration and amputation. In the neuropathic foot at risk, the patient requires management with a combination of accommodative shoes and pressure-relieving insoles.

Diabetic shoes: in all cases diabetic patients need education to ensure shoes of the correct size and design are chosen. Shoes for the neuropath need to accommodate the foot, to prevent ulceration. The basic design features include (Figure 4.18):

- soft, pliable leather uppers
- broad and deep toe box, such that there is excess vamp material when the patient stands in the shoe
- rocker sole
- bevelled heel for stability
- no stitching over the forefoot.

Total-contact orthoses (Figure 4.2): the essence of such orthoses is cushioning and accommodation of deformity. Attempts at correction will potentially lead to pressure and ulceration. The insoles reduce shear forces at the skin interface, redistribute pressure evenly over the maximal possible area, and absorb shock. These insoles have been shown to reduce the recurrence of ulceration in the neuropathic foot[13–14].

To make a total-contact orthosis, a closed-cell polyethylene foam is molded directly to the shape of the patient's foot. A positive model is produced. The total-contact orthosis is then constructed, employing four layers:

- The support layer. Usually made of a closed-cell polyethylene foam, such as Plastazote®. This must be easily moldable and cushioning.
- A shock-absorbing layer. This is usually made of an open-cell polyurethane rubber, commonly Poron®.
- A layer incorporating any additions, such as a metatarsal pad or arch support.
- The interface layer sits directly on the shoe and is the most durable. This layer is commonly made of ethylene vinyl acetate (EVA) due to its resilient and elastic properties.

The shoe will need to be deep enough to accommodate the foot and the insole. After a short period of ambulation the foot should be inspected for pressure areas. Areas of increased temperature and redness are indicators of increased shear, and adjustments should be made.

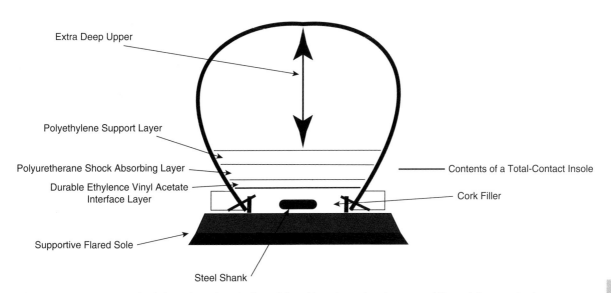

Extra Deep Upper

Polyethylene Support Layer

Polyuretherane Shock Absorbing Layer

Durable Ethylence Vinyl Acetate Interface Layer

Supportive Flared Sole

Steel Shank

Contents of a Total-Contact Insole

Cork Filler

Figure 4.18 The structure of a diabetic shoe. Note the flare of the mid- and outsole to increase stability, and the extra depth to accommodate a total-contact insole.

Total-Contact Casting (TCC)

The first descriptions of total-contact casting originate from the Indian subcontinent in the 1930s. The initial indication in these case studies was for neuropathic foot ulceration in patients with leprosy. The 1960s saw the widespread adoption of this practice to treat diabetic neuropaths. The total-contact cast is still considered the "gold standard" treatment for neuropathic ulceration, as demonstrated in multiple studies showing shorter healing time than other methods[13–17]. The cast closely conforms to the limb and sole of the foot, reducing shear and rotational stress across the skin, which would propagate any skin defect and prevent healing. The total-contact cast also redistributes force over a broader area during stance phase by transferring load evenly under the sole of the foot. In addition, immobilizing the ankle allows protection of the forefoot from point loading at toe off. A secondary beneficial effect of TCCs is a reduction of stride length so that with each step less force is transferred through the foot.

In the United States and the UK, TCCs are widely used in the treatment of neuropathic deformity and ulceration. This is not so across Europe[18]. Recently removable, commercially available, boots have begun to gain popularity and replace TCCs. The evidence to support the use of these devices is contradictory but one study suggested that all forms of protection were equal, as long as the patient wore the device. In the UK, the guidance from the National Institute for Health and Care Excellence (NICE) stipulates the application of a non-removable offloading device to the ulcerated limb as the initial treatment for all neuropathic ulceration.

The forefoot is the most common site of neuropathic ulceration and application of a TCC has been shown to reduce contact pressures across the fifth, fourth, and first metatarsal heads by 32%, 63%, and 69% respectively[19]. Heel ulcers are less effectively offloaded by TCC. Many clinicians favor a patellar tendon-bearing orthosis to offload the heel.

A trained individual should apply the TCC. Extreme care must be taken to protect bony prominences and avoid pressure points and ridges during casting. The stages of application include:

- application of a non-adhesive dressing over the ulcer
- gauze placed between the toes to avoid maceration
- cotton stockingette above the knee
- plaster felt pads over standard pressure points (tibial crest, malleoli, and points of deformity)
- total contact plaster layer
- fiberglass shell.

The first plaster change should be at five to seven days, as there is an initial, rapid change in shape as a result of the rapid reduction in peripheral edema. Thereafter cast changes can be performed at one- to two-week intervals. Whether to allow the patient to weight bear or not is controversial. However, in our practice we allow weight bearing.

Once the ulcer is healed, the foot can be transitioned into diabetic specification footwear, as described above.

Charcot Neuroarthropathy

The treatment of Charcot neuroarthropathy is aimed at maintaining foot shape, with the avoidance of deformity, until the foot has healed. Total contact casting is the gold standard for protection. The average healing times are six months in the forefoot, nine months in the midfoot, and twelve months in the hindfoot.

Once the foot has healed, it is usually placed into diabetic specification footwear. In the occasional patient instability persists, and if surgical stabilization cannot be undertaken devices such as the Charcot restraint orthotic walker (CROW) can be used (Figure 4.19). The CROW has been shown to allow early mobilization and healing of Charcot of the foot[20–21].

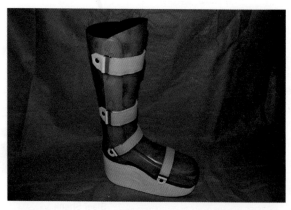

Figure 4.19 A Charcot restraint orthotic walker (CROW). Note the rocker sole and the stiff wellington construct, designed to give maximal control. In this case there was also a leg-length discrepancy.

Poliomyelitis

The word poliomyelitis is of Greek derivation and means "nerve inflammation of gray matter." Polio is a viral infection, which causes degeneration of the anterior horn cells of the spinal cord. It is highly contagious and spread via the fecal–oral route. The acute infection results in motor deficits in the trunk and limbs in 0.5% of patients contracting the virus. This condition is referred to as paralytic polio-myelitis. Ninety percent of these cases involve the lower limb[22]. Since the widespread introduction of vaccination, in 1954, new cases are rarely seen in the developed world.

Three distinct phases of the disease are identified.

1. *Acute phase* – this is characterized by a spectrum of symptoms ranging from multiple- or single-limb involvement (known as spinal polio), to loss of swallow reflex with respiratory embarrassment and diaphragmatic paralysis. Fifty percent of patients suffering from spinal polio can expect full recovery within the first four months, 25% have minor residual deficits, and the remaining 25% have severe functional loss. Recovery may be seen for up to two years.
2. *Chronic phase* – this is characterized by motor deficits. Weakness in this phase is clinically detectable when a threshold of 60% of motor neurons to a muscle group are affected.
3. *Post-polio syndrome* – 30 to 40 years after the initial infection, usually when the patient reaches the fifth or sixth decade of life, there is a gradual weakening of those muscles chronically affected by partial denervation. There is a gradual conversion of muscles to a Type 1 population, leading to early fatiguability[23].

In the polio patient, orthoses are used to stabilize the limb and normalize gait. The specific orthosis employed is determined by the pattern and extent of motor loss.

Treatment principles include:

- treating muscle pain by improvement of the efficiency of gait
- reducing eccentric joint forces caused by motor weakness
- maintaining range of movement and static alignment of the limb
- correcting any leg-length discrepancy
- maximizing loadbearing during stance phase
- decreasing asymmetry in gait.

The specific orthotic intervention varies depending on the phase of the viral infection encountered and the deformity present.

Acute Phase

This may involve a period of flaccid paralysis, during which time the patient is typically managed with bed rest and splinting, for example with an AFO, to prevent contracture formation.

Chronic Phase

The pattern of deformity is dictated by the spinal level affected. Weakness around the hip is common and results in a flexion, abduction, and external rotation deformity. In the leg the most commonly affected muscle is the tibialis anterior, followed by the tibialis posterior, and the quadriceps femoris[24]. Patients require quadriceps MRC grade 3 power, or above, to ambulate unaided.

The knee may have either a flexion or an extension (recurvatum) deformity.

- Flexion deformity may require serial casting or surgical release.
- Recurvatum, if mild, can help to stabilize the knee in stance phase. The hyperextension is usually accompanied by ankle equinus, which should be accepted if the foot, with the compensatory recurvatum, reaches plantigrade.

The foot manifestation is typically a hindfoot or forefoot cavus. In hindfoot cavus paralysis of the gastrocnemius–soleus complex, with sparing of the other muscles of the deep compartment, results in an excessive calcaneal pitch. The long flexors depress the metatarsal heads and the intrinsics contract to raise the calcaneal pitch.

Forefoot cavus is seen where a higher lesion in the spinal cord selectively affects tibialis anterior. The function of peroneus longus is unopposed resulting in depression of the first ray, and forefoot-driven cavus.

Principles of Bracing

There are four principles.

1. As many joints as possible should remain unbraced.
2. The device should be as light as possible.

3. Orthoses should be padded to prevent rubbing over atrophic soft tissues.
4. When children begin to ambulate, consideration should be given to extending the device to the knee or hip.

A small range of devices are typically used in the lower limb in the post-polio patient.

Thermoplastic AFO

- Indicated in flaccid equinus.
- If there is no dynamic varus or valgus the trim lines pass posterior to the malleoli, otherwise they are brought anterior to the malleoli.

Ground Reaction Force Orthosis (GRAFO)

- In patients with grade 3 power or below in their quadriceps, an anterior tibial shell is used (Figure 4.11).
- For patients with passively correctable recurvatum, a posterior extension, or high popliteal trim line may be added. This assists knee flexion, and is known as the Lehneis modification of the GRAFO.

Knee–Ankle–Foot Orthoses with a Drop–Lock Hinge (KAFO)

- A KAFO is indicated in bilateral quadriceps weakness with marked knee instability.
- Older devices locked the knee joint, but newer devices allow flexion of the knee in swing, yet lock and provide stability in stance.

KAFO with Bail Lock Knee Hinges and Quadrilateral Ischial Bearing Sockets (HKAFO)

- For patients presenting with grade 3 power or less about the hip, the HKAFO is indicated.

- The proximal disease usually coexists with marked instability of the knees and ankles, requiring bail lock hinges, which provide stability in knee extension and are manually unlocked by the patient using a spring-loaded mechanism.

Key Points

An orthosis is defined as "an externally applied device used to modify the structural and functional characteristics of the neuromuscular and skeletal systems."

Materials

- Materials require different properties depending upon application.
- They may be classified as hard or soft.
- Plastics fall into two main groups: thermoforming and thermosetting.
- Traditional materials such as steel and leather are important and still in widespread use.

Manufacture

- The process of custom orthosis manufacture involves assessment and casting.
- Manufacture of a positive model of the limb.
- Manufacture of the orthosis around this model.
- Fitting to the patient and adjustment as required.

Orthoses

- Orthoses are classified by the anatomic region the device supports.
- Foot orthoses may be corrective or accommodative.
- Ankle–foot orthoses are constructed of either metal and leather, or thermoformed plastic.

References

1. Shih Y-F, Wen Y-K, Chen W-Y. Application of wedged foot orthosis effectively reduces pain in runners with pronated foot: a randomized clinical study. *Clin Rehabil.* 2011; 25, 913–23. doi:10.1177/0269215511411938.

2. Hawke FE, Burns J, Radford JA, Du Toit V. Custom-made foot orthoses for the treatment of foot pain. *Cochrane Database Syst Rev.* 2007; 4. doi:10.1002/14651858.CD006801.

3. Pfeffer G, Bacchetti P, Deland J, et al. Comparison of custom and prefabricated orthoses in the initial treatment of proximal plantar fasciitis. *Foot Ankle Int.* 1999; 20:4, 214–21. doi:10.1177/107110079902000402.

4. Kearney R, Costa ML. Insertional achilles tendinopathy management: a systematic review. *Foot ankle Int/Am Orthop Foot Ankle Soc [and] Swiss Foot Ankle Soc.* 2010; 31:8, 689–94. doi:10.3113/FAI.2010.0689.

5. Sayana MK, Maffulli N. Insertional Achilles tendinopathy. *Foot Ankle Clin.* 2005; 10:2, 309–20. doi:10.1016/j.fcl.2005.01.010.

6. Wiegerinck JI, Kerkhoffs GM, van Sterkenburg MN, Sierevelt IN, van Dijk CN. Treatment for

insertional Achilles tendinopathy: a systematic review. *Knee Surgery, Sport Traumatol Arthrosc.* 2013; 21:6, 1345–55. doi:10.1007/s00167-012–2219–8.

7. Manoli A, Graham B. The subtle cavus foot, "the underpronator." *Foot Ankle Int/Am Orthop Foot Ankle Soc [and] Swiss Foot Ankle Soc.* 2005; 26:3, 256–63. doi:10.1177/107110070502600313.

8. Staheli LT. Planovalgus foot deformity. Current status. *J Am Podiatr Med Assoc.* 1999; 89:2, 94–9. doi:10.7547/87507315–89-2–94.

9. Pascual Huerta J, Ropa Moreno JM, Kirby KA. Static response of maximally pronated and nonmaximally pronated feet to frontal plane wedging of foot orthoses. *J Am Podiatr Med Assoc.* 2009; 99:1, 13–19. doi:10.7547/0980013.

10. Pascual Huerta J, Ropa Moreno JM, Kirby KA, et al. Effect of 7-degree rearfoot varus and valgus wedging on rearfoot kinematics and kinetics during the stance phase of walking. *J Am Podiatr Med Assoc.* 2009; 99:5, 415–21. doi:99/5/415 [pii].

11. Trotter LC, Pierrynowski MR. The short-term effectiveness of full-contact custom-made foot orthoses and prefabricated shoe inserts on lower-extremity musculoskeletal pain: a randomized clinical trial. *J Am Podiatr Med Assoc.* 2008; 98:5, 357–63. doi:98/5/357 [pii].

12. Trotter LC, Pierrynowski MR. Changes in gait economy between full-contact custom-made foot orthoses and prefabricated inserts in patients with musculoskeletal pain: a randomized clinical trial. *J Am Podiatr Med Assoc.* 2008; 98:6, 429–35. doi:98/6/429 [pii].

13. Uccioli L, Faglia E, Monticone G, et al. Manufactured shoes in the prevention of diabetic foot ulcers. *Diabetes Care.* 1995; 18:10, 1376–8. doi:10.2337/diacare.18.10.1376.

14. Paton J, Bruce G, Jones R, Stenhouse E. Effectiveness of insoles used for the prevention of ulceration in the neuropathic diabetic foot: a systematic review. *J Diabetes Complications.* 2011; 25:1, 52–62. doi:10.1016/j.jdiacomp.2009.09.002.

15. Armstrong DG, Nguyen HC, Lavery LA, Van Schie CHM, Boulton AJM, Harkless LB. Off-loading the diabetic foot wound: a randomized clinical trial. *Diabetes Care.* 2001; 24:6, 1019–22. doi:10.2337/diacare.24.6.1019.

16. Cavanagh PR, Bus SA. Off-loading the diabetic foot for ulcer prevention and healing. *J Vasc Surg.* 2010; 52:3 Suppl. doi:10.1016/j.jvs.2010.06.007.

17. Katz IA, Harlan A, Miranda-Palma B, et al. A randomized trial of two irremovable off-loading devices in the management of plantar neuropathic diabetic foot ulcers. *Diabetes Care.* 2005; 28:3, 555–9. doi:10.2337/diacare.28.3.555.

18. Prompers L, Huijberts M, Schaper N, et al. Resource utilisation and costs associated with the treatment of diabetic foot ulcers. Prospective data from the Eurodiale Study. *Diabetologia.* 2008; 51:10, 1826–34. doi:10.1007/s00125-008–1089–6.

19. Wertsch JJ, Frank LW, Zhu H, Price MB, Harris GF, Alba HM. Plantar pressures with total contact casting. *J Rehabil Res Dev.* 1995; 32:3, 205–9.

20. Mehta JA, Brown C, Sargeant N. Charcot restraint orthotic walker. *Foot Ankle Int.* 1998; 19:9, 619–23. doi:10.1177/107110079801900909.

21. Morgan JM, Biehl WC, Wagner FW. Management of neuropathic arthropathy with the Charcot Restraint Orthotic Walker. *Clin Orthop Relat Res.* 1993; 296, 58–63.

22. Joseph B, Watts H. Polio revisited: reviving knowledge and skills to meet the challenge of resurgence. *J Child Orthop.* 2015; 9:5, 325–38. doi:10.1007/s11832-015–0678–4.

23. Tiffreau V, Rapin A, Serafi R, et al. Post-polio syndrome and rehabilitation. *Ann Phys Rehabil Med.* 2010; 53:1, 42–50. doi:10.1016/j.rehab.2009.11.007.

24. Sharma JC, Gupta SP, Sankhala SS, Mehta MN. Residual poliomyelitis of lower limb-pattern and deformities. *Indian J Pediatr.* 1991; 58:2, 233–8.

Amputations, Prostheses, and Rehabilitation of the Foot and Ankle

Chapter 5

Stephen G. B. Kirker and James F. S. Ritchie

Introduction

This chapter describes surgery and prosthetic options for lower limb amputations in foot and ankle practice, covering immediate traumatic, planned essential (e.g., diabetic necrotic ulcers), and elective amputations (e.g., painful fused ankle), but not the management of congenital abnormalities or stump revision surgery.

Amputation is one of the oldest procedures in surgery. Evidence of digital amputations, perhaps performed for religious purposes, is present in cave art from 36 000 years ago found in modern-day France and New Mexico[1]. The first medical text on amputation, found in the Hippocratic text *On Joints*, however, is much more recent, dating from the latter half of the fifth century BC. The Hippocratic author describes the practice of amputating an ischemic limb below the "boundaries of blackening" as a measure of last resort[2]. The concept of amputating more proximally, through healthy tissue, did not appear for another four hundred years when Aulus Cornelius Celsus, a Roman encyclopedist who may or may not have practiced medicine, published his *De Medicina* in around 50 BC. In many ways, the principles he outlines hold true to this day:

> between the sound and the diseased part, the flesh is cut through with a scalpel down to the bone, but this must not be done actually over a joint, and it is better that some of the sound part should be cut away than that any of the diseased part be left behind. When the bone is reached, the sound flesh is drawn back from the bone and undercut from around it, so that in that part also some bone is bared; bone is then to be cut through with a small saw as near as possible to the sound flesh which still adheres to it, next the face of the bone, which the saw has roughened, is smoothed down, and the skin drawn over it; this must be sufficiently loosened in an operation of this sort to cover the bone all over as completely as possible[3].

Celsus was familiar with the use of ligatures on blood vessels, and may have used them during amputations but, interestingly, does not describe them in this context. Barring minor refinements, the technique of amputation remained largely unchanged for nearly 1800 years, until Jean-Louis Petit, who also invented the tourniquet, advocated dividing the skin and muscle at one level and the bone more proximally, the "two-stage circular cut," in 1718[4]. The use of a soft tissue flap for skin closure, meanwhile, had been described by James Yonge in 1679, a naval surgeon, although he attributed the innovation to "a very ingenious surgical brother, Mr. C. Lowdham of Exeter"[5].

The history of prosthetics is similarly ancient, with the first literary account, that of the warrior-queen Vishpla losing a leg in battle and having it replaced with an iron limb, being found in the Sanskrit *Rig Veda* of around 1800 BC[6]. Simple prostheses were used in the classical world, but during the renaissance some prostheses of quite remarkable sophistication, such as those designed by the surgeon Ambroise Paré, were made. At this time prostheses were individually bespoke, and the emphasis was upon producing a prosthesis that replicated the anatomy of the missing limb, rather than replacing its function. The pragmatic approach of designing cost-effective, functional prosthetic limbs that could be mass produced did not achieve currency until the battlefields of World War I saw amputations carried out in unprecedented numbers.

The word "amputation" is derived from the Latin "amputatio," meaning to cut or prune around. Although used in the classical Latin texts, the word did not appear in English until Peter Lowe's "Discourse on the Whole Art of Cirurgerie" of 1597. Lowe was a Scottish surgeon who traveled to the continent to study medicine in the late 1560s. He completed his training in Paris at a time when the legendary Ambroise Paré dominated the surgical life of the city. Paré had been using the word "amputation" since the 1550s, and although it is not clear whether Lowe studied under Paré, so great was the latter's stature that it is difficult to see how Lowe could not have been familiar with his work and teaching.

Annual statistics for patients newly referred to the 43 artificial limb clinics in the UK have been collected and published since 1996: initially under the National Amputee Statistical Database (NASDAB) heading and, since 2013, by Salford University[7]. The proportion of amputations performed for different causes has remained relatively stable although the proportion of below-knee, compared to above-knee, amputations has increased.

The NASDAB 2004[8] report identified 7000 amputations of the foot or lower limb from hospital activity data. Of these 4800 were referred to artificial limb clinics, of which 75% were due to vascular causes, 9% infection, and just 7% trauma, of which 80% were at trans-tibial or trans-femoral level. Although the incidence of traumatic amputations and congenital abnormalities is relatively low, as the patients have a long life expectancy their prevalence in amputee clinics is relatively high – 36% in the Cambridge unit.

The 2013 British documentation of amputations[9] concluded that the incidence of lower limb amputation is up to 8 to15 times higher in diabetic patients, compared to non-diabetic patients. Further, the number of people with diabetes in the UK has increased from 1.4 million to 2.9 million since 1996 and is likely to reach 5 million by 2025. Furthermore, up to 70% of people die within five years of having an amputation as a result of diabetes. The risk of death within 30 days of a lower limb amputation may be as high as 17%, reflecting the patients' multiple comorbidities.

Principles of Amputation

In planning an amputation, the primary aim is to produce a stump that will heal well and comfortably, and will accept the prosthesis best suited to the patient's functional needs. At what level and by what technique this is best achieved will, of course, depend upon many factors: age, health and functional demands of the patient, the pathology necessitating amputation, the state of the limb in question, the state of the patient's other limbs, and so on. In general, however, more distal amputations allow better function with higher walking speeds and lower energy consumption, while more proximal amputations offer more generous soft tissue cover, better tissue perfusion and therefore more reliable wound healing. As a rule of thumb, therefore, amputations should be carried out at the most distal level that offers a high probability of wound healing. Preserving limb length should not prejudice successful soft tissue cover. To do so, especially in diabetics, can often lead to "nibbling up the leg" in a series of unsatisfactory, and ever-more proximal, amputations.

There is, of course, more to planning an amputation than the technicalities of producing a satisfactory residual limb. Planning for the prosthesis is also of crucial importance, not just in terms of prosthesis fitting and suspension, but in determining the level of the amputation. This is because there is an inherent tension between limb preservation and prosthetic options. In simplistic terms, the more limb that is retained, the less length available to accommodate prosthetic components if the limb–prosthesis composite is to match the length of the contralateral limb. There is, of course, also the profound psychological impact of the procedure to be considered. For these reasons patients considering undergoing elective amputation surgery should ideally be assessed by a multidisciplinary team including a specialist in amputee rehabilitation and a psychologist, as well as the surgeon. Good communication between the different members of the team is essential to optimize patient outcome. Some patients find meeting amputees in a support group helpful in setting their expectations of the journey upon which they are to embark.

It is also important that patients considering undergoing an amputation, as opposed, perhaps, to limb reconstruction, should be aware that amputation is seldom the final procedure to be performed on the limb. Further surgery and stump revision may be required with the passage of time.

Elective amputations should be planned in collaboration with the prosthetic service that will be providing amputee rehabilitation in the long term, as there may be local variation in prescribing and limb-fitting practice. Contact should be made with that service as soon as possible after emergency amputations to allow patient expectations to be managed in a consistent way from the earliest stage. There are 43 NHS prosthetic and amputee rehabilitation services in the UK, many with satellite clinics[10], and a small number of private firms, which mainly cater for people with compensation claims following injury.

Technical Points

Skin and Muscle

Flaps should be kept thick with ample vascular supply. Excessive soft tissue dissection and undermining should be avoided. The aim should be to produce a sturdy soft tissue envelope for the stump. The various flap options at each level have been defined, but an atypical or unusual flap may be preferable to a more proximal level of amputation.

As a general rule, resection of muscles at least 5 cm distal to the level of bone resection will allow sufficient cover for the stump. Myodesis (suturing of muscle to bone) or myoplasty (suturing of muscle to its antagonist or fascia) confers greater soft tissue stability of the stump, reduces the risk of contractures, and reduces the rate of muscle wasting following the amputation.

Hemostasis

Most amputations are performed under tourniquet, except for cases of severe infection or ischemia where assessment of tissue viability is crucial.

Small vessels may be cauterized, but major structures should be ligated. It can be a useful practice to undertake this proximal to the level of bone resection to facilitate re-exploration of the stump and revision surgery if necessary. The tourniquet should be deflated and careful hemostasis carried out prior to skin closure.

Nerves

By definition, any transected nerve will form a stump neuroma. A variety of techniques have been described in the hope of preventing formation of painful neuromas: electrocautery, perineural closure, silastic capping, and burying the nerve stump in bone or muscle, to name but a few. None has won widespread acceptance and most surgeons now content themselves with pulling the nerve gently down into the wound and cutting it cleanly – well proximal to the level of bone resection – and allowing the nerve to retract into the stump.

Bone

Bone resection is classically carried out with a Gigli-type saw to avoid osteonecrosis, although a power saw with saline cooling may also be used. Periosteal stripping should be kept to a minimum to avoid bone overgrowth. Sharp bone edges and prominences should be resected and rasped to a smooth edge, especially in areas of poor soft tissue cover, such as the anterior tibia.

In an emergency, such as trauma or overwhelming infection, amputation of all or part of a limb may be carried out to save life or to preserve as much of the viable segment of the limb as possible. In such circumstances the luxury of detailed prosthetic and reconstructive planning is seldom available and the tissues available often determine the operative technique.

Even under these conditions some general principles should be followed:

1. All non-viable tissue should be removed.
2. The limb stump should be of sufficient length to accept a prosthesis easily but not so long as to make it difficult to accommodate a prosthesis distal to it.
3. The stump should be stable but well padded with good soft tissue cover over bony prominences.
4. If possible the stump should be sensate and motor control of the residual limb maintained with, for instance, a stable working knee joint.

In some cases in which trauma or sepsis has rendered the attainment of satisfactory soft tissue cover with good primary wound healing over a stump of satisfactory length unlikely, open amputation may offer an alternative to the fashioning of a short residual limb or amputation at a higher level. In an open amputation full wound closure is not attempted at the first operation. Rather the soft tissues are closed at a second procedure, with tissue transfer by a plastic surgeon, or the wound healed by secondary intention usually with a negative pressure dressing. This reduces the likelihood of persistent infection and wound failure but leads to a more protracted recovery with delayed ambulation.

Surgery and Prostheses at Each Level of Amputation

Forefoot and Toe Amputations

Forefoot amputations for diabetes, infection, or trauma are common. They require little or nothing in the way of prostheses and, as a rule, amputation of a single toe causes little disability. In the long run it may facilitate the development of malalignment of adjacent digits, such as hallux valgus arising after second toe amputation. In theory, this could be prevented by ray amputation, but against that one has to weigh the risk of transfer metatarsalgia developing as a result of the loss of a metatarsal head. In contrast to the hand, therefore, the role of central ray amputation in the foot is relatively limited: the interdigital gap caused by loss of a toe is largely cosmetic but loss of a load-sharing metatarsal head may cause significant functional problems secondary to the disruption of the metatarsal arcade. The exception is the lateral border amputation of the fifth metatarsal, such as for an ulcer of the fifth metatarsal head. In this procedure the fifth toe and most of the fifth metatarsal can be excised through a laterally based tennis-racquet incision. It is important that the insertion of peroneus brevis is not sacrificed, as this will lead to the development of hindfoot varus. Skin viability can be an issue, so the flaps should be kept as thick as possible.

Amputation of the great toe, or of all the lesser toes, with preservation of the metatarsal heads, usually causes little difficulty with slow walking, but can cause problems with brisk walking or running due to a loss of push-off in terminal stance. In the first ray, in particular, it is therefore desirable to try to preserve the proximal 1 cm of the proximal phalanx, and therefore some function of flexor hallucis brevis (FHB), if possible.

The level of amputation of an individual toe is usually determined by the extent of tissue damage, be it by trauma or infection. All non-viable tissue should be removed and a long plantar and shorter dorsal flap should be fashioned of healthy tissue. The flexor and extensor tendons should be cut cleanly and allowed to retract into the proximal tissues. The bone end should be smoothed after resection and the flaps closed traditionally with non-absorbable sutures.

A large proportion of forefoot amputations are carried out in diabetics, usually with infected ulcers and often osteomyelitis. Traditionally full primary closure, with or without a delay, has tended to be avoided in favor of healing by secondary intention, split skin grafting, or even the use of free-tissue transfer. In recent years vacuum-assisted closure, also known as negative-pressure wound therapy (NPWT), has been increasingly used and has been reported to increase the amount of the foot that can be usefully retained and to be less expensive and less labor intensive than conventional dressings[11]. More

recently, however, Shaikh et al.[12] showed good results following amputation combined with primary closure in infected diabetic feet so long as meticulous tissue handling was observed and the surgery was combined with judicious use of antibiotics and tight diabetic control.

The transmetatarsal amputation can produce a highly acceptable functional and cosmetic result if tissue perfusion is reasonable, but is not recommended in the face of ischemia, unless combined with vascular reconstruction. Ideally the bones should be contoured to replicate the anatomic forefoot cascade as far as possible to facilitate even weight bearing. The bone ends should be beveled to prevent irritation and breakdown of the underlying soft tissue due to excessive pressure. A long plantar flap is most commonly performed, but equal dorsal and plantar flaps can be effective. The flaps should be fashioned slightly longer on the medial side to provide cover for the greater depth of the foot on that side.

Many forefoot amputees manage well without prosthetics, but if an amputee chooses a toe filler and insole can be supplied: this may be molded to provide total contact, if pressure relief under the first metatarsal head is the priority, or be chosen from a range of thin, flat carbon fiber plates if energy return while wearing normal shoes is more important. A bespoke silicone toe (Figure 5.1) may be attached to an insole for patients who wish to have normal-looking feet in open-toed sandals. All diabetic forefoot amputees should be referred for custom insoles to reduce the risk of further diabetic ulceration or pressure points.

Partial Foot Amputations

Lisfranc and Chopart documented their techniques for partial amputations 200 years ago. The advantages of such amputations include the preservation of normal limb length, knee and some ankle function, as well as the production of a good end-bearing residual limb. These procedures can be carried out under regional anesthesia with a popliteal block. Disadvantages include the late development of equinovarus contractures, poor wound healing, particularly in diabetics and vasculopaths, and limited prosthetic options.

Evidence comparing the outcome of partial foot amputations to trans-tibial amputation (TTA) is poor. In many series, partial foot amputations have

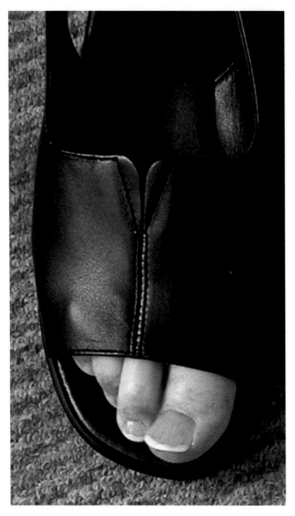

Figure 5.1 Bespoke high-definition silicone toes, fixed to sandals, following forefoot amputation.

scores in diabetics who had undergone midtarsal amputation for osteomyelitis or non-healing ulcers compared to matched controls who had undergone TTA. Neither group did really well, but the partial foot amputations seemed to be the best of a bad lot[15].

On balance, partial foot amputations are perhaps most useful following acute, unreconstructable, forefoot trauma, in which cases it is difficult to justify a trans-tibial amputation as a primary procedure. They can also be used for frail, high-risk patients of low functional demand to whom the greater range of prosthetic options offered by a TTA are of little benefit, and in whom it is desirable to minimize the surgical and anesthetic insult.

In the non-diabetic partial foot amputation, only bone that is protected by innervated plantar skin should be preserved. Insensate plantar skin is of limited functional usefulness and vulnerable to ulceration. Grafted skin is insufficiently durable to survive long term on the sole of the foot.

Jacques Lisfranc de St Martin described disarticulation through the TMTJs, and the crucial step of dividing the plantar ligament running from the medial cuneiform to the base of second metatarsal, in 1815. It is widely believed that Lisfranc's work was inspired by his service in Napoleon's ill-fated Russian campaign of 1812, during which he observed a large number of fracture-dislocations of the midfoot, particularly in cavalrymen in whom the foot could easily be twisted violently in the stirrup. Sadly the reality is a little more prosaic. Lisfranc did not join the army until 1813, and served not in Russia but Germany at the Battle of the Nations. Moreover, when he presented his paper[16] in May 1815 he identified "decay" and "crush injuries" as the main indications for his procedure.

Tarsometatarsal amputation can provide adequate functional outcome in some patients. Careful evaluation of the muscle balance around the foot is essential, specifically tendo Achillis tightness, and the function of the tibialis anterior and peronei should be assessed. Midfoot amputations significantly shorten the lever arm of the foot, so intraoperative tendo Achillis (TA) lengthening is often required. The insertions of tibialis anterior and the peronei should be preserved, or reattached if they have been removed during bone resection. These measures should prevent the muscle imbalance that, over time, can lead to progressive equinovarus deformity, difficulty in prosthetic fitting, and eventual loss of function. Special

not been shown to result in better functional outcome than TTA, but amputees are such a heterogeneous group that it is difficult to draw any definitive conclusions[13]. Moreover, Millstein and colleagues reported retrospectively that in a group of 260 partial-foot amputations resulting from industrial accidents, tarsometatarsal and midtarsal levels gave the most successful outcomes[14]. Despite this, functional outcome from amputation at this level is often disappointing as the residual foot is large enough to limit the prosthetic options but too small to function as a foot. These poor outcomes may just reflect the problems of the patient cohort for whom this amputation is selected, rather than of the procedure itself. Brown found similar mortality rates but better ambulation postoperative clamshell-type orthoses are useful during recovery to achieve maximal function. Postoperative immobilization of the limb in a cast may be necessary to allow the tendon reattachments to heal, as well as reducing edema and wound problems.

Chopart's amputation through the talonavicular and calcaneocuboid joints was described a decade prior to Lisfranc's. It removes the forefoot and midfoot while preserving the talus and calcaneus. Amputation through the midtarsal joint produces a foot with a very short lever arm, so rebalancing the TA, peroneal tendons, and tibialis anterior and posterior is especially important if long-term deformity is to be avoided. As with other partial foot amputations, plantar weightbearing skin is best used as a flap for closure; it is secured to bone to prevent shear, with bursa formation.

Prosthetic options following partial foot amputations are inevitably constrained by the limited space available in a shoe. The body weight is taken through the remaining sole of the foot, usually on a molded total-contact insole with a foam toe filler. This may be held in place on the stump by a soft leather bootee, which may fit inside the amputee's ordinary shoes. Few of these amputees walk outside the house, but for those with greater ambitions, a stiff, full-length sole plate can be added to improve push off at the end of stance phase. This has only a modest effect unless supported by a rigid lever arm extending up the lower leg, in the form of an AFO (Figure 5.2) or, more effectively, a full prosthetic socket, which is necessary to climb stairs or ladders. There is no space for any energy-storing prosthetic components, and the socket is so bulky that shoes usually have to be supplied as well. An alternative approach, for cosmesis rather than function, is a bespoke solid silicone foot (Figure 5.3). These may be sculpted and colored to look very lifelike, but are much heavier and more expensive than the other devices. Fit people hoping to regain high activities after forefoot trauma may wish to consider the greater prosthetic options and performance of a TTA.

Syme Amputation

James Syme described his amputation in 1843[17], to avoid the considerable dangers of TTA in the nineteenth century. Harris[18] subsequently revisited it. The Syme amputation is an ankle disarticulation, with removal of the calcaneus and talus and preservation

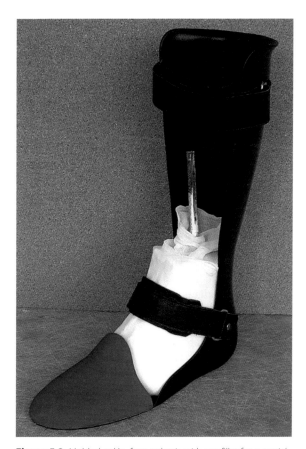

Figure 5.2 Molded ankle–foot orthosis with toe filler for a partial foot amputation. This provides maximum stability at the end of stance phase and when climbing stairs. It may require a larger shoe than on the remaining foot.

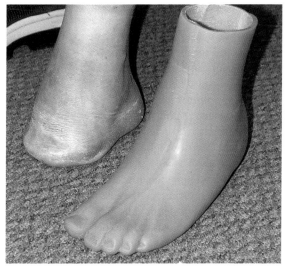

Figure 5.3 Low-definition silicone prosthesis for hind-foot amputation.

of the heel skin and fat pad. This highly specialized tissue is used to form a durable end-bearing flap for ambulation. The heel skin is sutured to the distal tibia to prevent posterior and medial migration of the fat pad, which can compromise function. Construction of a successful Syme stump allows ambulation for short distances without a prosthesis.

Anterior and posterior flaps provide soft tissue cover in a Syme amputation. The posterior flap is marked on the sides of the foot by lines dropped from the tips of the medial and lateral malleoli to the sole of the foot. An oblique line joins these lines across the sole, as the lateral malleolus lies posterior to the medial. The tissues are divided down to bone. The anterior flap is marked with a line taking the shortest distance across the front of the ankle. The extensor tendons are divided, the ankle entered, and the medial and lateral collateral ligaments divided from inside the joint. The posterior flap is then developed by subperiosteal dissection along the plantar surface of the os calcis as far as possible, taking care not to buttonhole the skin. On the dorsal surface, the posterior capsule of the ankle is divided and dissection continued along the superior surface of the os calcis staying close to the bone. A bone hook may be used to draw the os calcis forward to facilitate this process. Alternating dorsal and plantar dissection of the calcaneum is continued until the foot has been removed. The medial and lateral plantar and anterior tibial vascular bundles are ligated and divided, and the nerves are cut under tension. The malleoli are removed with an oscillating saw to produce a flat distal tibia, and the edges of the bone smoothed with a rasp. Some malleolar flare should be maintained for cosmesis and to allow suspension of the prosthesis. The posterior flap should be sutured to the tibia so that the heel pad is held centrally under the tibia. This can be accomplished in several ways, including tenodesis of the tendo Achillis to the posterior margin of the tibia through drill holes, transfer of the tibialis anterior and extensor digitorum tendons to the anterior aspect of the fat pad, or removal of the cartilage and subchondral bone to allow scarring of the fat pad to bone with suturing of the plantar fascia to the anterior tibial periosteum. The flaps are closed and a rigid dressing applied and molded to hold the fat pad centrally.

Although reported outcomes are adequate at this level, many investigators emphasize the need for frequent and accurate prosthetic fitting and unloading of the "weightbearing" stump for comfort[19]. Prosthetic fitting can be challenging, as the distal stump may have a larger circumference than the proximal part, particularly after muscle wastage. Thus the socket must be close fitting around a thin proximal calf, but it must expand distally to allow the wider tibial flare through when it is applied. Historically this was achieved by leaving a large window in the hard socket, which was closed by lace-up leather flaps or by a rigid plate held on with straps. It is now usually achieved with a molded hard foam liner, made from Pe-Lite®. The external surface is built up over the thin middle section to make it cylindrical. It is also split longitudinally to allow it to gape while being pulled over the stump.

These prostheses are cosmetically unpopular as they are much bulkier around the ankle than a trans-tibial prosthesis. The small space available between the end of the stump and the ground limits the options for prosthetic ankles and feet, which reduces function compared to a trans-tibial prosthesis. Ideally, all the body weight should be taken through the heel pad at the end of the stump. If this is not tolerated and the end has to be offloaded, the socket has to be longer and the proximal socket will have to be a patellar tendon bearing at the knee. To accommodate the extra length, the contralateral shoe may have to be built up, further impairing the overall appearance.

Trans-Tibial Amputation

Trans-tibial amputation is by far the most common of the major lower limb amputations. Historically it was mainly used in trauma and peripheral vascular disease, the transfemoral amputation being favored for diabetics because of supposedly better wound healing. In recent years, however, diabetes has become the most common indication for TTA.

The rise in popularity of the TTA is perhaps best explained by the fact that it is the most proximal level of amputation in the lower limb at which most amputees can expect to attain near-normal function. This is largely because preservation of the knee joint and limb length mean that when walking energy consumption, in both children and adults, is significantly less than following a transfemoral amputation[20–21]. Moreover, ambulant energy consumption has been shown to be no different in trans-tibial amputees to those who have undergone more distal amputations, such as a Syme. Overall use of prostheses and functional outcomes are significantly better in trans-tibial than transfemoral amputees.

In order for a TTA to be successful, certain preconditions should be met. The patient should have control of knee movement, particularly the quadriceps, the knee should be stable and pain free, and the stump will need to well perfused, preferably sensate, and of appropriate length. The use of free tissue transfer and microvascular techniques to improve soft tissue cover should be considered to allow a trans-tibial, as opposed to a more proximal, amputation.

There is no consensus as to the optimum level for TTA and, of course, the state and viability of the local tissues should be taken into consideration. In general, amputation through the distal third of the tibia is best avoided as the soft tissue cover will be poor and there are reduced prosthetic options. Traditionally, the optimum level for a TTA in an adult was regarded as preserving one inch of tibia per foot in height (= 2.5 cm per 30 cm). In most adults, therefore, bone sectioning will occur at 10 to 15 cm distal to the tibial tubercle. This remains our preferred practice, if the soft tissues allow. If there is doubt we recommend close liaison between the surgeon and prosthetist as to the minimum stump length required for the planned prosthesis. If a short trans-tibial stump is felt to be the best option, excision of the head of the fibula may allow the stump to fit more snugly within the socket. If it is not feasible to fashion a stump of acceptable length then through-knee or transfemoral amputation has to be considered.

A variety of techniques for TTA have been described but the long posterior flap remains the most widespread. With this a long posterior myocutaneous flap, based upon the blood supply from the gastrocnemius, provides the soft tissue cover. In most cases, particularly vasculopaths, this is the most reliably perfused flap, but in some instances alternative flap arrangements, such as skew and sagittal flaps, may be considered. In general, however, these alternative techniques have not been shown to improve outcome when compared to the posterior myocutaneous flap[22].

In the long posterior flap technique, the junctions of the flap bases are marked, medial and lateral, just under two-thirds of the way back to the mid-posterior line at the level of planned bone resection. From these points a short anterior flap measuring 2 cm and a long posterior flap are mark. The posterior flap should be 1 cm longer than the diameter of the limb

at the planned level of amputation and should have parallel, not tapering, sides when laid out flat. To avoid tapering the flap it is useful to elevate the limb and check the flap from behind before starting the dissection. The anterior flap should be raised with the skin, deep fascia, and the anterior tibial periosteum as a single composite layer at the level of the tibial section. The anterior tibial vessels should be ligated. The tibia can be sectioned with a short bevel on the anterior surface. The cut surface should be smoothed with a rasp as any sharp edges may cause pain. The fibula is sectioned 1 to 2 cm proximal to the level of tibial resection. In trauma cases with comminuted or segmental fractures, internal fixation can be useful to preserve length. The tibia is then retracted anteriorly and the posterior soft tissues are divided with an oblique cut running distally. When the desired level is reached, the cut is turned through 90° to divide the deep fascia and skin. The major vessels should be identified, transfixed, and ligated at a level proximal to the tibial bone cut, while nerves should be cut cleanly under gentle tension and allowed to retract into the soft tissues. The posterior flap is then fashioned with the skin and fascia left adherent to the underlying gastrocnemius. In most cases the soleus is removed from the flap, but some or all of its fibers can be retained if the flap would otherwise lack muscle bulk. The flap is wrapped around the distal tibia to gauge length; it should reach the anterior periosteum. The optimum length is marked and the flap cut to it under no tension. If necessary the corners of the flap can be tapered to prevent a bulbous shape. The tourniquet should be deflated at this point and meticulous hemostasis achieved. In order to stabilize the soft tissue envelope, and reduce muscle migration, the gastrocnemius can be sutured to the anterior periosteum or a formal myodesis with transosseous sutures performed. The flap should be secured with the knee in full extension to prevent flexion contractures.

In recent years, there has been interest in bone-bridging techniques to achieve a synostosis between the distal tibia and fibula. This can be a useful technique in revision surgery for those amputees suffering from tibiofibular instability and has the theoretical advantage of producing a better end-bearing limb. For primary amputations, however, the practical advantages appear limited: Kingsbury et al. could demonstrate no improvement in gait[23], while Keeling et al. found no improvement in running or walking distance, prosthesis wearing, or general well-being[24]. Moreover, complication rates, particularly infection and non-union of the bone-bridge, are higher than for a standard technique[25]. A synostosis may also complicate subsequent revision surgery. If it is considered desirable to use a bone-bridging technique, the synostosis can be created either using a periosteal sleeve or fibular strut graft. The latter may be anchored with screws or transosseous sutures with or without a compression device.

Trans-Tibial Prostheses

Prostheses are made up of a liner and socket, a shin tube, which may incorporate an alignment device, and a foot. The prosthesis is "suspended" from the limb.

Two main designs of socket are used for transtibial amputees:

- A patellar tendon bearing socket, in which body weight is supported by the tibial flare and patellar tendon, and only enough pressure is applied at the end of the stump to prevent tissue edema. Patellar tendon bearing sockets generally have a molded liner of hard foam (Pe-Lite®) and are worn over cotton, wool, or gel socks (Figure 5.4). They are easily modified and are more appropriate for new stumps, which change shape a lot over the first year.

- A total-contact design, in which weight is more evenly distributed. A total-contact socket offers much less scope for modification and is worn over a silicone or gel liner. These liners come in standard sizes, and rarely need to be custom made. These materials provide better protection from shear forces and rubbing, but with added weight, cost, heat retention, and awareness of sweating.

Sockets are made from polypropylene, or a laminate of layers of nylon, carbon fiber, or Kevlar® impregnated with acrylic resin. Polypropylene is a thermoplastic draped over a positive model of the stump. Polypropylene sockets have the advantages of speed of manufacture and ease of later modification, but laminates are stronger, more rigid, thinner, and cooler, and can be reinforced in places to allow windows to be cut out. While 3D scanning of the stump and carving of a positive model in hard foam by a computer-controlled mill is becoming more widespread, direct 3D printing of sockets is not yet practical.

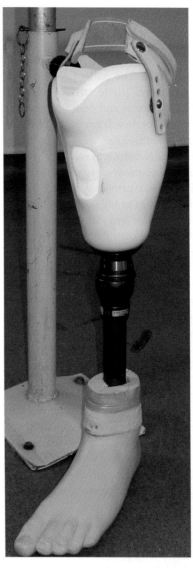

Figure 5.4
A modular endoskeletal transtibial prosthesis, with a patellar tendon bearing polypropylene socket, a window to offload the end of the tibia, Pe-Lite® liner, leather cuff suspension, and an alignment device between the socket and shin tube.

The prosthesis may be suspended, held on to the stump, by several techniques. Leather-cuff suspension has largely been replaced by "suction suspension" within an airtight, silicone-lined suspension sleeve, with a one-way valve in the distal socket. Suction may be enhanced with a pump to maintain sustained lower pressures within the socket, in which case it is called "vacuum" suspension. This is said to have the added advantage of reducing stump shrinkage and maintaining optimal socket fit, all be it at considerable extra expense (Figure 5.5). The link between the liner and socket may be with a metal pin embedded in the liner, which can engage with a locking mechanism

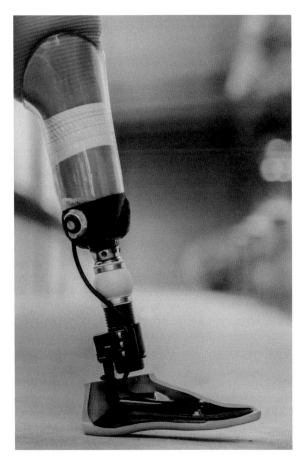

Figure 5.5 Trans-tibial amputation, transparent test socket over a Seal-In® liner, vertical and torsion shock absorber, carbon fiber energy storing foot with gait-activated pump to maintain low pressure ("vacuum") in the distal socket. (Unity system, Ossur.)

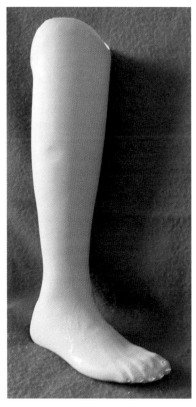

Figure 5.6 Trans-tibial prosthesis with sculpted foam to give shape and "off-the-shelf" silicone cosmesis. The shallow indentation overlies the button to release the pin lock suspension.

("pin lock") (Figure 5.6). An alternative is silicone ribs or fins, which form an airtight seal against the socket wall ("seal-in"). Some people find pin lock suspension tugs on loose soft tissue at the end of the stump. This is less of an issue with seal-in liners.

The socket is connected to the aluminum or carbon fiber shin tube by an alignment device, which allows the socket to be flexed, adducted, and shifted backward or forward over the shin.

There has been an increase in the variety and performance of prosthetic feet and ankles. For many vascular amputees, whose mobility may also be impaired by contralateral claudication, ischemic heart disease, and other comorbidities, the mobility goal may be just to transfer independently. In these patients the priority will be light weight and comfort, and they will often be supplied with the simplest type with a solid ankle and cushioned heel (SACH) foot. Limited community ambulators, who walk at a home, to their car, and 50 meters or so, may benefit from a more modern design, with a more flexible ankle (multiaxial ankle, e.g., Endolite Multiflex) and keel. Higher activity amputees, such as people working full time, or walking longer distances at different speeds, are usually supplied with a foot with greater energy return from carbon fiber keel (e.g., College Park Foot, Flex Walk, Esprit).

Amputees who run, jump down from tractors, or carry loads will need stiffer, stronger components to withstand these loads, and return much more of the energy stored at heel strike to toe off. Components have been developed to facilitate specific activities: the running blade, which has no heel; a cycling limb with a pedal cleat replacing the foot; the adjustable ankle that is locked at the best angle for different heel heights. The more recent hydraulic ankle adjusts automatically to inclines or declines; the torque absorber facilitates some rotation for golfers; the vertical shock absorber reduces forces transmitted up to a painful knee or hip at heel strike. There is even an ankle that can be locked in full plantar flexion for scuba diving. All of these components have a maximum weight limit, which includes any loads the amputee in carrying; so all the components in the limb for a fit 100 kg laborer who routinely carries 50 kg will need to be CE marked for 150 kg. A foot strong enough for carrying 50 kg at work may feel too stiff when walking round at home, and high-activity amputees will benefit from having several prostheses, optimized for different tasks or footwear.

Through-Knee Amputation

Through-knee amputation and above-knee amputation are relatively uncommon procedures in civilian orthopedic practice, although they are more common in vascular and military practice. Both procedures incur considerably greater penalties in terms of energy consumption and rate of locomotion than a trans-tibial amputation[20] and are associated with poorer functional outcomes and less frequent use of the prosthesis. In general, therefore, TTA is preferred.

If a more proximal procedure is required, knee disarticulation offers a quicker and simpler operation than above-knee amputation. Moreover, as the medullary canal is not breached, the intact articular cartilage and subchondral bone reduce bacterial colonization and may act as a barrier to bone infection. Other long-term advantages of the procedure are better end-bearing on the distal femur, which allows the prosthesis brim to be left lower, improving sitting comfort and reducing rubbing in the groin. It also allows preservation of limb length and the adductor muscle insertion, thus allowing better control of a powerful long lever in the residual limb. Suspension with "a self-suspending socket" by narrowing the Pe-Lite® liner above the femoral condyles is also an advantage.

The major disadvantage of knee disarticulation is the difference of prosthetic knee height from the contralateral limb. This leads to asymmetric gait as well as significant cosmetic problems, with the socket often appearing bulky above the knee (Figure 5.7) and the prosthetic knee protruding beyond the contralateral knee, even when a 4 bar or 6 bar knee, with a higher center of rotation than a single-axis knee, is used (Figure 5.8). While there are hydraulic 4 bar knees, all the sophisticated microprocessor-controlled knees are of single-axis design. If the amputee cannot tolerate taking all their weight through the end of the

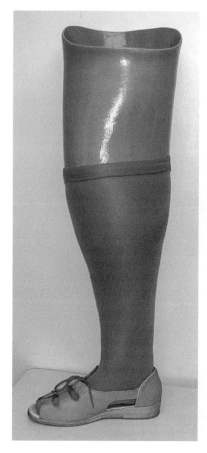

Figure 5.7
Prosthesis for a Gritti–Stokes knee disarticulation: the brim does not support the ischial tuberosity, so all weight must be taken at the end of the stump and diffusely through the soft tissues of the stump. The socket is much wider above the knee than a transfemoral prosthesis.

stump, this area must be offloaded by taking the weight through the ischial tuberosity and the knee will protrude even further. If the femoral condyles are poorly defined, or have been shaved off in a Gritti–Stokes amputation, the limb will have to be suspended by a waist belt or perhaps a Seal-In® liner, adding weight, girth, length, heat retention, and cost.

In children the considerable advantages of avoiding disruption of the growth plate, the tendency of the amputated femur to grow less than the other side, and the avoidance of bony spur growth from the cut end of the femur make disarticulation a better choice than transfemoral amputation.[26–27] In other situations, the disadvantages tend to outweigh any benefit. A meta-analysis of trauma patients noted that patients with a through-knee amputation wore their prosthesis significantly less, and had significantly more pain than those with an above-knee amputation[28]. This problem may be ameliorated by shortening the femur, ideally by 7 to 10 cm, to bring the center of prosthetic knee rotation to the same level myocutaneous flap based on gastrocnemius, analogous to that used for a TTA, has gained favor as it provides better tissue padding and improved vascular supply[31]. However, the flaps are raised, the incisions are carried down to bone, and the limb is removed by sharp dissection through the knee joint. The patellar tendon is resected from the tibial tubercle and the patella is excised from the quadriceps mechanism to prevent patello-femoral pain. The knee is flexed and the collateral ligaments divided. The femoral attachments of the cruciate ligaments should be left intact and sutured to the patellar tendon to help stabilize the quadriceps and improve muscle balance. The popliteal vessels are transfixed and ligated, and the tibial and common peroneal nerves cut cleanly under tension. The tourniquet is released and hemostasis secured. Judicious trimming of the femoral condyles, particularly the posterior condyles, may well be needed to produce a stump of optimal contour, but this should be discussed with the rehabilitation team preoperatively as it may prejudice suspension of the prosthetic limb.

Above-Knee Amputation

Above-knee amputation can be carried out at any level, but as the level becomes more proximal more muscle attachments are disrupted and the lever arm of the residual limb is reduced, thus compromising limb function. Similarly the increasing need for more complex proximal suspension systems reduces the likelihood of successful use of a prosthesis. To all intents and purposes amputation with bone sectioning at, or proximal to, the level of the lesser trochanter functions as a hip disarticulation. Preservation of femoral length is therefore of great importance in above-knee amputation and in traumatic cases internal fixation of fractures may be required to achieve this. On the other hand, amputation within 10 cm of the knee joint is usually best avoided, to allow room for a knee mechanism.

Osseo-integration has been developed for transfemoral amputation stumps by several groups to allow the prosthetic knee and distal components to be attached directly to a titanium abutment. This avoids the need for any socket, but very few centers have extensive experience and it should still be regarded as experimental[32–35].

Soft tissue cover for transfemoral amputations is usually provided by equal anterior and posterior

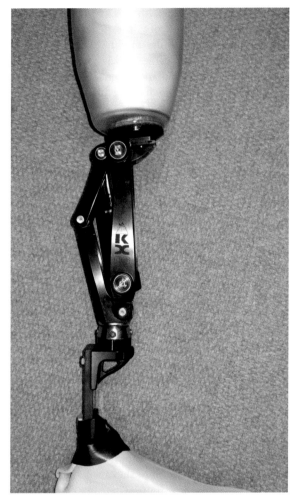

Figure 5.8 Transfemoral socket for a knee disarticulation with a very strong KX06 4 bar knee and carbon fiber strut to the energy-storing foot, for very high activities.

as the natural knee, although this technique has not become widespread[29–30]. The issue, of course, does not arise for bilateral amputees, or for those who are not going to use their limbs, for whom sitting balance is a higher priority and the longer the stump the better.

Traditionally, knee disarticulation is carried out with either anterior and posterior flaps or medial and lateral flaps, the bases of which should be level with the lower pole of the patella. If anterior and posterior flaps are used, the anterior flap should be as long as the knee is wide; the posterior flap should be about half this length. If medial and lateral flaps are used the medial flap should be 2 cm longer than the lateral, to allow sufficient tissue to cover the medial femoral condyle. More recently a long posterior semicircular skin flaps, each of which should be greater than half the diameter of the thigh at the level of planned bone resection. The use of atypical flaps, however, is quite acceptable and preferable to resorting to a higher level of amputation. For symmetrical flaps, the base should be at the level of planned bone resection in adults, perhaps 3 cm higher in children to allow for tissue elasticity and prevent undue laxity in the soft tissues. The flaps are traditionally cut from apex to base, and the subcutaneous tissues divided with a raking cut so that slightly more fat than skin is removed. The cut should transect the quadriceps so that it reaches the periosteum at, or slightly proximal to, the level of bone resection. In fashioning the posterior flap, the deep fascia should be cut sufficiently distally to allow it to cover the distal end of the bone. The sartorius should be mobilized by blunt dissection and divided at the level of bone resection. This allows access to the femoral vessels, which should be ligated individually and divided. The periosteum is divided and the bone sectioned with a Gigli saw or power saw with cooling. The femur can then be retracted anteriorly with a bone hook and the sciatic nerve visualized and cut well proximal to the level of bone resection. The anterior femur should be beveled with a rasp. Maintaining the balance of antagonistic muscle groups through myodesis is important in optimizing limb function, and in general the aim is to have each muscle group in slight tension with the femur in neutral. This is particularly important with regards to the adductors, and when these are being secured to the femur, usually through transosseous sutures, care must be taken to ensure that the femur is in neutral rotation; the linea aspera on the posterior surface may be of help with this. To avoid overtensioning of the adductors, the femur should be adducted slightly past the midline with the hip in neutral extension while the muscles are secured. As with a trans-tibial amputation meticulous hemostasis is needed and a pressure dressing applied.

Transfemoral Prostheses

The prostheses used for transfemoral amputees differ greatly from trans-tibial prostheses. Unlike the below-knee stump, there are no bony prominences to be offloaded in a well-fashioned above-knee amputation stump and the soft tissue can be modeled by measurements, cast by hand, or scanned over a silicone liner. The socket may be shaped to compress the soft tissue from side to side or back to front to reduce rotation. The brim, on which the body weight is taken through the ischial tuberosity, may be made in a range of standard shapes, of which the quadrilateral (Hosmer, "H") and ischial containment designs are most common (Figure 5.9). Most new amputees use a soft waist belt to suspend the leg – this is known as total elastic suspension or TES (Figure 5.10), although those with a very short stump or weak abductor muscles may benefit from the additional support of a rigid pelvic band. Fluctuations in stump volume may be accommodated by wearing more or less cotton or, rarely, wool socks. More agile amputees with muscular, rather than flabby, stumps of stable volume, may progress to suction suspension. These sockets have an inner wall of flexible plastic, worn next to the skin, and a removable one-way valve distally. This method provides more secure suspension, with less pistoning

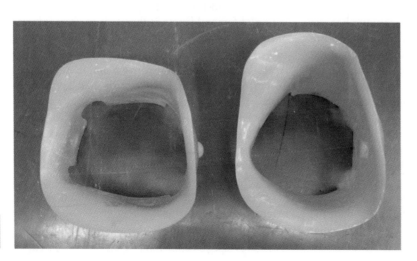

Figure 5.9 View from top of brims for casting two common styles of sockets for transfemoral amputees. The older quadrilateral design (left) has a flatter posterior shelf. The ischial containment style (right) is more triangular in shape and is molded around the ischial tuberosity, which reduces rotation of the socket.

back on the posterior brim: this may be very uncomfortable for the obese when sitting. To overcome these problems, new designs are being developed. The Marlo Anatomical Socket[36] is more flexible posteriorly, permitting a greater range of movement, and improved cosmesis, but requires great skill and usually many check sockets to achieve good results. The High Fidelity[37] socket applies pressure through more distal soft tissue and controls rotation, but is a patented design, requiring purchase of dedicated equipment and training. The Sub-Ischial[38] design distributes body weight through the soft tissue of the stump, with lower trim lines over a fin-type gel liner.

Prosthetic knees are designed to balance function with cost. Their cost ranges from £600 ($800) to £60 000 ($80 000). The prosthetist will select the knee based upon the patient's weight, mobility, degree of stability required, and the space available between the end of the stump and the contralateral knee-joint line. Amputees with weaker muscles or poor stump control may only be safe walking on a locked knee, which is released before sitting by pulling a lever (Semi-automatic Knee Lock, SAKL). Most amputees walk with a stabilized free knee, which stays extended when the body weight goes through the hindfoot at heel strike but releases and passively flexes when the body weight moves forward onto the toe. The rate of flexion and extension during swing phase may be controlled by pneumatic or hydraulic cylinders, which in turn may be controlled by microprocessors in the most sophisticated knees. These allow the rate of swing to vary, step by step, to give a smooth symmetrical gait at different speeds. Hydraulic knees may also permit controlled flexion under load ("yielding"), allowing the amputee to walk down slopes and stairs with a reciprocating gait. Microprocessor-controlled knees may become more rigid if they detect a stumble.

Postoperative Management

Postoperative care of an amputee is best undertaken by a multidisciplinary team including the surgeon, physiotherapist, and prosthetist. Close liaison with the rehabilitation center is required.

Dressings may be soft or rigid at the surgeon's discretion. As well as keeping the wound clean, and offering some protection from falls and external trauma, stump dressings are also used to control stump swelling and promote a conical, or at least cylindrical, shape to facilitate fitting of the first socket.

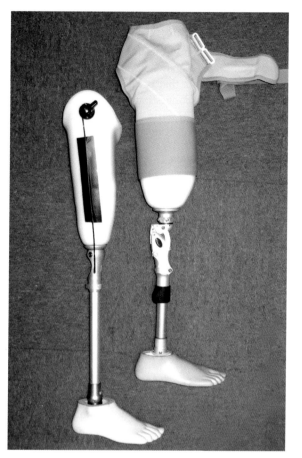

Figure 5.10 Transfemoral prostheses with polypropylene thermoplastic sockets and SACH feet for low-activity users. The left has a semi-automatic knee lock (SAKL) with a release lever; the right has total elastic suspension (TES) pelvic belt and 4 bar knee, set well back for maximum stability.

and rotation of the prosthesis, but stump shrinkage cannot be accommodated and the socket has to be refashioned. Pin lock suspension is particularly useful for short stumps. As the socket is only attached distally it may rotate easily if it becomes loose. Seal-In® liners have the advantages of firm contact between the silicone fins and the inside of the socket, which reduces rotation, as well as spreading the suspension force over more of the distal stump; this may be more comfortable if the soft tissues are mobile distally. Active and passive pumps may be used in above-knee sockets, as described for TTAs.

The brim of the common socket designs is rigid and may be uncomfortable when sitting. It may also be visible through close-fitting clothes. The anterior brim needs to be high enough to hold the ischial tuberosity

Application of Tubigrip™ or an elastic stump shrinker sock, after one to two weeks, when the wound is strong enough and tenderness reduced so that the patient can tolerate the pressures, is the commonest approach in the UK. A rigid plaster may be applied immediately after a trans-tibial amputation. This may control edema better in the first two weeks and may reduce time to first socket fitting[39–40] but it makes wound examination more difficult and may lead to delayed treatment of a complication. A plaster holding the knee extended may also help prevent a flexion contracture of the knee.

Once the patient is medically stable, physiotherapy can begin to teach the amputee to roll safely, to transfer, and to position and exercise the residual limb to prevent contractures.

Amputees may begin weight bearing on a pneumatic post-amputation mobility aid (PPAMAid) or Femurett early walking aid from two to four weeks post amputation, depending on healing, tenderness, and comorbidities. Techniques for immediate postoperative limb fitting have been described but are rarely attempted in the UK. A "primary" prosthesis is fabricated when the patient walks with the early walking aid, typically at five to eight weeks. This will usually have a simple "non-definitive" cosmesis or cover, as the socket shape, limb length and alignment often require alteration several times in the first few months. This first socket and other components are strong enough for everyday long-term use and should be regarded as definitive, although there is an expectation that adjustments to the socket and cosmesis will be required throughout the limb's, and patient's, life.

Complications

Wound Failure

This is particularly common in diabetics and vasculopaths. Conservative measures with dressings, including topical negative-pressure dressings, usually suffice to achieve wound closure; if not then stump revision with a wedge excision of soft tissue and bone, and closure without skin tension is required.

Joint Contractures

These may be caused by poor tensioning and anchoring of muscles intraoperatively, but can also arise in the postoperative period if the residual limb is not positioned and exercised correctly.

Edema

Postoperative swelling is common after amputation and can impede wound healing. Rigid dressings and elastic compression may help to reduce this. Chronic edema in soft tissue that is unsupported in the distal socket ("terminal congestion") may result in verrucous hyperplasia, a warty overgrowth of the skin, which usually responds to socket modifications.

Heterotopic Ossification

Heterotopic ossification is a relatively uncommon problem in elective civilian practice, except in patients with concomitant head injuries. It is much more common in military practice where it may affect 50 to 60% of traumatic amputees. The mechanism of its formation is not fully understood, but risk factors appear to include amputation through the zone of injury, blast injury, and the use of negative-pressure dressings. Fortunately, in most cases, the heterotopic bone can be accommodated within the prosthesis socket. Surgical excision, if required, usually leads to resolution[41]. Radiotherapy has been proposed as a prophylactic measure, but evidence for this remains equivocal.

Pain

Localized stump pain is often due to bone or soft tissue problems. This may be resolved with prosthesis modification but ultimately may require stump revision. In some patients, however, stump pain may have a neuropathic quality, analogous to phantom limb pain. In these cases it should be managed as phantom limb pain.

Phantom limb sensation, the feeling that all or part of the amputated limb is still present, is experienced by almost all adult amputees, but may not be problematic and usually decreases with time.

The earliest written description of phantom limb pain is from Ambroise Paré[42]. It is uncommon in pediatric amputees, but may occur in 60 to 80% of adult patients. It is most commonly felt in the most distal part of the missing limb and is often burning in quality. In most cases it starts soon after the surgery, but delayed onset years later is not unknown.

The precise mechanism by which phantom limb pain arises is unclear. It seems likely, however, that a cascade of events is initiated by sensitivity of damaged peripheral nerves to chemical and mechanical stimuli. This leads to hyperexcitability of spinal cord neurons and, with time, plasticity of the synapses within the spinal cord. Ultimately cortical brain structures are recruited.

Prevention of phantom limb pain is controversial. The initial promise shown by the use of perioperative epidurals has proved disappointing, and recent trials have shown no convincing evidence of benefit[43]. Latterly attention has shifted to the potential role of postoperative perineural infusions of local anesthetics and clonidine. These techniques show some potential, but remain unproven.

Treatment of phantom limb pain is usually medical with anti-neuropathic pain drugs such as amitriptyline, gabapentin, or pregabalin as well as standard opiate analgesics. Non-medical adjuncts such as transcutaneous electrical nerve stimulation (TENS), acupuncture, metallic socks, bio-feedback techniques, and hypnosis may be of help. Surgery is usually best avoided as it carries a significant risk of increased postoperative pain. While almost all amputees get some phantom pain, it remains a long-term problem for very few, and most stop taking medication for it within a few months of surgery.

Outcome of Amputation

Age itself is not a barrier to good function after an amputation, but comorbidities, cognitive impairment, and limited cardiovascular reserve all compromise the results in the elderly. Only half of elderly major lower limb amputees learn to walk at home[44]. Pre-amputation mobility and the ability to stand on one leg are important predictive factors of function[45].

Long-term functional outcomes after primary amputation or salvage surgery for trauma are similar up to seven years[46], although salvage patients have more surgery and episodes of hospitalization. When writing medico-legal reports, surgeons should consider the need for late amputation, which will encourage the solicitor to include costs of private prostheses in their compensation calculation. With the most sophisticated knees and ankles now costing up to £60 000 ($80 000) each, lifetime cost for private limbs can reach £500 000 ($650 000).

How a Prosthesis is Prescribed

There is little published trial evidence[47–51] on which to base details of prosthetic prescription and prosthetists will generally work from a short local "formulary," branching out from this only when specific patient demands arise, such as weight over 125 kg, frequent walking up hills, or demands of certain

leisure pursuits. People whose walking is limited to the house (level K1[1]), or who only use a prosthesis to help with transfers, will generally be fitted with simple feet and knees, which are as light as possible. People who can walk around outdoors (level K2) are usually supplied with more modern components, which accommodate uneven ground or control the rate of knee flexion and extension during the swing phase of gait. People with unrestricted mobility, but limited to walking and relatively sedate activities, are usually offered more energy-efficient feet and knees, which can control swing phase while walking at different speeds (K3) or which can flex slowly under load ("yielding") to allow them to descend stairs in the normal way. People who run, jump, carry heavy loads, and take part in sport (K4) may be offered stronger feet, which can store more energy at heel strike for return at toe off, perhaps with torque or vertical shock absorbers.

Recent reports suggest that less able or less fit K2 amputees may benefit from the more sophisticated and energy-efficient feet, which are usually only supplied to K3 amputees, if they are given additional training in their use[52–54]. This may not be apparent from self-reported measures[55].

---

[1] *Footnote:*

K0 – No mobility. This base level is assigned to amputees who do not have the ability or potential to ambulate or transfer safely with or without assistance. A prosthesis does not enhance the quality of life or mobility of the amputee.

K1 – Very limited mobility. The amputee has the ability or potential to use a prosthesis for transfers or ambulation on level surfaces at a fixed walking pace. Walking at various speeds, bypassing obstacles of any kind are out of the K1 class.

K2 – Limited mobility. The amputee has the ability or potential to use a prosthesis for ambulation and the ability to adjust for low-level environmental barriers such as curbs, stairs, or uneven surfaces. K2 level amputees may walk for limited periods of time, however, without significantly varying their speed.

K3 – Basic to normal mobility. The amputee has the ability or potential to use a prosthesis for basic ambulation and the ability to adjust for most environmental barriers. The amputee has the ability to walk at varying speeds.

K4 – High activity. The amputee exceeds basic mobility and applies high impact and stress to the prosthetic leg. Typical of the prosthetic demands of the child, active adult, or athlete.

Further Reading

www.orthobullets.com/trauma/1052/amputations

www.cirrie.buffalo.edu/encyclopedia/en/article/251/

www.oandp.health.usf.edu/Pros/pros_knees_class/Final%20Prosthetic%20Knees.pdf

References

1. Padula PA, Friedman LW. Acquired amputation and prosthesis before the sixteenth century. *Angiology*. 1987; 38: 133–41.

2. Hippocrates. *On joints*, LXIX.

3. Celsus C. *De Medicina* 6 VII 33.

4. Petit J-L. De l'amputation des membres. In Jean Louis Petit, *Trait´e des Maladies Chirurgicales et des Op´erations qui Leur Vonviennent (Vol. III)*. Paris, P. Fr. Didot, 1774, pp. 126–235, LXXIX.

5. Yonge, J. Currus triumphalis ex terebinthina (Londini 1679). In *Acta Eruditorum Lipsiensium*. Anno MDCXCVI. Lipsiae (1696), pp. 119–23.

6. *Rigveda* (RV) 1.112, 116, 117, 118 and RV 10.39.

7. www.limbless-statistics.org

8. www.cofemer.fr/UserFiles/File/Amput2004_05.pdf

9. www.ncepod.org.uk/pdf/current/LLA/LLAprotocol.pdf

10. www.limbless-association.org/index.php/directory

11. Armstrong DG, Lavery LA. Negative pressure wound therapy after partial diabetic foot amputation: a multicentre, randomised controlled trial. *Lancet*. 2005; 366, 1704–10.

12. Shaikh N, Vaughan P, Varty K, Coll AP, Robinson AHN. Outcome of limited forefoot amputation with primary closure in patients with diabetes. *Bone & Joint Journal*. 2013; 95:8, 1083–7.

13. Quigley M, Dillon MP. Quality of life in persons with partial foot or transtibial amputation: a systematic review. *Prosthet Orthot Int*. 2014 Sep 2. pii: 0309364614546526. [Epub ahead of print].

14. Millstein SG, MacCowan SA, Hunter GA. Traumatic partial foot amputations in adults: a long term review. *J Bone Joint Surg Br*. 1988; 70:2, 251–4.

15. Brown ML, Tang W, Patel A, Baumhauer JF. Partial foot amputation in patients with diabetic foot ulcers, *Foot Ankle Int*. 2012; 33:9, 707–16.

16. Lisfranc J. *Nouvelle méthode opératoire pour l'amputation partielle du pied dans son articulation tarso-métatarsienne: méthode précédée des nombreuses modifications qu'a subies celle de Chopart*. Paris, 1815.

17. Syme J. Amputation at the ankle joint. *London and Edinburgh Monthly Journal of Medical Sciences*. 1843; 3, 93.

18. Harris RI. Syme's amputation: the technical details essential for success. *J Bone Joint Surg Br*. 1956; 38B, 614–32.

19. Hornby R, Harris R. Syme's amputation: follow-up study of weight bearing in 68 patients. *J Bone Joint Surg Am*. 1975; 57:3, 346–9.

20. Waters R, Perry J, Antonelli E, Hislop, H. Energy cost of walking amputees. *J Bone Joint Surg Br*. 1976; 58A:1, 42–6.

21. Jeans KA, Browne RH, Karol LA. Effect of amputation level on energy expenditure during over ground walking by children with an amputation. *J Bone Joint Surg Am*. 2011; 93:1, 49–56.

22. Tisi PV, Than MM. Type of incision for below knee amputation. *Cochrane Database Syst Rev*. 2014; 8:4, CD003749. doi: 10.1002/14651858.CD003749.pub3.

23. Kingsbury T, Thesing N, Collins JD, Carney J, Wyatt M. Do patients with bone bridge amputations have improved gait compared with patients with traditional amputations? *Clin Orthop Relat Res*. 2014; 472:10, 3036–43. doi: 10.1007/s11999-014-3617-7.

24. Keeling JJ, Shawen SB, Forsberg JA, Kirk KL, Hsu JR, Gwinn DE, Potter BK. Comparison of functional outcomes following bridge synostosis with non-bone-bridging transtibial combat-related amputations. *J Bone Joint Surg Am*. 2013; 95, 888–93.

25. Tintle SM, Keeling JJ, Forsberg JA, Shawen SB, Andersen RC, Potter BK. Operative complications of combat-related transtibial amputations: a comparison of the modified Burgess and modified Ertl tibiofibular synostosis techniques. *J Bone Joint Surg Am*. 2011; 93, 1016–21.

26. Weiner DS. Prosthetic stimulation of femoral growth following knee disarticulation. *Inter-Clin Info Bull*. 1976; 15, 15–16.

27. Herring JA. Limb deficiencies. In *Tachdjian's Pediatric Orthopaedics: From the Texas Scottish Rite Hospital for Children*. (Elsevier, 2013).

28. Penn-Barwell JG. Outcomes in lower limb amputation following trauma: a systematic review and meta-analysis. *Injury*. 2011; 42:12, 1474–9.

29. Wendt KW, Zimmerman KW. [Shortening osteotomy of the femur after knee joint exarticulation]. [Article in German] *Unfallchirurg*. 1994; 97:12, 652–4.

30. Ateşalp AS, Yildiz C. Results of supracondylar osseous shortening in knee disarticulation. *Prosthet Orthot Int*. 2001; 25:2, 144–7.

31. Bowker JH, San Giovanni TP, Pinzur MS. North American experience with knee disarticulation with use of a posterior myofasciocutaneous

flap. Healing rate and functional results in seventy-seven patients. *J Bone Joint Surg Am.* 2000; 82-A:11, 1571–4.

32. Nebergall A, Bragdon C, Antonellis A, Kärrholm J, Brånemark R, Malchau H. Stable fixation of an osseointegated implant system for above-the-knee amputees: Titel RSA and radiographic evaluation of migration and bone remodeling in 55 cases. *Acta Orthopaedica.* 2012; 83:2, 121–8.

33. www.stanmoreimplants.com/itap-implant.php

34. www.royalfree.nhs.uk/services/services-a-z/plastic-surgery/prosthetic-limbs-and-body-parts/prosthetic-implants/

35. www.osseointegrationaustralia.com.au/the-ogap-opl-prosthesis

36. www.amputee-coalition.org/first_step_2003/marlo-anatomical-socket.html

37. www.biodesigns.com/hifi.html

38. www.oandp.org/olc/course.asp?course_id=8E117078-AC6F-446C-BE3B-62E1560FCE5D

39. Churilov I, Churilov L, Murphy D. Do rigid dressings reduce the time from amputation to prosthetic fitting? A systematic review and meta-analysis. *Ann Vasc Surg.* 2014; 28:7, 1801–8.

40. Punziano A, Martelli S, Sotgiu V, Giovannico G, Rahinò A, Cannone M, Bullo M, Maselli F. [The effectiveness of the elastic bandage in reducing residual limb volume in patients with lower limb amputation: literature review]. *Assist Inferm Ric.* 2011; 30:4, 208–14.

41. Potter BK, Burns TC, Lacap AP, Granville RR, Gajewski DA. Heterotopic ossification following traumatic and combat-related amputations. *J Bone Joint Surg Br.* 2007; 89-A:3, 476–86.

42. Paré A. *La maniere de traicter les playes faictes par hacqeubutes, que*

par flèches: & les accidentz d'icelles, cōme fractures & caries des os, gangrene & mortification: avec les traictz des instrumentz necessaires pour leur curation. Et la methode de curer les combustions principalement faictes par la pouldre a canon. 1552; Paris, Par Arnoul l'Angelié. fol. 45 r.

43. Nikolajsen L, Ilkjaer S, Christensen JH, Krøner K, Jensen TS. Randomised trial of epidural bupivacaine and morphine in prevention of stump and phantom pain in lower-limb amputation. *Lancet.* 1997; 350, 1353–7.

44. Fortington LV, Rommers GM, Geertzen JH, Postema K, Dijkstra PU. Mobility in elderly people with a lower limb amputation: a systematic review. *J Am Med Dir Assoc.* 2012; 13:4, 319–25.

45. Sansam K, Neumann V, O'Connor R, Bhakta B. Predicting walking ability following lower limb amputation: a systematic review of the literature. *J Rehabil Med.* 2009; 41:8, 593–603.

46. Busse JW, Jacobs CL, Swiontkowski MF, Bosse MJ, Bhandari M; Evidence-Based Orthopaedic Trauma Working Group. Complex limb salvage or early amputation for severe lower-limb injury: a meta-analysis of observational studies. *J Orthop Trauma.* 2007; 21:1, 70–6.

47. Gholizadeh H, Abu Osman NA, Eshraghi A, Ali S. Transfemoral prosthesis suspension systems: a systematic review of the literature. *Am J Phys Med Rehabil.* 2014; 93:9, 809–23.

48. van der Linde H, Hofstad CJ, Geurts AC, Postema K, Geertzen JH, van Limbeek J. A systematic literature review of the effect of different prosthetic components on human functioning with a lower-limb prosthesis. *J Rehabil Res Dev.* 2004; 41:4, 555–70.

49. Versluys R, Beyl P, Van Damme M, Desomer A, Van Ham R, Lefeber D. Prosthetic feet: state-of-the-art review and the importance of mimicking human ankle-foot biomechanics. *Disabil Rehabil Assist Technol.* 2009; 4:2, 65–75.

50. Cumming JC, Barr S, Howe TE. Prosthetic rehabilitation for older dysvascular people following a unilateral transfemoral amputation. *Cochrane Database Syst Rev.* 2006; 18:4, CD005260.

51. Hofstad C, Linde H, Limbeek J, Postema K. Prescription of prosthetic ankle-foot mechanisms after lower limb amputation. *Cochrane Database Syst Rev.* 2004; 1, 1–78.

52. Agrawal V, Gailey RS, Gaunaurd IA, O'Toole C, Finnieston A, Tolchin R. Comparison of four different categories of prosthetic feet during ramp ambulation in unilateral transtibial amputees. *Prosthet Orthot Int.* 2014; pii: 0309364614536762 [Epub ahead of print].

53. Agrawal V, Gailey R, O'Toole C, Gaunaurd I, Finnieston A. Influence of gait training and prosthetic foot category on external work symmetry during unilateral transtibial amputee gait. *Prosthet Orthot Int.* 2013; 37:5, 396–403.

54. Graham LE, Datta D, Heller B, Howitt J. A comparative study of oxygen consumption for conventional and energy storing prosthetic feet in transfemoral amputees. *Clin Rehabil.* 2008; 22:10–11, 896–901.

55. Gailey RS, Gaunaurd I, Agrawal V, Finnieston A, O'Toole C, Tolchin R. Application of self-report and performance-based outcome measures to determine functional differences between four categories of prosthetic feet. *J Rehabil Res Dev.* 2012; 49:4, 597–612.

Forefoot Pathology

Daniel Z. Goldbloom and John P. Negrine

Hallux Valgus

Introduction

Hallux valgus is a forefoot deformity comprised of lateral deviation of the great toe with medial deviation of the metatarsal head. This can occur with or without subluxation of the first metatarsophalangeal joint (MTPJ). The term was first introduced in the 1870s by Carl Heuter, a German surgeon. He recognized that the deformity was due to joint angulation, rather than simple enlargement.

The term "bunion" is derived from the Latin word *bunio*, meaning a turnip. The "turnip" describes the prominent medial eminence of the first MTPJ, and so hallux valgus is just one of the causes of a bunion. The management of hallux valgus has advanced significantly, as we have better understood the nature of the deformity and the biomechanical consequences of surgery.

Pathogenesis: Etiology, Epidemiology, and Pathophysiology

The prevalence of hallux valgus is unclear. It is probably around 2% in unshod populations, but is much higher in the shoe-wearing population[1]. Women comprise the majority of sufferers as they tend to wear narrow shoes with, or without, high heels. There are about nine women to every man presenting for surgical treatment of hallux valgus[2].

The etiology is unclear. There is an underlying genetic basis, which is activated by lifestyle factors. In one study, a family history was documented in 94%[2]. Genetic factors that have been implicated, but are as yet unproven, can be divided into bone, joint, and soft tissue factors (Table 6.1)

Hallux valgus deformity has four components. These are not necessarily sequential[4].

1. *Valgus* of the first MTPJ – always.
2. *Metatarsus primus varus* – nearly always.
3. *Pronation* of the proximal phalanx – often.
4. First metatarsal *elevation* – particularly in cases with a long first metatarsal.

In the normal foot, the first MTPJ is stabilized by *static* and *dynamic* structures, which normally prevent deformity. The static structures are the ligaments, capsule, and the crista of the first metatarsal head, and the dynamic structures are the musculotendinous structures.

In the development of hallux valgus the first structures to fail are the medial capsule and medial collateral ligament, which is essentially a thickening of the capsule. Failure of the medial structures leads to the first metatarsal moving into varus, *metatarsus primus varus*. The hallux moves into valgus. Figure 6.1 demonstrates, in the axial plane, how the deformity progresses.

Table 6.1 Genetic and lifestyle factors in the etiology of hallux valgus

Genetic factors	Lifestyle factors
Rounded metatarsal head	Narrow shoes
Rounded first metatarsocunieform joint	High heels
Medial-facing first metatarsocuneiform joint	Excessive loading (e.g., ballet dancers)
Single-faceted proximal first metatarsal articular surface	
Lateral exostosis of the first metatarsal base	
First metatarsal that is longer than the second metatarsal[3]	
Calf tightness with ankle dorsiflexion <10°	
Pes planus	
First-ray hypermobility	
Generalized ligamentous laxity	

(a)

(b)

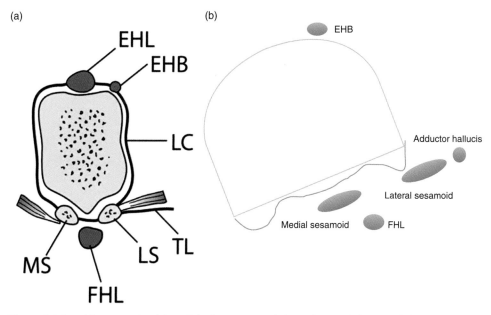

Figure 6.1 An axial, cross-sectional view of the first metatarsophalangeal joint. (**a**) The normal alignment; (**b**) as the metatarsal head moves medially the sesamoid mechanism remains and consequently appears to sublux laterally and superiorly. EHL: extensor hallucis longus; EHB: extensor hallucis brevis; FHL: flexor hallucis longus; LS: lateral sesamoid; MS: medial sesamoid.

It is important to understand that it is the metatarsal head that moves medially, with the sesamoid mechanism remaining essentially unmoved. The medial and lateral sesamoids lie in the respective heads of flexor hallucis brevis (FHB) (Figure 6.2). In remaining in situ, the sesamoids sublux laterally and superiorly relative to the first metatarsal head. The subluxation of the sesamoids causes the crista of the first metatarsal head to become flattened, as a result of abrasion by the medial sesamoid. As a result of the pull of the adductor hallucis tendon on the inferior part of the base of the proximal phalanx, the great toe also pronates.

The abductor hallucis moves inferolaterally and loses its ability to abduct the hallux. It should be remembered that the ab/adduction of the toes is described relative to the second metatarsal longitudinal axis. The long and short flexor and extensor tendons also come to lie lateral to the joint, and their line of pull is no longer neutral, but as partial adductors. Thus in correcting hallux valgus the first metatarsal head is relocated over the sesamoids, rather than the sesamoids being relocated under the metatarsal.

The result of the hallux valgus deformity is to defunction the first ray, consequently overloading the lesser rays. This overload leads to lesser MTPJ instability and lesser toe deformities, such as clawing (Figure 6.3).

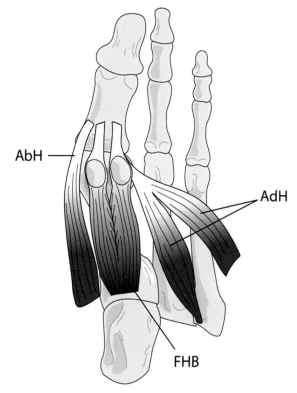

Figure 6.2 The sesamoid mechanism viewed from the plantar aspect. AbH: abductor hallucis; AdH: adductor hallucis; FHB: flexor hallucis brevis.

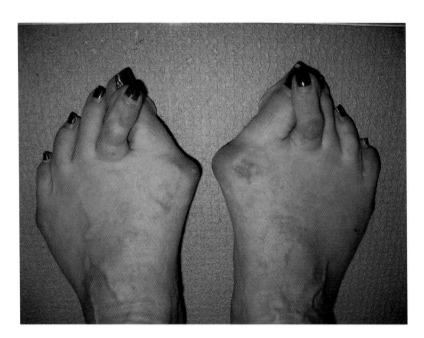

Figure 6.3 Bilateral hallux valgus, with secondary deformity of the lesser rays.

Table 6.2 Classification of hallux valgus

	Hallux valgus angle (HVA)	Intermetatarsal angle (IMA)
Normal	<15°	<9°
Mild	<20°	<11°
Moderate	<40°	<16°
Severe	<50°	<20°
Very severe	>50°	>20°

Classification

There are *two* important classification systems for hallux valgus. The first relates to severity (Table 6.2). This classification, for the most part, dictates surgical treatment. It relies on both the hallux valgus angle (HVA) and the intermetatarsal angle (IMA) (Figure 6.4).

The second classification depends on the congruency or incongruency of the MTP joint. This terminology is to some degree a misnomer, as an incongruent joint is in fact a joint that is subluxed. A congruent hallux valgus is one in which the distal metatarsal articular angle (DMAA) is increased, with the first metatarsal head being angulated laterally. Consequently the two joint surfaces are "congruent" (Figure 6.5a). Congruent hallux valgus is more likely

to be associated with juvenile onset hallux valgus and is often seen in combination with conditions such as Down's syndrome. The congruent joint is also more stable and the hallux valgus is less likely to progress. The incongruent hallux valgus (Figure 6.5b) is much commoner, is less stable, and more likely to progress.

Clinical Presentation

History and Examination

Patients with hallux valgus usually present with pain and deformity. The pain has often been present for years. It can be localized to the "bunion," or may be experienced more globally around the MTPJ. The patient is usually restricted in the style of shoes that can be worn. Metatarsalgia may also be reported with painful callosities under the lesser metatarsal heads; these are often called "transfer lesions." There is also often dorsal pain and callosities over the proximal interphalangeal joints (PIPJs) of the second and third toes.

Some patients describe a progressive deformity of the second MTPJ, which initially becomes synovitic, with tenderness and swelling of the joint. The second toe then deforms and may eventually cross over the big toe.

In considering hallux valgus it is important to consider the forefoot as a whole, as rebalancing all of the aspects of forefoot deformity is important in

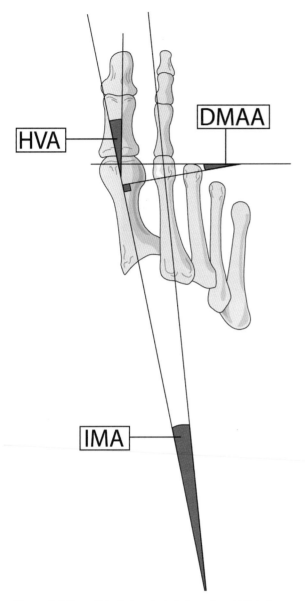

severity of the valgus; pronation of the toe; correctability of the MTPJ deformity; pain on movement of the MTPJ; MTPJ range of movement – a stiff joint will remain so after correction; erythema and tenderness; and size of the medial eminence. A neurovascular examination should be recorded, in particular the dorsomedial branch of the superficial peroneal nerve should be examined, as sensation is often reduced at the time of presentation and reduced sensation postoperatively may not be the result of surgical damage.

While an assessment is made for tendo Achillis (TA) tightness, pes planus, and first ray hypermobility, the role of these features in hallux valgus is poorly understood.

Investigations

Weightbearing AP and lateral plain radiographs are the primary, and usually only, investigation. The HVA, IMA, and DMAA are measured. The DMAA, also known as the proximal articular set angle (PASA), is the angle between the articular surface of the first MTPJ and the longitudinal axis of the first metatarsal (Figure 6.4), It is normally less than 10°. A high DMAA is seen in congruent hallux valgus and will need to be corrected by surgery. The plain radiographs may also show MTPJ arthritis, lesser MTPJ subluxation or dislocation, and TMTJ arthritis.

Treatment

Non-surgical. The non-surgical management of hallux valgus is not corrective, it is supportive and consists of:
- accommodative shoes with a deep and wide toe box, which can be bought off the shelf, or customized
- a toe separator can decrease pressure on the medial capsule and also relieve pain between toes
- padding, with or without a cut out, can be used to offload pressure from a corn or callus.

Custom-made orthoses do not play a significant role and, at best, provide short-term symptomatic relief.

Surgical. There are over 130 procedures described for the management of hallux valgus, as such no single operation is a panacea.

The indication for surgery has long been pain, which may prevent the wearing of shoes. We believe the indication should be extended to include progressive and severe deformity. The severe deformity, if left untreated, affects the lesser rays and makes eventual surgical management more complex.

Figure 6.4 The radiological angles in hallux valgus. HVA: hallux valgus angle; IMA: intermetatarsal angle; DMAA: distal metatarsal articular angle.

treatment. For example, in treating a claw second toe in the presence of hallux valgus it is necessary to correct both the hallux and the second toe, indeed on occasions all of the toes may need to be addressed. Management of lesser toe deformity is discussed later in this chapter.

Generalized ligamentous laxity should be noted, for example by recording a Beighton score. Local examination of the first MTPJ should record: the

(a) (b)

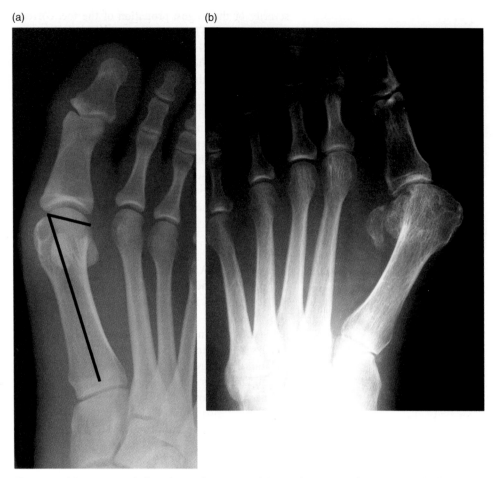

Figure 6.5 (a) A congruent hallux valgus with an increased DMAA; the joint articulates congruously. (b) An incongruent hallux valgus. Note the first MTP and sesamoid articulations are subluxed. The proximal phalanx is also rotated.

Bunionectomy with capsular plication has been shown to lead to recurrence and worsening of the deformity. It should not be undertaken for correction of hallux valgus. Surgically the HVA, DMAA, and IMA must be addressed. The aim of surgical treatment is to reduce the first metatarsal head over the sesamoids. Barouk described four components in correction of hallux valgus:

1. Distal soft tissue release
2. Osteotomy of the first metatarsal
3. Medial capsular plication
4. An Akin osteotomy to correct hallux valgus interphalangeus.

While not every patient needs all four of these components they should be considered in a stepwise fashion – for example, step four can be omitted if there is no hallux valgus interphalangeus. We will describe these steps in sequence.

1. **A distal soft tissue release** involves dividing the lateral structures, which prevent correction of the deformity. The adductor hallucis is released from its attachment to the lateral sesamoid. The lateral joint capsule, also known as the lateral sesamoid suspensory ligament, is released along the line of the sesamoid to allow the sesamoid to reduce under the head of the first metatarsal. Sectioning of the lateral collateral ligament is controversial. It allows a greater correction, particularly in cases of severe deformity, but also leads to a higher risk of hallux varus. As part of this procedure the medial capsule is opened and a bunionectomy, preserving the sulcus, is undertaken.

2. **An osteotomy** of the metatarsal may allow the head of the metatarsal to be translated laterally and

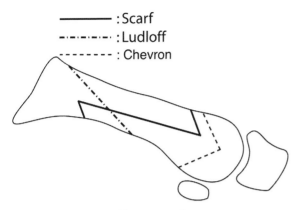

Figure 6.6 A selection of first metatarsal osteotomy patterns.

reduce the IMA. First metatarsal osteotomies are classified as distal, shaft, or basal.

In cases of a congruent joint with a high DMAA, an extra element is required, with rotation of the articular surface medially. This can be achieved by a medial closing wedge osteotomy of the shaft or by adding medial rotation to a translational shaft osteotomy – we prefer the latter.

The choice of osteotomy is determined by the severity of the deformity:

Mild deformity can be managed with a soft tissue procedure combined with a distal or shaft osteotomy of the first metatarsal.

The chevron osteotomy (Figure 6.6) is a distal osteotomy in which a "V" shaped cut of the metatarsal is made. This allows lateral translation of the capital fragment. It is stable, but can be fixed. We use a 2 mm absorbable rod. The results are satisfactory for mild deformity. When combined with a lateral release its indications can be stretched without an increased incidence of avascular necrosis[5].

Moderate to severe deformities can be managed with a number of techniques (Figure 6.6). Osteotomies can be classified as basal (e.g., basal chevron, crescentic) or shaft osteotomies (e.g., Scarf, Ludloff). In modern practice they are usually combined with a lateral release and offer a more powerful correction than distal osteotomy. Good results have been reported for all of the above osteotomies.

The Scarf osteotomy (Figure 6.7) is a shaft osteotomy. It is very versatile and can be used for mild, moderate, and severe deformities with success[6]. It has a large surface area, which almost eliminates the risk of non-union and has been shown to be a stronger construct than a proximal

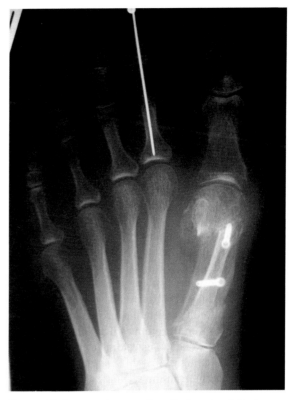

Figure 6.7 Postoperative correction of hallux valgus following a Scarf osteotomy.

crescentic osteotomy[7]. It is a technically demanding procedure, but allows:

– the IMA to be reduced
– plantar translation of the metatarsal head
– slight shortening of the first ray
– medial rotation of the articular surface to correct the DMAA, should this be necessary.

3. **Capsular plication** is important, but not always necessary. In some cases the sesamoids lie under the metatarsal head following the lateral release and osteotomy. In these cases the capsule needs simple closure. In others the sesamoids remain laterally displaced, in which cases the capsule is plicated.

4. **The Akin osteotomy** is an extra-articular medial-closing wedge osteotomy of the base of the proximal phalanx. Although often used to augment a hallux valgus correction, we believe its true indication is for the case of hallux valgus interphalangeus, which often coexists with hallux valgus. The deformity is due to different articulation angles between the proximal and distal articular surfaces of the proximal phalanx. Many surgeons use an Akin osteotomy in

80% or so of cases, as the fourth stage of hallux valgus correction. The decision as to whether to add an Akin osteotomy on the table is a clinical one, based upon the appearance of the foot after completion of the first three stages.

The more severe deformities, with a greater than 50° HVA, are more difficult to correct successfully with osteotomy. Arthrodesis of either the MTPJ or TMTJ is a safer option.

Fusion of the first TMTJ to correct hallux valgus is eponymously known as a Lapidus procedure. As well as severe deformity, other indications for a Lapidus type procedure are hallux valgus with TMT arthritis and TMTJ instability. The arthrodesis of the TMTJ includes excision of a laterally based wedge, to close the IMA. Distally the lateral soft tissue release, bunionectomy, and medial capsular plication are undertaken. The postoperative management requires six weeks of non-weight bearing to allow union. Reported satisfaction rates of the Lapidus procedure are generally lower than with osteotomies. Thus the majority of surgeons prefer to use an osteotomy as routine.

Arthrodesis of the first MTPJ will be discussed later in the chapter, in the section on hallux rigidus. Nevertheless it is worth noting that fusion of the first MTP leads to a reduction in the IMA.

Excisional arthroplasties in the form a Keller–Brandes, with excision of the basal half of the proximal phalanx, or a Mayo, with excision of the metatarsal head, have been used as a salvage for severe deformity with poor tissue quality, such as in rheumatoid arthritis. These procedures can lead to poor outcomes as they defunction the first ray, risking the development of transfer lesions to the lesser rays. They have largely been abandoned.

An algorithm for surgical decision making is shown in Table 6.3.

Table 6.3 An algorithm for surgical decision making in hallux valgus surgery

Mild	DSTR + distal or shaft osteotomy +/− Akin
Moderate	DSTR + shaft osteotomy +/− Akin
Severe:	Systemic disease – first MTPJ fusion No systemic disease – DSTR + shaft or basal osteotomy +/− Akin
Very severe	First MTPJ or TMTJ fusion

DSTR: distal soft tissue release.

Complications

The complications of hallux valgus surgery are commonly related to technical failure. It is important that the surgery is well planned, and the principles adhered to. Selection of the osteotomy is important.

- If the first metatarsal is excessively shortened or elevated there is a risk that the lesser rays will be overloaded, and the patients develop painful callosities under the lesser metatarsal heads. In time the lesser toes will deform.
- Stiffness can be a result of failure to shorten the first metatarsal and decompress the first MTP joint.
- Recurrence of the hallux valgus may be the result of a failure of correction, or choosing a procedure of limited corrective power.
- Hallux varus is usually resultant on being overly aggressive with corrective components – in particular the lateral release.

Avascular necrosis of the first metatarsal head has been reported, in particular with a chevron osteotomy. The blood supply of the metatarsal head has been well described[8]. On the lateral side, there are both dorsal and plantar networks of vessels from the continuation of the dorsalis pedis artery. They supply the metatarsal head via the capsule. Probably most important is the plantar plexus of vessels, which enter the head just proximal to the capsule. There is also a nutrient artery to the metatarsal shaft. Avascular necrosis is very rarely seen with a Scarf osteotomy, despite the routine performance of a lateral release. In a Scarf osteotomy much play is made on keeping the plantar blood supply to the metatarsal head intact. Thus we recommend keeping the inferior limb of a chevron osteotomy long, to maintain the plantar vascularity, if a lateral release is undertaken

Minimally Invasive Hallux Valgus Surgery

The advent of minimally invasive surgery in orthopedics has led to increasing numbers of correction options in hallux valgus[9]. The basics are similar in that a lateral release and distal osteotomy of the first metatarsal are performed. The difference is that the aims are achieved through percutaneous approaches with the use of a 2 to 3 mm diameter burr to perform the osteotomy. Large studies have been reported using various techniques. These techniques are technically demanding at the outset and, while they may become more popular, the important point to make is that

Type 1   Type 2   Type 3

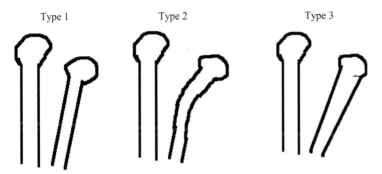

Figure 6.8 The Coughlin classification of bunionettes. (From left to right) type 1: enlarged metatarsal head; type 2: lateral deviation of the metatarsal shaft; type 3: increased fourth–fifth intermetatarsal angle.

one should not stray from the principles of deformity correction outlined above.

Bunionettes

Introduction

A bunionette is a deformity characterized by a prominence of the head of the fifth metatarsal. The overall incidence is difficult to determine, as many cases are asymptomatic, although they often present in joggers and Alpine skiers. The pressure of shoes causes pain from both bursitis and the formation of lateral or plantar keratoses. The female to male ratio may be as high as 9:1[10].

Coughlin's classification[11] is simple to use and helps to guide management (Figure 6.8). Type 1 can be due to a dumbbell-shaped head or a hypertrophied lateral condyle. Different studies show type 2 or 3 to be the most common.

Presentation

The patient presents with pain over the lateral, dorsolateral, or plantar aspect of the fifth metatarsal head, with associated swelling and erythema. If chronic there may be a lateral or plantar lateral hyperkeratosis. The fifth toe is often medially deviated and there may be an associated claw or hammer deformity.

Pes planus is commonly associated with symptomatic bunionettes[12]. There are two reasons for this: firstly, the planus loads the lesser metatarsal heads; and, secondly, it leads to forefoot pronation, which causes apparent widening of the fifth metatarsal head.

The investigation of choice is an AP and lateral weightbearing plain radiograph. The AP view determines the type of deformity. As with hallux valgus the MTPJ angle and IMA are measured. The MTPJ angle is normally $<14°$ and the IMA is $<8°$. The width of

the metatarsal head should be <13 mm. These measurements are not as useful or reliable as they are in hallux valgus.

Treatment

Most cases are treated non-operatively with comfortable shoes to accommodate the toes. Padding can be used to relieve pressure. Hyperkeratoses can be trimmed. Orthoses with a medial arch support to reverse forefoot pronation and a cut-out to accommodate the prominence may be helpful.

Surgical treatment is reserved for cases that are refractory to non-operative management, usually with intractable keratotic lesions. There are over 30 different procedures described. The aim of surgery is to relieve pressure by narrowing the width of the forefoot and, in some cases, elevate the metatarsal head.

Lateral condylectomy is commonly suggested for a type 1 deformity. It reduces the width of the forefoot, but just as with bunionectomy for hallux valgus, the recurrence rate is high and there is an incidence of medial subluxation of the MTPJ. We do not recommend this procedure.

Resection of the entire head and increasing amounts of the shaft have been suggested for salvage, in conditions such as rheumatoid arthritis and infection with ulceration. Unfortunately resection can lead to unsatisfactory biomechanics and poor function postoperatively.

We prefer osteotomy for most bunionettes requiring surgery. Type 1 and mild to moderate type 2 conditions can be treated with a distal osteotomy. A Weil osteotomy[13] is an extra-articular oblique cut of the metatarsal neck from dorsal distal to plantar proximal. Although it is more commonly used to shorten the metatarsal in cases of lesser MTPJ instability, in bunionettes the osteotomy can be used to translate the head medially to realign the fifth ray[14].

The osteotomy can be directed "uphill" from lateral to medial to offload the metatarsal head, in cases with plantar pressure.

The limitation of the Weil osteotomy is the width of the metatarsal. A larger deformity requires a proximal osteotomy. The tenuous blood supply to the watershed area at the proximal metaphyseal/diaphyseal junction is well described[15], as it is thought to inhibit the Jones fracture healing. Therefore the "proximal" osteotomy has to be more distal than its first ray equivalent. A well described option is the "oblique sliding osteotomy." It is similar to the Ludloff for the first ray (Figure 6.6) in that is a based around an oblique cut from dorsal proximal to plantar distal. The osteotomy is rotated to achieve correction. There is a real risk of inadequate fixation due to the width of the metatarsal. This can be offset by predrilling the screw hole. There is a paucity of studies on which to base surgical management of symptomatic bunionettes.

Hallux Rigidus

Hallux rigidus is the term used to denote the stiffness associated with osteoarthritis of the first MTPJ. It is present in 2.5% of the population aged over 50 years.

Etiology

Most cases arise spontaneously, although hallux rigidus has been associated with hallux valgus interphalangeus, a flat metatarsal head, a history of trauma, and female gender. Bilateral involvement is associated with a family history. Coughlin found no association with elevatus, first-ray hypermobility, a long first metatarsal, Achilles or gastrocnemius tendon tightness, abnormal foot posture, symptomatic hallux valgus, adolescent onset, shoes, or occupation[16].

History and Examination

The diagnosis is made from history, physical examination, and x-rays. There is usually a history of pain in forced dorsiflexion, such as during toe off. Nonweightbearing pain implies advanced disease.

On examination there is a reduced range of motion, particularly in dorsiflexion. It is important to note whether there is pain in the midrange on passive movement, as this has implications for treatment. Pressure areas dorsally and sometimes medially may be present as a result of osteophyte formation. The same osteophytes can cause paresthesia if they lead to pressure on the dorsal cutaneous nerve.

Imaging and Classification

Weightbearing AP, lateral, and oblique foot radiographs will show the typical changes of osteoarthritis: joint space narrowing, subchondral sclerosis, subchondral cysts, and osteophytes. In the case of a normal radiograph, an MRI may be helpful to look for early changes.

Coughlin and Shurnas classified this condition into five stages, 0 to 4[17], which helps to guide management (Table 6.4).

Table 6.4 Coughlin and Shurnas classification of hallux rigidus

Grade	Dorsiflexion	X-ray finding	Pain and stiffness
0	40–60° total *or* 10–20% loss compared to normal side	Normal	Stiffness but no pain
1	30–40° total *or* 20–50% loss compared to normal side	Dorsal osteophyte, minimal joint-space narrowing, or subchondral sclerosis	Mild or occasional pain at extremes of range
2	10–30° total *or* 50–75% loss compared to normal side	Dorsal and lateral osteophytes give flattened appearance to metatarsal head, dorsal 25% involvement. Mild to moderate osteoarthritic changes	Moderate to severe pain at extremes of range
3	<10° total *or* 75–100% loss compared to normal side	More severe than usual changes and more than dorsal 25% involved Sesamoids involved	Nearly constant pain and stiffness at extremes of range
4	As grade 3	As grade 3	As grade 3, with midrange pain

Treatment

Non-operative therapy is based around pain relief rather than restoration of movement. It consists of analgesia medication and shoe modification. Simple analgesia and NSAIDs have only a minor role to play, as they do not provide lasting relief. Corticosteroid and hyaluronic acid injections have been reported to give transient pain relief.

A shoe with a deep or wide toe box allows room to prevent pressure from osteophytes. A "Morton's extension" on an insole, or shank inside the shoe bridging the MTPJ will prevent movement. However, they are poorly tolerated. A rocker-bottom sole may also reduce pain.

Operative options for joint disease are traditionally divided into joint-preserving and joint-sacrificing procedures. Another way to classify the options is according to procedure type – cheilectomy, osteotomy, arthroplasty, and arthrodesis. Cheilectomy and arthrodesis are the mainstays of treatment.

Cheilectomy involves excision of the dorsal osteophyte and the dorsal 30% of the articular surface of the metatarsal head. We also release adhesions between the sesamoids and metatarsal head. Cheilectomy has the advantage of being a simple procedure, which preserves joint stability and restores mobility. There is a risk of dorsal subluxation of the proximal phalanx if the ostectomy is too aggressive. It has been shown to improve both pain levels and range of motion for grade 1 to 3 disease, where more than 50% of the metatarsal head cartilage remains. It also improves ankle push-off power[18]. If there is pain in the first MTPJ in the midrange, dorsal cheilectomy is relatively contraindicated, whereas dorsal impingement pain is an ideal indication.

Periarticular osteotomies have been advocated on both the metatarsal and phalangeal side. Their various aims are:

- to realign the joint
- to decompress the joint
- to bring better preserved parts of the articular surface into the load-bearing area.

A Moberg[19] osteotomy is probably the most commonly used periarticular osteotomy[20]. It is used in conjunction with a cheilectomy. It consists of a dorsal closing wedge near the base of the proximal phalanx to dorsiflex the phalanx.

On the metatarsal side, a number of osteotomies have been described but are rarely used. A Weil osteotomy, where the first metatarsal is cut parallel to the floor to allow proximal translation of the metatarsal head and decompression of the joint, has been described, especially when the first metatarsal is long. Malerba showed promising results for this particular technique[21]. When hallux valgus and rigidus are both present, realignment in conjunction with a cheilectomy can be used.

Arthroplasties can be excisional, interpositional, hemi-, or total replacements. None of the above options has provided consistently satisfactory results.

Excision arthroplasty, much as for hallux valgus, consists of a Keller–Brandes procedure, which involves excision of the proximal third of the proximal phalanx. The complications of the Keller procedure include shortening, cock-up deformity of the hallux, and late recurrence of pain in the pseudarthrosis. Nevertheless the major problem of the Keller is that it defunctions the great toe, and can lead to transfer metatarsalgia to the lesser rays, which is difficult to treat. Thus the Keller procedure should not be undertaken in active patients.

A variation of the Keller is by excision of a dorsally based wedge of the proximal phalanx, leaving the plantar aspect of the phalanx to preserve the FHB attachment and the windlass mechanism. The dorsal capsule and EHB are then interposed into the joint.

Total and hemiarthroplasties have consisted of Silastic® type implants, as well as cementless metal implants using press fit and porous coatings for fixation.

Hemiarthroplasties have been implanted on either side of the joint. Results are variable, often with unacceptably high implant complication rates. Subsidence, implant debris, and macrophage reaction leading to periarticular lysis and loosening are all reported.

Arthrodesis can be achieved with "cup and cone" style reamers or flat cuts. The strongest method of fixation is a headless compression screw and a dorsal plate. This goes against the orthopedic principle of placing fixation on the tension side, but it is obviously impractical to place a plate on the plantar aspect of the first ray.

The position of arthrodesis is critical in terms of varus/valgus, rotation, and particularly flexion/extension. In general we aim for 15° valgus and 20° dorsiflexion with respect to the metatarsal shaft. If the toe is too flexed the patient will catch it on the ground, if it is too extended the patient will be uncomfortable in shoes with unacceptable pressure beneath the lesser metatarsal heads. The key principles of arthrodesis must be adhered to[22]. These include compression of well prepared, cancellous bony surfaces with rigid fixation.

Success rates are consistently above 90% for arthrodesis and studies have shown that a high proportion of patients are able to return to their desired level of activity, such as hiking and tennis[23].

Lesser Toe Abnormalities

Lesser toe abnormalities comprise a number of deformities, which can be a significant cause of disability – particularly in the shoe-wearing population. This section will concentrate on the common mallet, hammer, and claw deformities, although other deformities are possible.

Mallet toe is defined as a flexion deformity of the distal interphalangeal joint (DIPJ). It only accounts for 5% of lesser toe deformities, with a much higher incidence in women than men[24]. It usually involves a single toe and its causes include:

- traumatic avulsion of the extensor tendon
- inflammatory arthritis
- flexor digitorum longus tendon tightness
- a long toe deformed by shoes.

The patients present with nail deformity and callus formation over the DIPJ and tip of the toe. On examination it is important to note whether the deformity is fully correctable, as this, although rare, may alter management.

Weightbearing radiographs should be performed, but usually provide little further insight into the management.

All cases should be treated non-operatively initially. Box 6.1 shows the non-operative options for treating mallet, hammer, and claw toes.

Box 6.1 Non-operative treatment for lesser toe deformities

Gel toe sleeve
Felt pad at toe tip
Toe crest – extends DIPJ
Shaving callus
Nail trimming
Deep toe box shoe
Low heel
Metatarsal dome or bar

If non-operative treatment fails surgical options are considered. These include: flexor tenotomy, resection arthroplasty, DIPJ arthrodesis, and distal phalangectomy. Our preferred technique is to perform a DIPJ arthrodesis, combined with a long flexor tenotomy. Both procedures are undertaken through a dorsal approach. In some patients the skin becomes part of the deforming force in chronic situations, and therefore may need to be released or allowed to tear on the plantar surface. It is then left open to heal.

The options for methods of fixation in arthrodesis of either the PIP or DIP joints include K-wires and a variety of metal and plastic implants. The K-wires are usually brought out through the skin, whereas the new implants are entirely internal and designed to be left in situ (Figure 6.9). We use K-wire fixation as the technique is simple and they are cheaper. We leave the wire prominent from the end of the toe and remove it after six weeks.

Hammer toe and claw toes have slightly overlapping definitions.

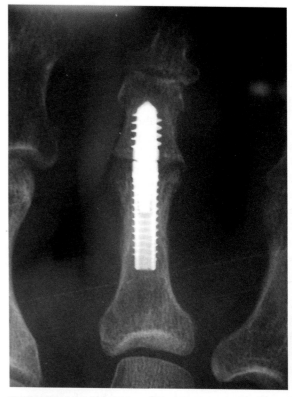

Figure 6.9 Intraosseous Stayfuse® device (Tornier, France) for internally fixing a PIPJ fusion.

Constricting shoes
Plantar plate degeneration
Hallux valgus
Neurological – cerebral palsy, lumbar disk
Charcot–Marie–Tooth
Inflammatory arthritis
Diabetes
Trauma – compartment syndrome

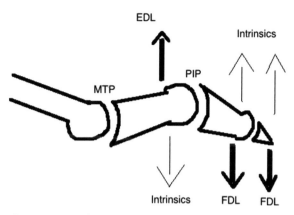

Figure 6.10 The forces acting on the lesser toes. EDL: extensor digitorum longus; FDL: flexor digitorum longus; MTP: metatarsophalangeal joint; PIP: proximal interphalangeal joint.

- A *hammer toe* is a flexion deformity of the *PIPJ*.
- A *complex hammer toe* also involves hyperextension of the *MTPJ*.
- A *claw toe* is primarily hyperextension of the *MTPJ* with flexion deformity of the *PIPJ*.

The difference between a claw toe and complex hammer toe is that claw toes usually involve more than one digit. The causes are outlined in Box 6.2.

In order to understand the pathophysiology of hammer and claw toes, one needs to understand the principal forces acting on the MTP and PIP joints of the lesser toes (Figure 6.10). The extensor digitorum longus (EDL) tendon is an extensor of all three joints; it divides over the proximal phalanx into three slips. The medial and lateral slips pass to a common insertion on the distal phalanx, while the central slip inserts onto the middle phalanx[25]. Its only attachment to the proximal phalanx is via the aponeurotic sling along the medial and lateral aspects of the proximal phalanx, which attach to the phalanx's plantar surface. The strongest action of the EDL, assisted by the extensor digitorum brevis (EDB), is MTPJ dorsiflexion. The weaker intrinsic muscles, interossei and lumbricals, *flex* the MTPJ, as they pass inferior to the MTPJs axis of rotation. However, the same intrinsic muscles *extend* the PIP and DIP joints. The FDL tendon provides the main flexion force on the DIP and PIP joints.

The normal action of walking encourages the MTPJ to dorsiflex. In this position the action of EDL is unopposed. When combined with tight-fitting shoes, or intrinsic dysfunction, it leads to attenuation of both the plantar plate and collateral ligaments, which are the main static stabilizers of the MTPJ. The MTPJ will eventually sublux and dislocate. The PIP and DIP joints also flex, producing the typical complex hammer, or claw, deformity.

History and Examination

The usual patient history is of pain and callosities in three areas:

- under the metatarsal heads
- over the dorsum of the PIPJ
- under the tip of the toe.

On examination sensation, blood supply, skin quality, the correctability of the deformity, and the presence and location of callosities should be recorded. Tendo Achillis tightness and cavus foot posture are associated with claw toes. Hallux valgus should be noted for two reasons: firstly, it may, as a result of first ray insufficiency, be the cause of the lesser toe deformity; and, secondly, it is important to note whether there will be room for the toe to sit comfortably, if the deformity is corrected.

Toe alignment should be recorded with the foot in a weightbearing, plantigrade position. In particular if the adjacent toe has interphalangeal joint flexion, but is otherwise normal, this is a good indication that the involved toe has FDL tightness, which should be released at the time of surgery. If the adjacent toe is not flexed the FDL can be left[26].

Weightbearing radiographs should be performed, in particular noting whether the MTPJ is enlocated, or not. The length of the lesser rays should also be noted. The ideal length is dictated by Maestro's formula (Figure 6.10).

Operative Treatment

The technique for *hammer toe* correction varies, depending on whether the toe is correctible or not.

For a correctible, or flexible, deformity we suggest a flexor to extensor tendon transfer[27], or Girdlestone–Taylor procedure. The FDL is released from the distal phalanx and transferred into the extensor tendon on the dorsum of the proximal phalanx. Thus the deforming long toe flexor is converted into a plantar flexor of the MTPJ.

Non-correctible deformity is treated with an arthrodesis of the PIPJ, with or without a flexor tenotomy. In treating a complex hammer toe the MTPJ should be addressed in the same way as is described for the claw toe, below.

Claw toe surgery involves addressing the MTPJ as well as the PIPJ. The MTPJ may be hyperextended, subluxed, or dislocated. The aim of surgery is to realign, or relocate, the MTPJ.

A flexible deformity is treated in the same way as a hammer toe, with a flexor to extensor tendon transfer.

The PIPJ requiring surgery is almost always fixed and requires arthrodesis. Traditionally a K-wire was used and left in situ for six weeks. The wire could then be removed in the clinic without anesthesia. However, newer "internal" implants for arthrodesis have been developed. Intramedullary screws, bioabsorbable implants, and temperature-sensitive devices are all documented in the literature (Figure 6.9). The advantage is principally the ease of care for patients. Their drawback appears to be the surgical learning curve, difficulty in removal if they fail, and increased cost.

The MTPJ will also need addressing. When simply hyperextended the extensor tendon is lengthened with a dorsal capsulotomy and a release of the collateral ligaments.

The subluxed and dislocated MTPJ are dealt with in the next section.

Lesser MTPJ Instability and the Plantar Plate

In 1985, seven patients with pain and swelling of the second and third MTPJs were described. The etiology was uncertain, but the suggested treatment was synovectomy[28]. In 1993, understanding of the condition was furthered by Michael Coughlin who described rupture of the plantar capsule[29]. Plantar plate injury is now known to be an important cause of pathology in the second and, less commonly, the third MTPJ.

Plantar Plate Anatomy

The plantar plate is a rectangular or slightly trapezoidal structure that supports the metatarsal head without strong attachment to it. On average it is 19 mm long and 11 mm wide; it is up to 5 mm thick[30]. It is similar to the menisci of the knee, being fibro-cartilaginous, of which 75% is type 1 collagen. It is firmly attached to the base of the proximal phalanx and blends laterally with the collateral ligaments, as well as the deep transverse metatarsal ligaments. The plantar aponeurosis blends with it. This explains the "windlass mechanism" – look at your foot and note that the plantar fascia tightens when dorsiflexing your toes.

Although early studies suggested that the collateral ligaments were more important than the plantar plate in resisting dorsal translation[31], it is now felt that the principal restraint to dorsal translation of the lesser MTPJ is the plantar plate.

Pathogenesis

As with the intervertebral disk, the knee-joint meniscus, and the rotator cuff, the plantar plate degenerates with age. In a study of 20 cadaver feet, the incidence of plantar plate tears was 50% in males with a mean age of 57, and 79% in females aged 71[32]. Most consider that the wearing of high-heeled shoes leads to attenuation of the plantar plate, hence the higher incidence in women. As the plantar plate degenerates it lengthens, the toe dorsiflexes, and the interossei and lumbricals, which were the principal flexors of the MTPJ, pass dorsal to the axis of rotation and become extensors. Thus the MTPJ extends.

Clinical Presentation

Patients present either acutely, following trauma, or with the insidious onset of pain and swelling, most commonly of the second MTPJ. They often describe walking on a stone. Neuritic symptoms are not uncommon. The condition is frequently misdiagnosed as a 2, 3 Morton's neuroma. Varus deviation and extension of the second toe are also observed. Eventually the plantar plate ruptures, the deformity worsens but, paradoxically, the pain lessens. In the later stages the MTPJ subluxes or dislocates. If associated with hallux valgus, the dislocated second toe sometimes crosses over the hallux.

Physical examination reveals deformity, with a gap between the second and third toes (Figure 6.11).

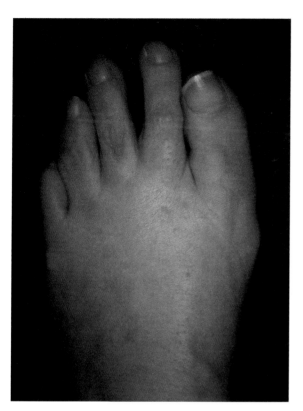

Figure 6.11 Patient with a plantar plate tear. Note the hallux valgus and deviation of the second toe into varus, creating a gap between the second and third toes.

There may be swelling and tenderness of the MTPJ, with a callosity beneath the second metatarsal head. Range of motion in the joint is preserved, as is sensation. This should be contrasted to a Morton's neuroma, where the tenderness is in the interspace and sensation in the toes may be reduced. Thompson and Hamilton described the drawer sign of the MTPJ[33]. This is similar to the Lachmann test for the anterior cruciate ligament, where one hand is used to stabilize the metatarsal head, and the other hand is used to translate the proximal phalanx of the toe dorsally. The affected toe is dorsiflexed 30° and the amount of translation is compared to the opposite side. A positive test shows laxity and reproduces the patient's pain.

Investigation

Plain weightbearing x-rays including AP, internal rotation oblique, and lateral views are obtained. Changes range from subtle subluxation to frank dislocation of the joint. More sensitive tests include ultrasound scanning, which is useful, but operator dependent. MRI does not detect the early stages of plantar plate attenuation, but can detect a tear. MRI is also useful in the exclusion of arthropathy, stress fractures, and the occasional tumor, which can present with MTPJ pain. Some use arthroscopic assessment of the joint to show plantar plate pathology.

Classification

Plantar plate tears can be classified clinically, radiologically, arthroscopically, and intraoperatively. Various staging and grading systems have been used to help plan management[34].

In essence, a prodromal phase is recognized with pain and swelling, but no deformity. The condition then progresses through malalignment, subluxation, and finally dislocation. Clinically the joint is said to be stable, less than 50% subluxatable, more than 50% subluxatable, dislocatable, and, finally, there is fixed dislocation.

Treatment

Initially, in the absence of deformity, the avoidance of high-heeled shoes, anti-inflammatory medication, taping the toe into plantar flexion, and use of a metatarsal offloading device can be helpful. Although intra-articular steroid is used extensively for inflammatory arthropathy, we do not believe that it is indicated for plantar plate injury.

Once the toe has extended and no longer touches the ground, surgery is the only way to restore its position. Until recently surgery to address this did not dealt directly with the plate itself – extensor tendon lengthening, capsulotomy, flexor to extensor tendon transfers, and metatarsal (Weil) osteotomies were used.

In current practice plantar plate repair from a dorsal approach using a Weil osteotomy for exposure has been a major advance[35]. The technique was described by Tim Schneider from Melbourne. Although published reports contain relatively few cases with relatively short follow-up, the proponents believe that plantar plate repair from a dorsal approach will significantly improve treatment. A Weil osteotomy of the metatarsal head is cut, proximally translated, and temporarily fixed with a 1.6 mm K-wire. The joint is then distracted with a second wire in the base of the proximal phalanx. The exposure is improved as a result of release of the collateral ligaments from the base of the phalanx.

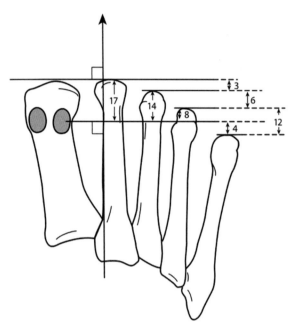

Figure 6.12 The ideal metatarsal parabola has been described by Maestro. The first and second rays are of identical length. The third, fourth, and fifth rays are progressively shorter, by 3, 6, and 12 mm.

The plantar plate is then carefully dissected off the base of the phalanx taking care not to injure the flexor tendons, and the plate is mobilized. Two sutures of O-FiberWire® (Arthrex Inc., Naples, FL) are placed in the healthy proximal portion of the plantar plate. The degenerate distal 5 mm of the plate is excised and the sutures passed through drill holes into the freshened base of the proximal phalanx. The Weil osteotomy is then fixed with 2 mm of shortening.

Excessive shortening must be avoided: according to the Maestro formula[36] the first and second metatarsals should be of approximately equal length, the third 3 mm shorter than second, the fourth 6 mm shorter than the third, and the fifth 12 mm shorter than the fourth (Figure 6.12). This is to maintain the metatarsal parabola and to decrease the chance of a transfer lesion.

The patient is placed in a postoperative shoe for six weeks. A range of motion exercises, especially plantar flexion, are commenced at two weeks.

Sesamoid Disorders of the Great Toe

Sesamoid disorders comprise 9%[37] of foot and ankle disorders. Their prevalence is skewed toward the

active population rather than the elderly. There are three sesamoid bones around the great toe. Two are related to the MTPJ and are constant. The third is single and related to the interphalangeal joint; it is not always present and will not be discussed further. They are named for their likeness to the shape of the sesame seed, which was thought to be indestructible.

In the anatomical position the sesamoids are located plantar and slightly proximal to the metatarsal head. The plantar surface of the metatarsal head has a medial and lateral groove for each sesamoid. The two grooves are separated by a central crista, or ridge. The sesamoids have articular cartilage on their dorsal surface and articulate with the first metatarsal head. They are encased in a fibrous envelope, which contains the plantar plate and the confluence of specific tendons:

tibial sesamoid – medial slip of the FHB and abductor hallucis

fibular sesamoid – lateral slip of the FHB and adductor hallucis.

The FHL runs on the plantar aspect between the two sesamoids (Figures 6.1 and 6.2).

Pathogenesis

The sesamoids increase the lever arm of both the FHL and FHB across the MTPJ. They take high loads, up to three times body weight, during the toe-off phase of gait. Most sesamoid conditions are associated with their inability to tolerate these high forces over a prolonged period.

The term sesamoiditis is frequently used; it implies inflammation of the sesamoid. This is misleading. The sesamoids suffer the same pathologies as any articular bone: fracture, with or without avascular necrosis of the proximal fragment; stress injury; osteoarthritis in its articulation with the first metatarsal; and diastasis of a bipartite bone. The sesamoids can also be prominent, leading to an intractable plantar keratosis, or at times ulceration, with or without osteomyelitis of the sesamoid.

The differential diagnosis of sesamoid pain includes FHL tenosynovitis, MTPJ arthritis, and digital nerve pain. Pain from the medial digital nerve to the hallux is known eponymously as Joplin's neuritis.

Presentation

Whatever the underlying cause of the sesamoiditis, patients present in the same fashion. Pain can be

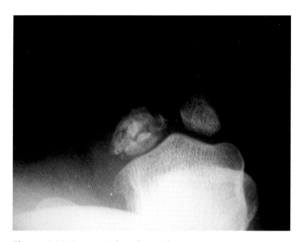

Figure 6.13 A sesamoid axial view demonstrating fragmentation of the fibular sesamoid.

diffuse or focal, but maximal tenderness is felt on palpation and compression of the affected sesamoid against the metatarsal head. A history of a snapping sensation during running is sometimes felt with acute injury.

MTPJ motion is usually reduced as sesamoid pathology often results in FHB tightness. Biomechanical abnormality, in particular a plantar flexed first ray, should be noted.

Imaging

An AP standing radiograph may demonstrate a bipartite sesamoid, fracture, osteophytes, or fragmentation consistent with avascular necrosis. The most useful radiographic view is the sesamoid view (Figure 6.13), which is an axial view of the foot with the MTPJ in maximal dorsiflexion. This shows the bone, its alignment, and its articulation with the first metatarsal head.

MRI scanning can demonstrate bone edema, stress fractures, and arthritic change, and is the most helpful modality. Technetium bone scanning may highlight stress fractures and other pathology not seen on plain radiographs. Unfortunately, while bone scanning has high sensitivity it has low specificity.

Treatment

Non-operative options for most painful sesamoid conditions include: rest, ice, compression, and elevation (RICE); NSAIDs; shoes with a cushioned sole; and orthoses with a gel-filled cut out under the sesamoid.

The treatment of sesamoiditis depends on the cause of the pathology.

Fracture. The commonest cause of sesamoid pain is a non-united fracture, with or without avascular necrosis of the proximal fragment. Acute fractures can be difficult to differentiate from a bipartite sesamoid. To further complicate matters a bipartite sesamoid can separate, and the resulting diastasis is painful. Sesamoid fracture is initially treated non-operatively. If this fails, internal fixation and partial or complete sesamoidectomy have been described. If the sesamoid is excised it is important to repair the resulting defect in the FHB tendon, as failure to do this can lead to hallux valgus after tibial sesamoid excision or varus after fibular sesamoid excision. Sesamoidectomy is effective and usually allows a return to full activity, including high-level sport.

Osteoarthritis of the sesamoid metatarsal articulation is most commonly associated with hallux valgus, as the sesamoids are dislocated. Surgical treatment involves managing the hallux valgus and then excising any prominent osteophytes. In some cases, the well-aligned hallux develops arthritis of the sesamoid/metatarsal head articulation. If this does not settle with non-operative management sesamoidectomy is effective.

An **intractable plantar keratosis** under the tibial sesamoid is often the result of high pressure from a plantar flexed first ray. This is usually managed non-operatively with callus debridement and orthoses. Occasionally surgical treatment is required, with either excision of the plantar half of the sesamoid or correction of the underlying mechanical abnormality, with a dorsiflexion osteotomy of the first metatarsal. Barouk, Rippstein, and Toullec described a dorsal closing wedge of the first metatarsal – the "BRT osteotomy."

If left untreated, especially in neuropaths, the plantar skin can ulcerate and osteomyelitis can ensue. These patients may require excision or shaving of the sesamoid, which may be accompanied by a BRT osteotomy.

Interdigital "Morton's" Neuroma

Interdigital Morton's neuroma is a painful condition of the common plantar digital nerves. It is not a tumor, or a tumor-like condition, and the name is therefore a misnomer. In 1876, Morton noted the clinical condition, but wrote of hypertrophy of the

Box 6.3   Possible pathogenic factors in Morton's neuroma

- Communication branches between the lateral and medial plantar nerves, increasing nerve volume
- Increased mobility at the 3/4 space
- Decreased volume of the 2/3 intermetatarsal space
- MTP capsule degeneration causing toe deviation and compression
- Constricting shoes
- High-heeled shoes
- Accessory branches in cases of recurrence
- Aberrant bands of the transverse metatarsal ligament
- Trauma

Table 6.5 Differential diagnosis of Morton's neuroma

Local	MTPJ disease
	Plantar plate injury
	Freiberg's infraction
	Stress fracture
	Tumor (either causing compression or a primary nerve tumor)
Neural	Lumbar disk disease
	Medial or lateral plantar nerve injury
	Tarsal tunnel syndrome

branches of the lateral plantar nerve, an explanation that has since been proven to be false. Gauthier discussed the theory of "entrapment" in his series of over 300 procedures, which involved release, without excision of the nerve[38]. Thus we consider Morton's neuroma to be primarily resultant on nerve entrapment at the anterior edge of the deep transverse metatarsal ligament. It is often combined with bursal irritation, leading to perineural fibrosis.

The anatomy of the web space helps us to understand the disease. The metatarsal heads are stabilized by the deep transverse metatarsal ligament. The MTPJ capsule and bursa both lie above the ligament, whereas the nerve, along with the lumbrical tendon and common plantar digital artery, are *plantar* to the ligament.

There are multiple theories as to the pathogenesis (Box 6.3).

History and Examination

Patients report neural pain, especially when walking and wearing constrictive shoes[39]. The classic history is a woman who is walking and has to take off her shoe and rub her foot to relieve the pain. The pain often radiates to the toes, with associated paresthesia. The differential diagnosis is shown in Table 6.5.

On examination there is web-space tenderness on the plantar aspect of the foot, between and just proximal to the metatarsal heads. Compression of this area between the examiner's thumb and index finger should reproduce the patient's pain. A positive Mulder's click is strongly suggestive, but not diagnostic. To elicit the click, the forefoot is compressed mediolaterally by one of the examiner's hands. The thumb of the examiner's other hand is then used to sublux the neuroma between the metatarsal heads, producing the characteristic "click." While numbness at the adjacent borders of the third and fourth toes is sought, it is not invariably present.

Imaging

The diagnosis of Morton's neuroma remains clinical. Plain standing radiographs should be performed. MRI scanning is useful to exclude other diagnoses. US can be helpful, but is operator dependent. Nevertheless clinical assessment has been shown to be superior over both of these imaging modalities[40]. The difficulty with imaging is that it detects nerve enlargement, which is not necessarily present in symptomatic patients, and furthermore may be present in asymptomatic patients.

A local anesthetic injection has been shown to be of variable diagnostic benefit. Given that there are a number of structures in close proximity that can be also be responsible for the patient's symptoms, the needle needs to be positioned precisely, with no fluid leak from the perineural area.

Treatment

Non-operative treatment is always preferable; however, it is not always successful. Comfortable shoes with a metatarsal bar decrease the pressure under the metatarsal head.

A multicenter randomized controlled trial of US-guided corticosteroid injections gave good short-term results at three months[41]. Another series demonstrated 66% positive results at nine months[42]. The side effects of a poorly directed injection include fat atrophy and MTP capsular degeneration. We recommend no more than a single attempt at a steroid injection.

Radiofrequency ablation has been reported to give satisfactory short-term results. This is performed by a radiologist under local anesthetic with US guidance. Satisfactory results at six months have been reported[43].

Operative treatment is controversial, in particular what operation to do and from which approach. Releasing the transverse metatarsal ligament has been shown to be effective, although there is a theoretical risk of metatarsal instability. Excision of the nerve leaves an area of anesthesia in the distal web space. A dorsal approach avoids a scar in the weightbearing plantar skin while a plantar approach is more anatomically direct.

We prefer a dorsal approach with division of the transverse metatarsal ligament combined with excision of the nerve. Coughlin performed a review of his series using this operation and reported 85% good or excellent results at an average of six years post surgery[44].

Risks of surgery include recurrence, with a stump neuroma, and arterial injury.

Key Points

Hallux Valgus

- Indications for surgery include pain and progressive deformity.
- Aim to reduce the sesamoids beneath the metatarsal head.
- The four basic elements are lateral release, osteotomy, capsular plication, and an Akin osteotomy.
- A congruent joint with high DMAA requires de-rotation of the metatarsal intraoperatively.

Hallux Rigidus

- Hallux rigidus is an osteoarthritic process, which progresses from dorsal to plantar.

- It is present in 2.5% of the population after the age of 50 years and genetics play a major role in its prevalence.
- Severity is classified from 0 to 4 by Coughlin and Shurnas, according to range of motion, pain, and radiological changes.
- Treatment is usually surgical with the mainstays being cheilectomy for early disease and arthrodesis for advanced disease.

Lesser Toes

- Mallet, hammer, and claw toes usually arise as a result of constricting footwear.
- Flexible deformities are managed by soft tissue release and tendon transfer.
- Fixed deformity requires arthrodesis or osteotomy.

Plantar Plate

- It is often associated with hallux valgus – first-ray insufficiency.
- Synovitis of the lesser MTPJs may be the presentation of inflammatory arthropathy.
- New instruments make plantar plate repair easier from a dorsal approach.

Sesamoiditis

- Sesamoiditis is caused by a number of pathologies, most commonly fracture, with or without avascular necrosis of the proximal fragment.
- Non-operative treatment with cushioned insoles is often successful.
- Surgery in the form of a sesamoidectomy usually returns individuals to sport.
- The plantar flexed first ray can lead to painful callosities under the sesamoid.

Morton's Neuroma

- Morton's interdigital neuroma is a painful entrapment condition with perineural fibrosis.
- The diagnosis is clinical.
- Surgical treatment is usually with a neurectomy.
- Controversies relate to whether to use a plantar or dorsal approach.

References

1. Sim-Fook L, Hodgson AR. A comparison of foot forms among the non-shoe and shoe-wearing Chinese population. *J Bone Joint Surg Am*. 1958; 40-A, 1058–62.

2. Coughlin MJ. Juvenile hallux valgus: etiology and treatment. *Foot Ankle Int*. 1995; 16, 682–97.

3. Mancuso JE, Abramow SP, Landsman MJ, Waldman M, Carioscia M. The zero-plus first metatarsal and its relationship to bunion deformity. *J Foot Ankle Surg*. 2003; 42, 319–26.

4. Perera AM, Mason L, Stephens MM. The pathogenesis of hallux valgus. *J Bone Joint Surg Am*. 2011; 93, 1650–61.

5. Trnka HJ, Zembsch A, Weisauer H, et al. Modified Austin procedure for correction of hallux valgus. *Foot Ankle Int*. 1997; 18, 119–27.

6. Weil LS. Scarf osteotomy for correction of hallux valgus: historical perspective, surgical technique and results. *Foot Ankle Clin*. 2000; 5, 559–80.

7. Newman AS, Negrine JP, Zevovic M, Stanford P, Walsh WR. A biomechanical comparison of the Z step-cut and basilar crescentic osteotomies of the first metatarsal. *Foot Ankle Int*. 2000; 21, 584–7.

8. Jones KJ, Feiwell LA, Freedman EL, Cracchiolo A 3rd. The effect of Chevron osteotomy with lateral capsular release on the blood supply to the first metatarsal head. *J Bone Joint Surg Am*. 1995; 77:2, 197–204.

9. Bauer T, de Lavigne C, Biau D, De Prado M, Isham S, Laffenétre O. Percutaneous hallux valgus surgery: a prospective multicenter study of 189 cases. *Orthop Clin North Am*. 2009; 40, 505–14.

10. Kitaoka HB, Holiday AD Jr. Lateral condylar resection for bunionette. *Clin Orthop*. 1992; 278, 183–92.

11. Coughlin MJ. Treatment of bunionette deformity with longitudinal diaphyseal osteotomy with distal soft tissue repair. *Foot Ankle Int*. 1991; 11:4, 195–203.

12. Diebold PF, Bejjani FJ. Basal osteotomy of the fifth metatarsal with intermetatarsal pining: a new approach to tailor's bunion. *Foot Ankle Int*. 1987; 8, 40–5.

13. Barouk LS. Weil's metatarsal osteotomy in the treatment of metatarsalgia. *Der Orthopäde*. 1996; 25, 338–44.

14. Barouk LS. Some pathologies of the fifth ray: tailor's bunion. In Barouk LS ed. *Forefoot Reconstruction*. (Paris: Springer-Verlag, 2002), pp. 276–83.

15. Shereff MJ, Yang QM, Kummer FJ, et al. Vascular anatomy of the fifth metatarsal. *Foot Ankle Int*. 1991; 11:6, 350–3.

16. Coughlin MJ, Shurnas PS. Hallux rigidus: demographics, etiology, and radiographic assessment. *Foot Ankle*. 2003; 24:10, 731–43.

17. Coughlin MJ, Shurnas PS. Hallux rigidus: grading and long-term results of operative treatment. *J Bone Joint Surg Am*. 2003; 85:11, 2072–88.

18. Smith SM, Coleman SC, Bacon SA, Polo FE, Brodsky JW. Improved ankle push-off power following cheilectomy for hallux rigidus: a prospective gait analysis study. *Foot Ankle Int*. 2012; 33, 457–61.

19. Moberg E. A simple operation for hallux rigidus. *Clin Orthop*. 1979; 142, 55–6.

20. Waizy H, Czardybon MA, Stukenborg-Colsman C, et al. Mid- and long-term results of the joint preserving therapy of hallux rigidus. *Arch Orthop Trauma Surg*. 2010; 130:2, 165–70.

21. Malerba F, Milani R, Sartorelli E, Haddo O. Distal oblique first metatarsal osteotomy in grade 3 hallux rigidus: a long-term follow up. *Foot Ankle Int*. 2008; 29:7, 677–82.

22. Kelikian AS. Technical considerations in hallux metatarsophalangeal arthrodesis. *Foot Ankle Clin*. 2005; 10:1, 167–90.

23. Brodsky JW, Passmore RN, Pollo FE, Shabat S. Functional outcome of arthrodesis of the first metatarso-phalangeal joint using parallel screw fixation. *Foot Ankle Int*. 2005; 26:2, 140–6.

24. Coughlin MJ. Lesser toe deformities. In *Mann's Surgery of the Foot and Ankle*, 9th edn. (Mosby, 2014), p. 324.

25. Sarrafian SK, Toprizian WK. Anatomy and physiology of the extensor apparatus of the toes. *J Bone Joint Surg Am*. 1969; 51:4, 669–79.

26. Coughlin MJ. Lesser toe deformities. In *Mann's Surgery of the Foot and Ankle*, 9th edn. (Mosby, 2014), p. 349.

27. Coughlin MJ. Lesser toe abnormalities. *J Bone Joint Surg*. 2002; 84A, 1446–69.

28. Mann RA, Mizel MA. Monoarticular non-traumatic synovitis of the metatarso-phalangeal joint: a new diagnosis. *Foot Ankle*. 1985; 6, 18–21.

29. Mann RA, Coughlin MJ (eds) *Surgery of the Foot and Ankle*, 6th edn. (Mosby, 1993), p. 373.

30. Johnston RB, Smith J, Daniels T. The plantar plate of the lesser toes: an anatomical study in human cadavers. *Foot Ankle Int*. 1994; 15, 276.

31. Fortin P, Myerson M. Second metatarsophalangeal joint instability. *Foot Ankle Int*. 1995; 16:5, 306–13.

32. Weil LS Jr. *The incidence of plantar plate tears in normal feet*. Presented at the Annual Meeting Australian Orthopaedic Foot and Ankle Society. Hobart. August 2012.

33. Thompson FM, Hamilton WG. Problems of the second metatarso-phalangeal joint. *Orthopaedics* 1987; 10, 83–9.

34. Coughlin MJ, Baumfeld DS, Nery C. Second MTP instability: grading of the deformity and description of the surgical repair of capsular insufficiency. *Phys Sports Med.* 2011; 29:3, 132.

35. Gregg J, Silberstein M, Clark C, Schneider T. Plantar plate repair and Weil osteotomy for metatarsophalangeal joint instability. *Foot Ankle Surg.* 2001; 13:3, 116.

36. Maestro M, Besse JL, Ragusa M, Berthonnaud E. Forefoot morphotype study and planning method for forefoot osteotomy. *Foot Ankle Clin.* 2003; 8, 695–710.

37. Dedmond BT, Cory JW, McBryde A. The hallucal sesamoid complex. *J Am Acad Orthop Surg.* 2006; 14:13, 745–53.

38. Gauthier, G. Thomas Morton's disease: a nerve entrapment syndrome. A new surgical technique. *Clin Orth Rel Res.* 1979; 142, 90–2.

39. Mann RA, Reynolds JD. Interdigital neuroma: a critical clinical analysis, *Foot Ankle Int.* 1983: 3, 238.

40. Sharp RJ, Wade CM, Hennessy MS, Saxby TS. The role of MRI and ultrasound imaging in Morton's neuroma and the effect of size of lesion on symptoms. *J Bone Joint Surg (B).* 2003; 85:7, 999–1005.

41. Thomson CE, Beggs I, Martin DJ, et al. Methylprednisolone injections for the treatment of Morton neuroma: a patient-blinded randomized trial. *J Bone Joint Surg.* 2013; 95:9, 790–8–S1.

42. Markovic M, Crichton K, Read JW, Lam P, Slater HK. Effectiveness of ultrasound-guided corticosteroid injection in the treatment of Morton's neuroma. *Foot Ankle Int.* 2008; 29:5, 483–7.

43. Chuter GSJ, Chua YP, Connell DA, Blackney MC. Ultrasound-guided radiofrequency ablation in the management of interdigital (Morton's) neuroma. *Skeletal Radiology.* 2013; 42:1, 107–11.

44. Coughlin MJ, Pinsonneault T. Operative treatment of interdigital neuroma. A long-term follow-up study. *J Bone Joint Surg Am.* 2001; 83:9, 1321–8.

Midfoot and Forefoot Arthritis

Caroline J. Lever and Andrew "Fred" Robinson

Introduction

Arthritis of the mid- and forefoot is frequently encountered in foot and ankle practice. Primary osteoarthritis is common and the prevalence increases with age. In one epidemiological study the population prevalence of symptomatic radiographic arthritis of the mid- and forefoot in those over the age of 50 was 16.7%, with the first metatarsophalangeal joint being the most frequently involved[1]. The overall population prevalence of symptomatic mid/forefoot arthritis is probably lower than this, and around 4% according to most studies. This chapter offers an overview of arthritis in the mid- and forefoot and is a guide toward the various treatments.

Midfoot Arthritis

Anatomy and Mechanics

During normal gait the movement of the foot and ankle joints is linked. Thus disease, deformity, and stiffness in one part of the foot impacts on the other parts. An understanding of the normal anatomy and biomechanics of the midfoot helps in appreciating the effects of midfoot arthritis.

The midfoot can be divided into three main longitudinal columns: medial, central, and lateral (Figure 7.1). The medial column consists of the first metatarsal and the medial cuneiform. The central column consists of the second and third metatarsals, which articulate with the middle and lateral cuneiforms. The fourth and fifth metatarsals articulate directly with the cuboid, and make up the lateral column. The less mobile columns are more stable, and vice versa. The central column has the least movement and is therefore the most stable, taking the greatest load during weight bearing with the highest contact forces. The lateral column TMTJs are the most mobile, although they only have about 10° of motion in the sagittal plane. The mobility of the lateral column is

thought to be important for shock absorption and allowing the foot to accommodate to uneven ground. Overall the midfoot moves little, allowing it to act as a rigid lever arm throughout stance phase, transferring forces from the hindfoot to the forefoot.

The stability of the midfoot is achieved in part as a result of its bony architecture, and in part from the strong ligaments around the joints. The second TMTJ is highly restrained, as the base of the second metatarsal is recessed between the medial and lateral cuneiforms. In the coronal plane the cuneiforms and metatarsal bases are trapezoid in shape, with wider dorsal than plantar surfaces. Thus they act as keystones in the transverse tarsal arch (Figure 7.2). Dorsal, interosseous, and plantar ligaments support the bony structure. The intermetatarsal interosseous ligaments between the bases of the second to fifth metatarsals are the strongest of all the ligaments.

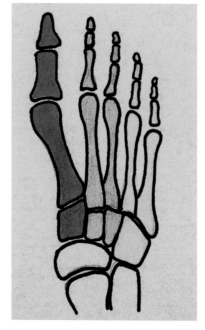

Figure 7.1 The three longitudinal columns of the foot (red: medial; green: central; yellow: lateral).

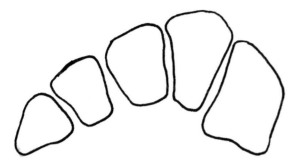

Figure 7.2 Line drawing of a cross-section through the level of the base of the metatarsals, showing the keystone configuration of the transverse tarsal arch.

The second metatarsal relies upon the Lisfranc ligament, which runs from the plantar aspect of the base of the second metatarsal to the medial cuneiform. There is no intermetatarsal ligament between the first and second metatarsals.

Although the amount of movement in the midfoot joints is limited they are ideally adapted to provide rigidity at some phases of the gait cycle, while allowing suppleness and shock absorption at other phases.

Pathogenesis: Etiology, Epidemiology, and Pathophysiology

Arthritis can affect any of the midfoot joints. Arthritis of the TMTJ, particularly the second, is the most common. This is a reflection of the high loads that pass through the joint and its central role in stability. The talonavicular, naviculocuneiform, and first TMT joints develop arthritis with decreasing frequency. Arthritis in the lateral column joints is also uncommon.

Midfoot arthritis has a number of etiologies including primary osteoarthritis, post-traumatic degeneration, inflammatory arthropathy, crystal disease, and neuroarthropathy. Primary osteoarthritis is the usual cause in patients presenting over the age of 60 years[2]. Post-traumatic arthritis is more often seen in younger age groups, where it is usually the result of a Lisfranc injury. Lisfranc injuries can occur even after low-energy trauma and subtle injuries are often missed at initial presentation. Rarer fractures of the cuneiforms, navicular, and cuboid with articular involvement can also cause arthritis. Symmetrical polyarthropathy with widespread change across the midfoot and collapse of the medial arch is seen in rheumatoid disease.

Extensive joint destruction and subluxation with a typical rocker-bottom foot deformity raises the concern of a Charcot neuroarthropathy.

Presentation

History and Examination

The symptoms of midfoot arthritis are typically pain and swelling. Pain can be dorsal or plantar. It is mechanical in origin and is usually worse with weight bearing. Swelling is seen dorsally and can be either soft tissue, with synovitis or a ganglion, or bony osteophytes. Occasionally the deep or superficial peroneal nerve branches are irritated by prominent swellings leading to radiating pain. Typically the deep peroneal nerve is affected with pain radiating down the foot to the web space between the hallux and second toe.

As always with orthopedic examination the mantra of "look, feel, move" should be followed.

Look

Examination begins with review of the shoes to identify abnormal wear patterns. When deformity exists it typically consists of flattening of the medial arch with midfoot abduction and supination of the forefoot on the hindfoot. In advanced cases, the plantar medial bony prominence under a deformed first TMTJ can be the cause of discomfort.

The patient is stood to assess foot position under load. Inspect the longitudinal medial arch for any midfoot collapse and look from behind to identify any heel deformity, in particular valgus. When pes planus exists the tibialis posterior tendon function should be assessed, although this may be difficult, as a single heel raise is difficult as a result of the loss of the medial longitudinal arch, and the pain, from the TMTJ arthritis.

Feel

Palpation of the foot identifies areas of tenderness, and this in itself is the best clinical indicator of the source of symptoms. A Tinel's test may indicate nerve irritation, in particular of the deep peroneal nerve over the second TMTJ.

Move

Movement of the midtarsal joint is limited, but deformity of the midfoot or the hindfoot should be noted. When midfoot deformity is present it is important to assess its location and to what degree it can be corrected. Tightness of the calf

121

musculature can increase midfoot symptoms, so any ankle equinus must be identified.

At the TMTJ the individual metatarsal heads are grasped between the thumb and index finger of one hand. The corresponding TMTJ is palpated between the thumb and index finger of the other hand. Each of the TMTJs should be individually stressed in a dorsal/plantar motion and any discomfort noted. The degree of motion achieved is usually minimal – the second and third having least movement, and the fourth and fifth the most. In cases where deformity or swelling is disproportionate to pain, a Charcot neuroarthropathy should be considered. Assessment of sensibility with a 10 g Semmes–Weinstein monofilament should be undertaken routinely. Assessment of the vascular status is imperative if surgery is being considered.

Investigations

Weightbearing AP and lateral foot radiographs are the workhorse of radiological diagnosis. An oblique 30° view allows assessment of all the midfoot joints. Medial and central column joints can be viewed more easily on the AP, while the oblique provides a good view of the lateral column joints. The lateral is useful to assess the second TMTJ space, which is seen parallel, but proximal, to the first TMTJ (Figure 7.3). When arthritic, narrowing of the joint can make it difficult to see on the lateral radiograph. Dorsal osteophytes are also often seen.

In cases in which there is doubt, a CT or MRI scan can be helpful in localizing the arthritic joints. Diagnostic injections with local anesthetic can also be helpful, but they should be carried out with an arthrogram, as there are numerous communications between the joints of the foot and if pain relief from the local anesthetic is used as a diagnostic criterion, it is important to know which joints have been anesthetized. If localization of pathology remains a problem, a single photon-emission computed tomography bone scan combined with CT (SPECT-CT) has been shown to help[3].

A previous history of trauma with malalignment of the TMTJs on radiographs may indicate an old Lisfranc injury.

On the lateral x-ray there should be no dorsal subluxation/translation of the metatarsals. The standing lateral film allows the level of deformity to be assessed in the planus foot. This is important for surgical planning. Meary's line, a line drawn longitudinally down the midaxis of the talar neck, should be collinear with the midaxial line of the first metatarsal. Where deformity exists the lines are not parallel and their intersection point indicates the apex of the deformity (Figure 7.4). The apex may be at the TMTJ or further proximally at the naviculocuneiform or talonavicular level.

Treatment of TMTJ Arthritis

Non-Operative

The mainstay of treatment is simple analgesic medication and in-shoe orthoses with a medial-arch support. Weight loss also helps to reduce load. Occasionally an AFO with a shoe rocker may be of help, but many patients are reluctant to accept this. Where dorsal osteophytes are the main issue, alternative lacing patterns on shoes can relieve pressure. Cut outs, stretching of the shoe upper, or padding over the area may also be helpful.

Surgical

Operative intervention should be reserved for cases that fail conservative management over a prolonged period, usually a minimum of six months. The surgical procedure depends upon the cause of the discomfort. It may simply involve removal of the dorsal osteophyte with release of the deep peroneal nerve.

More commonly, the pain arises from the joint. Arthrodesis is the mainstay of surgical treatment. As discussed above, surgical planning starts with determination of which joints are involved. This is usually based upon a combination of clinical examination and plain radiographs, although diagnostic local anesthetic injections with an arthrogram, MRI scanning, and SPECT-CT may be helpful.

The basis of all fusions includes joint preparation to bleeding bone and stable fixation. It is important to consider whether the fusion is in situ, or requires deformity correction. Even a fusion in situ requires care, for example avoiding excessive shortening or dorsiflexion in a TMTJ fusion.

The workhorse for surgery in the midfoot is a TMTJ fusion; however, not all TMTJ fusions are in situ. Deformity correction may include fusion of the foot with a rocker bottom, correction of a hallux valgus (Lapidus procedure), and TMTJ fusion as part of a flat-foot correction. It has been shown that if deformity is present, correction of that deformity in association with the TMTJ fusion gives better results than simple in situ fusion[4]. The aim is to achieve a stable, pain-free, plantigrade foot without bony prominences, which fits comfortably into standard shoes. Deformity correction should proceed from proximal to distal to ensure that the foot is plantigrade at the end of surgery, thus tendo Achillis lengthening and correction of hindfoot alignment should be addressed first. It is not until a neutral

(a)

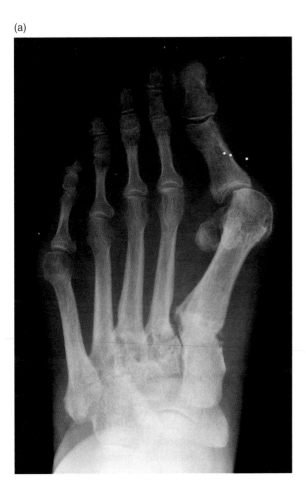

(b)

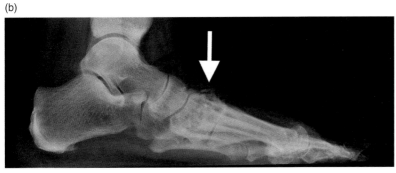

Figure 7.3 Tarsometatarsal joint arthritis in a patient with inflammatory arthritis. Note the loss of the second TMTJ space (arrow) on the lateral, weightbearing radiograph.

(a)

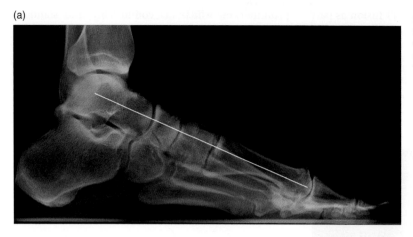

(b)

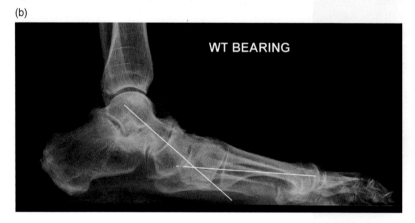

WT BEARING

Figure 7.4 (a) Meary's line, along the midaxis of first metatarsal, should pass centrally up the talar neck. **(b)** A broken Meary's line indicates a complex break at the naviculocuneiform and TMTJ.

hindfoot position has been achieved that the midfoot is positioned.

The technique of TMTJ fusion varies depending on the indication. The first ray can either be approached through a dorsal or medio-plantar approach. In all cases the joint is denuded of cartilage and taken back to bleeding bone. Minimal bone resection is usually required, even if deformity correction is required. This prevents shortening of the first ray and the consequent development of transfer metatarsalgia in the lesser rays. Thus with a Lapidus procedure only the most minimal laterally based wedge is excised, and even then the first metatarsal is translated plantarward and held in place with a stepped plate to hold the ray in this position.

One of the commoner deformities is of TMTJ collapse with abduction; this is often associated with a rocker-bottom type deformity. The patient complains of prominence and callosity under the midfoot. A corrective first TMTJ fusion with a closing plantar-medial wedge is required. This is best undertaken through a plantar-medial approach, which allows plantar plating of the joint (Figure 7.5). Cadaveric studies show plantar plating to be more biomechanically stable than dorsomedial plating, with greater initial and final stiffness and a greater load to failure[5].

The lesser TMTJs are approached through a dorsal incision, taking care not to damage the deep peroneal nerve and the dorsalis pedis artery. When a plantar medial approach is used to reach the first TMTJ a second dorsal incision can be made slightly more laterally between the second and third TMTJs to access these joints. This leaves a good skin bridge and the incision is not directly over the neurovascular bundle. Joint preparation needs to be undertaken with care. As the TMTJs are approached through a dorsal incision there is a tendency to remove more bone dorsally than plantarly, which can lead to fusion in a dorsiflexed position. In many cases, lesser metatarsal length will remain unaltered, in these cases one

(a)

(b)

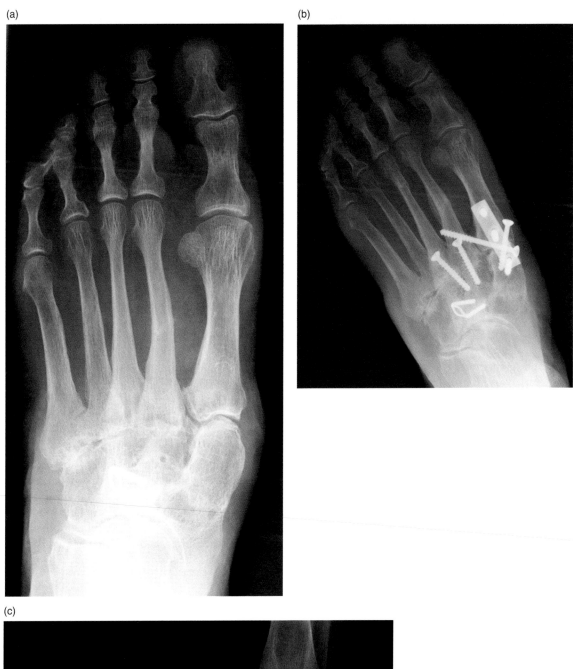

(c)

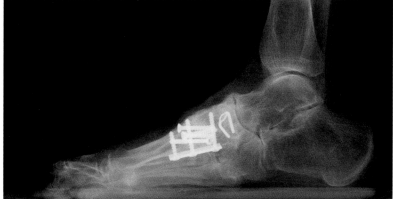

Figure 7.5 Plantar plating for TMTJ arthrodesis, in a patient who has had a previous naviculocuneiform fusion. The foot is often abducted and the arch collapsed, this should be corrected at the time of arthrodesis. There is a second metatarsal stress fracture.

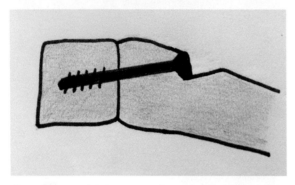

Figure 7.6 Manoli holes: a recessed countersink is burred from the metatarsal cortex to accommodate the head of the screw. If this is not undertaken there is a risk of the dorsal cortex of the metatarsal fracturing, as a result of upward pressure from the screw.

approach is to leave the plantar cortex intact. This creates a dorsal "trough," which can be filled with local bone graft from the os calcis.

A variety of internal fixation methods have been described including staples, screws, and locked and non-locked plates. The approach and degree of fixation are dependent on the combination of joints involved and the amount of bone loss or deformity that coexists. An isolated in situ fusion can be adequately stabilized with screws, although plating, particularly of the first ray, is commonly undertaken. If a screw is used from distal to proximal, countersinking the metatarsal shaft with a burr is useful to prevent the screw head pushing upward and cracking the dorsal cortex – so-called Manoli holes (Figure 7.6).

Bone Grafting

Not every case requires a bone graft. Nevertheless, even if it is required, the amount is often small and can be taken locally from the os calcis or proximal tibia. Graft from the calcaneus is easy through a short lateral incision. Proximal tibial bone can be accessed through a lateral cortical window. Complications, such as sural nerve injury, are rare although up to 13.8% of patients report some residual symptoms along the lateral border of the calcaneus[6]. One study that looked at pain outcome scores across multiple sites for autologous bone-graft harvest showed 12% of subjects reported clinically significant pain at the harvest site at 24 weeks and 8.5% at 52 weeks postoperatively, with each of the lower extremity harvest sites (calcaneum, distal tibia, and

proximal tibia) having greater rates of persistent pain at one year than the iliac crest bone-grafting group[7]. It is therefore important to remember that bone grafting is not without morbidity, and to consider this both in surgical planning and when obtaining consent.

Results and Complications

When restricted to patients who have failed conservative therapy for degenerative and inflammatory arthropathy, long-term overall operative results of arthrodesis of the midtarsal and TMTJs have shown 93% satisfaction at six-year follow-up[2]. Union rates between 92 and 98% for primary fusions are quoted[2,8–9]. A study of 72 patients showed that union occurred in the majority, 74%, by nine weeks – although 4% of patients took up to 16 weeks[9].

The complication rates vary from 4 to 17%[8–9]. The most frequent complication reported, in 13%, is malunion – with pain and prominence under the lesser metatarsal heads[2]. This does not always require further operative intervention, although Komenda found the need to perform a dorsal closing metatarsal wedge osteotomy to correct this in 2 out of 32 patients[10]. In the first ray, pain under the sesamoids is also reported as a result of the lack of flexibility[4]. Wound-healing problems, superficial infection, nerve injury with painful neuroma formation, stress fractures, and chronic regional pain syndrome are also reported[2,10].

Neuropathic Deformity

Midfoot fusions for Charcot neuropathic deformity are more challenging and prone to more complications than a standard midfoot fusion. The aim is to achieve a stable, plantigrade, shoeable foot, which is stable (Figure 7.7). In patients with diabetes mellitus this can be satisfactorily achieved in about 60% non-operatively. The remaining patients are at increased risk of amputation, although Pinzur detailed a 92% salvage rate with correction and ring fixation in this group[11]. There are a number of factors that need to be taken into consideration in operating upon these patients, these include the blood supply, ulceration and infection, the magnitude of the deformity, techniques of fixation, and the length of immobilization.

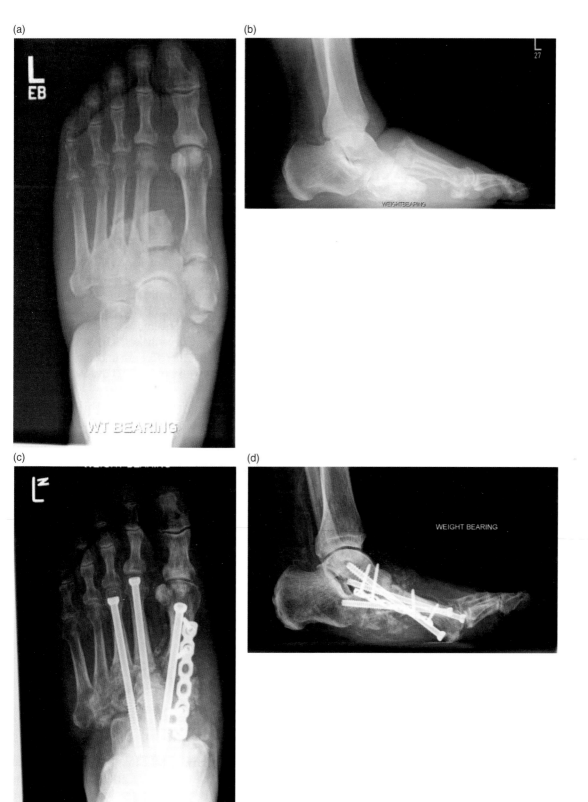

Figure 7.7 (**a**, **b**) Pre- and (**c**, **d**) postoperative radiographs of reconstruction of Charcot neuropathy with midfoot collapse. Both intramedullary screws and plantar plating have been used in combination. There has been loss of position of the first metatarsal screw, although this was asymptomatic.

- Ulceration and infection may necessitate that surgery is staged, with primary debridement and exostectomy to heal the ulcer, followed by reconstruction with arthrodesis. External, rather than internal, fixation may also be chosen.
- The magnitude of the deformity is often extreme, requiring significant bony resection. It is important at the end of surgery to be left with a relaxed soft tissue envelope, which can be easily closed.
- Fixation techniques will need to vary from the standard. In the presence of persisting ulceration and infection, a ring fixator may be chosen. Internal fixation has to be robust. Multiple axially placed intramedullary screws have been proposed as providing a stable construct to achieve and maintain correction of the deformity[12]. However, the insertion of intramedullary screws is technically demanding, and failures have been reported[13]. Furthermore, when tested biomechanically, plantar plating and intramedullary screw fixation show equal stiffness and load to failure with no notable biomechanical difference between the techniques[14].
- The duration of immobilization needs to be increased to reflect that, on average, complete osseous union takes six months in the neuropath. Consequently, protection and weightbearing limitations need to be prolonged. The old adage, of taking the standard time for treatment and doubling it, is a start.

Isolated Lateral Column Arthritis

The fourth and fifth TMTJs are the most mobile, and symptomatic arthritis is rare. Unsurprisingly, the literature is sparse with only small case series. It is usually advised that arthrodesis of these joints should be avoided and that fourth and fifth TMTJ arthritis should be treated with excisional arthroplasty. Raikin reviewed 28 patients undergoing midfoot arthrodesis: six had an isolated lateral column fusion and the others had a combined medial, central, and lateral-column arthrodesis. At two-year follow-up the fusion rate was 92% with pain levels improving from 8.2 to 2.4 in those with isolated lateral column disease. Thus despite the concern that arthrodesis of the lateral column is ineffective it has been reported with good results[15].

Excisional arthroplasty with tendon interposition has also been shown to be effective. In a small series of 12 patients, three-quarters were satisfied with the result of surgery[16]. In an attempt to maintain movement of the fourth and fifth TMTJs, interpositional arthroplasty with ceramic components has also been tried. Despite reported improvement in pain levels the study sizes are very small and the follow-up less than three years[17–18].

Isolated Talonavicular Arthritis

Isolated talonavicular fusion has a 93% satisfaction rate and is most commonly carried out for adult-acquired flat foot, isolated osteoarthritis, or rheumatoid arthritis. It should be borne in mind that isolated fusion of the talonavicular joint almost completely abolishes subtalar movement; nevertheless, it is less invasive than a triple fusion and is therefore not uncommonly undertaken in patients with isolated TNJ disease[19].

Isolated Naviculocuneiform Arthritis

Arthrodesis of the naviculocuneiform joints may form part of a medial-column stabilization, although isolated fusion of this joint complex is uncommon. Isolated fusion may be indicated in a small group of patients with a degenerate naviculocuneiform joint (Figure 7.8) or as part of a planovalgus foot correction. One retrospective analysis of 33 fusions, undertaken for a mixture of degeneration and planovalgus deformity, showed it to be safe and reliable with 97% union rates. Union did, however, take slightly longer than fusions elsewhere in the foot with an average of 22 weeks. The patient who had a non-union was revised and subsequently went on to have a successful union[20].

Forefoot Arthritis

Hallux Rigidus

Introduction

Degenerative arthritis of the first MTPJ is manifested as a stiff and painful great toe, and is often known as hallux rigidus. It was originally described by Davies Colley in 1887.

The normal first MTPJ is a cam-shaped, hinge joint with a greater range of dorsiflexion (40–100°) than plantar flexion (3–43°). The maximum standing

(a)

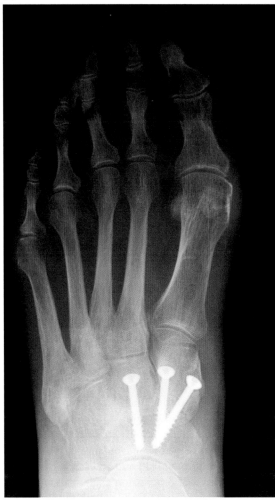

(b)

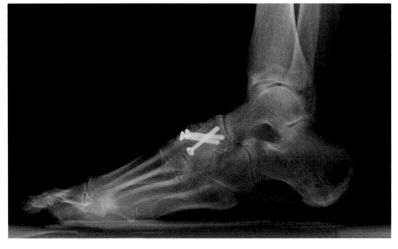

Figure 7.8 Isolated naviculocuneiform arthrodesis with screws.

Table 7.1 The Hattrup and Johnson classification of first MTPJ degeneration

Grade 1	Mild changes with a maintained joint space and minimal spurring
Grade 2	Moderate changes, joint space narrowing, bony proliferation of the metatarsal head and proximal phalanx, and subchondral sclerosis or cysts
Grade 3	Severe changes with moderate to severe joint space narrowing, extensive bony proliferation, and loose bodies or a dorsal ossicle

range of movement on tiptoe stance averages 65°, but the functional range of motion during walking is only 38°. In running a range of 60° may be needed.

Pathogenesis

Hallux rigidus is commoner in women and its prevalence increases with age. In the over 50s, there is a 7.8% prevalence of symptomatic first MTPJ arthritis. Bilateral disease is common, affecting up to 80% of patients, although the severity of symptoms differs on each side[21].

The majority of cases of hallux rigidus are idiopathic, although it can be secondary to trauma, inflammatory arthropathy, or crystal arthropathy. There have been many theories as to the etiology of idiopathic hallux rigidus with a number of authors looking at anatomical variations as the underlying mechanical factor leading to disease. Metatarsus primus elevatus, metatarsus primus varus, a flattened first metatarsal head, hypermobility, increased first metatarsal length, and calf tightness have all been implicated, but none has been proven to be the definitive cause.

With *metatarsus primus elevatus* the elevation may be idiopathic, secondary to malunion of a fracture, or iatrogenic, following a first metatarsal osteotomy. It is postulated that elevation of the first metatarsal head leads to the proximal phalanx being relatively plantarly subluxed. Therefore during early toe-off the base of the proximal phalanx impinges against the dorsal metatarsal head, causing osteochondral damage of the dorsal aspect of the metatarsal head[22]. This fits with the pattern of wear that is seen in hallux rigidus with early loss of the dorsal articular cartilage. Opposing the view that elevatus is etiological is evidence that the elevatus is a secondary change in joints that are already degenerative.

Furthermore a study by Meyer has shown that the elevated first metatarsal is a normal finding in midstance[23].

Classification

A number of grading systems for hallux rigidus exist. In general, they assess both the range of movement and the radiographic features of the joint. The most widely used classification is that described by Hattrup and Johnson[24] (Table 7.1), which has subsequently been modified by Coughlin[25] (Table 7.2).

Presentation

History and Examination

The typical symptoms of a degenerative first MTPJ are of a reduced range of movement with pain in the early stages at the extremes of movement, particularly in maximal dorsiflexion. Symptoms may be exacerbated by running or wearing high heels. As the disease progresses, pain becomes more severe with day-to-day activities, while wearing non-heeled shoes, and even at rest.

Look

Dorsal swelling of the joint is a good indication of first MTPJ arthritis (Figure 7.9), giving rise to the term "dorsomedial bunion." Subtle alterations in gait can be observed with avoidance of full dorsiflexion of the MTPJ and an early toe-off or an increased foot progression angle. The foot supinates, taking more load through the lesser rays leading to lateral metatarsalgia, which is not uncommonly secondary to a Morton's neuroma.

Feel

Dorsal osteophytes are usually palpable, even in the early stages. Palpation will also reveal tenderness over the dorsolateral joint.

Move

Joint range of movement is restricted. Dorsiflexion is reduced more than plantar flexion. Pain in the mid-range or pain on "grind" testing is an indication that arthrodesis is likely to be a more reliable treatment than a cheilectomy. The interphalangeal joint can develop compensatory hyperextension, with a callosity underneath it.

Occasionally the main complaint is of pressure from footwear on the dorsal osteophyte. The dorsal osteophyte can also impinge upon the dorsomedial cutaneous nerve, causing neuritic pain and reduced

Table 7.2 Coughlin's Modified Clinical–Radiographic classification of first MTPJ degeneration

Grade	Dorsiflexion	Radiographic findings	Clinical findings
0	40 to 60° 10 to 20% loss compared to normal side	Normal	No pain Only stiffness and loss of motion
1	30 to 40° 20 to 50% loss compared to normal side	Dorsal osteophyte Minimal joint-space narrowing Minimal subchondral sclerosis	Mild or occasional pain and stiffness Pain at extremes of dorsiflexion or plantar flexion
2	10 to 30° 50 to 75% loss compared to normal side	Osteophytes Flattened appearance of metatarsal head Up to 25% of dorsal joint involved on lateral radiograph Mild to moderate joint-space narrowing	Moderate to severe pain and stiffness, which may be constant Pain occurs just before maximum dorsiflexion or plantar flexion
3	≤10° 75 to 100% loss compared to normal side Loss of MTP plantar flexion as well (often ≤10° of plantar flexion)	Same as grade 2 but with substantial narrowing, subchondral cysts Over 25% of dorsal joint involved on lateral radiograph Sesamoids enlarged +/− cystic +/− irregular	Nearly constant pain, substantial stiffness, pain at extremes but not at midrange
4	As in grade 3	As in grade 3	As grade 3 *but* with pain in the midrange with passive motion

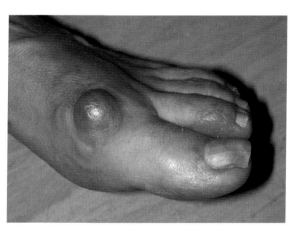

Figure 7.9 Dorsal osteophyte in hallux rigidus: often called a "dorsomedial bunion."

sensation along the dorsum of the great toe. Often patients are more aware of reduced sensation following surgery; it is therefore important to document any altered sensitivity at the initial assessment.

Investigations

Anteroposterior and lateral weightbearing radiographs are usually all that is required (Figures 7.10 and 7.11). Typically, loss of joint space, subchondral sclerosis, cysts, and osteophytes are evident. The alignment of the toe should be assessed along with lesser toe deformity. Assess the medial-arch alignment and whether there is coexisting TMTJ arthritis. Cysts in the metatarsal head should be noted, as fixation techniques may need to be altered and bone graft may be necessary if arthrodesis is being considered.

Treatment

Non-Surgical

The majority of hallux rigidus can be successfully managed non-operatively. In the early stages, patients should be counselled with regard to activity modification, simple analgesia, weight loss, and shoe modification. Training shoes or walking boots with a forefoot rocker and a stiffer sole offer comfort. An

(a)

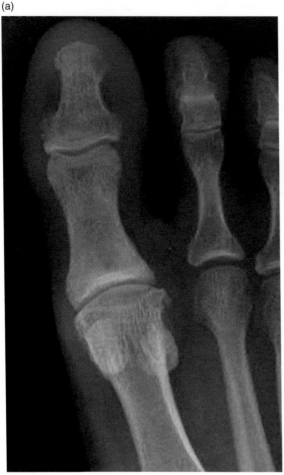

(b)

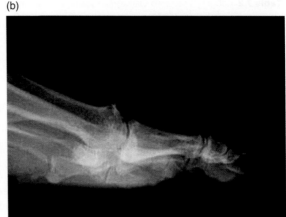

Figure 7.10 Radiograph of early hallux rigidus. Note the loss of joint space and the characteristic dorsal osteophyte.

orthosis with a Morton's extension under the first ray can be of benefit, but their use is often limited in those with dorsal osteophytes as the thickness of the insole can exacerbate the pressure from the osteophyte on the shoe. Non-operative measures often make the symptoms manageable for many years.

Manipulation and joint injection may give some relief in the earlier stages. Relief for up to six months was reported in those with grade 1 changes, with only one-third progressing to surgery versus two-thirds of those with grade 2 change. Joint injections give little symptomatic benefit in grade 3 arthritis and are not advised in this group.[26]

Surgical

The main surgical options for the majority of cases are either a cheilectomy or first MTPJ arthrodesis.

Both have been shown to be reliable and safe procedures. Arthroplasty of the first MTP joint has not shown reliable long-term results but patients will still often enquire about this.

Cheilectomy

A dorsal cheilectomy involves resection of the dorsal third of the articular surface of the metatarsal head. Cheilectomy gives good results in the early stages of degenerative disease in Coughlin grades 1, 2, and selected patients with grade 3 disease. In these groups, Coughlin has shown that cheilectomy offers pain reduction and good function in 92% of cases, at nine-year follow-up[25]. Those with grade 3 changes and over 50% cartilage loss on the metatarsal head along with all grade 4 cases are better treated with a fusion.

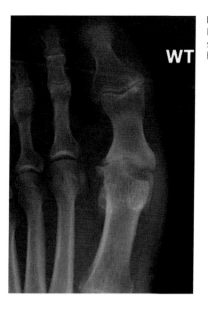

Figure 7.11
Radiograph showing advanced hallux rigidus.

Cheilectomy is traditionally carried out as an open procedure with the level of osteophyte and metatarsal head resection being the dorsal margin of articular cartilage loss. This level removes the dorsal osteophyte and 30% of the metatarsal head. The osteophytes on the proximal phalanx are also cleared. Resection of more than 50% is not advised as it can lead to instability of the joint and increased pain. An adequate resection should allow 70° of dorsiflexion intraoperatively. The final postoperative range is usually less than that achieved on the table. Once the wound has healed, early movement is the key and it is important to encourage the patient to mobilize the toe and stop using a rigid-soled shoe.

Minimally invasive dorsal cheilectomy is undertaken using one or two portals and a specialized burr. The portals are small and hence recovery from the soft tissue aspect of the surgery is quicker. Nevertheless, such surgery does not extend the Coughlin grade of arthritis treatable by cheilectomy.

Many patients are averse to the idea of great toe fusion, and hence the usual cause of failure of cheilectomy is ongoing arthritic pain as a result of an extension of the indications to the higher Coughlin grades in an attempt to avoid fusion. Some patients are agreeable to an intraoperative decision of cheilectomy or fusion by the surgeon, dependent on the degree of arthritis found. A painful joint in the early stages post-cheilectomy can sometimes be helped to settle by a steroid injection and manipulation under anesthesia.

Arthrodesis

First MTPJ fusion is the gold standard surgical procedure for symptomatic, advanced arthritis of the first MTPJ. When performed correctly it achieves high rates of union with little functional restriction in 77 to 100% patients. The surgical principles are to adequately prepare the joint surfaces without significantly shortening the toe, to align the toe in a functional position, and to stabilize the toe until fusion is achieved. There are many different methods of joint preparation and stabilization, and hence technique will vary from individual to individual.

A medial or dorsal approach is used. A dorsomedial approach should be avoided as it risks damaging the cutaneous nerve. The line of the medial corner of the nail bed is a useful anatomical landmark for the position of the cutaneous nerve. Joint preparation can be carried out by hand, planar cuts, crescentic saw cuts, or ball and cup reamers. When preparation is carried out by hand, care must be taken to form congruent surfaces with good bony apposition. Ball and cup reamers produce two highly congruent surfaces but can lead to excessive shortening and do require greater exposure to allow reamer access. With planar cuts it is important to get the correct alignment with the resection, as there is no flexibility of toe position after the cuts have been made.

The joint should be fixed. There are numerous techniques using plates, screws (Figure 7.12), and staples. A cadaver biomechanical study has shown that dorsal plating is stronger than crossed screws in both force to failure and initial stiffness[27]. Nevertheless, importantly, clinical studies have not shown statistical differences in time to fusion between the two constructs, although there is a large difference in hardware costs, with screws being much less expensive[28].

The position of the arthrodesis is also important to a successful outcome. The position of fusion is referenced to the floor, and not the first metatarsal, as there is considerable variation in the metatarsal's declination angle between individuals. At the time of surgery a load-simulation test is undertaken with the ankle in neutral and using a flat surface placed under the foot to simulate the floor. It is a good idea, before commencing the dissection, to note the position of the toe referenced to the flat surface. This gives a good idea of the great toe position to which the patient has become accustomed. An ideal position is where the toe just touches the flat surface, but has enough

(a)   (b)

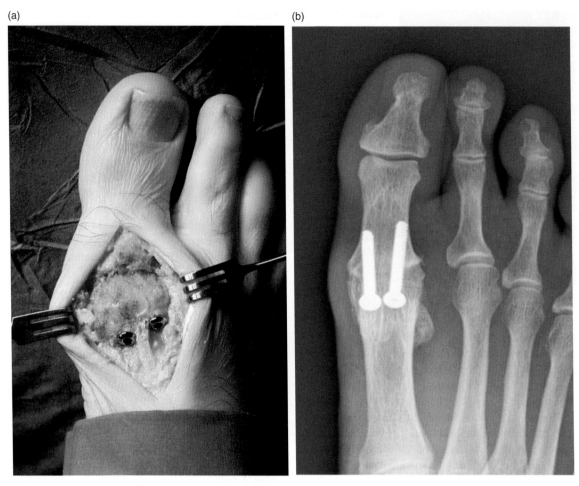

Figure 7.12 (**a**) Clinical and (**b**) radiological images of one method of screw fusion of the first MTPJ.

interphalangeal joint extension to allow the surgeon's finger to pass under the pulp. The varus/valgus position of fusion must also be correct and is best assessed relative to the second toe. There should be a small gap between the great and second toes to avoid impingement. The hallux should be in slight valgus to avoid rubbing on the shoe medially. Finally, it is important to ensure the correct rotation of the toe prior to fixation. In hallux rigidus the toe often pronates. This needs to be corrected intraoperatively, otherwise the patient will develop a callosity under the medial condyle of the proximal phalanx at the interphalangeal joint. The toe nail is used perioperatively as a reference to assess the rotational alignment.

It is important to remember that when hallux valgus coexists the intermetatarsal angle reduces spontaneously; it is not necessary to undertake a first

metatarsal osteotomy or soft tissue release to correct this.

Standard recovery involves mobilizing weight bearing in a heel-bearing or rigid-soled postoperative shoe for six weeks following surgery. Reported complications include infection, non-union, malunion, metalwork prominence, scar sensitivity, and nerve damage. Reported non-union rates are 2 to 23%, although non-union is sometimes asymptomatic and does not need revising[29]. A systematic review, in 2011, of 37 studies with 2818 first MTPJ arthrodeses showed an overall non-union rate of 5.4% (153 of 2818), of which only 33% were symptomatic, thus the incidence of symptomatic non-union was 1.8%. The incidence of malunion was 6%, with dorsal malunion accounting for 87% of these. Hardware removal was required in 8%[30]. If the toe is fixed in

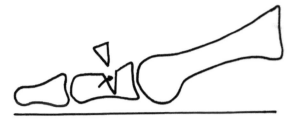

Figure 7.13 Diagram demonstrating the dorsally based wedge Moberg osteotomy.

excess plantar flexion the patient complains of pain under the condyles of the proximal phalanx. With excessive dorsiflexion the patient develops a thickened painful callus under the metatarsal head and clawing of the interphalangeal joint of the great toe, which rubs dorsally on shoes.

Female patients need to be aware that the comfortable heel height will be limited post-fusion to 5 cm, or less. This is an operation for pain control and not the ability to wear fashionable shoes. Attempts to fuse the toe in greater degrees of dorsiflexion to allow for a higher heeled shoe should be avoided as this affects barefoot walking and the dorsiflexed great toe often becomes symptomatic.

Moberg Procedure

The Moberg procedure is a dorsiflexion closing wedge osteotomy of the proximal phalanx of the hallux (Figure 7.13)[31]. Preoperatively the patients need to have an adequate range of plantar flexion of the MTPJ as the osteotomy alters the arc of motion of the joint, decreasing plantar flexion to improve dorsiflexion. The Moberg osteotomy is usually used in combination with a cheilectomy of the first metatarsal head. The only outcome studies have reported small numbers of patients. One study reviewing 24 toes treated with a dorsal cheilectomy and extension osteotomy of the proximal phalanx showed 96% patient satisfaction, despite improvement of only around 7° of dorsiflexion[32].

Metatarsophalangeal Joint Replacement Arthroplasty

Metatarsophalangeal joint arthroplasty relieves pain while maintaining motion. Various designs have been used with total or hemiarthroplasty of the joint, using polyethylene, silastic, ceramic, metal, and even hydrogel implants. A cheilectomy with resection of the osteophytes is required to maximize the range of movement. The medullary canals are reamed and

the implant is fixed, normally in an uncemented fashion with a press or screw-fit technique.

Although a systematic meta-analysis of the literature documenting first MTPJ arthroplasty has shown patient satisfaction levels of 95%, the meta-analysis does not document other outcomes[33]. Other studies have repeatedly shown disappointing clinical results. The ceramic Moje total replacement was reported with a 26% re-operation rate and 52% of the prostheses becoming radiologically loose at two- to eight-year follow-up[34]. Similar poor radiological results with high revision rates have been noted by other authors using the ceramic MOJE replacement[35]. McGraw agreed that loosening and subsidence are problematic with the MOJE, despite reasonable patient satisfaction[36]. A 12-month follow-up of 160 patients with a Toefit™ metal/polyethylene bearing total joint again showed good overall functional improvement with AOFAS scores which rose from 38 preoperatively to 83 postoperatively. However, there was a 29% revision rate and 20% aseptic loosening[37].

Furthermore two comparative studies with fusion have both favored arthrodesis. Raikin compared hemiarthroplasty with fusion. The AOFAS score improved more in the arthrodesis group. Five of 21 hemiarthroplasties were revised, while there was only one non-union among the 27 fusions[38]. A randomized controlled trial by Gibson, comparing total joint replacement and fusion, showed significantly better improvement in pain score and higher patient satisfaction with a fusion when compared to a metal/polyethylene bearing replacement[39].

Unlike other weightbearing joints that undergo successful arthroplasty, the orientation of the MTPJ means that it encounters mainly shear forces during gait. It is likely that the small surface area of the joint, with large forces going through it, make it a biomechanically difficult joint to replace successfully. Interestingly, a recent study using a hydrogel first MTPJ replacement in a prospective, randomized non-inferiority study showed equivalent pain relief and functional outcomes for the implant compared to arthrodesis in patients who wished to maintain first MTPJ motion[40].

Keller Procedure

Excision arthroplasty of the base of the proximal phalanx is known as a Keller procedure. With the success of arthrodesis, the Keller procedure is rarely undertaken. The procedure leads to weakness of the forefoot at toe-off and the patients are prone to develop an extension, or "cock-up," deformity of the hallux. With time, the first-ray insufficiency leads to transfer lesions of the lesser toes. This may even progress onto subluxation and dislocation of the lesser MTPJs with metatarsalgia. Treatment of this is complicated and requires fusion with a bone graft (see below). For these reasons the Keller procedure is now reserved for low-demand patients who would not be able to manage the postoperative rehabilitation for an arthrodesis, or who have infection that precludes other procedures[41].

Salvage Procedures

In cases of failed fusion or arthroplasty a revision arthrodesis may be necessary. Interposition bone grafting from the iliac crest is required if there is shortening of the metatarsal or significant bone loss from lysis or a previous excision arthroplasty (Keller). In these cases a tri-cortical pelvic bone graft is stabilized with dorsal plating. Lengthening of up to 29 mm has been achieved, although 10 mm is more usual (Figure 7.14). Grafts larger than this risk increased skin tension and wound breakdown over the dorsal plate. Union rates of 73 to 93% have been reported with iliac crest bone-graft fusions. Union normally occurs within 12 to 15 weeks; the fusion between the distal graft and the remnants of the proximal phalanx is the usual site of non-union. Complication rates are relatively high at around 40%, with wound healing, superficial and deep infection, and non-union being most troublesome. Nevertheless the overall reported patient satisfaction rates are good[42–43].

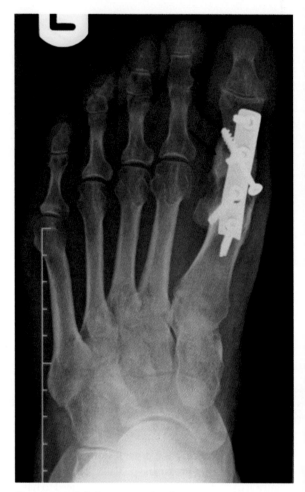

Figure 7.14 Keller's excision arthroplasty, converted to an arthrodesis with a tricortical iliac crest bone graft (arrow).

Gout

Gout is a crystalline arthropathy caused by the intra-articular precipitation of monosodium urate crystals. It most commonly affects the first MTPJ; over 75% of patients with gout will have an episode affecting the hallux at some time. It is commoner in males and tends to affect those over the age of 30 years. A typical history of recurrent intermittent episodes of a hot, painful, and swollen joint should raise clinical suspicion. Blood urate levels can be normal in those with gout, and high in those without. A joint aspirate that demonstrates needle shaped, negatively birefringent crystals under polarized light confirms the diagnosis. In chronic cases the typical radiographic features are of destructive joint changes and peri-articular erosions at the capsular attachments can be seen.

Treatment of the acute attack is aimed at settling the episode with non-steroidal anti-inflammatory medication or colchicine. Allopurinol may be introduced when acute symptoms have subsided to try and prevent recurrent episodes. Surgery may be required in long-standing cases due to pain from the secondary degenerative change. Arthrodesis of the joint is usually required.

Hallux Interphalangeal Arthritis

Occasionally degenerative change can occur in the hallux interphalangeal joint. This can be secondary to a previous hallux MTPJ fusion, trauma, or

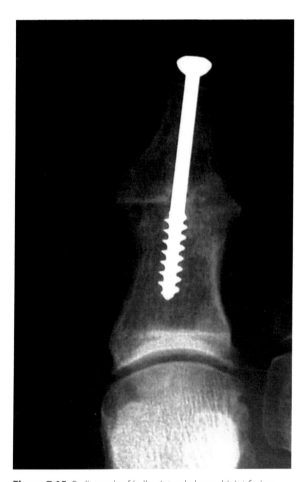

Figure 7.15 Radiograph of hallux interphalangeal joint fusion.

inflammatory arthropathy, specifically psoriatic arthropathy. If symptoms cannot be controlled with conservative measures and adjustment to shoes then an interphalangeal joint fusion can be undertaken. This is done via a dorsal L-shaped incision over the interphalangeal joint to allow joint surface preparation prior to passing a partially threaded cancellous screw from the tip of the distal phalanx longitudinally down the phalanx (Figure 7.15). Complications include non-union, malunion (commonly a rotational deformity), and the need for metalwork removal.

Lesser Toe Arthritis

Lesser toe arthritis is uncommon. It may be secondary to inflammatory arthropathy, trauma, and occasionally following lesser toe deformity with dislocated MTPJs. Arthritis of the lesser MTPJs is rare and has been treated with debridement, fusion, osteotomy,

and replacement. The authors prefer either debridement or a Weil's osteotomy to decompress the joint. Again isolated IPJ arthritis is rare, but is easily treated with fusion.

Freiberg's Disease

Freiberg's disease, or "infraction," is thought to be caused by avascular necrosis of the lesser metatarsal heads. It is most commonly seen in the second metatarsal head as, presumably, this metatarsal is the longest and most susceptible to repetitive trauma. Freiberg's infraction typically affects athletic, adolescent females and presents with a painful, stiff MTPJ.

The disease progresses through the stages typical of all avascular necrosis pathologies. Initially no changes can be seen on plain radiographs, although MRI scan shows edema or subchondral fracture. Dorsal articular surface collapse and fragmentation then becomes visible on plain radiographs (Figure 7.16). The disease progresses to arthritis with joint-space narrowing and osteophytes, which may present in middle age.

The initial management is non-operative with rest, NSAIDs, and avoidance of aggravating activities. Orthoses with a metatarsal bar to offload the MTPJ in combination with a rigid-soled shoe may also be helpful. A short period in a walking cast may help to settle an acute painful episode.

Surgical options are debridement of the joint with removal of loose bodies, osteochondral drilling, and removal of osteophytes. More invasive options include decompression of the joint with a shortening and rotational osteotomy to rotate the preserved plantar articular dorsally. When severe degenerative changes exist, and if other surgeries fail, then either a Weil osteotomy or an excision arthroplasty in the form of a Stainsby procedure may be used.

Inflammatory Arthropathy

Patients with rheumatoid feet present with forefoot, midfoot, and hindfoot pathology. The usual symptoms are of pain and deformity. In general it is better to treat proximal limb disease before foot and ankle disease, and to treat the hindfoot before the forefoot. Clearly, if there is ulceration and infection, this may require treatment before surgery with implants.

As with the rheumatoid hand, the forefoot is normally symmetrically affected. Synovitis causes hallux

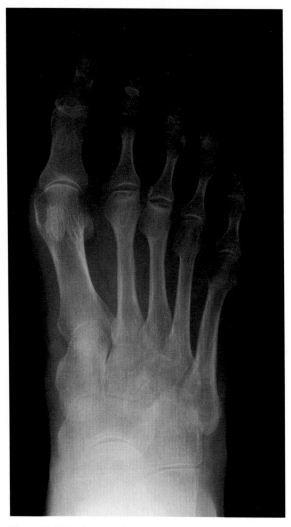

Figure 7.16 Radiograph showing Freiberg's disease with articular collapse of the second and third metatarsal heads.

valgus and deformity of the lesser toes. The synovitis results in incompetent collateral ligaments and plantar plate destruction, leading to dorsal subluxation and eventual MTPJ dislocation. This results in increased plantar pressure with the development of plantar callosities and bursae under the lesser metatarsal heads (Figures 7.17 and 7.18).

Non-operative treatment of the "rheumatoid forefoot" includes total contact insoles and rocker-bottomed shoes to decrease the pressures under the forefoot. Intra-articular corticosteroid injections of the rheumatoid forefoot should be used with caution, as they are associated with joint instability, and even dislocation of the MTPJs.

If surgical treatment of the forefoot is chosen, the forefoot needs to be considered as a whole, and it is necessary to correct both the hallux and the lesser toes, balancing the forefoot. For clarity we will discuss the first and lesser rays separately.

First ray. Excision of the base of the proximal phalanx (Keller's procedure) and excision of the first metatarsal head (Mayo's procedure) have been shown to give initial patient satisfaction, but usually lead to late recurrent deformity, pain, and functional deterioration, as they defunction the first ray and increase the pressure under the lesser rays, which deform, dislocate, and become symptomatic[44].

Arthrodesis of the first MTPJ offers reliable relief of pain and predictable outcomes. It refunctions the first ray and offloads the lesser metatarsals. Hence, arthrodesis is preferred to excision for pain relief, cosmetic appearance, shoe fitting, maintenance of alignment, and the restoration of weight bearing under the hallux[45].

Realignment osteotomies may be used in the rheumatoid patient as they maintain movement and reduce pain. They are relatively contraindicated if the patient has osteopenic bone or secondary degeneration. The choice of osteotomy depends on the surgeon's preference. A Scarf osteotomy gives good results in patients with medically well-controlled disease, and a well-preserved joint space.

Arthroplasty of the MTPJ of the hallux has been proposed as an alternative to resection arthroplasty or arthrodesis, but there are the same limitations as have been discussed in the hallux rigidus section.

Lesser rays. The aim of surgery to the lesser toes is to reduce the MTPJs and realign the toes, thereby reducing the plantar pressure under the MTPJs and the dorsal pressure over PIPJs. It is rare for a single ray to require surgery in isolation. In planning a forefoot reconstruction all four rays should be considered with the aim to produce a balanced forefoot. Reduction of the MTPJ is the most important aspect of surgery, and can be addressed by metatarsal head excision[46], Weil's metatarsal osteotomy, or proximal phalangectomy.

Excision of the metatarsal heads, in a cascade, cut parallel to the floor, is still widely used and effectively reduces pain. Joint-preserving surgery with shortening and realignment osteotomies is an alternative approach[47]. Weil's osteotomy allows shortening without plantar flexion of the metatarsal

(a)

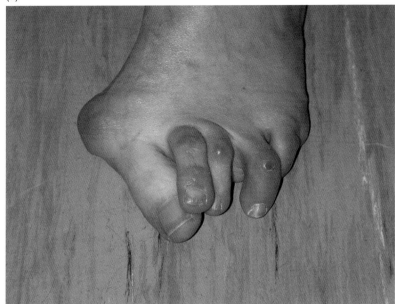

(b)

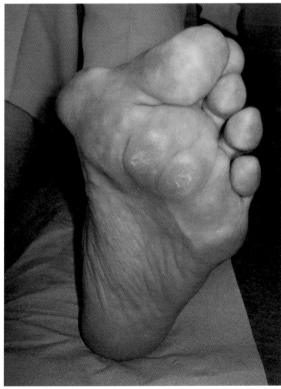

Figure 7.17 Rheumatoid forefoot. Note the marked hallux valgus, lesser toe deformities, and callosities under the dislocated lesser MTPJs.

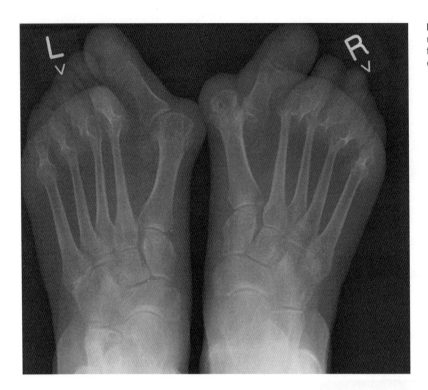

Figure 7.18 Bilateral forefoot rheumatoid arthritis. This was treated by a first MTPJ fusion and metatarsal head excision, as the disease is so advanced.

heads. This reduces the plantar pressure by reducing the joint and the plantar plate.

The final option is the Stainsby procedure[48]. Through a dorsal approach an extensor tenotomy and generous proximal phalangectomy are performed, excising the proximal half to two-thirds of the proximal phalanx. The plantar plate is mobilized and the toe is held reduced with an axial K-wire. Stainsby originally recommended tenodesis of the extensor to the flexor tendon, through the phalangeal resection, although this is not universally performed. The Stainsby procedure has been shown to be associated with good functional, if not cosmetic, results[49].

Distal deformities in the lesser toes at the proximal and distal IPJs may be addressed by either fusion or excision arthroplasty. We prefer to undertake an arthrodesis as we feel this gives a more durable result.

Key Points

- The mainstay of treatment for TMTJ arthritis is analgesic medication with in-shoe orthoses with a medial arch support.

- The differing indications for TMTJ fusion include a rocker-bottom foot, hallux valgus (Lapidus procedure), flat foot correction, and an in situ fusion for arthritis or for first TMTJ instability. The technique varies depending upon the indication.

- The lateral column is more mobile, and fusion of it is controversial.

- In the treatment of hallux rigidus, dorsal cheilectomy gives good results in Coughlin grade 1, 2, and selected patients with grade 3 disease. Grade 3 patients with over 50% cartilage loss and all grade 4 cases are usually treated with a fusion.

- Arthroplasty of the first MTPJ is controversial, and can be difficult to revise.

- Freiberg's disease is thought to be caused by AVN of the lesser metatarsal heads. It is most commonly seen in the second ray in adolescent females.

- The rheumatoid forefoot should be rebalanced. The first ray may be fused or realigned with an osteotomy. The lesser MTPJs can be treated by metatarsal head excision, Weil osteotomy, or a Stainsby procedure.

References

1. Roddy E, Thomas MJ, Marshall M, Rathod T, Myers H, Menz HB, Thomas E, Peat G. The population prevalence of symptomatic radiographic foot osteoarthritis in community-dwelling older adults: cross-sectional findings from the Clinical Assessment Study of the Foot. *Ann Rheum Dis*. 2015; 74(1):156–63.

2. Mann RA, Prieskorn D, Sobel M. Mid-tarsal and tarsometatarsal arthrodesis for primary degenerative osteoarthrosis or osteoarthrosis after trauma. *J Bone Joint Surg Am*. 1996 Sep; 78(9):1376–85.

3. Singh VK, Javed S, Parthipun A, Sott AH. A radionuclide bone scan with single photon-emission computed tomography and CT (SPECT-CT). *Foot Ankle Surg*. 2013 Jun;19(2):80–3.

4. Jung HG, Myerson MS, Schon LC. Spectrum of operative treatments and clinical outcomes for atraumatic osteoarthritis of the tarsometatarsal joints. *Foot Ankle Int*. 2007 Apr;28(4):482–9.

5. Klos K, Simons P, Hajduk AS, Hoffmeier KL, Gras F, Fröber R, Hofmann GO, Mückley T. Plantar versus dorsomedial locked plating for Lapidus arthrodesis: a biomechanical comparison. *Foot Ankle Int*. 2011 Nov; 32(11):1081–5.

6. O'Malley MJ, Sayres SC, Saleem O, Levine D, Roberts M, Deland JT, Ellis S. Morbidity and complications following percutaneous calcaneal autograft bone harvest. *Foot Ankle Int*. 2014 Jan;35(1):30–7.

7. Baumhauer J, Pinzur MS, Donahue R, Beasley W, DiGiovanni C. Site selection and pain outcome after autologous bone graft harvest. *Foot Ankle Int*. 2014 Feb;35(2):104–7.

8. Nemec SA, Habbu RA, Anderson JG & Bohay DR. Outcomes following midfoot arthrodesis for primary arthritis. *Foot Ankle Int* 2011;32(4): 355–61.

9. Filippi J, Myerson MS, Scioli MW, Den Hartog BD, Kay DB, Bennett GL, Stephenson KA. Midfoot arthrodesis following multi-joint stabilization with a novel hybrid plating system. *Foot Ankle Int*. 2012 Mar;33(3):220–5.

10. Komenda GA, Myerson MS, Biddinger KR. Results of arthrodesis of the tarsometatarsal joints after traumatic injury. *J Bone Joint Surg Am*. 1996 Nov;78 (11):1665–76.

11. Pinzur MS. Neutral ring fixation for high-risk nonplantigrade Charcot midfoot deformity. *Foot Ankle Int*. 2007;28:961-966.

12. Sammarco VJ, Sammarco GJ, Walker EW Jr, Guiao RP. Midtarsal arthrodesis in the treatment of Charcot midfoot arthropathy. Surgical technique. *J Bone Joint Surg Am*. 2010 Mar;92 Suppl 1 Pt 1:1-19.

13. Butt DA, Hester T, Bilal A, Edmonds M, Kavarthapu V. The medial column Synthes Midfoot Fusion Bolt is associated with unacceptable rates of failure in corrective fusion for Charcot deformity. *Bone Joint J*. 2015 Jun;97-B(6):809–13.

14. Pope EJ, Takemoto RC, Kummer FJ, Mroczek KJ. Midfoot fusion: a biomechanical comparison of plantar planting vs intramedullary screws. *Foot Ankle Int*. 2013 Mar;34(3):409–13.

15. Raikin SM, Schon LC. Arthrodesis of the fourth and fifth tarsometatarsal joints of the midfoot. *Foot and Ankle Int*. 2003 Aug;24(8):584–90.

16. Berlet HC, Hodges Davis W, Anderson RB. Tendon arthroplasty for basal fourth and fifth metatarsal arthritis. *Foot Ankle Int*. 2002 May;23(5):440–60.

17. Shawen SB, Anderson RB, Cohen BE, Hammit MD, Davis WH. Spherical ceramic interpositional arthroplasty for basal fourth and fifth metatarsal arthritis. *Foot ankle Int*. 2007 Aug; 28(8):896-901.

18. Viens NA, Adams SB Jr, Nunley JA 2nd. Ceramic interpositional arthroplasty for fourth and fifth tarsometatarsal joint arthritis. *J Surg Orthop Adv*. 2012 Fall; 21(3):126–31.

19. Ma S, Jin D. Isolated talonavicular arthrodesis. *Foot Ankle Int*. 2016, EPub ahead of Publication

20. Ajis A, Geary N. Surgical technique, fusion rates, and planovalgus foot deformity correction with naviculocuneiform fusion. *Foot Ankle Int*. 2014 Mar;35 (3):232–7.

21. Coughlin & Shurnas. Hallux rigidus: Demographics, etiology and radiographic assessment. *Foot Ankle Int*. 2003;24(10):731–43.

22. Lambrinudi C. Metatarsus primus elevatus. *Proc. Roy. Soc. Med*. 1938; 31(11):1273.

23. Meyer JO, Nishon LR, Weiss I, Docks G. Metatarsus primus elevatus and the etiology of hallux rigidus. *J Foot Surg*. 1987; 26(3):237–41.

24. Hattrup SJ, Johnson KA. Subjective results of hallux rigidus following treatment with cheilectomy. *Clin Orthop Relat Res*. 1988;226:182–91.

25. Coughlin MJ, Shurnas PS. Hallux rigidus. Grading and long-term results of operative treatment. *J Bone Joint Surg Am*. 2003 Nov;85-A(11):2072–88.

26. Solan MC, Calder JD, Bendall SP. Manipulation and injection for hallux rigidus. Is it worthwhile? *J Bone Joint Surg Br*. 2001 Jul; 83(5):706–8.

27. Rongstad K, Miller G, Vander Griend R, and Cowin D. A biomechanical comparison of four fixation methods of first

metatarsophalangeal joint arthrodesis. *Foot Ankle*. 1994; 15:415–9.

28. Hyer CF, Glover JP, Berlet GC, Lee TH. Cost comparison of crossed screws versus dorsal plate construct for first metatarsophalangeal joint arthrodesis. *J Foot Ankle Surg*. 2008 Jan-Feb;47(1):13–8.

29. McKeever DC. Arthrodesis of the first metatarsophalangeal joint for hallux valgus, hallux rigidus and metatarsus primus varus. *JBJS Am*. 1952;34(1):129–34.

30. Roukis TS. Non-union after arthrodesis of the first metatarsal-phalangeal joint: a systematic review. *J Foot Ankle Surg*. 2011 Nov-Dec;50(6):710–3.

31. Moberg E. A simple operation for hallux rigidus. *Clin Orthop* 1979;142:55–56.

32. Thomas PJ, Smith RW. Proximal phalanx osteotomy for the surgical treatment of hallux rigidus. *Foot Ankle Int*. 1999 Jan;20(1):3–12.

33. Cook E, Cook J, Rosenblum B, Landsman A, Giurni J, Basile P. Meta-analysis of first metatarsophalangeal joint implant arthroplasty. *J Foot Ankle Surg*. 2009 Mar-Apr;48(2):180–90.

34. Dawson-Bowling S, Adimonye A, Cohen A, Cottam H, Ritchie J, Fordyce M. MOJE ceramic metatarsophalangeal arthroplasty: disappointing clinical results at two to eight years. *Foot Ankle Int*. 2012 Jul;33(7):560–4.

35. Nagy MT, Walker CR, Sirikonda SP. Long term outcome of first MTPJ replacement using ceramic prosthesis with press fit design. *Bone Joint J*. 2013;95-B:21.

36. McGraw IWW, Jameson SS, Kumar CS. Mid-term results of the Moje hallux MP joint replacement. *Foot Ankle Int*. 2010 July;31(7):592–99.

37. Al-Maiyah M, Rice P & Schneider T. Outcome of first metatarsophalangeal total joint replacement (Toefit): A clinical outcome and survival analysis. *Bone Joint J*. 2013;95-B no. SUPP 21:32

38. Raikin SM, Ahmad J, Pour AE, Abidi N. Comparison of arthrodesis and metallic hemiarthroplasty of the hallux metatarsophalangeal joint. *J Bone Joint Surg Am*. 2007 Sep;89(9): 1979–85.

39. Gibson JN, Thomson CE. Arthrodesis or total replacement arthroplasty for hallux rigidus: A randomised control trial. *Foot Ankle Int*. 2005 Sep;26(9): 680–90.

40. Baumhauer JF, Singh D, Glazebrook M, et al. Prospective, randomized, multi-centered clinical trial assessing safety and efficacy of a synthetic cartilage implant versus first metatarsophalangeal arthrodesis in advanced hallux rigidus. *Foot Ankle Int*. 2016;37(5):457–69.

41. Keller W. The surgical treatment of bunions and hallux valgus. *N Y Med J*. 1904;80:741–2.

42. Myerson MS, Schon LC, McGuigan FX, Oznur A. Result of arthrodesis of the hallux metatarsophalangeal joint using bone graft for restoration of length. *Foot Ankle Int*. 2000 Apr;21(4):297–306.

43. Brodsky JW, Ptaszek AJ, Morris SG. Salvage first MTP arthrodesis utilizing ICBG: clinical evaluation and outcome. *Foot Ankle Int*. 2000 Apr;21(4):290–6.

44. Majkowski RS, Galloway S. Excision arthroplasty for hallux valgus in the elderly: a comparison between the Keller and modified Mayo. *Foot Ankle*. 1992;13:317–20.

45. Mulcahy D, Daniels T, Lau J, Boyle E, Bogoch E. Rheumatoid forefoot deformity: a comparison study of 2 functional methods of reconstruction. *J Rheumatol*. 2003;30:1440–50.

46. Hoffmann P. An operation for severe grades of contracted or clawed toes. *Am J Orthop Surg*. 1911;9:441–9.

47. Barouk LS, Barouk P. Joint preserving surgery in rheumatoid forefeet: Preliminary study with more than two year follow up. *Foot Ankle Clinics*. 2007;12(3): 435–54.

48. Briggs PJ, Stainsby GD. Metatarsal head preservation in forefoot arthroplasty. *Foot Ankle Surg*. 2001;7:93–101.

49. Hossain S. Stainsby procedure for non-rheumatoid claw toes. *Foot Ankle Surg*. 2003;9:113–18.

8

Ankle and Hindfoot Arthritis

Jacob R. Zide and James W. Brodsky

Introduction

Ankle and hindfoot arthritis have a significant impact on patient function. Saltzman et al. evaluated the impact of ankle osteoarthritis on physical function and quality of life. They prospectively compared 195 patients with ankle osteoarthritis to 95 matched controls. The SF-36 physical impairment score of patients with ankle osteoarthritis was found to be equivalent to that of patients with severe medical problems, including end-stage kidney disease and congestive heart failure. This striking finding underscores our understanding of the disability that ankle osteoarthritis causes to patients on a daily basis[1].

The goal is to decide which of the treatment alternatives is appropriate for each patient, based upon a thorough assessment of the nature and extent of the arthritis, the deformity of the leg and foot, and any associated soft tissue pathology, all of which may affect the results of treatment.

Etiology, Pathogenesis, and Epidemiology

There are numerous etiologies that cause arthritis of the ankle and hindfoot, including primary osteoarthritis, post-traumatic arthritis, chronic ligamentous instability, the inflammatory arthropathies, deformity of the leg or foot, neurological disease, and Charcot neuroarthropathy.

Post-traumatic ankle arthritis, as a result of prior fracture or chronic ligamentous ankle instability, causes approximately 78% of all ankle arthritis[2]. The low rate of primary osteoarthritis of the ankle, compared to hip and knee arthritis, has not been explained. The cartilage of the ankle joint is thinner, 0.95 to 1.45 mm, than that of the tibial plateau and distal femur, 1.99 and 3.51 mm respectively. However, its tensile stiffness and tensile fracture stress decline at a slower rate than that of the hip. This may explain the lower rate of primary osteoarthritis of the ankle[3–4]. One clinical study demonstrated that knee osteoarthritis has an incidence approximately 9.4 times that of ankle arthritis[5].

The true prevalence of ankle osteoarthritis is unknown. This may be related to the variable level of symptoms among patients with advanced radiographic degeneration of the tibiotalar joint. Radiographs are also relatively insensitive in identifying even large areas of full-thickness cartilage loss.

The prevalence of hindfoot osteoarthritis is also unknown. Hindfoot arthritis may be primary, but most commonly is secondary to hindfoot valgus as a result of longstanding tibialis posterior tendon rupture. Post-traumatic arthritis following fractures of the talus, calcaneus, navicular, or cuboid is self-evident, but arthritis as a late presentation of unrecognized talocalcaneal or other tarsal coalitions is not uncommon, and the etiology of some cases of hindfoot arthritis is not obvious.

Hindfoot and ankle arthritis commonly coexist, one being resultant upon the other, or the other's treatment. It has been postulated that the restricted motion of one joint results in an increase in the forces in the adjacent joint. A laboratory study in cadaver specimens showed increased contact pressures at the talonavicular and calcaneocuboid joints following simulated ankle arthrodesis[6].

There are numerous reports of progressive arthritis in the hindfoot joints distal to the ankle following tibiotalar arthrodesis, but the extent to which this preexists the arthrodesis, or is accelerated by it is unproven. Certainly post-traumatic arthritis of the ankle and hindfoot frequently coexist. One study documented subtalar arthritis in 32.5% of patients who had undergone an ankle fusion. The degenerative changes were exacerbated in patients in whom the changes were present before surgery[7]. Another study reported radiographic evidence of preoperative hindfoot arthritis in 68 of 70 patients who underwent ankle arthrodesis[8]. On the other hand, using high-resolution techniques in the gait lab, a study of patients undergoing ankle arthrodesis pre- and post-operatively showed that total sagittal motion barely changed after tibiotalar arthrodesis, perhaps signifying that almost all of the sagittal-plane motion in patients with severe ankle arthritis occurs in the talonavicular joint, even prior to ankle arthrodesis[9].

Two studies investigated the effect on gait of ankle arthrodesis compared to total ankle arthroplasty. The studies showed that both operations improved the patients' gait in comparison to pre-surgery, but that neither restored the gait parameters to normal. These studies demonstrated that the stiffness of arthrodesis has little impact on function compared to the inhibitory effect of pain. These objective functional data corroborated the clinical axiom that patients with ankle arthrodesis have a high satisfaction rate and excellent walking[9–10].

Classification of ankle and hindfoot arthritis is far less important than putting the patient's arthritis into the proper context of her or his lifestyle and physical activity level, in order to advise regarding treatment choices. It is valuable to identify deformities proximal and distal to the ankle and hindfoot, such as tibial malunion, or fixed supination of the forefoot as a result of chronic hindfoot valgus, because these can affect treatment choices and surgical results. While it is possible to grade the severity of ankle and hindfoot arthritis radiographically, these systems are not sufficiently sensitive, or meaningful, to guide practical decision-making[11]. Moreover, in the subtalar joint, radiographs and even CT scanning are notoriously insensitive as measures of the severity of arthritis. Many patients with severe pain and complete loss of motion have only moderate joint-space narrowing, or have narrowing in only a portion of the subtalar joint on CT.

Presentation

The predominant location of pain is an important indicator of the location of pathology. Pain along the anterior ankle joint is the most common location for symptomatic tibiotalar arthritis, while pain over the medial or lateral hindfoot is indicative of subtalar arthritis. However, there are pitfalls: isolated talonavicular arthritis, which is common in patients with rheumatoid arthritis, is frequently mistaken for ankle pain as a result of its proximity to the ankle; tibialis posterior tendon or peroneal pathology may cause medial and lateral hindfoot pain.

The patient will often describe a deep ache, which is exacerbated by use of the joint. Typically, arthritic pain in any joint is worse on initiation of the activity – so called "start-up pain" – and subsides or diminishes with activity, although the pain usually becomes more severe after activity. Frequently, patients feel at their best in the morning and report that their pain progressively worsens throughout the day. Arthritic pain is characteristically variable and inconsistent, but the key in the history is its worsening following activity. Pain exacerbated by forward motion is typical of ankle pain, while pain on side-to-side and twisting activities, or walking over uneven or slanted surfaces, is indicative of pathology in the three more distal hindfoot joints. Beware of pain that is not activity related, especially if it is worse at night, or while resting in bed, as this is typical of peripheral neuropathy.

Physical Examination

It is important to examine both lower extremities of every patient, on every occasion. It is quick, and you will never be a first-rate surgeon if you do not. Secondly, the musculoskeletal unit of the foot and ankle includes the musculature; it is therefore important to examine the lower limb at least to the level of the knee. Finally, the arthritic patient must be examined non-weight bearing as well as standing and walking.

The patient is examined for a knee-flexion contracture or tibial-shaft deformity. Coronal-plane deformities of the knee are particularly important because severe arthritic varus or valgus of the knee must be surgically corrected prior to deformity correction at the ankle or hindfoot.

In the seated, or supine, position follow an examination routine and record the findings, including: pulses, skin color and capillary refill, light touch sensation, swelling, tenderness, and scars. Examine and simultaneously try to develop a differential diagnosis, so that you can consider and record the appropriate, relevant data, that are needed. For example, a patient with known or suspected peripheral neuropathy can be assessed with Semmes–Weinstein monofilaments. All the tendons should be palpated for continuity and function, and the joints of the ankle and hindfoot individually palpated for tenderness, effusion, and osteophytes.

Swelling of the ankle and hindfoot is not a prominent or consistent physical finding in arthritis of these joints. Unlike other joints, such as the hip, the loss of motion of the tibiotalar joint is not necessarily proportional to the severity of the arthritis. Some patients with very severe arthritis of the ankle have an extensive, but painful, range of motion. This has been one of the indications for the recent increase in interest in total ankle arthroplasty.

Next, record the range of motion for both limbs including ankle dorsiflexion and plantar flexion, hindfoot inversion and eversion, and abduction and abduction through the talonavicular and calcaneocuboid joints. Examination of hindfoot motion can be subtly deceptive unless one is careful to measure hindfoot inversion/eversion while the ankle is held in maximum dorsiflexion. This is aided by flexing the knee. Otherwise, plantar flexion of the talus in the mortise allows rocking of the ankle in the coronal plane. While holding the ankle in maximal dorsiflexion with one hand, selectively dorsiflex and plantar flex the forefoot at the talonavicular joint (TNJ) to identify the contribution of the TNJ to sagittal-plane motion. Increased motion of the TNJ frequently occurs in the setting of decreased motion through the arthritic ankle, especially when the ankle is limited by anterior oteophytes. One can also distinguish the TNJ as a source of pain, compared to the ankle, which is particularly important in rheumatoid arthritis (RA), due to the predilection of the latter for the TNJ.

It is essential to check for contracture of the tendo Achillis and also gastrocnemius by utilizing the Silfverskiöld test. Holding the hindfoot locked in inversion while undertaking the Silfverskiöld test is important, as hindfoot eversion is multiplanar and includes an element of dorsiflexion.

Strength testing is important in identifying the weakness associated with tendinopathy and neurological disease, which is common in this population, and needs treatment to obtain a satisfactory result. Commonly, tendinosis or ruptures of the tendon can lead to weakness, as a result of either tendon discontinuity or pain. The tibialis posterior and peroneal tendons are particularly important in maintaining balance of the hindfoot.

Examination of Stance and Gait

Standing examination of the foot and ankle includes assessments of ankle and hindfoot varus/valgus, arch height, forefoot position, and toe deformity. View the feet from front, back, and sides to note varus and valgus deformities (Figure 8.1).

Observe the patient's gait for antalgia, weakness, contracture, and asymmetry between the left and right legs. Walking with the foot in an externally rotated position is a reliable, but non-specific, indicator of severe pain, and to a lesser degree of stiffness in a heel-to-toe gait. Functionally, this compensatory external rotation, which occurs at the hip, allows limb progression without ankle or hindfoot motion.

Investigations

Proper evaluation requires weightbearing radiographs of the ankle and foot, without which accurate diagnosis is not possible. When standing films are precluded because of severe pain or acute injury, simulated weightbearing radiographs with the patient seated and holding the foot in a position as close to plantigrade as possible are taken. Radiographic evaluation of the foot and ankle is discussed elsewhere, but it is important to understand the radiographic appearance of hindfoot valgus and varus, including calcaneal pitch, talonavicular coverage, AP and lateral talocalcaneal angles, and that special ankle–hindfoot alignment views are described[12–14]. It is important to look for subchondral sclerosis, cyst formation, and marginal osteophytes, which are a reaction to cartilage damage.

Computed tomography is an invaluable adjunct in the evaluation of the arthritic ankle and hindfoot, as it shows alignment, bone loss, and bone quality. Sagittal and axial images are easiest to acquire, but proper CT of the ankle and hindfoot should include coronal images, either primarily acquired or created through reformatting *perpendicular* to the plane of the posterior facet of the subtalar joint.

Magnetic resonance imaging is helpful in the evaluation of avascular necrosis and osteochondral lesions not shown on plain radiographs. MRI can also identify soft tissue pathology, such as tears of the tibialis posterior and peroneal tendons.

Technetium-99 bone scans are too sensitive and too non-specific to be warranted or helpful, although indium-labeled white-cell scans can help distinguish between infection and arthritis, and especially between infection and Charcot neuroarthropathy.

(a)

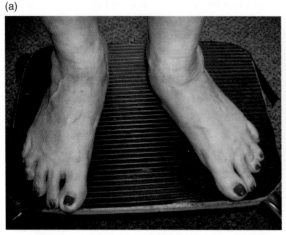

(b)

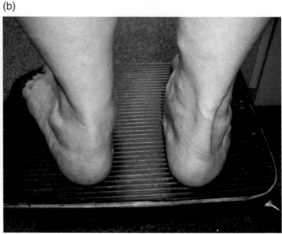

(c)

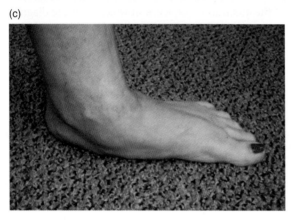

Figure 8.1 Clinical photographs of a patient with posterior tibial tendon dysfunction. Viewed from the front (**a**), note the abducted position of the left foot compared to the normal right foot. From the back (**b**), one can appreciate the increased hindfoot valgus and the "too-many-toes" sign of the left foot. Viewing the medial side of the foot (**c**), shows the loss of arch height.

Treatment

Non-Surgical Treatment

The mainstays of non-operative treatment are immobilization and anti-inflammatory medications. Injection of corticosteroids provides only transient relief, of diminishing effect with repetition and, as yet, there is no consensus on the role of visco-supplementation in arthritis of the ankle and hindfoot.

The effectiveness of bracing for arthritis of the ankle and hindfoot is largely proportionate to the restriction of motion it provides. More rigid braces such as the Arizona or posterior AFO are effective, but sometimes have poor patient acceptance due to the limitations in the shoes that accommodate them.

Surgical Treatment

While the focus of this chapter is on arthrodesis and total ankle arthroplasty (TAA), there are reports of early and mid-stage ankle arthritis treated with extra-articular realignment procedures, although the role and indications for this are not widely agreed. Examples include supramalleolar and calcaneal osteotomies undertaken for coronal-plane deformity. Realignment procedures aim to counterbalance overload of the medial or lateral portion of the ankle.

The resurgence of TAA has spawned new awareness and understanding of the biomechanical effect of hindfoot and forefoot deformities on the outcome of ankle surgery, and the need to correct foot deformity to prevent failure of TAA. To successfully reconstruct varus or valgus malalignment of the ankle and hindfoot with surgery requires an understanding of its relation to associated fixed deformities of the midfoot or forefoot.

Neither open nor arthroscopic debridement is a reliable procedure for "conservative" treatment of "early" arthritis of the ankle.

Ankle Arthritis

The two most commonly performed procedures for the treatment of end-stage ankle arthritis are ankle fusion and TAA. Ankle arthrodesis is the well-established procedure with a high success and satisfaction rate. Total ankle arthroplasty was first attempted in the 1970s, but poor results led to it being abandoned. Subsequently TAA has enjoyed a revival. While TAA continues to grow in popularity and frequency, there are still many indications for fusion, which remains an excellent treatment[15].

The resurgence of TAA has come as a result of new implant designs and improved surgical techniques that have lengthened implant survival. While a consensus has yet to be reached with regard to the advantages and disadvantages of TAA compared to arthrodesis, TAA has been firmly established in the current armamentarium of treatments for ankle arthritis.

A wealth of experience has shown the effectiveness of ankle arthrodesis in relieving the pain of ankle arthritis. While obtaining osseous union is of vital importance, it is not the only measure of success. Careful apposition of the bone surfaces and appropriate alignment are essential to a successful outcome. The principles for arthroplasty are more complex, because correction of the associated deformities of the foot is also required for successful long-term results.

One of the major concerns that many patients express is the worry of losing motion after an arthrodesis. It is important to advise patients, as well as remembering yourself, that most patients have already lost a great deal of their motion once the arthritis has progressed to the point of reconstruction. Recent data have shown a less than 5° loss of sagittal-plane motion after ankle arthrodesis[9]. Nevertheless, the debate about the relative advantages and disadvantages of arthrodesis compared to arthroplasty continues at the current time. Fortunately, new studies are underway to prospectively compare the two treatments, although the likely result will be to distinguish among the indications for each, rather than the superiority of one over the other.

Ankle Arthrodesis

Ankle arthrodesis is well established in producing pain relief and patient satisfaction. Much has been written regarding hypermobility of the joints adjacent and distal to the ankle joint following fusion. This hypermobility is thought to be compensatory for the stiffness of the arthrodesis. However, it has never been proven that this is a result specifically of the arthrodesis, as opposed to the stiffness of the tibiotalar joint from the ankle arthritis that necessitated the fusion. It has been noted that after fusion of the ankle, motion in the subtalar and medial column joints is increased. Again, we do not have prospective studies to prove when and how much of this change precedes or follows the surgery. One study showed a difference in subtalar range of motion of about 4° and medial column motion increased by 2°. This study found that an improved quality of life was associated with the increased secondary hindfoot and midfoot motion after ankle arthrodesis. The authors postulated that statistically significant increases in motion of the foot joints distal to the fusion may be necessary to develop a functional gait after fusion[16]. In any case, it is well established that patients with ankle arthrodesis have a functional and painless gait that is often clinically indistinguishable from normal.

Arthrodesis can be undertaken through a variety of approaches (anterior, posterior, lateral (transfibular), medial), mini-arthrotomies, or arthroscopically[7, 17–28]. Likewise, a wide range of fixation techniques are reported to be successful, including crossed or parallel screws, external fixation, and plating. There are no convincing data as to which technique is best. The decision is left to the surgeon as to which method is most appropriate.

However, four principles are common to all techniques: careful articular surface preparation, rigid fixation, protected non-weightbearing postoperatively, and proper alignment of the arthrodesis. Surface preparation requires complete removal of cartilage and soft tissue, and exposure of cancellous, or bleeding, bone surfaces.

Sagittal alignment should be within 5° of neutral (plantigrade), coronal alignment should be mild valgus of approximately 5°, and external rotation should be about 5 to 10°[29]. Slight dorsiflexion is better tolerated than plantar flexion, which causes knee extension ("back-knee" gait).

For uncomplicated, primary arthrodesis, the authors prefer an anterior mini-arthrotomy of about 5 cm; preparation of the opposing surfaces of the tibia and talus with both malleoli and the medial and lateral sides of the talus being prepared; fixation is with three large cannulated screws, placed under fluoroscopic control. The first is directed from the posterior tibia, through the center of the talar dome, and into the talar neck; the second is from the infero-lateral talus in a superior direction, through the sinus tarsi into the posteromedial tibia; the third is from the anterior tibia into the posterior talar body. Any two screws are perpendicular to each other, producing maximum stability. A bone graft of the surgeon's choice is placed to fill small voids, especially in the gutters between the talus and malleoli (Figure 8.2).

The initial splint is replaced with a cast at 10 to 14 days postoperatively. The patient is maintained non-weightbearing for six to eight weeks, followed by four to six weeks of weight bearing in a cast or removable boot.

Total Ankle Arthroplasty

Two concepts have propelled the resurgence of TAA. Firstly, the preservation of tibiotalar motion, with presumed greater normality of function; and, secondly, the hope that maintenance of tibiotalar motion will delay the onset, or at least decrease the progression, of arthritic changes in the adjacent hindfoot and midfoot joints.

Most TAA is performed through an anterior approach, although one recent design uses a lateral approach through a fibular osteotomy. While the details of the surgical technique vary according to the specific prosthesis, five principles are universal and of paramount importance: minimal soft tissue handling; excellent press-fit between bone and implant; correction of deformity at the ankle, primarily coronal-plane alignment; concomitant ligament and tendon reconstruction; and correction of any foot deformity that would adversely affect longevity of the implant.

Not just meticulous, but minimal, soft tissue handling dramatically decreases the wound-healing complications of the anterior incision, effected by using a long incision to minimize tension, retracting only when and where actively working, and avoidance of self-retaining retractors. Creating an excellent bone–implant interface requires familiarity with the instrumentation and improves with surgeon experience. Meticulous attention to detail cannot be substituted.

Correction of coronal-plane deformity requires a combination of both bone and soft tissue techniques. Intraoperative radiographic control is used to assure that the tibial jig creates the transverse tibial cut in the appropriate varus–valgus alignment. Most

prostheses then reference the horizontal cut of the talus from the tibial cut and its jig, so that the tibial and talar cuts are parallel. After performing the tibial cut, but before the talar cut, talar balancing with the tibial cut is achieved by debriding the gutters, medial soft tissue release of the deltoid ligament, and even bone debridement of the margins of the talus or malleoli. Alignment is confirmed radiographically so that the talus is level in the coronal plane and not extruded anteriorly.

Ligamentous reconstruction is usually the last step, once the implants have been inserted. Experience has shown that lateral instability may exist both with varus and valgus deformities of the ankle. Ligamentous reconstruction is most commonly required on the lateral side. A number of techniques can be used, which include a modified Broström method using a bone anchor in the fibula, or use of a part of the peroneus brevis tendon tensioned through a hole in the fibula. Peroneal tendon reconstruction may also be required, as some patients with severe ankle arthritis have chronic instability and associated peroneal tendon tears or instability.

Coronal plane deformities greater than 15 to 20° were once thought to be a contraindication to TAA, but newer literature suggests that successful TAA is a possibility, even in the presence of more severe deformity. Varus deformity of the ankle is likely to cause early failure of the implant. Authors vary in their approach to the correction of combined ankle and foot deformity. The first decision is whether to fix the ankle and foot at the same time or sequentially; and, if sequentially, in which order. Some authors have temporarily realigned the ankle by placing methyl methacrylate cement in the ankle joint after soft tissue release. The hindfoot is then corrected around the realigned talus, with a triple arthrodesis or extra-articular procedures. The TAA is then undertaken as a secondary procedure with removal of the cement. Others subscribe to the principle of correction from proximal to distal, beginning with the total ankle replacement and returning at a subsequent surgical session to correct the fixed deformity of the hindfoot and forefoot.

Postoperative care includes non-weightbearing and immobilization in a splint or cast for four to six weeks, or at least until the incision heals. The patient is then transitioned into a removable boot to begin progressive weight bearing and range of motion exercises of the ankle (Figure 8.3).

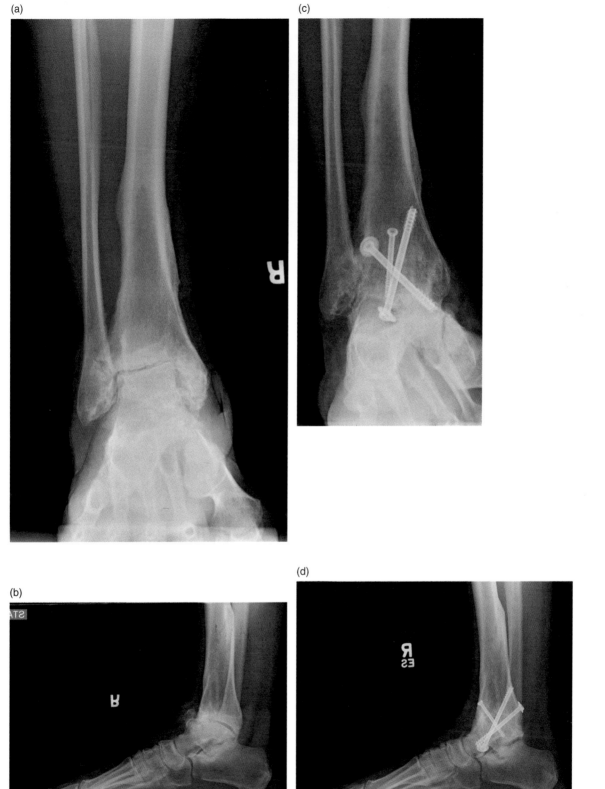

Figure 8.2 (a) Mortise, and (b) lateral radiographs demonstrating end-stage ankle arthritis. Notice the varus deformity in the mortise view. Also note the anterior translation of the talus relative to the tibial plafond on the lateral view. (c) Mortise, and (d) lateral views after successful ankle fusion. Notice the correction of ankle alignment in the coronal plane and the correction of talar alignment in the sagittal plane.

(a)

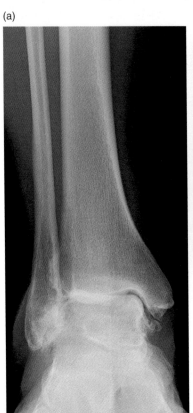

(c)

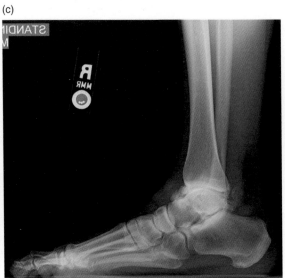

(b)

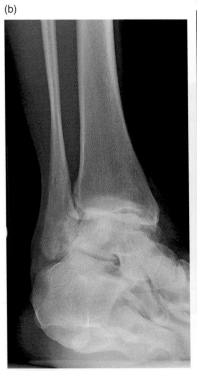

(d)

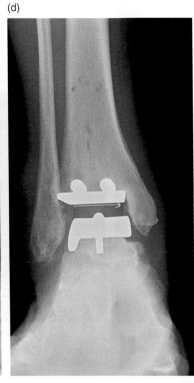

Figure 8.3 (**a**) Anteroposterior, (**b**) oblique, and (**c**) lateral views of an ankle with end-stage arthritis. Notice that the oblique view is an over-rotated mortise. We often obtain this view in practice as it provides a helpful assessment of the posterior facet of the subtalar joint. Mortise (**d**) and lateral (**e**) views of the ankle after total ankle replacement.

(e)

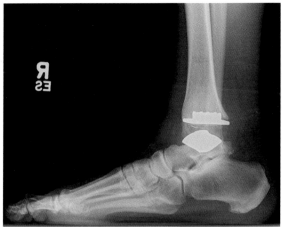

Figure 8.3 *(cont.)*

Contraindications to TAA include active infection, prior osteomyelitis, peripheral neuropathy, Charcot neuroarthropathy of the foot or ankle, and avascular necrosis of the talus.

Triple Arthrodesis

Triple arthrodesis is a workhorse operation performed for a multitude of disorders presenting with hindfoot arthritis or deformity. As with ankle arthrodesis, a multitude of studies demonstrate an increase in radiographic arthritis of the ankle joint after triple or subtalar arthrodesis, but the clinical impact of this radiological change is not well quantified[30–35].

The reason triple arthrodesis is so important is that it allows realignment of the hindfoot in all three planes. However, the technical difficulty is such that it requires great skill and significant judgment in order to achieve satisfactory results; it is far more technically challenging than most joint arthroplasty, as there are no jigs to guide the surgeon.

Issues in triple arthrodesis include: surgical approach; method of surface preparation; type of fixation; order of joint fixation; and use of bone graft.

Surgical approaches can be combined medial and lateral, or extensile single-lateral incisions. In the cases of severe damage to the soft tissue envelope laterally, the procedure can be done through a medial incision[86]. The latter is technically challenging, not so much because of the medial neurovascular structures but because it is more difficult to visualize proper alignment from the medial side.

Articular surface preparation can be by a number of techniques. The surgical principle is to remove all cartilage, soft tissue, and sclerotic bone, while maximally preserving the native shape of the joints, especially the subtalar joint. It is important to understand that correction of deformity through joint rotation, as opposed to simple wedging into varus or valgus, maximizes bone contact and stability as well as correcting the deformity. Visualization is greatly enhanced by distraction with a laminar spreader. The authors use hand-instruments, namely, curettes and osteotomes, rinse the joints, then roughen the surfaces by wide and shallow drilling or fish-scaling with an osteotome.

The talonavicular joint is the most difficult to distract, see, and prepare. This leads to it having the highest non-union rate of the three joints. The authors always debride the navicular surface before the talus, to prevent accidental crushing of the talar head, which is softened by removal of the subchondral bone.

The subtalar joint is fixed first, in order to align the heel in valgus. Many techniques are acceptable. The authors prefer a screw from the neck of the talus into the body of the calcaneus, through the posterior facet, because it is rarely symptomatic, unless too long, and because one can use a screw with a long thread, thus gaining more secure fixation. We routinely use axial heel views in the intraoperative fluoroscopy to determine screw length. A second screw may be added for enhanced fixation and rotational control. We prefer a screw from the inferior portion of the lateral calcaneus into the body of the talus (shown in an isolated subtalar fusion in Figure 8.4). Care must be taken to avoid penetration of the ankle joint.

The talonavicular joint is fixed next. Techniques for fixation vary widely, with the use of screws or even plates. However, the most important thing is to understand how crucial it is to achieve proper alignment of the talonavicular joint before fixation. This may require provisional fixation with pins and radiographic confirmation of position before placement of definitive fixation. As their alignment is linked it is frequently necessary to make adjustments to the bony configuration of both the talonavicular and the calcaneocuboid joints, to achieve proper position in all three planes: pronation–supination, adduction-abduction, and plantar flexion–dorsiflexion. Correct positioning of the forefoot on the hindfoot, through

(a)

(b)

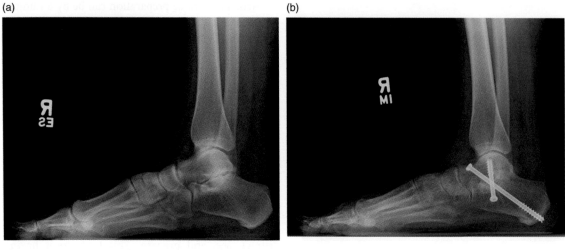

Figure 8.4 (a) An example of a patient with isolated subtalar arthritis. Note the joint-space narrowing of the subtalar joint and unaffected talonavicular and calcaneocuboid joints. (b) Following successful subtalar fusion. Note the orientation of the two screws with one placed from the talar neck across the posterior facet of the calcaneus and the other placed from the lateral calcaneus into the body of the talus.

the midfoot, is the most technically challenging portion of the operation.

The calcaneocuboid joint is fixed last. It is the most forgiving and the joint with the lowest non-union rate. It can be augmented with bone graft to accommodate changes in alignment. A technical pearl is to assure that the calcaneocuboid joint is fixed in mild flexion. Any extension at this location simulates hindfoot varus and will be painful once the patient resumes walking (Figure 8.5).

Of course, each step of the fixation is undertaken under fluoroscopic control in at least two orthogonal planes. The wound is closed in layers over a non-clotting silicone suction drain to reduce hematoma and wound-healing complications. The patient is kept non-weightbearing in a postoperative splint and then a cast for six to eight weeks, followed by walking casts, and then a walking boot, for a total of three months.

Single and Double Arthrodesis of the Hindfoot

The most common fusion undertaken in the hindfoot is an isolated subtalar arthrodesis (Figure 8.4). This is often performed for post-traumatic arthritis following calcaneal fracture and is highly successful at relieving pain. It is also commonly used in the correction of hindfoot deformity associated with varus or valgus. The most common technique involves debridement through an open incision and screw fixation. The fine points of surgical technique include consideration of inclusion of the anterior and middle facets of

the subtalar joint in the arthrodesis. The latter is required in the presence of severe deformity in order to achieve sufficient realignment. It is important to realize that intraoperative alignment of the arthrodesis is not only related to varus/valgus, but that rotation is the key element. External rotation of the calcaneus on the talus produces valgus; internal rotation produces varus. Indeed simple derotation can correct the alignment, and make bone grafting with structural grafts or implants unnecessary. This is, of course, true for triple fusions, as well as for simple subtalar fusion.

Double arthrodesis is used for less extensive arthritis of the hindfoot. Most commonly it is a combined talonavicular and calcaneocuboid fusion. This has the advantage of being a more durable construct than isolated talonavicular fusion because of the wider fusion mass and the ability to realign both in varus–valgus and adduction–abduction, which cannot be easily done with fusion of a single joint (Figure 8.6). Be prepared to use a bone graft in single or double fusion, because of the common disparity in medial and lateral column lengths, once the foot is realigned.

Double arthrodesis of the subtalar and talonavicular joints has been proposed as a procedure that can be performed in the setting of a relatively unaffected calcaneocuboid joint[36]. It can be performed through a standard two-incision approach or through a single medial incision[37]. The postoperative protocol is the same as that described for triple arthrodesis.

(a)

(b)

(c)

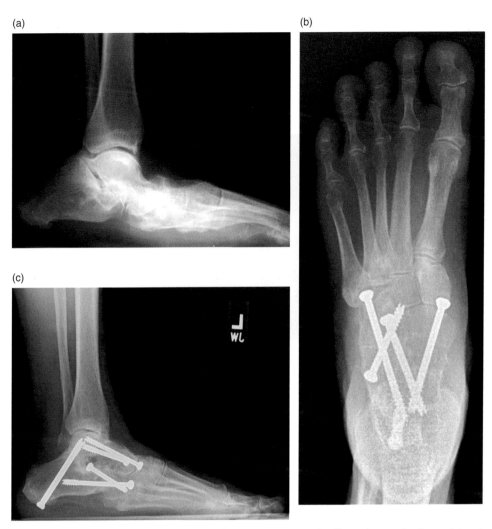

Figure 8.5 (a) A preoperative lateral radiograph of a patient with severe hindfoot arthritis and collapse of the talonavicular joint. Postoperative anteroposterior (b), and lateral (c), radiographs after successful realignment and fusion with a triple arthrodesis.

Tibiotalocalcaneal Arthrodesis

Combined arthritis of the both the ankle and subtalar joints is frequent and can be treated with a combination of TAA and subtalar arthrodesis, or with tibiotalocalcaneal (TTC) arthrodesis. TTC arthrodesis has been shown to have a high fusion rate and a high success rate for salvage of severe deformity, painful arthritis of both joints, and in cases with extensive bone loss[38–46].

The principles of the surgical approach and joint preparation, as well as deformity correction, are as described above for isolated arthrodeses. While any number of fixation techniques are possible, the authors prefer the use of a compressing, retrograde intramedullary nail, which has been shown to increase the rate of primary union[46].

Fixation with a retrograde intramedullary nail is facilitated by proper preparation of the joint surfaces, with good apposition of the bone surfaces. Alignment is made easier by medialization of the talus and foot at the ankle; this corrects the slight lateral offset of the longitudinal access of the calcaneus, compared to that of the tibia. Thus medialization of the ankle allows the guide wire entry point in the calcaneus to align with the medullary canal of the tibia. The alternative is to use a curved nail to allow for this offset. There are several nails available on the market. Both straight and curved nails have been shown to be successful[38–43,46]. The authors prefer the enhanced compression afforded by a straight nail (Figure 8.7).

Postoperative care is similar to ankle and triple arthrodesis, with slightly longer periods of immobilization and non-weightbearing.

Combined Ankle and Triple Arthrodeses (Pantalar Arthrodesis)

As with TTC arthrodesis, pantalar arthrodesis is considered a salvage procedure and is a reasonable

(a)

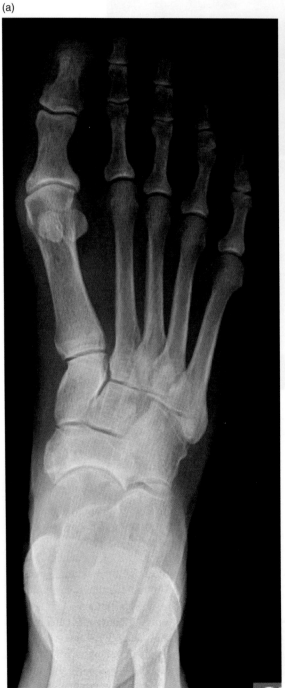

(b)

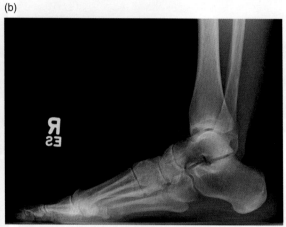

Figure 8.6 Preoperative anteroposterior (**a**), and lateral (**b**), radiographs demonstrating isolated talonavicular arthritis. Postoperative anteroposterior (**c**), and lateral (**d**), radiographs following successful double arthrodesis.

(c)

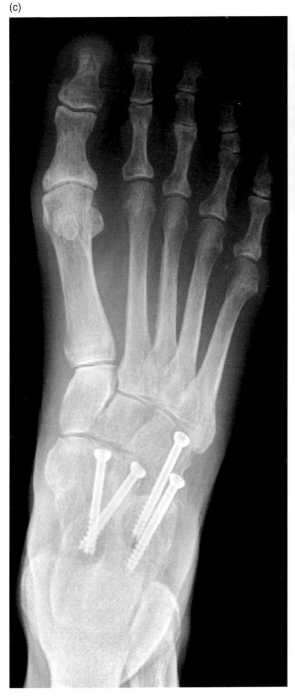

(d)

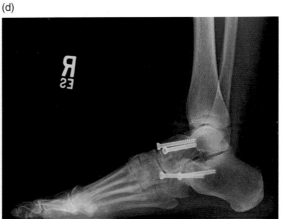

Figure 8.6 *(cont.)*

alternative to amputation[45]. Technically, pantalar arthrodesis involves all joints involved with the talus, but most often it is more accurately described as a combined ankle and triple arthrodesis. Outcomes of patients with inflammatory arthropathy,

post-traumatic arthritis, and diabetic neuropathy treated with pantalar arthrodesis generally result in significant symptomatic improvement[47–48]. An alternative treatment for patients with pantalar arthritis is triple arthrodesis combined with TAA, which can be

(a)

(c)

(b)

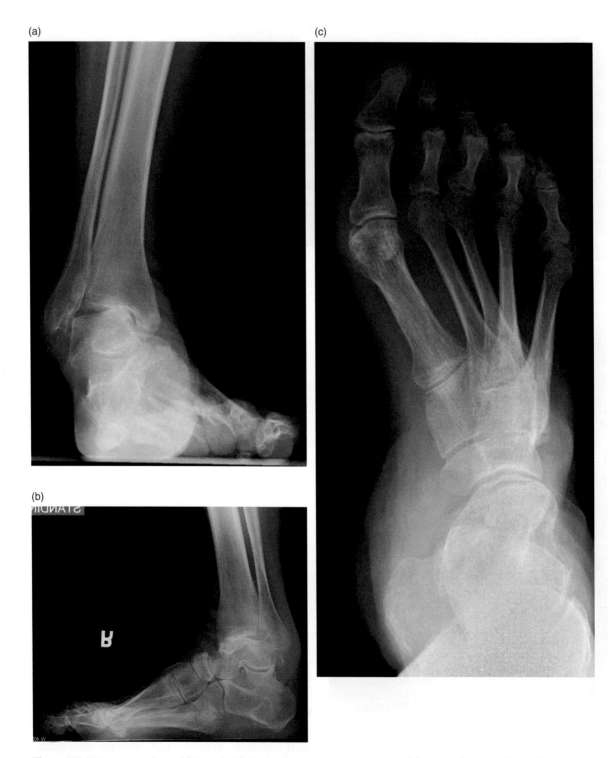

Figure 8.7 (a) Anteroposterior, and (b) lateral, radiographs of a patient with severe varus deformity and arthritis of the ankle joint. The AP radiograph (c) of the foot demonstrates significant supination of the midfoot and forefoot as a result of the ankle deformity. Images (d) and (e) demonstrate successful fusion after tibiotalocalcaneal arthrodesis with a straight hindfoot nail. Note the correction of coronal-plane alignment on the AP radiograph compared to the preoperative image.

(d)

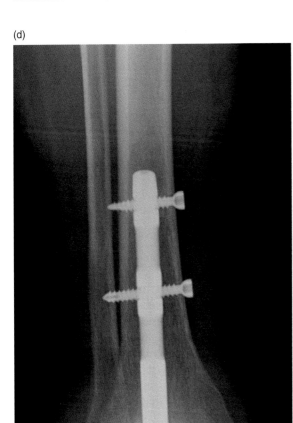

(e)

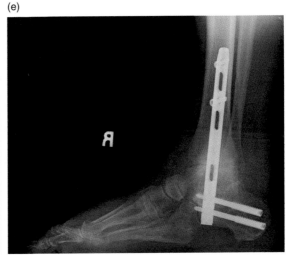

Figure 8.7 (cont.)

performed in a single setting or as a staged procedure. Much remains undetermined regarding the long-term results of combined extensive-arthrodesis and ankle arthroplasty. On one hand the clear advantage functionally is the preservation of ankle-joint motion in the absence of hindfoot motion. However, some surgeons believe there is increased stress on the implant as result of the hindfoot stiffness, potentially reducing the longevity of the total ankle implant.

Results and Complications

Ankle Arthrodesis

Ankle arthrodesis is a reliable procedure with union rates of between 80 and 100%[18–26,49–52]. Interestingly, very few studies actually document the position of the arthrodesis, so we lack information on the effect of biomechanical factors on fusion rates and functional

157

outcomes. The long-term success of arthrodesis has also proven durable, with 91% of patients reporting satisfaction at a mean follow-up of nine years[18].

The most common complication is non-union. Risk factors for the development of non-union include previous open fractures, fractures involving the talus, combined talar and tibial plafond fractures, AVN, neurologic deficits, infection, smoking, and patients with major medical problems[87].It is clinically accepted that non-union rate is increased by early weight bearing, extensive soft tissue stripping, poor surface preparation, and the presence of prior hindfoot arthrodesis.

Progression of subtalar arthritis has been identified in 33 to 37% of patients after ankle arthrodesis at final radiographic follow-up[7,50]. Despite the radiological findings, patients may not complain of subtalar pain with these changes[18].

Arthroscopic ankle arthrodesis has been shown to result in equivalent union rates, shorter hospital stays, and faster time to obtaining solid fusion in comparison to open arthrodesis[17,28]. While at least one study has shown deformity correction with the arthroscopic approach[19], most surgeons find deformity correction easier with open techniques.

Total Ankle Arthroplasty Outcomes

Good patient outcomes with improved quality of life and reduced pain following TAA are now documented. There are also longer term data demonstrating improvement in TAA survivorship[53–54]. One prospective controlled trial of TAA versus ankle arthrodesis was a non-inferiority study, which confirmed that at 24 months following surgery ankles treated with a Scandinavian total ankle replacement (STAR) ankle replacement had better function and equivalent pain relief, compared to ankles treated with fusion[55].

Other comparisons of TAA to arthrodesis have also been published. In a large non-randomized report, intermediate-term data comparing the two procedures demonstrated a major complication rate of 19% in the TAA group compared to 7% in the arthrodesis group. Both groups in the study had improvements in outcome measures. While the complication rates were higher in the TAA group, the study showed that the differences between the two groups were small after adjustment for baseline characteristics and surgeon[56].

Another study reported that rates of reoperation after ankle replacement were 9% at one year and 23% at five years. This was compared to 5% and 11% respectively in ankle arthrodesis. The arthrodesis patients had a higher rate of subtalar fusion at five years postoperatively of 2.8% compared with 0.7%. Regression analysis confirmed a significant increase in the risk of major revision surgery of 1.93 with TAA, but a lower risk of subtalar fusion of 0.28[57].

Data on the long-term implant survivorship for the STAR is generally positive. One study reported implant survival of 96% at five years and 90% at ten years[58]. In another study, STAR survivorship was reported as 90% at five years and 84% at eight years. In that study, 11% underwent component revision and two were converted to fusion. The overall complication rate was 21% and subsequent surgery (excluding component revision) was necessary in 17%[59]. The most recent data on the STAR demonstrated improvements in the disability, pain, and SF-36 score at intermediate to long-term follow-up. A 12% rate of metal component revision and 18% rate of polyethylene failure at a mean of five years was reported in this study[60].

Short-term data for a two-component fixed-bearing TAA (Salto Talaris) reported 67 patients with a mean follow-up of 2.8 years. Implant survival was 96%. This used revision of the metallic component, implant removal, or impending implant failure as the endpoint. Additional procedures at the time of the index surgery were performed in 45 patients, most commonly a deltoid ligament release. Eight patients underwent additional surgery after the primary procedure[61].

Wound-healing problems are the most common complication of TAA. A retrospective review of TAA patients showed that diabetes significantly increased the risk of wound-healing problems. Female sex, history of corticosteroid use, and underlying inflammatory arthritis were all associated with an increased risk. Inflammatory arthritis was the most significant risk factor for major wound complications requiring reoperation[62].

Gutter impingement is also a common complication; in one study it had an incidence of 7% in patients followed for at least one year[63], although it increases with time and varies according to the type of prosthesis.

Gait Studies for Ankle Arthroplasty and Arthrodesis

Ankle arthritis causes severe functional limitation[64]. In a study comparing patients with end-stage ankle arthritis to normal controls, the arthritic patients were found to take fewer total steps per day, to take fewer high-intensity steps, and to walk at a slower speed. Gait analysis in this study showed decreased total ankle motion, as well as decreased peak ankle plantar flexor moment, peak ankle power absorbed, and peak ankle power generated when compared to the normal ankle[65].

In a gait study evaluating patients who had undergone ankle arthrodesis, significant differences were identified between healthy controls and postoperative patients in cadence (steps per minute) and stride length. The arthrodesis group also showed significantly decreased sagittal, coronal, and transverse range of motion of the hindfoot and midfoot during the stance and swing phases of gait[52].

Only two studies have prospectively compared the gait of arthritic patients before and after TAA and arthrodesis[9–10]. Both studies showed that the majority of parameters of gait improved significantly following both arthrodesis and arthroplasty, when compared to their preoperative function. There were two other important findings: firstly, neither TAA nor arthrodesis showed conclusively better results and, secondly, neither group achieved gait parameters equivalent to the normal controls. Patients with TAA had a higher walking velocity and more normalized first and second gait rockers compared to the arthrodesis group. Patients with TAA also had significantly better dorsiflexion, whereas arthrodesis patients had better coronal-plane eversion. Total ankle arthroplasty produced a more symmetric vertical ground reaction force curve than the arthrodesis group[9]. One of the studies comparing arthroplasty and arthrodesis groups demonstrated improvements in both pain and gait function. There was an increased range of hip movement in the arthrodesis group and an increase in the range of ankle movement in the TAA group[10].

Postoperative gait analysis of TAA patients was compared to arthrodesis patients and to normal controls: TAA patients demonstrated greater postoperative sagittal-plane motion, with 18.1°, versus arthrodesis patients, with 13.7°. What is striking is how little difference there was in motion between the arthroplasty and arthrodesis groups. Neither treatment group had normalized gait patterns compared to the control group, and there was similar improvement in the ankle osteoarthritis scale and SF-36 in both treatment groups[66].

Hindfoot Arthrodesis

Triple arthrodesis has been reported to be a generally successful operation with high satisfaction rates of greater than 90% with few complications[67–68]. The most common complications are malunion, non-union, and wound-healing problems. Progression of surrounding joint arthritis is also commonly noted after triple arthrodesis and usually occurs in the midfoot joints[69]. Interestingly subtalar or triple arthrodesis has little adverse influence on the function of the tibiotalar joint, even after many years[88].

High union rates after double arthrodesis (talonavicular and subtalar joints) have also been reported. One study reported an overall satisfaction rate of 78%[37].

Not all studies demonstrate acceptable results after triple arthrodesis. In a study of patients with Charcot–Marie–Tooth disease who underwent the procedure, 15% of patients developed a talonavicular non-union[70]. In this study, there were a large number of unsatisfactory results with problems related to recurrent, progressive deformity. With these findings in mind, it has been postulated that tendon rebalancing with transfer of the posterior tibialis tendon will prevent the recurrence, or perhaps undercorrection, of the deformity[71–72].

Another complication that has been reported with some frequency in the literature is lateral wound dehiscence[73–76]. This is postulated to result from the tension placed on the lateral skin after deformity correction, specifically in cases of severe hindfoot valgus correction.

Gait outcomes after triple or double arthrodesis have been evaluated in patients who were an average of 5.2 years post-surgery. Of the 13 patients studied, ten rated their outcome as good or excellent. There was a 13% increase in flexion of the ipsilateral knee during third rocker. Ankle range of motion decreased by 33%. There was a 6° loss of plantar flexion at toe-off, which accounted for the decrease in ankle range of motion. There was a mean 13% reduction in the peak ankle dorsiflexion moment and 45% reduction in mean maximum power generation at the ankle[35,77].

Studies of isolated talonavicular arthrodesis have shown non-union rates of 10% in healthy patients and up to 37% in patients with inflammatory arthropathy[35,78–80] Despite this, clinical satisfaction is generally high in cases of isolated talonavicular arthrodesis[30].

High fusion rates have been reported after isolated subtalar arthrodesis. In one study, the use of a single lag screw resulted in 98% fusion rate[81]. In another, the rate of union of subtalar arthrodesis was found to be significantly diminished by smoking, more than two millimeters of avascular bone at the arthrodesis site, and the failure of previous subtalar arthrodesis. This study demonstrated primary fusion was achieved in 86% of patients. The rate of fusion among non-smokers, however, was 92% – as opposed to 73% for smokers. Seventy-one percent of patients undergoing revision achieved union[82].

Outcomes of TTC Arthrodesis

Overall union rates after TTC arthrodesis have been reported as being between 84 and 100%[38–40,42–44,83–84]. Gait evaluation after combined ankle and subtalar arthrodesis demonstrates significant increases in gait velocity, decreased total support time, and improvement in gait symmetry. There was only a small decrease in sagittal-plane ankle motion from 0.3° to 10°[85].

One study demonstrated an 82% satisfaction rate. Complications included deep infection, amputation, stress fracture, non-union, and prominent hardware[41]. Another study found that the use of a retrograde intramedullary nail was satisfactory for coronal-plane deformity correction (average correction 13°),with a demonstrated union rate of 97% and improved clinical outcomes with an increase in the AOFAS ankle/hindfoot score from 30 to 74, an increase in SF-36 score from 86 to 99, and a decrease in the visual analogue score (VAS) from 6.5 to 1.3.

Complications included three cases of tibial stress reaction, at the proximal extent of the nail, three of transient plantar nerve irritation, and three cases of wound infection[46].

A multicenter retrospective study on the use of a hindfoot nail for TTC arthrodesis evaluated results in 38 patients. The overall union rate was 84%. The complication rate was 24% and included a 16% non-union rate. Fifteen of the 19 employed patients in the group retained their working status[38].

Key Points

- Disability from ankle osteoarthritis is equivalent to that of end-stage kidney disease and congestive heart failure.
- Fracture or chronic ligamentous ankle instability causes 78% of all ankle arthritis.
- Ankle fusion should be with the foot plantigrade, in mild (5° of) valgus and with external rotation of about 5 to 10°.
- The long-term success of ankle arthrodesis has proven durable, with 91% of patients reporting satisfaction at a mean follow-up of nine years.
- The best results with TAA show implant survival of 96% at five years and 90% at ten years.
- Total ankle arthroplasty has a 1.93 times increased risk of major revision surgery compared to ankle arthrodesis, but a lower risk of subtalar fusion of 0.28.
- Total ankle arthroplasty has been shown not to be inferior to ankle arthrodesis at 24 months.
- In performing a triple fusion, the subtalar joint is fixed first, to establish heel valgus. The talonavicular and calcaneocuboid joints are fixed in sequence to position the forefoot in neutral relative to the hindfoot.
- In neuromuscular disease, rebalancing the foot with tendon transfers should be considered in combination with the fusion.

References

1. Saltzman CL, Zimmerman MB, O'Rourke M, Brown TD, Buckwalter JA, Johnston R. Impact of comorbidities on the measurement of health in patients with ankle osteoarthritis. *J Bone Joint Surg Am.* 2006; 88:11, 2366–72.

2. Valderrabano V, Horisberger M, Russell I, Dougall H, Hintermann B. Etiology of ankle osteoarthritis. *Clin Orthop Relat Res.* 2009; 467:7, 1800–6.

3. Ateshian GA, Soslowsky LJ, Mow VC. Quantitation of articular surface topography and cartilage thickness in knee joints using stereophotogrammetry. *J Biomech.* 1991; 24:8, 761–76.

4. Athanasiou KA, Niederauer GG, Schenck RC Jr. Biomechanical topography of human ankle cartilage. *Ann Biomed Eng.* 1995; 23:5, 697–704.

5. Cushnaghan J, Dieppe P. Study of 500 patients with limb joint osteoarthritis. I. Analysis by age, sex, and distribution of symptomatic joint sites. *Ann Rheum Dis.* 1991; 50, 8–13.

6. Jung HG, Parks BG, Nguyen A, Schon LC. Effect of tibiotalar joint arthrodesis on adjacent tarsal joint pressure in a cadaver model. *Foot Ankle Int.* 2007; 28:1, 103–8.

7. Takakura Y, Tanaka Y, Sugimoto K, Akiyama K, Tamai S. Long-term results of arthrodesis for osteoarthritis of the ankle. *Clin Orthop Relat Res.* 1999; 361, 178–85.

8. Sheridan BD, Robinson DE, Hubble MJ, Winson IG. Ankle arthrodesis and its relationship to ipsilateral arthritis of the hind- and mid-foot. *J Bone Joint Surg Br.* 2006; 88:2, 206–7.

9. Flavin R, Coleman SC, Tenenbaum S, Brodsky JW. Comparison of gait after total ankle arthroplasty and ankle arthrodesis. *Foot Ankle Int.* 2013; 34:10, 1340–8.

10. Hahn ME, Wright ES, Segal AD, Orendurff MS, Ledoux WR, Sangeorzan BJ. Comparative gait analysis of ankle arthrodesis and arthroplasty: initial findings of a prospective study. *Foot Ankle Int.* 2012; 33:4, 282–9.

11. Tanaka Y, Takakura Y, Hayashi K, Taniguchi A, Kumai T, Sugimoto K. Low tibial osteotomy for varus-type osteoarthritis of the ankle. *J Bone Joint Surg Br.* 2006; 88:7, 909–13.

12. Saltzman CL, el-Khoury GY. The hindfoot alignment view. *Foot Ankle Int.* 1995; 16:9, 572–6.

13. Sangeorzan BJ, Mosca V, Hansen ST Jr. Effect of calcaneal lengthening on relationships among the hindfoot, midfoot, and forefoot. *Foot Ankle.* 1993; 14:3, 136–41.

14. Saltzman CL, Brandser EA, Berbaum KS, et al. Reliability of standard foot radiographic measurements. *Foot Ankle Int.* 1994; 15:12, 661–5.

15. Pugely AJ, Lu X, Amendola A, Callaghan JJ, Martin CT, Cram P. Trends in the use of total ankle replacement and ankle arthrodesis in the United States medicare population. *Foot Ankle Int.* 2014; 35:3, 207–15.

16. Sealey RJ, Myerson MS, Molloy A, Gamba C, Jeng C, Kalesan B. Sagittal plane motion of the hindfoot following ankle arthrodesis: a prospective analysis. *Foot Ankle Int.* 2009; 30:3, 187–9.

17. Townshend D, Di Silvestro M, Krause F, et al. Arthroscopic versus open ankle arthrodesis: a multicenter comparative case series. *J Bone Joint Surg Am.* 2013; 95:2, 98–102.

18. Hendrickx RP, Stufkens SA, de Bruijn EE, Sierevelt IN, van Dijk CN, Kerkhoffs GM. Medium- to long-term outcome of ankle arthrodesis. *Foot Ankle Int.* 2011; 32:10, 940–7.

19. Dannawi Z, Nawabi DH, Patel A, Leong JJ, Moore DJ. Arthroscopic ankle arthrodesis: are results reproducible irrespective of pre-operative deformity? *Foot Ankle Surg.* 2011; 17:4, 294–9.

20. Guo C, Yan Z, Barfield WR, Hartsock LA. Ankle arthrodesis using anatomically contoured anterior plate. *Foot Ankle Int.* 2010; 31:6, 492–8.

21. Plaass C, Knupp M, Barg A, Hintermann B. Anterior double plating for rigid fixation of isolated tibiotalar arthrodesis. *Foot Ankle Int.* 2009; 30:7, 631–9.

22. Gougoulias NE, Agathangelidis FG, Parsons SW. Arthroscopic ankle arthrodesis. *Foot Ankle Int.* 2007; 28:6, 695–706.

23. Rippstein P, Kumar B, Müller M. Ankle arthrodesis using the arthroscopic technique. *Oper Orthop Traumatol.* 2005; 17:4–5, 442–56.

24. Ferkel RD, Hewitt M. Long-term results of arthroscopic ankle arthrodesis. *Foot Ankle Int.* 2005; 26:4, 275–80.

25. Winson IG, Robinson DE, Allen PE. Arthroscopic ankle arthrodesis. *J Bone Joint Surg Br.* 2005; 87:3, 343–7.

26. Cameron SE, Ullrich P. Arthroscopic arthrodesis of the ankle joint. *Arthroscopy.* 2000; 16:1, 21–6.

27. Paremain GD, Miller SD, Myerson MS. Ankle arthrodesis: results after the miniarthrotomy technique. *Foot Ankle Int.* 1996; 17:5, 247–52.

28. Myerson MS, Quill G. Ankle arthrodesis. A comparison of an arthroscopic and an open method of treatment. *Clin Orthop Relat Res.* 1991; 268, 84–95.

29. Buck P, Morrey BF, Chao EY. The optimum position of arthrodesis of the ankle. A gait study of the knee and ankle. *J Bone Joint Surg Am.* 1987; 69:7, 1052–62.

30. Pell RF 4th, Myerson MS, Schon LC. Clinical outcome after primary triple arthrodesis. *J Bone Joint Surg Am.* 2000; 82:1, 47–57.

31. Haritidis JH, Kirkos JM, Provellegios SM, Zachos AD. Long-term results of triple arthrodesis: 42 cases followed for 25 years. *Foot Ankle Int.* 1994; 15:10, 548–51.

32. Tenuta J, Shelton YA, Miller F. Long-term follow-up of triple arthrodesis in patients with cerebral palsy. *J Pediatr Orthop.* 1993; 13:6, 713–16.

33. Figgie MP, O'Malley MJ, Ranawat C, Inglis AE, Sculco TP. Triple arthrodesis in rheumatoid arthritis. *Clin Orthop Relat Res.* 1993; 292, 250–4.

34. Graves SC, Mann RA, Graves KO. Triple arthrodesis in older adults. Results after long-term follow-up. *J Bone Joint Surg Am.* 1993; 75:3, 355–62.

35. Bennett GL, Graham CE, Mauldin DM. Triple arthrodesis in adults. *Foot Ankle.* 1991; 12:3, 138–43.

36. Sammarco VJ, Magur EG, Sammarco GJ, Bagwe MR. Arthrodesis of the subtalar and talonavicular joints for correction of symptomatic hindfoot malalignment. *Foot Ankle Int.* 2006; 27:9, 661–6.

37. Anand P, Nunley JA, DeOrio JK. Single-incision medial approach for double arthrodesis of hindfoot in posterior tibialis tendon dysfunction. *Foot Ankle Int.* 2013; 34:3, 338–44.

38. Rammelt S, Pyrc J, Agren PH, et al. Tibiotalocalcaneal fusion using the hindfoot arthrodesis nail: a multicenter study. *Foot Ankle Int.* 2013; 34:9, 1245–55.

39. Budnar VM, Hepple S, Harries WG, Livingstone JA, Winson I. Tibiotalocalcaneal arthrodesis with a curved, interlocking, intramedullary nail. *Foot Ankle Int.* 2010; 31:12, 1085–92.

40. Pelton K, Hofer JK, Thordarson DB. Tibiotalocalcaneal arthrodesis using a dynamically locked retrograde intramedullary nail. *Foot Ankle Int.* 2006; 27:10, 759–63.

41. Hammett R, Hepple S, Forster B, Winson I. Tibiotalocalcaneal (hindfoot) arthrodesis by retrograde intramedullary nailing using a curved locking nail. The results of 52 procedures. *Foot Ankle Int.* 2005; 26:10, 810–15.

42. Anderson T, Linder L, Rydholm U, Montgomery F, Besjakov J, Carlsson A. Tibio-talocalcaneal arthrodesis as a primary procedure using a retrograde intramedullary nail: a retrospective study of 26 patients with rheumatoid arthritis. *Acta Orthop.* 2005; 76:4, 580–7.

43. Mendicino RW, Catanzariti AR, Saltrick KR, et al. Tibiotalocalcaneal arthrodesis with retrograde intramedullary nailing. *J Foot Ankle Surg.* 2004; 43:2, 82–6.

44. Chou LB, Mann RA, Yaszay B, et al. Tibiotalocalcaneal arthrodesis. *Foot Ankle Int.* 2000; 21:10, 804–8.

45. Papa JA, Myerson MS. Pantalar and tibiotalocalcaneal arthrodesis for post-traumatic osteoarthrosis of the ankle and hindfoot. *J Bone Joint Surg Am.* 1992; 74:7, 1042–9.

46. Brodsky JW, Verschae G, Tenenbaum S. Surgical correction of severe deformity of the ankle and hindfoot by arthrodesis using a compressing retrograde intramedullary nail. *Foot Ankle Int.* 2014; 35:4, 360–7.

47. McKinley JC, Shortt N, Arthur C, Gunner C, MacDonald D, Breusch SJ. Outcomes following pantalar arthrodesis in rheumatoid arthritis. *Foot Ankle Int.* 2011; 32:7, 681–5.

48. Herscovici D, Sammarco GJ, Sammarco VJ, Scaduto JM. Pantalar arthrodesis for post-traumatic arthritis and diabetic neuroarthropathy of the ankle and hindfoot. *Foot Ankle Int.* 2011; 32:6, 581–8.

49. Gordon D, Zicker R, Cullen N, Singh D. Open ankle arthrodeses via an anterior approach. *Foot Ankle Int.* 2013; 34:3, 386–91.

50. Strasser NL, Turner NS. Functional outcomes after ankle arthrodesis in elderly patients. *Foot Ankle Int.* 2012; 33:9, 699–703.

51. Kennedy JG, Hodgkins CW, Brodsky A, Bohne WH. Outcomes after standardized screw fixation technique of ankle arthrodesis. *Clin Orthop Relat Res.* 2006; 447, 112–18.

52. Thomas R, Daniels TR, Parker K. Gait analysis and functional outcomes following ankle arthrodesis for isolated ankle arthritis. *J Bone Joint Surg Am.* 2006; 88:3, 526–35.

53. Kofoed H. Scandinavian total ankle replacement (STAR). *Clin Orthop Relat Res.* 2004; 424, 73–9.

54. Nunley JA, Caputo AM, Easley ME, Cook C. Intermediate to long-term outcomes of the STAR total ankle replacement: the patient perspective. *J Bone Joint Surg Am.* 2012; 94:1, 43–8.

55. Saltzman CL, Mann RA, Ahrens JE, et al. Prospective controlled trial of STAR total ankle replacement versus ankle fusion: initial results. *Foot Ankle Int.* 2009; 30:7, 579–96.

56. Daniels TR, Younger AS, Penner M, et al. Intermediate-term results of total ankle replacement and ankle arthrodesis: a COFAS multicenter study. *J Bone Joint Surg Am.* 2014; 96:2, 135–42.

57. SooHoo NF, Zingmond DS, Ko CY. Comparison of reoperation rates following ankle arthrodesis and total ankle arthroplasty. *J Bone Joint Surg Am.* 2007; 89:10, 2143–9.

58. Mann JA, Mann RA, Horton E. STAR™ ankle: long-term results. *Foot Ankle Int.* 2011; 32:5, S473–84.

59. Karantana A, Hobson S, Dhar S. The Scandinavian total ankle replacement: survivorship at 5 and 8 years comparable to other series. *Clin Orthop Relat Res.* 2010; 468:4, 951–7.

60. Daniels TR, Mayich DJ, Penner MJ. Intermediate to long-term outcomes of total ankle replacement with the Scandinavian total ankle replacement (STAR). *J Bone Joint Surg Am.* 2015; 97, 895–903.

61. Schweitzer KM, Adams SB, Viens NA, et al. Early prospective clinical results of a modern fixed-bearing total ankle arthroplasty. *J Bone Joint Surg Am.* 2013; 95:11, 1002–11.

62. Raikin SM, Kane J, Ciminiello ME. Risk factors for incision-healing complications following total ankle arthroplasty. *J Bone Joint Surg Am*. 2010; 92:12, 2150–5.

63. Schuberth JM, Babu NS, Richey JM, Christensen JC. Gutter impingement after total ankle arthroplasty. *Foot Ankle Int*. 2013; 34:3, 329–37.

64. Agel J, Coetzee JC, Sangeorzan BJ, Roberts MM, Hansen ST Jr. Functional limitations of patients with end-stage ankle arthrosis. *Foot Ankle Int*. 2005; 26:7, 537–9.

65. Segal AD, Shofer J, Hahn ME, Orendurff MS, Ledoux WR, Sangeorzan BJ. Functional limitations associated with end-stage ankle arthritis. *J Bone Joint Surg Am*. 2012; 94:9, 777–83.

66. Singer S, Klejman S, Pinsker E, Houck J, Daniels T. Ankle arthroplasty and ankle arthrodesis: gait analysis compared with normal controls. *J Bone Joint Surg Am*. 2013; 95:24, e191(1–10).

67. Smith RW, Shen W, Dewitt S, Reischl SF. Triple arthrodesis in adults with non-paralytic disease. A minimum ten-year follow-up study. *J Bone Joint Surg Am*. 2004; 86-A:12, 2707–13.

68. Wapner KL. Triple arthrodesis in adults. *J Am Acad Orthop Surg*. 1998; 6:3, 188–96.

69. Knupp M, Skoog A, Törnkvist H, Ponzer S. Triple arthrodesis in rheumatoid arthritis. *Foot Ankle Int*. 2008; 29:3, 293–7.

70. Wukich DK, Bowen JR. A long-term study of triple arthrodesis for correction of pes cavovarus in

Charcot–Marie–Tooth disease. *J Pediatr Orthop*. 1989; 9:4, 433–7.

71 Wetmore RS, Drennan JC. Long-term results of triple arthrodesis in Charcot-Marie-Tooth disease. *J Bone Joint Surg Am*. 1989; 71:3, 417–22.

72. Zide JR, Myerson MS. Arthrodesis for the cavus foot: when, where, and how? *Foot Ankle Clin*. 2013; 18:4, 755–67.

73. Fortin PT, Walling AK. Triple arthrodesis. *Clin Orthop Relat Res*. 1999; 365, 91–99.

74. Graves SC, Mann RA, Graves KO. Triple arthrodesis in older adults: results after long-term follow-up. *J Bone Joint Surg Am*. 1993; 75, 355–62.

75. Pell RF, Myerson MS, Schon LC. Clinical outcomes after primary triple arthrodesis. *J Bone Joint Surg Am*. 2000; 82, 47–57.

76. Saltzman CL, Fehrle MJ, Cooper RR, Spence EC, Ponseti IV. Triple arthrodesis: twenty-five and forty-four-year average follow-up of the same patients. *J Bone Joint Surg Am*. 1999; 81, 1391–402.

77. Beischer AD, Brodsky JW, Pollo FE, Peereboom J. Functional outcome and gait analysis after triple or double arthrodesis. *Foot Ankle Int*. 1999; 20:9, 545–53.

78. Ljung P, Kaij J, Knutson K, Pettersson H, Rydholm U. Talonavicular arthrodesis in the rheumatoid foot. *Foot Ankle*. 1992; 13:6, 313–16.

79. Chen CH, Huang PJ, Chen TB, et al. Isolated talonavicular arthrodesis for talonavicular arthritis. *Foot Ankle Int*. 2001; 22:8, 633–6.

80. Chiodo CP, Martin T, Wilson MG. A technique for isolated arthrodesis for inflammatory arthritis of the talonavicular joint. *Foot Ankle Int*. 2000; 21:4, 307–10.

81. Haskell A, Pfeiff C, Mann R. Subtalar joint arthrodesis using a single lag screw. *Foot Ankle Int*. 2004; 25:11, 774–7.

82. Easley ME, Trnka HJ, Schon LC, Myerson MS. Isolated subtalar arthrodesis. *J Bone Joint Surg Am*. 2000; 82:5, 613–24.

83. Myerson MS, Alvarez RG, Lam PW. Tibiocalcaneal arthrodesis for the management of severe ankle and hindfoot deformities. *Foot Ankle Int*. 2000; 21:8, 643–50.

84. Mann RA, Chou LB. Tibiocalcaneal arthrodesis. *Foot Ankle Int*. 1995; 16:7, 401–15.

85. Tenenbaum S, Coleman SC, Brodsky JW. Improvement in gait following combined ankle and subtalar arthrodesis. *J Bone Joint Surg Am*. 2014; 96:22, 1863–9.

86. Saville P, Longman CF, Srinivasan SC, Kothari P. Medial approach for hindfoot arthrodesis with a valgus deformity. *Foot Ankle Int*. 2011; 32:8, 818–21.

87. Frey C, Halikus NM, Vu-Rose T, Ebramzadeh E. A review of ankle arthrodesis: predisposing factors to nonunion. *Foot Ankle Int*. 1994; 15:11, 581–4.

88. de Heus JA, Marti RK, Besselaar PP, Albers GH. The influence of subtalar and triple arthrodesis on the tibiotalar joint. A long-term follow-up study. *J Bone Joint Surg Br*. 1997; 79:4, 644–7.

The Cavus Foot

Paul H. Cooke and Thomas A. Ball

Historical Aspects and Modern Perspectives

Of the few articles written in the early days of ortho-pedics, a large proportion were about the clubfoot, including the adult clubfoot. One expert in the man-agement of cavus, Naughton Dunn from Birming-ham, England, wrote little by today's standards, but what he did write was mostly on the subject of calca-neocavus deformity of the feet in polio – a condition treated by his eponymous triple fusion and tendon transfer[1]. Dunn stated that paralytic cavus was one of the most crippling deformities of infantile paralysis. He noted that once deformity was established, treat-ment by splintage was difficult and usually ineffective. He observed that varus and valgus deformities tend to develop owing to the "faulty incidence of body weight or unequal muscular action." These comments on treatment and progression remain true and relevant today, but Dunn's outcome measure that "the results are nearly always excellent" would not pass the scru-tiny of modern peer review.

In drawing lessons from the past on the subject of cavus, we must remember that in his time spina bifida and polio were rife, aging and infirmity were accepted, and that fashionable shoes and road run-ning were the luxury of the few, not the right of all. So the etiology of the condition and the expectations of treatment have changed.

Today, overall we see fewer cases of neurological disease. In most countries patients are more likely to present with severe neurological cavus as part of Charcot–Marie–Tooth disease (CMT). Charcot–Marie–Tooth is a collection of neurological diseases and has many genetic variants. Some use the term hereditary motor and sensory neuropathy (HMSN), but most patients and clinicians prefer the eponym CMT. Other neurological diseases, such as polio and spina bifida, have all but disappeared over a generation, as a result of immunization, prenatal diagnosis, genetic counseling, and public-health measures such as the widespread prophylactic treat-ment of pregnant women with folic acid.

The range of patients presenting with cavus to an orthopedic clinic is wide. Nevertheless, the majority of patients with cavus are never referred for an ortho-pedic opinion; they either live with mild deformity and symptoms by simple modification or restriction of footwear and activity, or receive treatment from podiatrists and/or orthotists.

In tertiary practice, we mostly see patients with neurological disease as a result of CMT or cerebral palsy, who suffer the consequences of severe deform-ity. Nevertheless, in both specialist and general ortho-pedic practice, we also frequently see patients with subtle cavus and its consequences. They may com-plain of pain and varus instability when engaged in running and other physical pursuits, with limitation of the ability to wear more fashionable shoes, and secondary claw toes.

Definition, Classification, and Etiology

The definition of cavus is loose – being any foot with a high arch. Forefoot plantaris is the defining feature (Figure 9.1). Plantaris refers to plantar flexion of the forefoot relative to the hindfoot, and produces an increase in the height of the arch. Plantaris may occur in combination with any deformity of the hindfoot (calcaneus, equinus, varus, or valgus).

Cavus may be subdivided into physiological or pathological. Physiological cavus represents an extension of the normal range of arch elevation and is usually mild. Pathological cavus occurs sec-ondary to neuromuscular imbalance, and is usually more severe.

Cavus feet can also be divided anatomically into three groups, in order of severity:

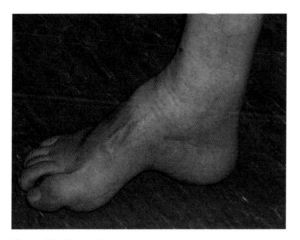

Figure 9.1 A case of a symptomatic moderate cavus foot showing forefoot plantaris.

Table 9.1 The causes of cavus foot

•	Idiopathic	
•	Congenital	residual talipes
		arthrogryposis
•	Traumatic	post-compartment syndrome
		nerve injury
		burn contracture
•	Neurological	hereditary sensorimotor
		neuropathy/Charcot–Marie–
		Tooth disease
		cerebral palsy
		spina bifida
		polio
		myelodysplasia
		diastematomyelia
		tumor
		syringomyelia
•	Muscular	muscular dystrophy

1. The "straight" cavus foot – where the arch is elevated but there is no other anatomical abnormality.
2. The inverted *cavovarus* foot – where the arch is high and the heel is inverted.
3. The complex foot – with multiple deformities affecting the whole foot. This includes feet with *equino-cavovarus* or *calcaneo-cavovarus* deformity.

Cavus feet tend to deteriorate, with increasing symptoms and deformity. Even those that start as mild cavus can deteriorate to a more severe anatomical and symptomatic group. This deterioration is much more likely in cases where there is an underlying neurological cause.

Deformity does not improve without treatment, so once symptoms arise there is no place for withholding treatment – whether by conservative or surgical means[2].

Cavus, in its mildest form, is common, occurring in between 7 and 15% of people[3–4]. The causes of cavus are shown in Table 9.1. The proportion of physiological cases appearing in an orthopedic clinic depends on geography and the special interest of the surgeon, with reports of up to 70% of cases being physiological. In the senior author's clinic, which has a special interest in neurological diseases, there are less than 20% of physiological cases, with the remaining 80% being pathological. The proportion of cases with a neurological diagnosis increases in the special interest or tertiary clinic, but also increases as the clinician becomes more diligent in seeking a neurological cause. All authors note a significant increase in the new diagnosis of neurological disease following neurological referral from the foot clinic[5].

The diagnosis of neurological disease is important so that treatment can be tailored to the future course of the disease and the known patterns of progression. Similarly, early diagnosis of spinal disorders, such as spinal dysraphism, diastematomyelia, and cord tumors, is important if progressive mono- or paraplegia and incontinence are to be avoided. It is not uncommon for a cavus foot to be the initiating referral of these spinal conditions.

Today, of the neurological causes of cavus (Table 9.1) the HMSNs and cerebral palsy are the commonest in the UK, with the decline of polio and spina bifida.

The types of CMT are summarized in Table 9.2, but there are many types and subtypes. Over 35 different genetic origins are described.

Clinically, CMT1 and CMT2 are the commonest subtypes, together accounting for around 80% of cases. They usually cause progressive lower motor neuron weakness in the limbs, with resultant deformities from adolescence or young adulthood onward.

CMT2 is often less severe and of later onset than CMT1. Some types of CMT2 present with weakness

Table 9.2 The types of Charcot–Marie–Tooth disease

Type	Subtype	Genetics	Chromosome abnormality	Age of presentation	Features
CMT1 Demyelinating	A	Autosomal dominant	Duplication Ch17	At 10 to 15 years. May be detected earlier in known families	Weakness, ataxia, distal sensory decrease, areflexia, cavus increases. May progress to cavovarus, equino cavovarus, or more often to calcaneo cavovarus
	B	Autosomal dominant			
	C	Autosomal dominant			
	D	X-linked (may also have preserved myelin – CMT2).			
CMT2 Myelin preserved	A	Autosomal dominant	Duplication Chr1	Often later onset up to 20 to 30 years	Each type may present like CMT1 or with stork-leg appearance, weakness, and flat foot (due to weakness)
	B		Partial deletion Ch3		
	C		?		
	D		Duplication Ch7		
CMT3 (Dejerine Sottas Syndrome) Demyelinating		Autosomal recessive	Variable	Presents in infancy or childhood	As CMT1, severe and progressive, associated with severe spinal deformity
CMT4, CMT5, CMT6, CMT7	All rare	Multiple	Multiple	Early – infancy or childhood	Often severe and generalized (including cranial nerves) neuropathy

For a detailed description refer to www.cmt.org.uk.

and flat foot, rather than cavus. These cases will continue with this pattern of deformity as they age, and do not go on to develop high arches – the pattern does not change. Sensory symptoms, including numbness (rare) and neuropathic pain (common), are variable.

CMT3, known as Dejerine–Sottas disease, is rare and results in limb weakness and disability in early childhood. Patients with CMT4 may suffer respiratory difficulty and hearing loss as well as weakness. The other types are extremely rare and beyond the scope of this chapter.

What Causes Cavus?

It used to be thought that cavus of the foot was secondary to idiopathic tightening of the plantar fascia. This explanation is attractive but inadequate to explain the primary and secondary problems. For example, if cavus resulted from tightness of the plantar fascia, the toes would be flexed at the metatarsophalangeal joints, and the extended MTPJs and claw toes, which nearly always accompany cavus, would not be seen.

Duchenne first suggested muscle imbalance as the cause of cavus as a result of his neurophysiological experiments[6]. This theory was later revived[7]. Price looked at patients with HMSN using computed tomography and showed intrinsic atrophy[8], particularly in the pedal lumbricals and interossei. Two years later the Liverpool group showed correlation between MRI and histological findings[9], finding hyperplasia of the peroneus longus and atrophy of the tibialis anterior. The sum of the anatomical, MRI, and CT studies of the leg and foot in cavus documents atrophy and contracture of the intrinsic muscles in pure cavus, and of both the intrinsic and calf muscles in some idiopathic cases and all the complex forms of cavovarus.

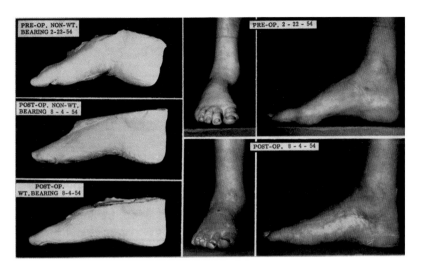

Figure 9.2 The carefully documented work of Garceau and Brahms[10] shows that intrinsic denervation before maturity allows collapse of a high arch.

The concept of dysfunctional intrinsic activity causing cavus is further supported by work by Garceau and Brahms who studied 47 patients with pure cavus[10]. They undertook selective division of the intrinsic motor branches of the plantar nerves. This reduced arch height and improved the shape of the footprint. They followed up these cases with pre- and postoperative plaster cast models to document foot shape over time. They noted improvement in shape in 46 of the patients (Figure 9.2).

The contradictory nature of this evidence – that cavus is associated with atrophic intrinsic muscles, but that denervation of the intrinsics leads to improvement of cavus, indicates that we do not fully understand the effects of denervation. It is likely that chronic denervation causes contracture and hence deterioration – especially when the skeleton is growing, whereas with acute denervation there is weakness, without contracture, which decreases the tendency of the arch to foreshorten.

The cause of cavus and its associated deformities in CMT is probably a complex combination of weakness and contracture of the pathologically affected muscles. This is especially marked if there is an imbalance of power between antagonistic muscles.

Thus contracture of the intrinsic muscles usually causes the plantaris and cavus. Weakness of the peroneal musculature and dorsiflexors causes inversion and equinus, respectively, as the relatively stronger, but also weakened, calf muscles and inverters continue to act. Equinus may result from the relative overactivity of the calf muscles. Calcaneus occurs when the calf muscles are weak.

In CMT the cavus is often associated with differential plantar flexion of the first ray. The etiology for plantar flexion of the first ray is controversial. One school holds that there is relative overactivity of the peroneus longus, which in combination with the weakness of the tibialis anterior, leads to plantar flexion of the first ray. The evidence for this is based upon surface electrophysiological studies undertaken during gait. Surface electrical activity may also be caused by passive stretching of muscles, so it is equally possible that this activity reflects passive stretching of a contracture of peroneus longus secondary to antagonistic activity of the stronger tibialis posterior. The tibialis posterior is relatively preserved in CMT. This seems a more probable explanation given that the peroneal muscles are always weakened in CMT.

Although difficult, understanding the cause of the deformity is necessary to treat it and avoid recurrence. Fortunately, once a pattern of muscle imbalance and contracture has presented, that pattern remains consistent and so we do not have the added complication of changing patterns of deformity and the forces causing it.

Clinical Presentation

The clinical presentations of the different patterns of deformity vary. In simple cavus the presentation relates to the shape of the foot, with problems in finding fashionable shoes, rubbing of the dorsal bumps of the tarsometatarsal joints, metatarsalgia, and clawing of the toes.

A study of 1047 veterans with diabetes found a highly significant correlation of cavus with prominent metatarsal heads, bony prominences, and hammer and claw toes[11]. High plantar pressures are correlated with metatarsalgia. In these cases the patients overcame the metatarsalgia by reducing activity and adopting a slow and cautious gait to avoid peak forefoot pressures[12].

The tarsus in a cavus foot is in a "close-packed" state, a state that is produced physiologically at the end of gait by means of the windlass mechanism. The windlass mechanism imparts rigidity to the foot at push-off, which is advantageous. However, the cavus foot is fixed in this rigid condition throughout the gait cycle, so shock absorption and adaption of the foot to unevenness in the floor are poor during early stance. Thus metatarsalgia, foot pain, and other more proximal disorders, including hip, knee, and back pain associated with high levels of transmitted shock, are more common in the patient with the cavus foot.

Crosbie showed that the diffuse foot pain in cavus feet was more closely related to the severity of the cavus than to any other variable, excepting body weight[13]. Thus athletic patients with cavus have low tolerance to the repeated shocks from running and jogging, while older people, with less compliant tissues, suffer with foot discomfort in everyday life. All of these problems are in turn commoner in overweight patients.

Despite this, and while the shape of the foot and the toes may be problematic, significant midfoot pain is surprisingly uncommon in pure cavus. It can usually be treated by insoles, with adequate accommodation in capacious shoes – although pressure from the dorsal boss, which commonly forms over the apex of the arch, may be problematic in fashionable shoes.

Cavus feet with a varus heel exhibit all of the problems described for cavus feet, often in a more severe form. However, the varus heel also leads to other, more disabling, symptoms, namely ankle instability and pain, as well as lateral foot pain with overload or fracture of the fifth metatarsal. These tendencies to lateral foot pain, fracture, ankle deformity, and ankle arthritis increase with the severity of the deformity.

The heel varus is significant not only because of the acute and chronic symptoms it causes, but also as the fifth metatarsal fractures and ankle instability

Table 9.3 The consequences of complex cavus foot deformities with CMT

• Limb pain	90%
• Rubbing toes	62%
• Metatarsalgia	52%
• Ankle instability	31%
• Lateral border pain	11%
• Ankle/hindfoot pain	9%
• Ulceration	1%

recur after treatment, unless the heel varus is recognized and corrected.

By the time we move on to the complex deformities, general features of the neurological disease are added to the local problems of the foot (Table 9.3).

In our unit 399 patients with CMT were surveyed: we found that the most common feature of the disease was low- to medium-level generalized lower limb pain. This did not improve with treatment and is probably a manifestation of the painful neuropathy[14]. The commonest problems caused by cavus were toe and footwear problems – often with superimposed metatarsalgia. Instability was also common, and was especially disabling as it is combined with the poor proprioception, as a result of the neuropathy. Lateral foot pain was seen in 11% of cases, with many having more than one focus of pain. Of the patients with lateral foot pain, over 50% of those who had no treatment went on to develop a fifth metatarsal fracture. Of those with a fracture, half went on to have two or more fractures before receiving definitive treatment. Ulceration was fortunately rare, occurring in less than 1% of all cases. Nevertheless, it was of huge significance when it did occur.

Management: Examination and Investigation

The management of the cavus foot requires the clinician to combine the skills of the physician and surgeon. An adequate history is essential. It is important to carefully establish the patient's symptoms, including pain, numbness, poor balance, and fatigue – as well as bladder and bowel dysfunction. Similarly the past history and the family history may give important clues as to the etiology of the deformity.

Examination starts with a general examination, including posture, and a visual examination of the back and lower limbs. Careful examination of both feet, including both the medial and lateral arch height, the posture, flexibility, and deformity of the foot, is undertaken (Figure 9.3). Callosities on the sole of the foot reflect areas of high pressure under the foot, and occur particularly under the metatarsal heads and down the lateral margin of the foot (Figure 9.3d). This is combined with examination of the soles, uppers, and inside of the shoes, which provides a simple but effective form of functional gait analysis.

The alignment and mobility of each joint from the ankle to the toe joints is assessed. It is then important to systematically examine and chart the power of foot and calf muscles (Figure 9.4). This can appear daunting within the time pressures of a clinic. However, it is easy to do, rapid to perform with practice, and vitally important, because failure to diagnose imbalance will lead to poor results with recurrent deformity. Special note should be made of muscle imbalance, which usually indicates a neurological origin of the cavus.

The neurological examination is completed by checking the reflexes and sensation. No examination of the cavus foot should be completed without testing fine touch with Semmes–Weinstein monofilaments and vibration sense with a tuning fork or vibrometer. Subtle neuropathy may only be revealed by these tests.

Finally, the Coleman block test (Figure 9.5) is performed in any case when inversion has been observed. Such inversion may be driven from varus at the heel or by a plantar flexed first ray, which drives the foot and produces secondary hindfoot varus. The patient stands on a block with the first ray unsupported. Provided that the hindfoot is flexible, if the varus comes from the heel the varus malalignment remains when the patient is standing on the block. Alternatively, if the heel now corrects, as the first ray is now defunctioned, it indicates a forefoot-driven varus.

It is tempting to be exhaustive and highly technical in a description of further medical investigations. For surgical planning, detailed investigation is rarely necessary, or is best done by others, especially when referral to a neurologist is required. As a rule of thumb, we refer unilateral cases, severe cases, cases that are deteriorating, and cases with muscle imbalance or sensory loss to a neurologist, but do not refer cases of apparent physiological cavus with no neurological history or signs.

Footprints can be useful to chart progress and the Harris and Beath footprint is a cheap and reliable technique, which gives adequate information. In the majority of cases in our clinics, investigation will be limited to radiographs and footprints, with magnetic resonance imaging of the spine ordered en route to the neurologist. Muscle biopsies, electromyograms, and blood tests to determine disease types are ordered by the neurologists.

In our unit, the radiological protocol for deformity is a standing lateral and AP x-ray of the foot with a mortise ankle view. The x-rays are taken AP to detect secondary structural and degenerative changes. Measurement of the radiological angles gives variable results as a result of the effects of rotation and positioning. Thus, pre and post surgery, sequential measurements should be interpreted with great caution. Measuring calcaneal pitch (Figure 9.6a) is important, as we are referred a number of tertiary cases in which the TA has been lengthened and weakened unnecessarily, in treating a calcaneocavus foot.

Meary's angle (Figure 9.6b) is measured by recording the angle between a line along the first metatarsal and a second line along the axis of the talus on the lateral standing radiograph. The normal result is less than 5° between the two lines.

A standing hindfoot view demonstrates alignment (Figure 9.6c), but varies as a result of rotation. Again specific views such as Cobey's view are difficult, or impossible, to standardize as a result of torsional deformity, and sequential measurements must be regarded with caution.

Treatment

The treatment of pure cavus is almost always non-operative, with orthoses. Surgery is reserved for the treatment of toe deformities. Insoles for the treatment of the cavus foot often have to be bespoke, as off-the-shelf insoles do not give adequate support to the high arch. Trials of different orthoses by Burns et al. have shown that custom-made foot orthoses are more effective than sham orthoses[3]. A study at the Nuffield Orthopaedic Centre, Oxford, confirmed that bespoke orthotics are more cost-effective than off-the-shelf, preformed insoles, which tend to be discarded as they are ineffective. LoPicollo showed in a retrospective, non-randomized study that foot pain and ankle instability were markedly reduced with custom-made corrective ethylene vinyl acetate (EVA) insoles in a series of subtle cavus feet[15].

Molloy has shown that mean plantar contact pressure is increased by 68% in high-arched feet. It can be

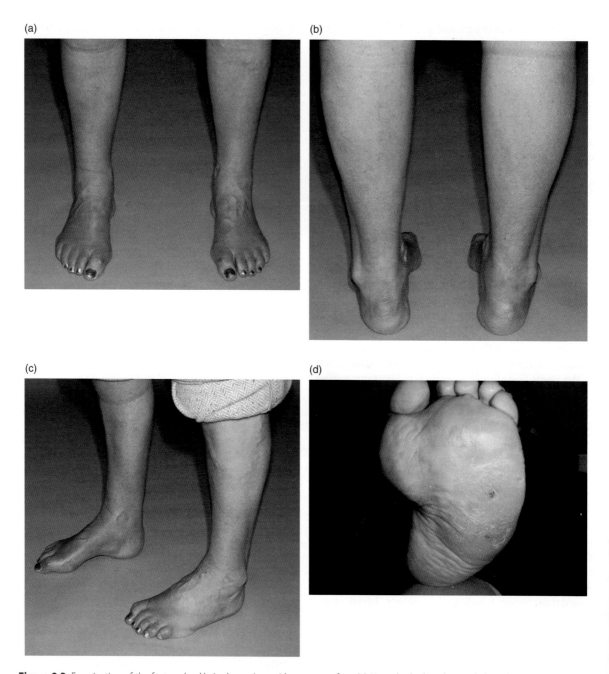

Figure 9.3 Examination of the foot and ankle in the patient with cavovarus feet. (**a**) Note the high arches and clawed great toes with callosities; (**b**) varus heels in association with the raised medial arch; (**c**) note the callosity beneath the fifth metatarsal head and the prominence of the lateral malleolus. (**d**) In a different patient, examination of the sole shows areas of callosity, which correspond to areas of peak pressure on standing and walking.

reduced by about 30% by wearing motion-control cushioned running shoes. Motion-control running shoes are more rigid and heavier duty than flexible running shoes. They typically have a firm midsole, a deep heel counter, and incorporate arch support and a rocker[16].

The foot pain and metatarsalgia of the cavus foot can be managed non-operatively using insoles and

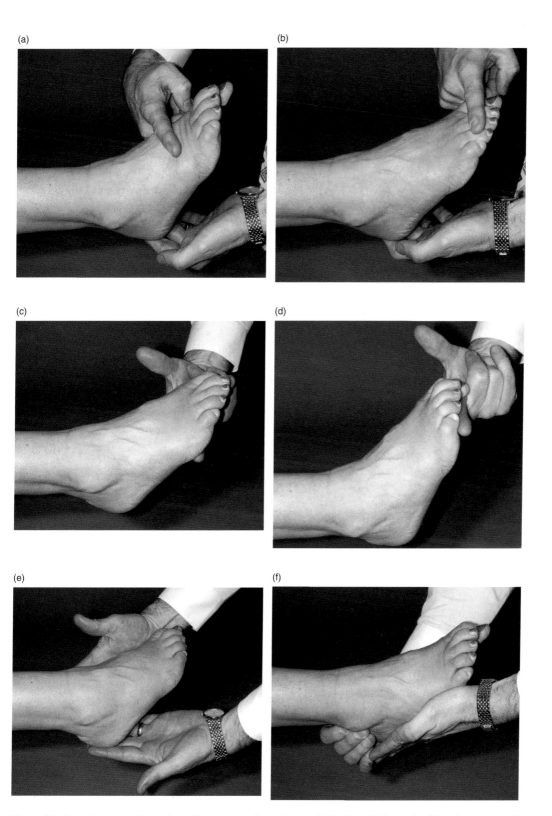

Figure 9.4 Power is assessed by testing active power against resistance. (**a**) Testing tibialis anterior; (**b**) testing extensor digitorum longus and extensor digitorum brevis; (**c**) testing the gastrocnemius/soleus power; (**d**) testing the long flexors of the toes. (**e**) The inverting power of the tibialis posterior is tested in plantar flexion, to neutralize the inversion power of the tibialis anterior. (**f**) The patient is asked to evert the foot against the examiner's hand to assess peroneal power.

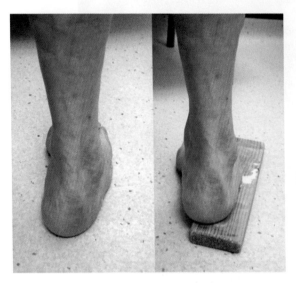

Figure 9.5 The Coleman block test shows forefoot-driven varus. (Photograph courtesy of Mr N. Geary.)

shoes in the majority of patients, provided they will accept the cosmetic limitations of the orthoses and shoes. Such management is dependent upon a good orthotic service and a good understanding of the components, materials, and design of the orthoses and shoes.

As soon as varus, as opposed to simple cavus, becomes an issue, the orthoses necessarily become larger and more structural. A typical insole for cavovarus would incorporate a recess for the first metatarsal head, with a small heel raise to accommodate the forefoot plantaris and pronation. Lateral heel posting will provide a pronatory moment to counter the supinatory moment of hindfoot varus, helping with ankle instability.

Surgical shoes custom made by an orthotist, typically extending above the ankle, are often necessary to accommodate such orthoses. Eventually, when orthotic management becomes either ineffective or too cumbersome, it is necessary to consider surgery.

Surgery for the cavus foot is reliant on the principles for correction of any major foot deformity:

1. The foot should be positioned in line with and squarely beneath the leg.
2. The foot should be square to the ground in all planes.
3. Muscle balance should be corrected.
4. The foot should be shoe shaped.

A choice of appropriate osteotomies and fusions are used to correct the cavovarus foot shape and position. Generally osteotomies are preferred for milder, correctable deformities, and fusions for severe uncorrectable deformities, or those where there is secondary degeneration of a joint.

Once the position and shape of the foot have been corrected, muscle imbalance needs to be addressed. On rare occasions realignment of the foot also realigns the tendon, and no further tendon transfers are required. An example is after a lateral displacement calcaneal osteotomy (Dwyer osteotomy) for varus deformity of the heel. As the heel shape is corrected with lateral displacement and angulation of the heel, the insertion of the tendo Achillis (TA) is transferred laterally. At the beginning of the procedure the TA will be exerting a varisizing effect, as well as producing plantar flexion. At the end of the procedure there will be a valgisizing effect, as the TA insertion is now lateral to the midline.

More often, in cases of neurological imbalance, such as CMT, cerebral palsy, and spina bifida, when the major deforming force has been corrected, appropriate tendon transfers are performed to rebalance the foot and prevent recurrence.

Table 9.4 lists the common combinations of procedures in different situations, for different diseases. It can be seen that tibialis posterior transfer is the commonest transfer in CMT, and a split tibialis anterior tendon transfer in cerebral palsy or after a cerebrovascular accident.

In the following sections we will describe corrective surgery to the foot and ankle by region: forefoot, midfoot, and hindfoot and ankle.

Forefoot Surgery

Claw toes are commonly associated with the cavus and cavovarus foot. They cause discomfort as a result of pressure, as well as making orthotic management difficult. It is important to record the location and direction of the deformity. There is usually a combination of extension of the metatarsophalangeal joint, and flexion of the interphalangeal joint(s).

Flexible deformities of the MTPJ can be treated by release of the MTPJ capsule and the extensor tendons. In physiological cases, simple release may be sufficient. In neurological cases, transfer of the flexor

(a)

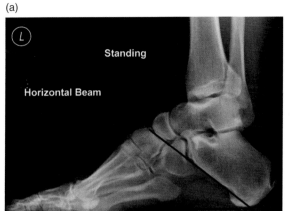

(b)

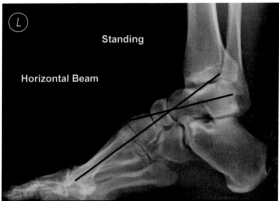

(c)

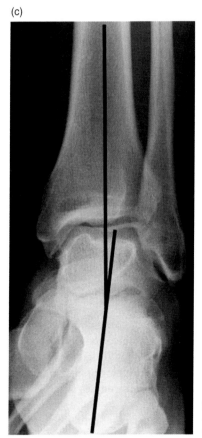

Figure 9.6 Measurements of (**a**) calcaneal pitch; (**b**) Meary's angle; and (**c**) hindfoot alignment are illustrated. These are not reproducible measurements for sequential use, as they will be affected by rotation.

digitorum longus into the extensor tendon (Girdlestone–Taylor) may be necessary. This transfer also corrects the interphalangeal joint flexion deformity. However, in severe neurological cases, or when the deformity is fixed, it is better to correct the deformity by extensor and MTPJ release in association with a fusion of the interphalangeal joint. Excision or interposition arthroplasty, as opposed to fusion, of the interphalangeal joints should be avoided, as they are associated with recurrence.

Table 9.4 Recipes for complex surgery. Toe surgery includes a Jones and Hibbs correction (see text)

Deformity	Disease	Surgical recipe
Cavus	Physiological	Toe correction
Cavus	Post-polio	Midfoot osteotomy for severe deformity, toe correction
Cavus	CMT	First metatarsal osteotomy for plantar flexed first ray +/− toe surgery
Early/moderate cavovarus	CMT	First metatarsal dorsiflexion osteotomy, lateral displacement calcaneal osteotomy, and toe surgery. Consider a tibialis posterior tendon transfer
Calcaneo-cavovarus or severe cavovarus	CMT	As above – or if severe triple fusion, tendon transfers, and toe surgery
Equino-cavovarus	CMT	As above – add tendo Achillis lengthening
Equino-cavovarus	Cerebral palsy	Triple fusion, split or total tibialis anterior tendon transfer, TA lengthening

In cases with severe extension of the MTPJ and metatarsalgia, the Jones procedure to the great toe, and its equivalent in the lesser toes, the Hibbs tenosuspension, are performed. In these procedures the extensor tendon is divided at the MTPJ and the MTPJ capsule is released. The proximal end of the divided extensor tendon is transferred into the distal metatarsal under tension, such that the extensors elevate the metatarsal heads, rather than extend the toes. The use of tissue anchors to fix the extensor tendon into the metatarsals has greatly simplified the Jones and Hibbs procedures, as previously the tendon was passed through a transvers hole in the metatarsal neck – tricky to achieve in the great toe, and even more difficult in the lesser metatarsals. This operation is performed with interphalangeal joint fusion of the toes, which is usually performed using a buried screw in the great toe and wires in the lesser toes. After fusion with wires, especially when combined with other major procedures in the foot, it is advisable to use a single cork to anchor the K-wires and maintain alignment (Figure 9.7).

There are no reliable reported results for the Jones procedure performed in isolation, but follow-up of tenosuspension of the lesser metatarsals shows 80% excellent or satisfactory results with improvement in both the toe alignment and metatarsalgia[17].

Midfoot Surgery

Correction of the arch height alone can be performed by osteotomy or arthrodesis at a variety of levels. For the foot with a plantar flexed first ray and a mild, mobile deformity of the rest of the midfoot, as is commonly seen in CMT, the deformity is addressed with a dorsiflexion osteotomy of the first ray, which is usually performed in combination with other procedures to the hind- or forefoot.

Dorsiflexion osteotomy of the first ray is performed through a straight medial incision centered over the proximal first metatarsal. The TMTJ is identified and a V-shaped osteotomy is performed with the base of the V on the dorsal aspect of the metatarsal. It is best to cut the osteotomy with a saw, leaving the inferior cortex intact. This allows the metatarsal to be dorsiflexed, closing the dorsal base of the wedge, while preserving a stable hinge on its inferior surface.

The metatarsal can be held in position using screws or plates, but we prefer to use a compression staple either dorsally or dorsomedially.

Nowadays, dorsiflexion osteotomy of the first ray is by far the most common operation performed, as the major pathology treated is CMT. In the past, when polio was more prevalent, multiple dorsiflexion osteotomies of the metatarsals or arthrodeses of the TMTJs were commoner.

Correction of severe cavus, affecting the whole width of the midfoot, can be achieved by osteotomy or arthrodesis at various levels, from the proximal metatarsals to the talonavicular/calcaneocuboid level. In general, osteotomy should be performed when the joints are preserved, with arthrodesis being kept for those cases that are degenerate. In reality any osteotomy performed through the midtarsal bones

(a)

(b)

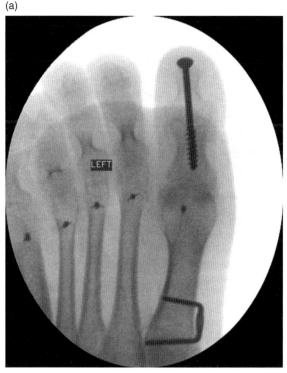

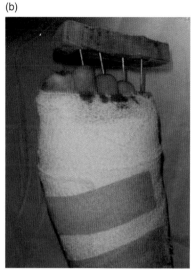

Figure 9.7 (**a**) Jones and Hibbs transfers have become simple to perform with the advent of modern internal fixation. (**b**) Wire fixation of multiple toes is maintained by a single cork to maintain alignment.

inevitably breaches at least one joint and stiffness may result.

Many different osteotomies have been performed and described. These include those described by:

- Swanson, who described multiple metatarsal osteotomies[18]
- Jahss described removing a dorsally based wedge and fusing the tarsometatarsal joint[19]
- Japas described a V-shaped osteotomy across the midfoot, with the apex in the navicular, and the two arms of the V ending in the medial cuneiform and cuboid. It therefore crosses several midfoot joints[20]
- Weiner described a domed or "Akron" osteotomy, which passes through the cuneiforms, cuboid, and fifth metatarsal[21,22].

The articles, which are mostly historical, describe a number of approaches – from multiple longitudinal incisions to a single transverse incision. The single transverse incision is no longer recommended as it is transnervous and may damage the nerves, in particular the small branches of the superficial peroneal nerve, and blood vessels. The description of the osteotomies often incorporates complex geometric cuts to provide stability. With modern fixation, the complexity of these osteotomies is no longer needed and they are only important for historical reasons. The results of midtarsal osteotomy are all reported in complex cases in historical series. All are level 4 or 5 evidence, and should be interpreted with caution. Nevertheless, they do help inform us as to the type of surgery that is appropriate today.

We use a V-osteotomy with the apex plantar, or arthrodesis straight across the foot, which is simpler and can be stabilized with screws, plates, or staples. The surgical approach is most commonly through a medial incision centered on the level of surgery, with a lateral incision based over the interval between the fourth and fifth metatarsals. On occasions a midline incision half way between medial and lateral incisions is also needed. Through these incisions a simple transverse V osteotomy or arthrodesis can be created and internally fixed.

Jahss described 34 osteotomies, with excellent results in all[19]. He also noted that patients were

(a)
(b)

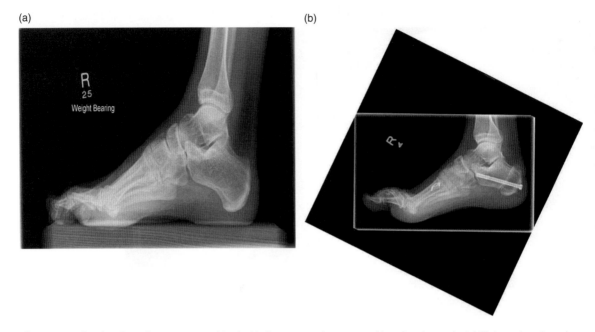

Figure 9.8 A "modern Dwyer" osteotomy combined with first metatarsal osteotomy. Note that the tendo Achillis is not lengthened, as the preoperative clinical examination and radiographs show calcaneus at the heel.

pleased, even when the correction was incomplete. Japas reported 70% good results[20]. Wilcox and Weiner reported early satisfactory results in 94% of patients[21] although later follow-up, 23 years later, suggested good results in less than 80%[22]. Wülker and Hurschler from Germany and Naudi from France suggested 70% satisfaction with osteotomy in a series of adults with mostly idiopathic cavus[23–24]. Consolidating these results, it seems that corrective osteotomy does not give good enough results in mild to moderate idiopathic disease. There is failure, or deterioration, in about a third of cases and corrective osteotomy should be restricted to only the most severe cases of pure cavus.

Osteotomies should, when possible, be performed at the apex of the deformity. Nevertheless, the most common fusions performed for cavus are performed at the level of the midtarsal joint, as part of a triple fusion for a complex deformity involving varus of the hindfoot (see below).

Hindfoot and Ankle Deformities

To correct the hindfoot, osteotomy is again favored over arthrodesis in most situations unless joint degeneration or very severe deformity demand radical excisions necessitating fusion.

Hindfoot Varus

For varus deformity of the heel, a lateral displacement calcaneal osteotomy will correct the majority of mobile deformities, and will restore a stable base in moderate fixed deformities. A version of this osteotomy was originally described by Dwyer, who performed the osteotomy through a direct lateral oblique approach, removing a lateral closing wedge, rather than translating the heel laterally[25].

Today the lateral displacement calcaneal osteotomy is most commonly performed as an open procedure, with an extended lateral approach, as for calcaneal fractures. A direct oblique approach to the calcaneum is best avoided because of risk of damage to the sural nerve. The calcaneum is divided transversely after protecting the medial soft structures (by passing spikes superiorly and inferiorly around the calcaneum). Chevron, step, and other geometric variations are described to increase the stability, but we find a simple, straight osteotomy allows displacement, which is then rigidly fixed using a stepped staple, a single screw passed from the posterior (Figure 9.8), or a stepped plate. Lateral translation of 8 to 10 mm of the calcaneal tuberosity should be possible. It is rarely possible to achieve more than 10 mm of displacement because of the medial soft tissue attachments. Thus if more correction is needed angulation of the posterior fragment is added to the translation, as was described by Dwyer.

More recently, lateralizing calcaneal osteotomies have been performed with a minimally invasive technique using a low-speed, high-torque burr[26]. It has been shown that both open and minimally invasive surgery achieve equivalent displacement, although with minimally invasive surgery the soft tissue envelope is preserved and an extensive scar is avoided.

Whether performed open or by minimally invasive surgery, the Dwyer-type osteotomy and its derivatives, with lateral displacement, correct bony structure and also realign the pull of the TA.

Dwyer described 63 cases, with one infection and six cases requiring further surgery because of recurrent deformity with age – his patients were mostly children. His results are mirrored in modern reports with confirmation of satisfactory surgical results in many articles[26].

Triple fusion is performed for severe uncorrectable deformity and in cases where there is degeneration in the hindfoot joints. Midfoot correction at the talonavicular and calcaneocuboid joints is used to produce a plantigrade foot with a neutral midfoot. A triple fusion is usually performed using a two-incision technique. One incision is lateral from the tip of the fibula toward the fourth metatarsal base; a second is medial or dorsal to expose the talonavicular joint. Transverse incisions, such as the Ollier incision, which sweeps across the top of the foot, are transnervous and consequently necessitate dividing the cutaneous nerves. They should no longer be used.

The bone cuts for the triple fusion should be designed, cutting out wedges from the bone around the joints to allow full correction. Through the lateral approach the subtalar and calcaneocuboid joints are exposed. A wedge that is narrow on the medial side and broad on the lateral side is cut to correct varus. Sagittal wedges are used to correct calcaneus or equinus. Shortening wedges through the talonavicular and calcaneocuboid joints can also be designed to correct plantaris. Figure 9.9 illustrates an example of the wedges drawn in preoperative planning.

Fusion for varus is now reserved for the treatment of patients with severe deformity. In historical series, fusion for varus has a poor reputation as a result of the high rate of recurrent deformity. However, recurrent deformity was often because simultaneous

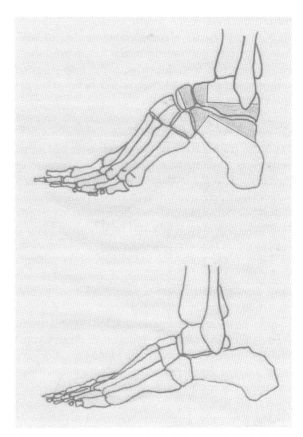

Figure 9.9 Planning pictures drawn before complex triple fusion showing the size of wedges to be excised.

tendon transfers were not performed to rebalance the foot[27]. Roper and Tibrewal (1989) and Gould (1984) showed that bony surgery must be accompanied by appropriate soft tissue surgery, with tendon releases and transfers to balance any deforming forces[28–29]. Thus even with fusion it is important to rebalance the foot and ankle; with such surgery the high rate of recurrent deformity can hopefully be substantially reduced.

In some cases of complex cavovarus deformity, especially if they have been longstanding, there is also severe deformity and degeneration of the ankle. In these cases the triple fusion will need to be extended to include the ankle. This is known as a "pantalar fusion." Thus a corrective fusion of the ankle joint is performed simultaneously with corrective fusions of the subtalar, talonavicular, and calcaneocuboid joints. This is usually best performed using an extended lateral incision carried down over the fibula and curving forward at the tip of the fibula toward the base of the fourth metatarsal. Although such surgery carries a considerable burden of stiffness, a correctly positioned pantalar fusion produces a stable, pain-free foot, which with the help of good orthoses, including full-length rocker bottoms on the shoes, allows reasonable gait.

The majority of the more recent reports concern the outcomes of complex hindfoot surgery for CMT. We know from a study of 399 people with CMT that surgery is commonly required in this group of patients[14]. Taylor also showed that the results of such surgery have been poor, with increased pain, although it has to be borne in mind that these results are largely historical. However, results can be improved upon if the principles of correcting deformity are adhered to. In 2008, Ward presented the results of 25 patients with CMT who had undergone first metatarsal osteotomy, plantar fascia release, a peroneus longus to brevis tendon transfer, and in selected cases a lateral transfer of the tibialis anterior tendon. With a mean follow-up of 26 years, they found that surgery combining deformity correction with tendon transfer gave lower rates of degenerative change, with only 20% of feet requiring further surgery, and no patient requiring a triple fusion[30].

More recently, Louwerens reported his series of 53 patients treated with osteotomies and tendon transfers, and found only two patients relapsed and needed a triple fusion at an average of five years follow-up. Ninety percent were satisfied with the outcome of their surgery[31].

In our unit we have corrected 58 feet in 46 CMT1 or CMT2 patients with calcaneo-cavovarus deformity. We added a tibialis posterior tendon transfer to bony procedures, which included osteotomy and fusion, in an attempt to rebalance the foot and also correct the drop foot. At between zero and 14 years follow-up we have had just three recurrent deformities, which required a revision procedure to a triple or pantalar fusion. In our opinion, it remains unclear whether the addition of the tibialis posterior transfer to treat the drop foot element of the deformity improves the results in the longer term.

Key Points

- The simple cavus – high-arched – foot is usually treated with orthoses. Surgery is reserved for the treatment of toe deformities.
- Heel varus is significant not only because of the acute symptoms it causes, but because fifth metatarsal fractures and ankle instability recur after treatment, unless the varus is corrected simultaneously.
- The commonest neurological causes of a cavus foot are HMSN, commonly known as CMT, and cerebrovascular accidents.
- Correctable deformities are corrected with soft tissue releases and tendon transfers.
- Fixed deformities are corrected with bony procedures – preferably an osteotomy, but in the severest deformities, or in the presence of arthritis, a fusion is required.
- In treating CMT the most frequently undertaken procedures for cavovarus include a first ray dorsiflexion osteotomy, a lateral displacement calcaneal osteotomy, and a tibialis posterior tendon transfer.
- In the most complex cases, a triple or even a pantalar fusion may be required.

References

1. Dunn N. Calcaneo cavus and its treatment. *J Bone Joint Surg.* 1919; 1, 711–21.

2. Aminian A, Sangeorzan BJ. The anatomy of cavus foot deformity. *Foot Ankle Clin.* 2008; 13, 191–8, v.

3. Burns J, Crosbie J, Ouvrier R, Hunt A. Effective orthotic therapy for the painful cavus foot: a randomized controlled trial. *J Am Podiatr Med Assoc.* 2006; 96, 205–11.

4. Scherer PR. Orthotic management of the pes cavus foot. *Lower Extremity Review Magazine.* 2011.

5. McCluskey WP, Lovell WW, Cummings RJ. The cavovarus foot deformity. Etiology and management. *Clin Orthop Relat Res.* 1989; 27–37.

6. Duchenne GB. Physiologie des mouvements démontrée à l'aide de l'expérimentation électrique et de l'observation clinique, et applicable à l'étude des paralysies et des déformations. https://archive.org/stream/physiologiedesm00duch#page/449: (J.-B. Bailliere et Fils, 1867) pp. 526–35.

7. Sabir M, Lyttle D. Pathogenesis of Charcot–Marie–Tooth disease. Gait analysis and electrophysiologic, genetic, histopathologic, and enzyme studies in a kinship. *Clin Orthop Relat Res,* 1984; 223–35.

8. Price AE, Maisel R, Drennan JC. Computed tomographic analysis

of pes cavus. *J Pediatr Orthop.* 1993; 13, 646–53.

9. Helliwell TR, Tynan M, Hayward M, Klenerman L, Whitehouse G, Edwards RH. The pathology of the lower leg muscles in pure forefoot pes cavus. *Acta Neuropathol.* 1995; 89, 552–9.

10. Garceau GJ, Brahms MA. A preliminary study of selective plantar-muscle denervation for pes cavus. *J Bone Joint Surg Am.* 1956; 38, 553–62.

11. Ledoux WR, Shofer JB, Ahroni JH, Smith DG, Sangeorzan BJ, Boyko EJ. Biomechanical differences among pes cavus, neutrally aligned, and pes planus feet in subjects with diabetes. *Foot Ankle Int.* 2003; 24, 845–50.

12. Burns J, Crosbie J, Hunt A, Ouvrier R. The effect of pes cavus on foot pain and plantar pressure. *Clin Biomech (Bristol, Avon).* 2005; 20, 877–82.

13. Crosbie J, Burns J, Ouvrier RA. Pressure characteristics in painful pes cavus feet resulting from Charcot–Marie–Tooth disease. *Gait Posture.* 2008; 28, 545–51.

14. Taylor A, Porter D, Cooke PL. Leg, foot and ankle pain in Charcot–Marie–Tooth disease. *J Bone Joint Surg Br.* 2003; 85-B, proceedings, 128.

15. LoPicollo Mea. Effectiveness of the cavus foot orthosis. *J Surg Orthop Adv.* 2010; 19, 166–9.

16. Molloy JM, Christie DS, Teyhen DS, et al. Effect of running shoe type on the distribution and magnitude of plantar pressures in individuals with low- or

high-arched feet. *J Am Podiatr Med Assoc.* 2009; 99, 330–8.

17. Vlachou M, Beris A, Dimitriadis D. Modified Chuinard–Baskin procedure for managing mild-to-moderate cavus and claw foot deformity in children and adolescents. *J Foot Ankle Surg.* 2008; 47, 313–20.

18. Swanson AB, Braune HS, Coleman JA. The cavus foot concept of production and treatment by metatarsal osteotomy. *J Bone Joint Surg Am.* 1966; 48, 1019.

19. Jahss MH. Tarsometatarsal truncated-wedge arthrodesis for pes cavus and equinovarus deformity of the fore part of the foot. *J Bone Joint Surg Am.* 1980; 62, 713–22.

20. Japas LM. Surgical treatment of pes cavus by tarsal V-osteotomy. Preliminary report. *J Bone Joint Surg Am.* 1968; 50, 927–44.

21. Wilcox PG, Weiner DS. The Akron midtarsal dome osteotomy in the treatment of rigid pes cavus: a preliminary review. *J Pediatr Orthop.* 1985; 5, 333–8.

22. Weiner DS, Morscher M, Junko JT, Jacoby J, Weiner B. The Akron dome midfoot osteotomy as a salvage procedure for the treatment of rigid pes cavus: a retrospective review. *J Pediatr Orthop.* 2008; 28, 68–80.

23. Wülker N, Hurschler C. Cavus foot correction in adults by dorsal closing wedge osteotomy. *Foot Ankle Int.* 2002; 23, 344–7.

24. Naudi S, Dauplat G, Staquet V, Parent S, Mehdi N, Maynou C.

Anterior tarsectomy long-term results in adult pes cavus. *Orthop Traumatol Surg Res.* 2009; 95, 293–300.

25. Dwyer FC. Osteotomy of the calcaneum for pes cavus. *J Bone Joint Surg Br.* 1959; 41-B, 80–6.

26. Kendal A, Ball T, Rogers M, Cooke P, Sharp R. Minimally invasive calcaneal osteotomy: a safe alternative to open calcaneal osteotomy with fewer complications. *Foot Ankle Int.* 2015; 36, 685–90.

27. Wetmore RS, Drennan JC. Long term results of triple arthrodesis in CMT disease. *J Bone Joint Surg Am.* 1989; 71, 417–22.

28. Roper BA, Tibrewal SB. Soft tissue surgery in Charcot–Marie–Tooth disease. *J Bone Joint Surg Br.* 1989; 71, 17–20.

29. Gould N. Surgery in advanced Charcot–Marie–Tooth disease. *Foot Ankle.* 1984; 4, 267–273.

30. Ward CM, Dolan LA, Bennett DL, Morcuende JA, Cooper RR. Long-term results of reconstruction for treatment of a flexible cavovarus foot in Charcot–Marie–Tooth disease. *J Bone Joint Surg Am.* 2008; 90, 2631–42.

31. Leeuwesteijn AEEPM, de Visser E, Louwerens JWK. Flexible cavovarus feet in Charcot–Marie–Tooth disease treated with first ray proximal dorsiflexion osteotomy combined with soft tissue surgery: a short-term to mid-term outcome study. *Foot Ankle Surg.* 2010; 16, 142–7.

Chapter 10

Adult Acquired Flat Foot Deformity

Ruairi F. MacNiocaill and Terence S. Saxby

Introduction

Pes planus, or flat foot, and its variations are a spectrum of foot and, occasionally, ankle disease. It is one of the core conditions treated by the foot and ankle surgeon. A clear understanding of the true nature of the spectrum of the disease is essential for the successful assessment and treatment of these patients. The adult-acquired flat foot is the commonest pathological cause of flat foot, and is illustrative of the anatomical, pathophysiological, and biomechanical principles of pes planus.

Flat foot is to some extent a maligned term. It has for many years received much attention in musculoskeletal screening, particularly in times of war, where otherwise fit and healthy people are given a "diagnosis" on the basis of having flexible flat feet on the assumption that this will limit their effectiveness. Thankfully, perhaps less so for the reluctant recruit, sense has prevailed with the recognition that the vast majority of flexible planus and planovalgus feet are part of the normal spectrum. In essence, young children are supposed to have flat feet, the bulk of which remain asymptomatic without orthoses or "special shoes." It is the stiff flat foot or the extreme deformity in the child and the acquired flat foot in the adult that represent true pathology, and it is on the acquired adult flat foot that we shall concentrate our efforts in this chapter.

Definition

Pes planus – flat foot – is a decrease in height of the medial longitudinal arch of the foot. It is often associated with a valgus deformity of the hindfoot – planovalgus.

Pathogenesis/Pathoanatomy

The apex of the medial longitudinal arch of the foot is at the midtarsal joint. The talonavicular joint (TNJ) is most commonly the fulcrum of hindfoot deformity. Classically in the flat foot there is sag at the TNJ with abduction of the forefoot and valgus of the hindfoot, with overall pronation of the foot. Despite this the forefoot is often supinated, to compensate, and produce a plantigrade foot[1].

The medial longitudinal arch of the foot has static and dynamic stabilizers.

Static stabilizers of the arch are:

- *The bony anatomy* of the foot, which interlocks to produce a degree of stability. Particular elements include the interlocking "ball and socket" relationship of the TNJ – the "acetabulum pedis" linking the hindfoot to the mid- and forefoot. The sustentaculum tali also supports the bony architecture of the normal arch, as does the "roman arch" arrangement of the tarsometatarsal joints (TMTJs).
- *Ligamentous structures* are also important. The plantar and plantar-medial elements of the talonavicular, naviculocuneiform and TMTJ capsules resist dorsiflexion and abduction of the forefoot on the midfoot. There are two main, named ligaments – the spring and Lisfranc ligaments. The plantar calcaneonavicular ligament (spring ligament) runs between the sustentaculum tali and the plantar surface of the navicular and acts as a check rein to the descent of the medial longitudinal arch in stance. The Lisfranc ligament, running between the base of the second metatarsal and medial cuneiform is also crucial to the maintenance of the tarsometatarsal arch. Failure of these plantar ligamentous and capsular structures leads to the arch sagging, and flattening under load.

Dynamic stabilizers of the arch:

The most important dynamic stabilizer is the *tibialis posterior*, which arises from the posterior aspect of the proximal third of the tibia, fibula, and the intervening interosseous membrane. Its tendon runs in a groove at the posterior aspect of the distal tibia and angles anteriorly and inferiorly to insert into the tuberosity of the navicular, with slips to the sustentaculum tali, plantar surface of the cuneiforms, cuboid, and the bases of second, third, and fourth metatarsals. The tibialis posterior plantar flexes and inverts the foot, in addition to inverting the subtalar joint and adducting the forefoot[2]. Importantly for diagnosis, it initiates hindfoot varus on heel rise.

Understanding the function of tibialis posterior is key to understanding the adult-acquired flat foot deformity. The line of pull of the posterior tibial tendon (PTT) is medial to the axis of the sagittal plane of rotation of the subtalar joint, giving it a mechanical advantage in inverting the heel. The line of the tendo Achillis (TA) pull is just lateral to the axis[2–3]. Should the tibialis posterior muscle or its tendon become abnormally lengthened this mechanical advantage may be lost. In addition, the excursion distance of the PTT is short and lengthening of 1 cm, or more, causes dysfunction. Defective PTT function results in its antagonist, the peroneus brevis, which everts the foot, becoming dominant and abducting the forefoot with resultant gradual attenuation of the TNJ capsule and the spring ligament, leading to a plantar flexion of the talus with a loss of arch height. Associated with this is the development of heel valgus, which lateralizes the insertion of the TA, which in turn worsens the heel valgus. The hindfoot valgus also leads to the development of gastrocnemius–soleus tightness and contracture[4].

Etiology

Pes planus has many causes (Table 10.1). The flexible flat foot is a normal variant and rarely, in itself, causes serious symptoms or disability. The infant is born with a flat foot, and the arch develops in the first decade, therefore flat foot is commoner in childhood and often resolves spontaneously. Nevertheless, the adult-acquired flat foot, which is usually caused by PTT dysfunction, is a cause of pain and disability. Planovalgus foot deformity in the adult may be caused by failure of any of the structures named above, but these are far less common than PTT dysfunction.

In normal gait the foot is supple at heel strike, as the subtalar joint is everted and the tibia is relatively

Table 10.1 The causes of flat foot. This is not an exhaustive list

Physiological, flexible flat foot

Pathological
- Tibialis posterior tendon insufficiency
- Degenerative and inflammatory arthritis: TMTJ, subtalar
- Tarsal coalition and congenital vertical talus
- Trauma: Lisfranc injury, spring ligament injury, plantar fascia
- Charcot neuroarthropathy
- Neuromuscular: cerebral palsy, polio
- Ligamentous laxity: Marfan, Ehler–Danlos

internally rotated, "unlocking" the transverse tarsal joint. Conversely, during toe-off the tibia is externally rotated and under the influence of the tibialis posterior the subtalar joint inverts locking the midtarsal joint, causing the foot to become more rigid. Thus the normal foot is "flatter" at heel strike, when it is positioned for shock absorption, whereas at toe-off it is stiffer with a varus heel and a locked midtarsal joint. The stiffer foot is more efficient for the transfer of muscle forces to the ground, which is better for an effective push-off; the supple foot is better for the shock absorption of heel strike. Thus the flat foot is ineffective for the transference of force in late stance phase, which leads to a feeling of weakness and fatigue in the foot.

Epidemiology

There is considerable disparity across the scientific literature as to the incidence and prevalence of pes planus. A population study of 75 000 people in the United States identified that adult pes planus was associated with being male, a military veteran, African American, having a high body mass index, and other foot abnormalities, such as bunions and hammer toes. Pes planus is associated with poverty, although this is thought to be through the association of poverty with ill health, with "ill health" having a strong association with pes planus[5–6]. There is also, rather surprisingly, an association between pes planus and white-collar work; this conflicts with the other socio-economic findings.

Posterior tibial tendon dysfunction occurs almost exclusively in feet that have an underlying planus morphology. There is a bimodal peak of occurrence of PTT dysfunction with age, with a subgroup of traumatic PTT dysfunction in the young and a second larger peak of degenerative PTT dysfunction in the older patient. The cause is thought to be hypovascularity of the tendon in the vascular watershed zone posterior and distal to the medial malleolus[7]. It is interesting to note that PTT dysfunction is associated with hypertension, obesity, diabetes, steroid exposure, and trauma or surgery to the medial side of the foot and ankle, with 60% of patients having one or more of these conditions[8]. Hypertension, obesity, diabetes, and steroids are all associated with an acceleration of the micro- and macrovascular degeneration seen with aging. The effect of local trauma or surgery to this area is probably also likely to be as a result of its effect on the vascularity of this critical tendon zone.

Classification

For a classification system to be accepted in clinical practice, it must reflect the natural history of the disease, identify specific clinical stages, and guide treatment. In general terms, pes planus can be thought of as being: congenital or acquired; symptomatic or asymptomatic; pediatric or adult; traumatic or atraumatic; and fixed or flexible.

Despite this the adult-acquired flat foot is most commonly caused by PTT dysfunction. It was initially described in 1969 by Kettelkamp et al.[1] and classified by Johnson and Strom (1989)[9]. The classification was modified by Myerson (1997), who added stage IV disease[10]. This classification is the most widely accepted and used, relating specifically to acquired PTT dysfunction.

Stage I: Inflammation and dysfunction of the intact PTT – minimal deformity with symmetrical heel shape – single heel rise is possible.

Stage II: Elongation or rupture of the tendon leading to established, but flexible or correctable, planus/planovalgus deformity – a single heel rise is usually possible, but is painful and the patient fatigues in comparison to the other side.

This is a large group with significant variation in severity, which Myerson's group[11] has further subdivided into subgroups:

Stage IIA-1: Upon correction of the hindfoot valgus, the remaining forefoot supination is either corrected completely or is minimal.

Stage IIA-2: Upon correction of the hindfoot valgus, the forefoot supination does not correct.

Stage IIB: There is abduction of the forefoot, either at the TNJ or TMTJ.

Stage IIC: The medial rays is unstable. This instability may occur at the TNJ, naviculocuneiform joint, or the TMTJ.

Stage III: Deformity that is usually more severe but, importantly, is fixed and the hindfoot valgus is no longer passively correctable.

Stage IV: In stage IV disease the ankle tilts into valgus as a result of the chronic planovalgus deformity of the foot. The ankle joint develops valgus degenerative change.

This group is further subdivided into (a) and (b), based on the correctability of the tibiotalar joint deformity and the presence or otherwise of ankle joint arthrosis:

Stage IVa: Correctable valgus tilt within the tibiotalar mortise without major degenerative changes.

Stage IVb: The more advanced stage with fixed deformity and established tibiotalar arthrosis.

Presentation

The history is usually of a gradual, or insidious, onset of pain and swelling on the medial side of the midfoot or ankle, below and behind the medial malleolus. There is often no specific traumatic incident and although some patients may recall an injury, only a small number of these represent a true, acute tendon injury. Many patients are overweight, older, and have a background of asymptomatic flat feet; many also have other medical conditions including diabetes mellitus and hypertension, as well as other foot conditions such as hallux valgus. Patients also often describe a vague "soreness" and "weakness" in the foot, which is increased by activity and limits their ability to exercise. As the condition progresses the patient may notice their foot "changing shape" with a progressive loss of the medial longitudinal arch.

Examination should commence as the patient walks into the office, assessing age, height, weight, and general health. This is followed by a more specific examination of the gait.

Patients should be inspected standing, with their lower limbs exposed above the knee. The shoe-wear pattern and any orthoses should be noted. Look for overall lower limb alignment and rotation, particularly knee valgus and lower limb internal rotation, both of which can be associated with the planovalgus foot. Observe the calves from behind for muscle bulk and symmetry. Swelling, scars, the quality of the skin, and a general impression of vascular status should be noted.

Observing from behind, the heel alignment is noted. Hindfoot valgus of 5 to 7° is normal. On a heel rise the heel moves to neutral or a few degrees of varus. The "too many toes sign" is observed from behind. This is a record of the number of lesser toes that are not obscured by the hindfoot and can be seen from behind – one and a half toes are considered normal. In reality the "too many toes sign" is of limited use as it is dependent upon the position of the examiner's head and the rotation of the patient's leg. After inspection ask the patient to walk toward a wall in the office and look for dynamic increases in deformity during gait.

The patient is instructed to face the wall and place the hands flat against it at approximately shoulder height. She is then asked to perform a double heel rise. Observe for restoration of medial longitudinal arch height and movement of the heel into varus. Restoration of the arch is a variation of Jack's test – the plantar fascia comes under tension with MTPJ extension, drawing the anterior and posterior extremes of the arch closer together with a resultant ascent of the apex of the arch. The patient is then asked to perform repeated single heel rises on both sides, in turn. If she gets pain, ask "is that the pain you get?" Patients may also complain of pain on the medial side of the ankle. In the presence of significant PTT dysfunction the patient is unable to repeatedly perform a single heel rise, as the tibialis posterior is the "initiator" of heel rise.

We prefer to complete the examination with the patient sitting on the edge of the examination couch with the legs hanging over the side and the examiner seated. Palpate over the course of the PTT with particular emphasis on the portion distal to the medial malleolus: there may be tenderness, thickening, or fullness. Palpate for tenderness in the other key structures of the ankle, hindfoot, and midfoot. Active and passive range of motion should be assessed in the ankle, subtalar, and midtarsal joints. Noting whether the deformity is fully correctable, or not, is important, as this has a bearing on treatment. Long-standing and severe deformities will tend to be uncorrectable, or "fixed."

The strength of the tibialis posterior muscle is best established with the patient sitting. Active

inversion or resistance to passive eversion is tested in plantar flexion. Plantar flexion defunctions the tibialis anterior muscle, which can function as an inverter if the ankle is dorsiflexed, masking tibialis posterior weakness. Placing a thumb firmly over the tibialis anterior tendon can diminish its action and one can also feel it working. In terms of quantifying weakness, a useful rule of thumb is simply that a lower limb muscle should be stronger than one in the forearm, and therefore the examiner should not be able to overpower the normal tibialis posterior.

Establishing the relationship between the forefoot and the hindfoot is important. If the subtalar joint position is corrected, and moved from valgus to neutral, the forefoot position should be noted. In some cases the forefoot supination does not correct; in these cases surgery to correct the subtalar joint may well be inadequate, and further surgery to correct the forefoot supination may be required.

In summary, the patient can be seen to progress through the stages outlined in Johnson and Strom's classification.

Stage I: Patients present with medial pain and swelling around the medial ankle along the distal course of the PTT. With the patient standing "square" they have no deformity and symmetrical hindfeet.

Stage II: As the tendon elongates hindfoot valgus develops and the medial arch descends. This is flexible and can be passively corrected by the examiner. In the later stages, abduction occurs through the midfoot with a progressive uncovering of the talar head. There may be medial midfoot callosities where patients have walked on the uncovered, flexed talar head. The forefoot also abducts with callosities under the medial border of the first ray.

Stage III: The deformity becomes more pronounced and with time there is joint degeneration, especially of the subtalar and TNJ, leading to the deformity becoming fixed.

Stage IV: Finally, with longstanding abnormal loading of the medial ankle joint, the medial soft tissue stabilizers of the ankle gradually fail, and valgus ankle arthrosis develops.

Finally, assessment of the patient's lower limb neurological and vascular function should be performed, particularly if surgery is being considered.

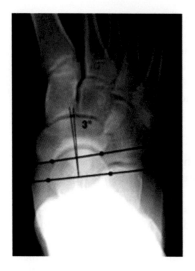
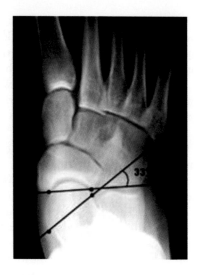

Figure 10.1 The talonavicular coverage angle. This is normally <7°.

(a)

(b)

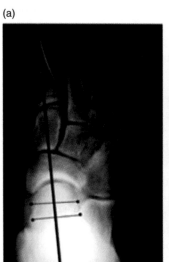
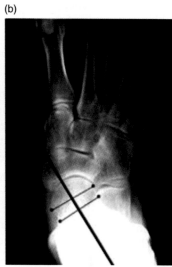

Figure 10.2 The AP talar–first metatarsal angle. (a) Normal; (b) abnormal.

Investigation

The first-line investigation of the acquired flat foot is good quality plain radiographs. Weightbearing views of the ankle mortise, and AP, lateral, and oblique views of the foot are obtained.

The **AP weightbearing radiographs** of the foot should be assessed for talonavicular coverage, talar–first metatarsal angle, talocalcaneal angle, degree of forefoot abduction, and joint degeneration.

Talonavicular coverage angle: the edges of the articular surface of the talar head are marked, and the two points joined by a line (Figure 10.1). A similar process is undertaken for the navicular. The angle between these two lines indicates the degree of talonavicular lateral subluxation. The coverage angle is normally less than 7°.

The AP talar–first metatarsal angle is a measure of forefoot alignment, by comparing the relative relationship of the long axes of the talus and the first metatarsal (Figure 10.2). The long axis of the talus should be almost parallel to that of the first metatarsal. If the talar axis passes medial to the first metatarsal axis the forefoot is abducted. Forefoot abduction is usually caused by pes planus.

The AP talocalcaneal or "Kite's" angle is a measure of hindfoot valgus and is an angle formed by the intersection of the long axis of the talus and the lateral border of the calcaneus (Figure 10.3). It can be

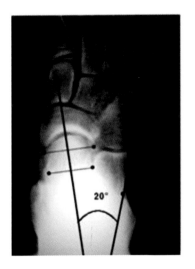
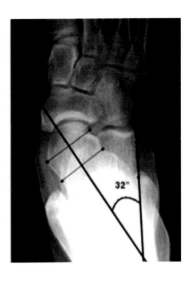

Figure 10.3 The AP talocalcaneal, or Kite's, angle. Normal 15 to 30°.

(a) (b)

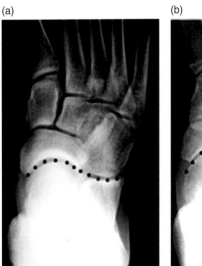
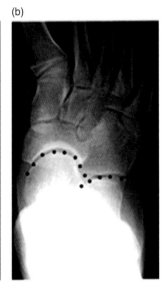

Figure 10.4 The cyma line, the broken line shown in (**b**) is abnormal.

difficult to measure, as under- or overexposure may obscure the calcaneal outline.

The AP cyma line (Figure 10.4) is a sigmoid line drawn through the midtarsal joint and should be smooth or unbroken. A broken line, or line with a step, suggests "shortening" of the lateral column or adduction or flexion of the talus. The term "cyma" is borrowed from the world of architecture where it refers to the junction of two differing curves as seen in the architrave of classical architecture.

Lateral weightbearing radiographs of the foot should be assessed for calcaneal pitch, Meary's angle, talocalcaneal angle, midtarsal, naviculo-cuneiform or tarsometatarsal joint "sag" or break, height of medial cuneiform from the ground, degree of talar flexion, and joint degeneration.

The calcaneal pitch is the angle between the undersurface of the calcaneus and the floor (Figure 10.5), in essence it is the angle of the "posterior portion" of the arch. Put simply, the flatter the angle or pitch, the flatter the foot.

Meary's angle (Figure 10.6) is the angle between the long axis of the talus and the first metatarsal, which should be linear. A "break" in the foot between the talus and the metatarsal is abnormal. An increase in Meary's angle may be caused by

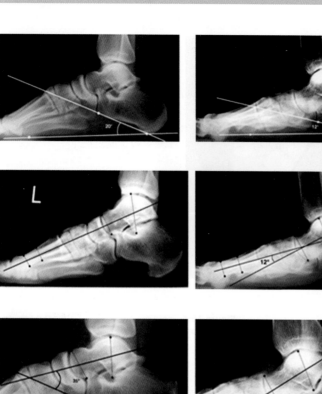

Figure 10.5 The calcaneal pitch angle. Normal 10 to 20°.

Figure 10.6 The lateral talo–first metatarsal angle. Normal 0 +/– 4°.

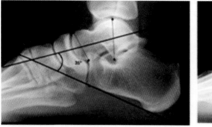
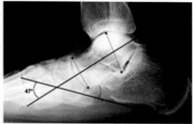

Figure 10.7 Lateral talocalcaneal angle. Normal 25 to 45°.

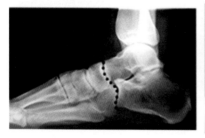
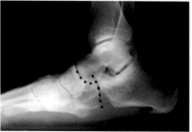

Figure 10.8 The lateral cyma line.

sagging of the midfoot joints with gapping on the plantar surface. On the lateral weightbearing view it is also possible to appreciate "descent" of the cuboid toward the floor when there is significant loss of arch height.

The lateral talocalcaneal angle is measured between the central axis of the talus and the undersurface of the calcaneus. An increase in the angle greater than 45° suggests hindfoot valgus (Figure 10.7).

The lateral cyma line (Figure 10.8) should be continuous, as on the AP radiograph.

When assessing the plain radiographs of the patient with adult-acquired flat foot, the presence or absence of degenerative change must be noted. This is for two reasons. Firstly, the flatness of the foot may be resultant on arthritis, in particular of the midtarsal joint, naviculocuneiform, or tarsometatarsal joints and, secondly, as the presence of degeneration, even if the primary diagnosis is PTT dysfunction, will alter management, with fusion surgery being favored.

A standing mortise view of the ankle should also be obtained. Valgus ankle tilt is seen in stage IV PTT dysfunction.

Ultrasound and MRI

MRI has a sensitivity of 95%, a specificity of 100%, and an accuracy of 96% in the diagnosis of disorders of the PTT[12]. The MRI findings have been classified by Conti et al.[13]. Ultrasound is cheaper and more widely available but is more operator dependent, albeit with sensitivity and specificity approaching that of MRI[14] in the best hands. Ultimately the diagnosis is very much clinical in nature with tests having a confirmatory role, also aiding in the quantification of structural damage, such as degenerative change.

Treatment

In most cases the treatment of PTT dysfunction is initially non-operative. If surgical treatment is required, the nature of the surgery depends on many factors. These include the patient's level of pain, physiological age, medical comorbidities, and their expectations and activity levels. The soft tissue, vascular, and neurological integrity of the foot and ankle are also important, as are the degree of deformity, its correctability, and which joints are involved. Degenerative joints are more likely to be fused. On balance treatment is principally dictated by the stage of disease.

Stage I: Tendinosis of PTT but no deformity.
Treatment: orthoses/physiotherapy/temporary immobilization/surgical debridement.

Stage II: Tendon rupture or functional failure leading to varying degrees of passively correctable pes planus.
Treatment: Corrective orthoses/physiotherapy/ surgical procedures to correct the deformity, but maintain joint motion. The commonest procedure is a flexor digitorum longus (FDL) tendon transfer to the navicular combined with a medial-displacement calcaneal osteotomy. Alternative and supplementary procedures include lateral column lengthening procedures, Cobb procedure, Cotton procedure, extended medial column fusion, and spring ligament repair.

Stage III: The planovalgus deformity becomes fixed as a result of a combination of joint degeneration with soft tissue contracture.
Treatment: Soft accommodative orthoses/ surgical treatment with realigning arthrodesis procedures – classically a triple arthrodesis is

used, although increasingly more selective fusion is being used[15–17].

Stage IV: In this stage there is failure of the medial ankle stabilizers leading to valgus arthrosis of the ankle joint proper.
Treatment: Surgical treatment at this stage may be ankle arthrodesis, which may form part of a pantalar arthrodesis; however, there are also procedures to reconstruct the deltoid ligament with tendon graft.

Non-Operative Treatment

Non-operative treatment is the first line of treatment for most with acquired pes planus. The degree of deformity and the flexibility of the foot are key factors. In Stage I patients with PTT pain, but symmetrical heel alignment, immobilization for six weeks, oral anti-inflammatory medication, followed by the use of an AFO is tried. Surgical debridement, open or tendonoscopic, is reserved for those patients who fail non-operative treatment.

In the patient with a flexible, stage II, deformity non-operative treatment is initially with corrective orthoses. The key elements of the deformity requiring correction are hindfoot valgus, forefoot abduction, and supination with first-ray dorsiflexion and loss of the medial longitudinal arch. The corrective orthosis is generally a shoe insert or insole. There should be a medial heel wedge to correct the subtalar joint valgus and a lateral forefoot post to correct the forefoot abduction. Incorporation of a medial-arch support can be useful, but care must be taken with the selection of the material used – in severe deformity there may be a sag at the talonavicular, naviculocuneiform, or tarsometatarsal joint, leading to a bony prominence in the medial-plantar foot, under which a callosity may form. In particular, a TNJ break, with uncovering of the head of the talus as a result of forefoot abduction, can lead to patients walking on the talar head. These patients need a cushioned, noncorrective insole. Trying to drive the medial arch back up with a rigid, corrective insole leads to pain under the prominence, making the orthosis unwearable. In summary, an uncorrectable deformity requires treatment with a soft, accommodative orthosis, with the harder, corrective orthoses being reserved for patients with correctable deformities.

More severe hindfoot and forefoot deformity may be addressed with the University of California

Biomechanics Laboratory (UCBL) orthosis. This has a deep heel cup, which grips the posterior calcaneus, controlling the heel valgus and arch height. It can also be molded about the lateral forefoot, reducing the forefoot abduction and controlling the first metatarsal.

Ultimately the severity of the deformity may outstrip the ability of in-shoe orthoses to control the foot and it is necessary to employ an AFO, which is more rigid and extends more proximally across the ankle, providing a more efficient and powerful lever to hold the hindfoot. Good results have been shown in the medium term for resolution of symptoms with the use of a low-articulating AFO. It has been shown that stage I and II PTT dysfunction, without tendon rupture, can be effectively treated non-operatively with an orthosis and a structured exercise program in over 80% of cases[18]. Nevertheless in younger patients and individuals with severe symptoms, refractory to non-operative treatment, surgery may be the only option[19].

Although some clinicians offer steroid and local anesthetic injection into the PTT sheath for symptomatic relief, most avoid injection as PTT dysfunction is a degenerative, not an inflammatory, condition. Furthermore steroid injections are associated with tendon rupture and therefore most feel that injection should be avoided.

Surgical Management

Surgical treatment of adult-acquired flat foot deformity gives good pain relief and a reasonable return in subjective foot strength and function in over 90% of patients[20]. The prerequisites for surgery include an adequate blood supply and skin condition to allow wound healing, neurological control of the foot, absence of active infection, and a patient capable of understanding and participating in the postoperative regime.

In common with many foot and ankle conditions, adult-acquired pes planus lends itself to an approach where multiple procedures are utilized from a "surgical shopping list," allowing an individualized approach for each patient. There is a large variation in practice. A survey of foot and ankle surgeons treating stage II disease in 2002 revealed that 97% would employ a bony procedure, with 88% preserving both the subtalar and talonavicular joints. A medializing

calcaneal osteotomy was used by 73%, and 41% used lateral column lengthening. A further 98% would use an additional soft tissue procedure, with 86% augmenting the PTT with the FDL, 53% repairing the spring ligament, and 70% releasing an equinus contracture[21].

Surgical Options
Tibialis Posterior Tendon Debridement

Surgical treatment for stage I is controversial and should be considered only after a minimum of three months' non-operative treatment. Tendon debridement is generally reserved for those with an inflammatory arthropathy, such as rheumatoid arthritis. Resection of the inflammatory pannus from around the tendon can relieve pain and may prevent progression to frank tendon failure. In the past this procedure was carried out on those with non-inflammatory tendinosis, but it has lost favor as it does not address mechanical or alignment-related factors. The healing potential of the PTT in the watershed zone is also questionable. There is therefore no compelling evidence that debridement alters the natural history of the condition, although one study with medium-term follow-up showed reduced pain but no objective enduring improvement in function[22].

Medial Displacement Calcaneal Osteotomy and FDL Tendon Transfer

Medial displacement calcaneal osteotomy and FDL tendon transfer constitute the workhorse in the surgical treatment of adult-acquired flat foot in our practice, as well as many centers worldwide. As previously outlined, failure of tibialis posterior leads to a loss of heel inversion through the subtalar joint in late stance phase and loss of the ability to initiate a heel raise. There is also a loss of the "suspensory" function of the PTT on the arch. A calcaneal osteotomy with medial translation and secure fixation medializes the pull of the TA, increasing the action of the TA as a foot inverter. It also reduces the pressure under the first and second metatarsals. Transfer of the FDL to the navicular allows the FDL to dynamically and statically maintain the medial longitudinal arch and forefoot adduction.

As these procedures are central to the treatment of adult-acquired flat foot we will describe them in detail. They are carried out under general

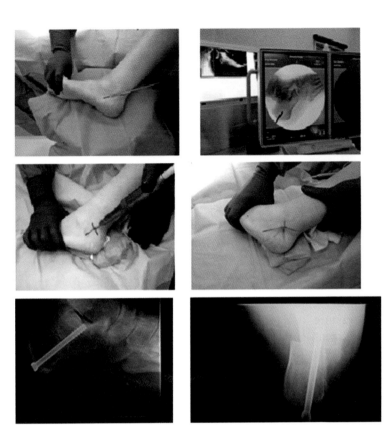

Figure 10.9 Percutaneous medial displacement calcaneal osteotomy – image intensifier guided.

anesthesia supplemented by an ankle block; the patient is positioned supine with a "sandbag" beneath the ipsilateral buttock, to make access to the lateral aspect of the calcaneus easier. The calcaneal osteotomy is carried out percutaneously with a burr (Figure 10.9), although many use an open technique. The entry point and the line of the osteotomy are marked on the lateral calcaneal skin, under image intensifier control. The line of the bony cut is marked at approximately 45°, linking the dorsal and plantar "bare areas" of the calcaneal tuberosity. The center of this line is then used as the entry point of the burr. The burr is used to penetrate both medial and lateral cortices, which gives an impression of the depth. The osteotomy is then completed along the marked line proximally and distally, first dividing the lateral cortex and most of the cancellous depth of the calcaneus. The osteotomy is then completed by dividing the medial cortex. The tuberosity fragment is then manually displaced to ensure that it is free. The tuberosity fragment is displaced medially by inserting a guide wire into the main fragment. This wire is then used as a lever to medially displace the tuberosity fragment. The wire is then advanced as a buttress, and the osteotomy is secured with a partially threaded 7 mm cannulated screw under image intensifier control.

The sandbag is then removed, to allow the leg to roll out, facilitating access to the medial ankle and PTT (Figure 10.10). A curved incision is made over the distal course of the PTT. The incision should be of sufficient length to allow adequate exposure of the navicular tuberosity and distal dissection of the FDL tendon. The PTT tendon sheath is opened. Clear fluid is usually present and the tendon is enlarged, flattened, and matt in appearance, often with longitudinal tears. At this point the plantar calcaneonavicular (spring) ligament is also exposed and inspected for tears. These should be repaired if present.

We like to retain the PTT if possible. There is debate as to when the PTT is worth retaining. There is no clear answer. Firstly, the tendon itself should be inspected. If it is in perfect condition one must look for other causes of the flat foot – in many cases

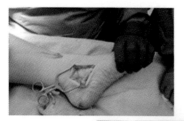
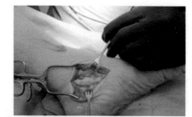
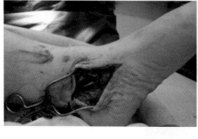

Figure 10.10 Flexor digitorum longus tendon transfer: the tibialis posterior tendon is exposed, debrided, and the FDL tendon transferred.

simply retracting the tendon will reveal a rupture of the spring ligament. A ruptured spring ligament should be repaired; in these cases we retain the PTT, but often augment it with an FDL transfer. Where there is clear tendinosis of the PTT we visually assess how much of the tendon is involved and whether the muscle functions. It is thought that with prolonged disuse the muscle fibroses and loses its elasticity, thus at surgery we pull in the tendon and watch for recoil from the muscle belly. Where there is little elasticity, or more than 50% of the tendon is diseased, the tendon is excised and replaced with the FDL. Even when the PTT is retained it is usually augmented with an FDL transfer.

The FDL tendon is identified. It lies posterior to the PTT. It must also be differentiated from the FHL, by gentle traction and observation of toe movement. The FDL is then dissected out along the medial/plantar aspect of the foot to a short distance beyond its intersection with the distal portion of the FHL tendon at the Knot of Henry. The tendon is divided under direct vision. A drill hole is made through the tuberosity of the navicular with a 4.5 mm drill. When placing the bone tunnel in the navicular it should be sufficiently lateral so as not to leave the medial bone susceptible to fracture. The tendon is then passed from plantar to dorsal and sutured back to itself. In those patients in whom the PTT is retained the FDL tendon is tenodesed side to side to the PTT, rather than through a navicular drill hole. There is no clear evidence on which to assess the efficacy of this

approach, or many other technical modifications of the surgery for that matter.

The wound is closed in layers and a below-knee backslab is applied. The patient is kept non-weightbearing for six weeks.

Arthroereisis

The concept of arthroereisis involves the use of a space-occupying implant in, or adjacent to, a joint with the aim of blocking "abnormal" motion. In the case of adult-acquired flat foot an arthroereisis screw is inserted into the sinus tarsi, where it occupies the space normally taken up by the everted lateral calcaneus. The arthroereisis screw acts as a mechanical block to hindfoot valgus. Arthroereisis is more commonly employed in the treatment of pathological pediatric flexible pes planus; however, the screws have been used in adult PTT dysfunction, in conjunction with other modalities, such as FDL tendon transfer and calcaneal osteotomy[23]. We mention arthroereisis here for the sake of completeness, rather than to suggest that it represents anything but a minor adjunct to treatment in some centers.

Lateral Column Lengthening

The fulcrum for the deformity of the adult-acquired flat foot is the TNJ. There is dorsolateral rotation, abduction of the forefoot, and loss of medial longitudinal arch height. As the TNJ is the fulcrum there is progressive uncovering of the talar head with abduction, which, at least theoretically, causes a relative lengthening of the medial and shortening of the lateral column of the foot. Procedures that lengthen the lateral column, relative to the medial, will de-rotate the foot, thereby covering the talar head, and re-establishing the talus–first metatarsal angle.

Lateral column lengthening can be achieved in two ways. Firstly, it may be achieved by an anterior calcaneal lengthening osteotomy, based on that described by Evans. In the Evans procedure, the anterior process of the calcaneus is osteotomized proximal to the calcaneocuboid joint. The lateral column is then lengthened by inserting a structural bone graft, which is internally fixed. This lengthens the lateral column and reduces the TNJ, while preserving the motion of the midtarsal joint. A concern is that the contact stress/load across the calcaneocuboid joint is increased, which may hasten the onset of calcaneocuboid degeneration.

An alternative to a lengthening osteotomy is a distraction fusion of the calcaneocuboid joint. This lengthens the lateral column, restoring alignment without risking later calcaneocuboid joint arthrosis. Unfortunately nothing in life is free, and the fusion significantly limits subtalar movement, which is not always a bad thing. Non-union is also common, which limits the technique's use. Consequently neither lateral column lengthening procedure is a mainstay of treatment; they are used as part of the "á la carte" approach to adult flat foot surgery.

Generally there is a preference for medial displacement calcaneal osteotomy over calcaneocuboid fusion. Both procedures have been shown to give excellent improvement in all the radiographic parameters and roughly equivalent clinical improvement, but the complication rates, with delayed union and non-union of the calcaneocuboid distraction arthrodesis, continue to tip the balance toward calcaneal osteotomy[24]. For those surgeons using lateral column lengthening procedures, most will combine these with a medial soft tissue balancing procedure such as a transfer of the FDL to the navicular.

Where there is a significant equinus contracture, lengthening of triceps surae should be considered. As in the majority of foot conditions, residual equinus leads to suboptimal gait biomechanics and therefore should be addressed where significant. In general terms, we will accept dorsiflexion to neutral – where this is not possible we tailor our intervention based on

cause and severity. Mild deformities are treated with simple "triple cut" percutaneous TA lengthening – this will be all that the bulk of patients require. Greater degrees of deformity may require more invasive procedures such as gastrocnemius recession or even open TA lengthening for the most severely affected.

The Cobb Procedure

The Cobb procedure is an alternative tendon transfer, of British origin. It involves the medial transfer of a split tibialis anterior tendon graft. The tibialis anterior is split, and the medial half is divided proximally. The divided half of the tibialis anterior tendon is passed through the medial cuneiform or the navicular and then back up through the PTT sheath, to be sutured to the PTT stump proximally. It is said to give a strong reconstruction. The limited number of papers suggest that it may be equivalent to FDL transfer. It is not in wide use and therefore is mentioned only for completeness.

Arthrodesis

In patients with advanced longstanding deformities, those with stiff degenerative painful joints, and those with progressive neurological conditions, arthrodesis is the most sensible approach. Joint fusion where applied appropriately and performed correctly should give predictable and enduring deformity correction and pain relief. Various patterns of fusion are undertaken, these include pantalar, triple, selective transverse tarsal, lengthening calcaneocuboid, and extended medial column. A pantalar fusion is a combined triple and ankle fusion.

The traditional approach to an adult-acquired flat foot in which there is fixed deformity and pain was to perform a "triple arthrodesis" of the subtalar, calcaneocuboid, and talonavicular joints. Indeed triple fusion continues to be a good option for many patients with a flat foot, but with a move toward more selective fusion the main indication for triple fusion is fixed deformity and painful arthritis affecting all three joints.

When considering selective fusion it is logical to consider which joints are deformed and which joints are painful. Weightbearing radiographs are used to localize any break or sag in the foot. On the lateral view, sag may be seen at the talonavicular, naviculo-cuneiform, tarsometatarsal, or a combination of these joints. The sag occurs as a result of the gradual attenuation of the plantar, midfoot ligaments and results in dorsiflexion of the forefoot.

In the advanced, degenerative flat foot it is almost always necessary to fuse the TNJ; the decision as to whether to fuse additional joints depends on their radiological appearance. When weightbearing lateral radiographs of the foot show that TNJ involvement is isolated it may be sufficient to fuse only the subtalar and talonavicular joints. Such a double fusion can be undertaken through a single medial incision, using the interval between the PTT and FDL to access both joints. The joints are fixed with image-intensifier guided 7 mm or 5.5 mm cannulated screws. The single medial incision (Figure 10.11) is said to give better visualization of the joints, allowing a more accurate reduction, and also leads to fewer wound problems, being on the shortening, as opposed to lengthening, side of the correction. Nevertheless a traditional two-incision medial and lateral approach fusing all three joints is also very acceptable.

In the rarer situations where there is a further break at the naviculocuneiform or tarsometatarsal joints an extended medial fusion might be considered, with the utilization of specialized locking plates

Figure 10.11 A subtalar and talonavicular fusion, undertaken from the medial side.

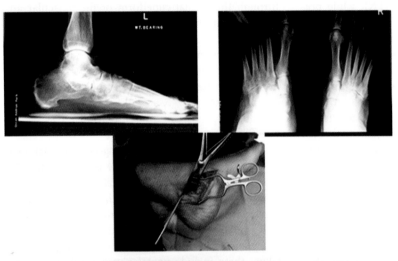

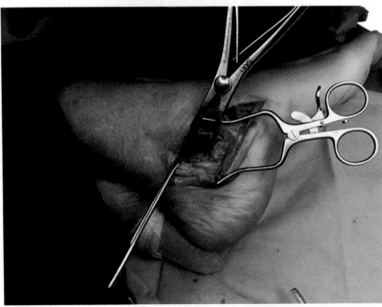

spanning the joints. In our practice all of these patients are discharged in a plaster slab, which is converted to a removable boot at ten days. They are treated with six weeks' non-weightbearing followed by a further six weeks' weight bearing in the boot.

Where other procedures have been performed and correction is incomplete one can add a dorsal opening, plantar flexion osteotomy of the medial cuneiform (Cotton osteotomy) or first ray to improve arch height and diminish residual heel valgus. If fusion procedures have been used and there is significant residual heel valgus a medial displacement calcaneal osteotomy may also be added to restore neutral alignment.

Which Combination of Procedures Should I Use?

There are various techniques available for the treatment of adult-acquired flat foot, implying that none is perfect. In our practice we plan each patient's surgery based upon their preoperative assessment, selecting a tailored combination of procedures from the available "menu" with the addition of minor modifications at the time of surgery as required. Our basic rule is to correct a flexible deformity though a combination of soft tissue and bony realignment procedures, and to fuse painful stiff joints. The most common presenting stage in our clinic is stage II with established, painful but flexible deformity. As a result medial displacement calcaneal osteotomy and FDL tendon transfer has become the workhorse for us and has given very satisfactory results. Lateral column lengthening can be considered where the lateral column is considered to be a driving factor, with significant talar head uncovering in conjunction with hypermobility. Nevertheless, the literature does not provide a systematic or scientific method for procedure selection, thus much of surgical decision making is based upon the surgeon's preference, which in turn is often determined by soft factors such as geography, fellowship training, and "schools of thought." Again, with fusion, a pragmatic approach is most sensible, with the most degenerative, painful, and deformed joints being fused. It is worth bearing in mind that TNJ fusion dramatically limits calcaneocuboid and subtalar movement, and vice versa.

Stage IV Disease

In stage IV disease there is ankle valgus, which must be addressed at surgery. Where the deformity is correctable and in the absence of established tibiotalar arthrosis, deltoid ligament reconstruction may be an option (stage IVa). In our practice this is a relatively rare scenario. When possible, however, stabilizing the ankle in conjunction with rebalancing the foot may act to halt the progression of frank ankle arthrosis. There are many techniques described for the reconstruction of the deltoid ligament, ranging from peroneus longus tendon transfer, through tendon allografts, to fully synthetic ligament replacements. All these procedures use tunnels in the talus and medial distal tibia with interference type fixation. One must emphasize that ankle joint preservation will only be successful where the driver of the ankle deformity is effectively addressed – i.e., correction of the coronal plane valgus moment about the ankle caused by the planovalgus foot.

In cases where there is fixed tibiotalar deformity or established arthrosis (stage IVb) fusion may be required. If the ankle is involved we prefer a tibotalar–calcaneal fusion to a pantalar fusion. Leaving the midtarsal joint mobile allows dorsi/plantar flexion movement. Generally an FDL tendon transfer is not required, as the stabilization of the subtalar joint partially addresses the planovalgus. An FDL tendon transfer should be considered where the midtarsal joint is deformed and correctable. In the case of widespread fixed arthrosis there is little alternative to a pantalar fusion. The role of total ankle replacement in stage IV disease has not yet been established, although there is no doubt that in severe cases the deformity mandates a pantalar fusion.

Results and Complications

Results

Non-Operative

There is no absolute evidence that orthotic devices slow or prevent the progression of the planovalgus deformity[25]. However, it has been shown that almost 83% of patients with stage I or II disease make a good subjective and functional recovery with non-operative treatment using a structured program of physiotherapy and orthoses[18]. In another study of patients with stage II disease treated with a double upright AFO, 70% avoided surgery and were brace free at seven to ten years. Therefore the results of non-operative treatments are satisfactory. As the majority of patients' symptoms resolve with non-operative management, especially those with lower stage disease and lesser degrees of deformity, surgery should be reserved for those who have failed conservative treatment, or who have little prospect of successful non-operative treatment[26–28].

Surgical Treatment

Stage I – Surgical treatment for stage I is controversial and although there is some evidence that surgical treatment provides short-term relief of pain, it is generally accepted that it does not substantially change the natural history of the condition[25,29].

Stage II – Flexor digitorum longus tendon transfer with a medial displacement calcaneal osteotomy has been shown to lead to excellent function and pain relief, with 92% satisfied with the procedure. Nevertheless the deformity correction was less good, with 25% rating the alignment as fair and 25% using orthoses at four years[30]. Lateral column lengthening procedures are of two types: a lengthening calcaneal osteotomy leaving the calcaneocuboid joint open[31–32], or a distraction arthrodesis of the calcaneocuboid joint with a structural bone graft. Both procedures led to an 84% success rate, with good improvement in the AOFAS score and radiographic parameters[33]. Nevertheless the lateral column lengthening procedures had high complication rates, with complications reported in 32 of 34 patients[33]. The complications differ depending on what type of lengthening is undertaken. The Evans procedure increases calcaneocuboid joint pressure and risks the later development of calcaneocuboid joint arthritis[34]. On the other hand, calcaneocuboid joint fusion in distraction has a significant delayed and non-union rate[34]. Nevertheless there is no clear consensus as to whether lateral column lengthening or calcaneal osteotomy is superior.

Stage III – The deformity is fixed here and arthrodesis is usually required. For many this will require at least TNJ fusion; for the more severe deformity triple arthrodesis is required. Correction of deformity is satisfactory in most fusions with the greater number of joints fused correlating with greater degrees of stiffness and functional limitation[35].

Stage IV – There is relatively little in the scientific literature to guide the surgeon on outcomes in operative treatment in stage IV disease. It has been shown that reconstruction of the deltoid ligament with tendon graft leads to a restoration of talar alignment within the ankle mortise in four of five patients at more than two years[36]. Where the foot is flexible, but the ankle is in valgus, the deformity can be corrected with joint sparing, as for stage II disease, with the addition of a deltoid ligament reconstruction. However, where the foot is stiff fusions provide better results up to and including pantalar arthrodesis[37]. As always the greater degree of joint degeneration and rigidity of the deformity, the more extensive the fusion, and the poorer the functional outcome.

Pitfalls

Non-Operative Management

- Although PTT dysfunction is the most common cause of adult-acquired flat foot, other diagnoses should be considered, including trauma (Lisfranc injury), TMTJ arthritis with collapse of the medial column, and rare conditions such as isolated spring ligament ruptures[39].

- In non-correctable deformity hard corrective orthoses are painful and patients will discard them. This group of patients requires soft conforming insoles to provide cushioned support.

- Low-profile in-shoe orthoses in the presence of significant foot pronation and tibial internal rotation may not be adequate. An AFO gives more powerful correction, but may be cosmetically unacceptable, impractical, or ineffective. In these cases surgery may be indicated.

Operative Management

Reconstruction

- Patients' expectations must be managed preoperatively. While case series with good results have been widely reported in the literature, the foot is not normal after surgery. In spite of this 97% of patients report pain relief, 94% improvement in function, 87% improvement in foot shape, and 84% being able to wear a shoe without an orthosis[38].

- The "workhorse" surgery of an FDL transfer and medial displacement calcaneal osteotomy (MDCO) can be used when the joints are supple and the deformity is correctable. It will not address a fixed and painful deformity with degenerate joints. A realigning calcaneal osteotomy may improve hindfoot alignment; however, if the midfoot is not correctable, fixed forefoot supination will remain. This may be corrected with fusion, or a Cotton osteotomy.

- Take time to examine and repair the spring ligament where necessary.
- Calcaneal osteotomy – the main pitfalls relate to fixation of the osteotomy. We generally use cannulated compression screws and care must be taken not to place the tip of the screw in the subtalar joint. Where large medial shifts of the tuberosity fragment are achieved a more lateral entry point in the heel may be required.

Arthrodeses

- Subtalar arthrodesis carried out though a lateral incision, where a large correction of hindfoot valgus may lead to difficulty closing the lateral wound, with potential wound-healing problems. A medial approach can be considered in cases in which the lateral skin is compromised, tight, or very large corrections are required.
- The majority of cases only require local bone graft[40].

Key Points

- The flexible flat foot is a variant of normal and rarely requires treatment.
- PTT dysfunction is the commonest cause of adult-acquired flat foot. Lisfranc injury, arthrosis,

Charcot neuroarthropathy, spring ligament rupture, and occult tarsal coalition are other causes.

- The classic patient is an obese woman in her fifties or sixties, often with diabetes mellitus and hypertension.
- Presentation is with medial pain and weakness in the ankle, with a loss of the medial arch, and asymmetrical heel valgus.
- The patient has an inability to undertake a repeated single heel raise.
- Non-operative management includes the use of in-shoe orthoses, University of California Biomechanics Laboratory (UCBL) orthoses, or an AFO.
- Understanding of PTT dysfunction is determined by the Johnson and Strom classification, with Myerson's addition of stage IV.
- Stage I – no deformity – cast for six weeks, followed by orthoses.
- Stage II – correctable deformity – over 70% satisfied with non-operative treatment. Operative treatment involves FDL tendon transfer and medial displacement calcaneal osteotomy.
- Stage III – non-correctable deformity – non-operative treatment with accommodative insoles; if this fails triple fusion is required.
- Stage IV – ankle tilt – if non-operative treatment fails consider either deltoid ligament reconstruction or pantalar fusion.

References

1. Kettelkamp DB, Alexander HHJ. Spontaneous rupture of the posterior tibial tendon. *Bone and Joint Surg.* 1969; 51-A:759–64.

2. Funk DA, Cass JR, Johnson KA. Acquired adult flat foot secondary to posterior tibial-tendon pathology. *J Bone Joint Surg.* 1986; 68-A:95–102.

3. Mann RA and Coughlin MJ eds. Flat foot in adults. In *Surgery of the Foot and Ankle*, 6th edn. (St Louis: C.V. Mosby, 1993), pp. 757–84.

4. Johnson JE, Harris GF. Pathomechanics of posterior tibial tendon insufficiency. *Foot and Ankle Clin.* 1997; 2:227–39.

5. Gould N, Schneider W, Takamara A. Epidemiological survey of foot problems in the continental United States: 1978–1979. *Foot Ankle.* 1980; 1:8–10.

6. Shibuya N, Jupiter DC, Ciliberti LJ, VanBuren V, La Fontaine J. Characteristics of adult flatfoot in the United States. *J Foot Ankle Surg.* 2010; 49:363–8.

7. Frey C, Shereff M, Greenidge NJ. Vascularity of the posterior tibial tendon. *Bone and Joint Surg.* 1990; 72-A:884–8.

8. Holmes GB, Mann RA. Possible epidemiological factors associated with rupture of the posterior tibial tendon. *Foot Ankle.* 1992; 13:70–9.

9. Johnson KA, Strom DE. Tibialis posterior tendon dysfunction. *Clin Orthop Relat Res.* 1989; 239:196–206.

10. Myerson MS. Adult acquired flatfoot deformity: treatment of dysfunction of the posterior tibial tendon. *Instr Course Lect.* 1997; 46:393–405.

11. Bluman EM, Title CI, Myerson MS. Posterior tibial tendon rupture: a refined classification system. *Foot Ankle Clin.* 2007; 12(2):233–49.

12. Rosenberg ZS. Chronic rupture of the posterior tibial tendon. *Magn Reson Imaging Clin N Am.* 1994; 2(1):79–87.

13. Conti S, Michelson J, Jahss M. Clinical significance of magnetic resonance imaging in preoperative planning for reconstruction of posterior tibial tendon ruptures. *Foot Ankle.* 1992; 3:208–14.

14. Nallamshetty L, Nazarian LN, Schweitzer ME, et al. Evaluation of posterior tibial pathology: comparison of sonography and MR imaging. *Skeletal Radiol.* 2005; 34(7):375–80. Epub 2005 May 14.

15. Graves SC, Mann RA, Graves KO. Triple arthrodesis in older adults. Results after long-term follow-up. *J Bone Joint Surg.* 1993; 75A:355–62.

16. Sennara H. Triple arthrodesis: a modified new technic. *Clin Orthop.* 1972; 83:237–40.

17. Vogler HW. Triple arthrodesis as a salvage for end-stage flatfoot. *Clin Podiatr Med Surg.* 1989; 6:591–604.

18. Alvarez RG, Marini A, Schmitt C, Saltzman CL. Stage I and II posterior tibial tendon dysfunction treated by a structured non-operative management protocol: an orthosis and exercise program. *Foot Ankle Int.* 2006; 27:2–8.

19. Saltzman CL. Stage I and II posterior tibial tendon dysfunction treated by a structured non-operative management protocol: an orthosis and exercise program. *Foot Ankle Int.* 2006; 27:2–8.

20. Wacker JT, Hennessy MS, Saxby TS. Calcaneal osteotomy and transfer of the tendon of flexor digitorum longus for stage-II

dysfunction of tibialis posterior. Three- to-five-year results. *J Bone Joint Surg.* 2002; 84B:4–58.

21. Hiller L, Pinney SJ. Surgical treatment of acquired flatfoot deformity: what is the state of practice among academic foot and ankle surgeons in 2002? *Foot Ankle Int.* 2003; 24(9):701–5.

22. Sharma P, Singh SK, Rao S. Is there a role for surgical decompression in stage I tibialis posterior tendon dysfunction? *J Bone Joint Surg Br.* 2003; 85:102 (suppl II).

23. Needleman RL. A surgical approach for flexible flatfeet in adults including a subtalar arthroereisis with the MBA sinus tarsi implant. *Foot Ankle Int.* 2006; 27:9–18.

24. Deland JT, Otis JC, Lee KT, Kenneally SM. Lateral column lengthening with calcaneocuboid fusion: range of motion in the triple joint complex. *Foot Ankle Int.* 1995; 16:729–33.

25. Deland JT. Adult-acquired flatfoot deformity. *J Am Acad Orthop Surg.* 2008; 16:399–406.

26. Bowring B, Chockalingam N. Conservative treatment of tibialis posterior tendon dysfunction: a review. *Foot (Edinb).* 2010; 20(1):18–26.

27. Logue JD. Advances in orthotics and bracing. *Foot Ankle Clin.* 2007; 12(2):215–32.

28. Lin JL, Balbas J, Richardson EG. Results of non-surgical treatment of stage II posterior tibial tendon dysfunction: a 7- to 10-year followup. *Foot Ankle Int.* 2008; 29(8):781–6.

29. Teasdall RD, Johnson KA. Surgical treatment of stage I posterior tibial tendon dysfunction. *Foot Ankle Int.* 1994; 15(12):646–8.

30. Wacker JT, Hennessy MS, Saxby TS. Calcaneal osteotomy and transfer of the tendon of flexor digitorum longus for stage-II

dysfunction of tibialis posterior. Three- to five-year results. *J Bone Joint Surg Br.* 2002; 84(1):54–8.

31. Evans D. Calcaneo-valgus deformity. *J Bone and Joint Surg.* 1975; 57-B(3):270–8.

32. Philips GE. A review of elongation of os calcis for flat feet. *J Bone Joint Surg.* 1983; 5-B(1):15–18.

33. Thomas RL, Wells BC, Garrison RL, Prada SA. Preliminary results comparing two methods of lateral column lengthening. *Foot Ankle Int.* 2001; 22:107–19.

34. Cooper PS, Nowak MD, Shaer J. Calcaneocuboid joint pressures with lateral column lengthening (Evans) procedure. *Foot Ankle Int.* 1997; 18(4):199–205.

35. Deland JT, Page A, Sung I-H, O'Malley MJ, Inda D, Choung S. Posterior tibial tendon insufficiency results at different stages. *Health Soc Serv J.* 2006; 2:157–60.

36. Deland JT, de Asla RJ, Segal A. Reconstruction of the chronically failed deltoid ligament: a new technique. *Foot Ankle Int.* 2004; 25:795–9.

37. Bluman EM, Myerson MS. Stage IV posterior tibial tendon rupture. *Foot Ankle Clin.* 2007; 12(2):341–62, viii.

38. Myerson, SM, Badekas A, Schon LC. Treatment of Stage II posterior tibial tendon deficiency with flexor digitorum longus tendon transfer and calcaneal osteotomy. *Foot Ankle Int.* 2004; 25:445–50.

39. Borton DC, Saxby TS. Tear of the plantar calcaneonavicular (spring) ligament causing flatfoot. A case report. *J Bone Joint Surg Br.* 1997; 79(4):641–3.

40. Rosenfeld PF, Budgen SA, Saxby TS. Triple arthrodesis: is bone grafting necessary? The results in 100 consecutive cases. *J Bone Joint Surg Br.* 2005; 87(2):175–8.

Sports Injuries of the Foot and Ankle

Brian S. Winters and Steven M. Raikin

Introduction

Sports injuries of the foot and ankle are a frequent reason for office visits to the orthopedic surgeon or non-operative sports medicine physician. No matter what the sporting event is or whether an individual is a professional athlete or a weekend warrior, the foot and ankle is likely needed in some capacity to participate and is therefore at risk of injury. This area of the body is extremely complex due to its unique biomechanics and 3D anatomy, with 28 bones, 33 joints, 107 ligaments, and 19 muscles and tendons. As these structures are all in close proximity, the various injuries can present with similar signs and symptoms, so understanding of the anatomy is essential. In this chapter our discussion is limited to injuries involving the lateral ankle ligamentous complex, the syndesmosis, the peroneal tendons, anterior and posterior ankle impingement syndromes, and turf toe.

Lateral Ankle Ligamentous Complex Injuries

Acute ankle sprains are among the most common musculoskeletal injuries[1–2]. The vast majority involve the lateral ankle ligament complex, which consists of the anterior talofibular ligament (ATFL), the calcaneofibular ligament (CFL), and the posterior talofibular ligament (PTFL). Fifteen to 20% of all sports injuries involve the lateral ankle ligament complex[3–4]. Nevertheless, despite their frequency, the injury is often considered an insignificant one with about 55% of individuals not even seeking treatment[5]. Therefore the true incidence is likely much higher. When diagnosed and treated in an appropriate manner, long-term sequelae are rare. The problem with this injury occurs when either the diagnosis is missed or the injury is undertreated. This often leads to chronic pain, muscular weakness, and instability.

Lateral ankle sprains most commonly occur following excessive inversion and internal rotation of the hindfoot while the leg is externally rotated. This puts the lateral ankle ligament complex under maximal tension[2,6]. The ATFL, the weakest of the three lateral ankle ligaments, is involved in nearly all lateral ankle sprains, either alone, or in combination with the CFL in 50 to 75% of such injuries. The PTFL is involved in only 10% of injuries[7]. The PTFL is not commonly injured because of the large amount of dorsiflexion and force that is required to put the ligament under significant tension. Increasing dorsiflexion in fact stabilizes the ankle, which further decreases the likelihood of a PTFL injury[8].

A patient with an acute lateral ankle ligament sprain will most often complain of pain and a sense of decreased stability. Assessment of the patient should begin with a thorough history and physical examination based on the Ottawa ankle rules for diagnosing a possible ankle fracture. When warranted, standard ankle radiographs must be obtained. Examination often reveals diffuse swelling, ecchymosis on the lateral side of the ankle, and heel and tenderness over the ATFL and CFL. Anterior talofibular ligament laxity is evaluated clinically by assessing the amount of anterior displacement of the talus from the ankle mortise using the anterior drawer test[9]. Here the hindfoot is held with the ankle in 15 to 20° of plantar flexion and the distal tibia is immobilized with the other hand. The hindfoot is then drawn anteriorly with slight internal rotation, and the amount of anterior translation and character of the endpoint are noted[10]. The talar-tilt test assesses the integrity of the CFL and is performed by inverting the hindfoot on the tibia, with the foot held in neutral dorsiflexion/plantar flexion. Again the amount of movement and character of the endpoint are estimated[11]. Both of these tests are subsequently compared to the contralateral, uninjured side and differences noted. Clinical examination is reasonably accurate in diagnosing a lateral ligament complex injury, but may be subject to false negatives[2]. It is important to note that in an acute injury the anterior drawer or talar-tilt test is painful, making it difficult to accurately assess the stability of the joint, as the patient may guard against examination. Once the swelling and tenderness subside, it is possible to perform a more accurate assessment of the joint. A local anesthetic ankle block an is option if an acute evaluation is necessary.

Lateral ankle ligament injuries are graded from I to III[12].

- Grade I: The ATFL is stretched with some tearing of the fibers, but no disruption. Clinically, the patient presents with mild swelling, ATFL tenderness, and no or mild restriction of active range of motion. Difficulty full weight bearing is sometimes seen. There is no laxity on examination.
- Grade II: A moderate injury, frequently with a complete tear of the ATFL and a partial tear of the CFL. Examination reveals a restricted range of motion with localized swelling, ecchymosis, and tenderness of the anterolateral aspect of the ankle. The ankle may be mildly lax or stable. A grade II injury may present with swelling and functional loss, making it indistinguishable acutely from a grade III injury.
- Grade III: Injury implies complete disruption of both the ATFL and CFL. A capsular or PTFL tear may also be present.

Malliaropoulos further subclassified grade III injuries into IIIA and IIIB, based on anterior drawer stress radiographs. According to Milliaropoulos' classification, grade III injuries lack more than 10° of movement and have more than 2 cm of measurable edema compared to the uninjured side. In a grade IIIA injury the stress radiographs are normal, as opposed to a grade IIIB injury where there is a 3 mm, or greater, measurable distance between the posterior articular surface of the tibia and the nearest point of the talus when compared to the normal side[13].

Although stress views are not required to establish the diagnosis of instability, they can be a helpful adjunct when the clinical presentation is unclear or to assess the severity of the injury. The standard stress views evaluate anterior draw of the talus beneath the tibia and a varus tilt of the talus within the mortise

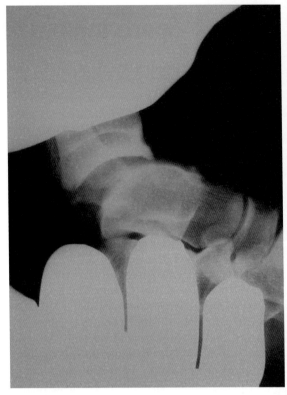

Figure 11.1 Positive anterior drawer stress radiograph as illustrated by the anterior translation of the talus on the tibial plafond due to anterior talofibular ligament incompetency.

(Figures 11.1 and 11.2). There is no absolute value that confirms instability, so comparison views with the opposite side can be very helpful and should be considered. In a stable ankle, the anterior drawer translation should measure less than 10 mm, or within 3 to 5 mm of the opposite side[11]. Normal talar-tilt values can range widely from 5 to 20°, although an absolute value of more than 10°, or a difference of greater than 3 to 5° compared to the uninjured side, is consistent with laxity[11]. Nevertheless laxity is common and often non-pathological, thus the numerical value of stress radiographs alone should never dictate your treatment.

MRI scanning has been shown to be an ineffective diagnostic modality for acute injuries and is of no value as a static test to determine dynamic instability[2,11]. Furthermore up to 60% of patients undergoing MRI scans for pathology other than instability have an ATFL tear as an incidental finding. Nevertheless, bearing in mind these limitations, MRI can be very useful in the subacute or chronic ankle sprain where

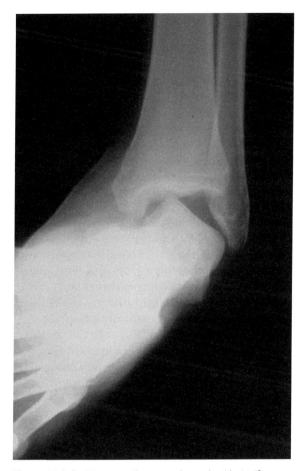

Figure 11.2 Positive varus tilt stress radiograph with significant instability of the lateral ankle ligament complex due to calcaneofibular ligament injury.

pain persists and is unresponsive to conservative measures. The MRI can demonstrate other causes of ankle pain, such as osteochondral lesions of the talus or tibial plafond, occult fractures, tendon tears, degeneration, and impingement lesions.

In the patient with an acute lateral ankle ligament complex sprain, the primary goals are to manage pain, control inflammation, and protect the joint. This involves early mobilization with an external support and a protocol of rest, ice, compression, elevation (RICE), and non-steroidal anti-inflammatory medication (NSAID) therapy. This is followed by a rehabilitation program, which consists of range-of-motion exercises, peroneal tendon strengthening, proprioception, and activity-specific training. Proprioception training is particularly important for the recovery of balance. In addition to providing mechanical stability,

external supports provide additional proprioceptive feedback and aid rehabilitation[2,4–5].

Ardèvol conducted a randomized controlled trial comparing cast immobilization with functional rehabilitation[14]. Functional management allowed an earlier return to sport, with fewer symptoms at three and six months post injury. There was also a greater reduction in radiographic laxity, although there was no difference in the re-injury rates between the two groups. A meta-analysis of randomized controlled trials comparing immobilization and functional rehabilitation of acute lateral ankle ligament injuries has demonstrated that functional management allows a higher proportion of patients to return to sport[15]. The functionally rehabilitated patients also demonstrated a higher rate of satisfaction, returned to work earlier, had less swelling, and their range of motion was improved when compared to those who were treated with cast immobilization[15]. Finally, in a systematic review of acute ankle ligament injuries, Kerkhoffs concluded that lace-up supports were most effective, while taping was found to be no better than semi-rigid supports. Of note, elastic bandages were the least effective form of treatment[16].

Treatment of the acute sprain is dependent on how quickly the patient wishes to return to athletic activity. In the elite athlete, an acute, severe sprain in an ankle, which is stable to clinical testing, can be treated symptomatically. An unstable ankle with a positive anterior drawer or talar tilt by clinical examination is further evaluated with stress radiographs[2,4–5,9,12]. If the stress radiographs are negative, then functional treatment is instituted. If they are positive, then surgical repair can be considered. It is important to understand that non-operative treatment is acceptable in the athlete and continues to demonstrate good results in approximately 90% of cases[2,4–5]. If non-operative treatment is unsuccessful, late reconstruction of the ligaments gives a good outcome[12]. In the non-elite athlete, non-operative treatment is pursued in the vast majority of cases. Acute operative intervention should be considered when an unstable ankle occurs in association with an osteochondral fracture, there is evidence of a syndesmotic injury, or in the presence of other associated injuries that would require surgical treatment, such as peroneal tendon injuries.

Chronically the main indication for surgery is failure of non-surgical management, with persistent, symptomatic ankle instability. Two subtypes of chronic instability have been described – mechanical and functional[9]. Patients with mechanical instability complain of giving way and have reproducible hyper-mobility of the tibiotalar joint on physical examin-ation. Individuals with functional instability present with a complaint of ankle instability but a lack of any objective signs of instability. Patients with mechanical instability are more likely to benefit from surgery than patients with functional instability.

Many surgical techniques are described for chronic lateral ankle instability; however, they fall into two basic categories: anatomic repair and tenodesis.

Anatomic repair: The goals of anatomic repair are to restore the normal anatomy and joint mechan-ics. Anatomical repairs are based upon the "Broström procedure,"[2,9] although the exact technique varies from surgeon to surgeon. Broström originally described a midsubstance imbrication of the lateral ligaments with sutures[17]. Gould subsequently aug-mented this with the posterior portion of the extensor retinaculum – the "Gould modification"[18]. In most procedures today the "Broström procedure" has been modified such that suture anchors are used to reattach the shortened and retensioned ATFL to its fibular insertion point. This is then reinforced with the Gould modification reefing the extensor retinaculum.

Tenodesis stabilization: Where the lateral liga-ments are irreparable tendon grafts can be used to reconstruct the ankle ligaments. The three classic reconstructions, all of which use the peroneus brevis tendon, are the Evans, Watson-Jones, and Chrisman–Snook procedures (Figure 11.3). All are well docu-mented with both the short- and long-term results reported[12,19–21]. One of the major drawbacks of all of the above procedures is that they are non-anatomic reconstructions and sacrifice normal structures. This is particularly concerning when utilizing the peroneus brevis tendon as it is the primary dynamic stabilizer of the ankle joint. Transfer of the peroneus brevis may in turn result in altered ankle kinematics, which could ultimately lead to degenerative changes of the ankle or subtalar joints.

- **The Watson-Jones** procedure reconstructs the ATFL, but not the CFL, by using a split peroneus brevis tendon transfer[21]. Several good short-term results have been reported, but long-term follow-up studies showed disappointing results[12].
- **The Evans** tenodesis is the least technically demanding, but biomechanically it does not reconstruct either the ATFL or the CFL, as the tendon graft is positioned in between these two ligaments[20]. Several investigators reported good short-term results after this reconstruction, but the long-term results have varied[12].
- **The Chrisman–Snook** procedure attempts to restore both the ATFL and CFL by routing the tendon through a complex system of bone tunnels, and probably is the most widely used tenodesis to reconstruct the ligaments[12]. In one study, satisfactory results were reported in 94% of patients with stress testing showing less residual laxity[2].

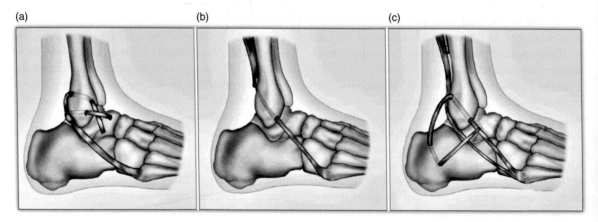

(a)   (b)   (c)

Figure 11.3 Three, largely historical, tenodesis procedures to reconstruct the lateral ankle ligaments: (**a**) Watson-Jones procedure; (**b**) Evans procedure; (**c**) Chrisman–Snook procedure.
(After Colville, MR. Surgical treatment of the unstable ankle. *J Am Acad Orthop Surg* 1998; 6: 368–377)

- **Semitendinosis tendon allograft** in a more recent study showed promising results where the ligament reconstructions were carried out with a near-anatomically placed graft to reconstruct the ATFL and CFL. Preservation of the peroneal tendons avoided loss of eversion strength and the reconstruction provided good ankle stability without sacrificing subtalar motion. There was also a decreased predisposition to subtalar arthritis in short-term follow-up[22].

Coexistent pathology should also be addressed at the same time as the ligament reconstruction. This is principally in two areas.

- In the cavovarus foot, correction of the deformity with a calcaneal or first-ray osteotomy, as dictated by the Coleman block test, should be considered at primary surgery to prevent recurrence.
- The patient with an underlying connective tissue disorder and global hypermobility also needs identifying. These patients are better treated with an augmented reconstruction. We use a semitendinosus allograft or autograft.

Studies show that wound problems, nerve injury, recurrent instability, and stiffness are not uncommon following surgery[2,23].

- **Wound complications** tend to be superficial in nature, while **nerve injuries** can range in severity from mild disturbances in sensibility to neuroma formation. Both tend to occur less commonly in the anatomic repairs. This has been attributed to the more extensive dissection required for the tenodesis procedures[2,12,23].
- **Instability** after surgical reconstruction can occur early or late. Several factors have been shown to predispose patients to operative failure, which include longstanding instability, high functional demand, reduced muscle strength, and slow muscle reaction time.

  The patient with recurrent instability needs to be carefully examined for a cavovarus deformity and hypermobility – these factors should ideally be assessed at the time of primary surgery as outlined above.

  Patients with recurrent instability should initially be treated with a proprioceptive-based physical therapy program. It has to be recognized that persistent functional instability in the setting of a structurally sound repair unfortunately can be very difficult and frustrating to treat. The outcome of revision surgery has been shown to be very unpredictable[2,9,12].

  The literature has consistently reported that patients with a previous history of lateral ankle sprain who wear ankle braces or tape have a lower incidence of re-injury than those who do not[2,5,12]. This reduction may be due to the mechanical support and enhanced proprioception that the brace offers.

- **Stiffness** is common after both anatomic and non-anatomic lateral ankle reconstruction procedures, although it occurs more frequently after tenodesis procedures as a result of overtightening the graft. Generally such stiffness is well tolerated[2,23] and considered to be an acceptable trade-off. Unfortunately, it can ultimately lead to impingement-type pain.
- **Major complications**, including deep venous thrombosis, pulmonary embolism, septic arthritis, and osteomyelitis, have been reported following the operative treatment of lateral ligamentous complex injuries[2,5,9,23]. They are fortunately rare.

Syndesmosis Injuries

An injury to the ankle syndesmosis, also referred to as a "high ankle sprain," is a significant injury, especially in the athlete. Literature dating back to 1773 has emphasized the importance of this ligamentous complex[24]. The diagnosis unfortunately is not always an easy one and requires a high index of suspicion as it constitutes a wide spectrum of injuries, ranging from a simple ligamentous sprain to frank diastasis with a concomitant osteochondral and medial ligament injury. Isolated syndesmotic sprains are reported to account for about 1% of all ankle sprains[25], although the prevalence may be much higher, as the injury is frequently misdiagnosed or missed completely. In one study 32% of professional football players were noted to have late calcification of the syndesmosis, signifying previous injury[25–26]. Mismanaged injuries can ultimately lead to chronic ankle pain, disability, and eventually arthritic change.

The ankle syndesmosis ligament complex consists of four main structures[4,24,27] (Figure 11.4).

- **The anteroinferior tibiofibular ligament** (AITFL) is the most frequently injured. It is often multifascicular, with the most inferior fascicle sometimes described as a separate structure

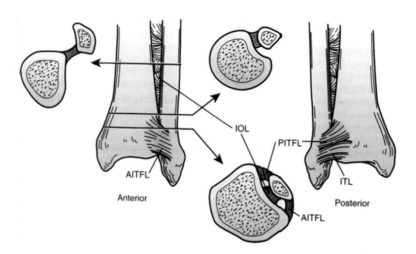

Figure 11.4 The four principal components forming the syndesmotic ligament complex. For abbreviations see text.
(After Rockwood and Green. *Fractures in Adults*, 7th edn. Philadelphia: Lippincott Williams & Wilkins; 2010. Figure 57-12)

entirely – Bassett's ligament. Bassett's ligament is a cause of anterior ankle impingement, and can impinge on the lateral talar dome[28].

- **The interosseous ligament** (IOL) connects the tibia and fibula from 0.5 cm to 2 cm above the plafond and surrounds the synovial recess, which extends upward from the ankle. At its superior margin, the IOL blends with the interosseous membrane (IOM). The IOM adds very little in terms of strength.

- Posteriorly there are two ligaments. The **inferior transverse ligament** (ITL) has a fibrocartilaginous appearance and functions, similarly to the glenoid labrum, to deepen the tibiotalar articulation. This is often continuous with the **posterior tibiofibular ligament** (PITFL). The ITL will be considered a part of the PITFL for the purposes of this chapter. Without these ligamentous restraints, the syndesmosis widens (Figure 11.5).

As a result of the unique shape of the talus, the fibula externally rotates and translates proximally and laterally during ankle dorsiflexion. It moves in the opposite direction with plantar flexion[29]. The syndesmotic ligaments, which accommodate this dynamic process, are most commonly injured in the setting of forceful external rotation and hyperdorsiflexion of the talus[29–31]. The talus external rotates against the fibula and in turn tensions the AITFL, which ultimately fails first (Figure 11.6). If the force is continued, disruption of the IOL and IOM occurs (Figure 11.7), followed by the PITFL. Isolated, complete ruptures of the syndesmosis were traditionally considered to be

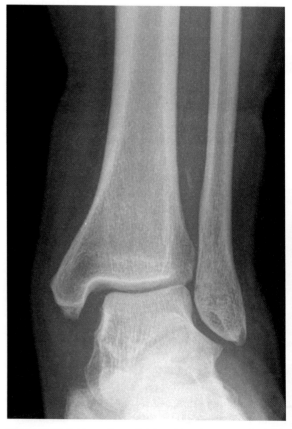

Figure 11.5 Ankle syndesmosis injury. Note the increased medial and tibiofibular clear spaces, as well as the decreased tibiofibular overlap.

a rarity, with syndesmosis injuries thought to more usually occur in conjunction with a distal fibula fracture. However, with increasing awareness and more

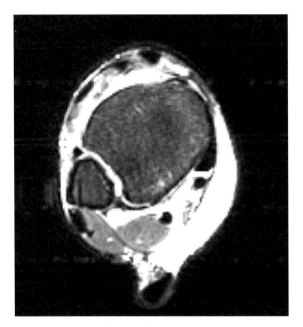

Figure 11.6 T2 weighted MRI demonstrating an AITFL tear.

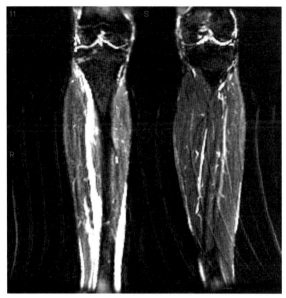

Figure 11.7 T2 weighted MRI in a patient with a Maisonneuve fracture variant and subsequent injury to the interosseous membrane. Note the substantial amount of soft tissue edema, demonstrating the severity of the injury.

sophisticated imaging isolated syndesmotic injuries are increasingly being recognized[26,32].

Numerous cadaveric studies have been performed to evaluate the relative contributions of each structure to ankle stability. Ogilvie-Harris determined that the AITFL contributes about 35%, the PITFL 40%, and the IOL 22% to overall stability. Injuring two of these structures decreases the syndesmotic resistance to lateral displacement by nearly 50%[33]. Xenos performed serial sectioning studies and found that cutting the AITFL alone resulted in an average 2.3 mm diastasis. Sectioning the distal 8 cm of the IOM/IOL resulted in an additional 2.2 mm, and sectioning the PITFL a further 2.8 mm. This equates to a total displacement of 7.3 mm[34]. These are large displacements as there is a 42% reduction in contact area, and consequent increase in pressure, with lateral translation of the talus of 1 to 2 mm, fibular shortening of 2 mm, and external rotation of 5° of the distal fibula with deltoid ligament strain[29-31]. This pathologic redistribution of pressures can result in the accelerated development of post-traumatic arthritis.

It is important to maintain a high index of suspicion as pain and difficulty with ambulation are common to both syndesmotic and lateral ankle ligament injuries. The physical examination of both injuries usually reveals ecchymosis and swelling over the anterolateral aspect of the ankle. The classic finding in acute syndesmotic, as opposed to a lateral ligament injury, is localized tenderness anteriorly over the syndesmosis, which is aggravated with forced dorsiflexion. The distance over which this tenderness extends proximally has been referred to as the "tenderness length." This is shown to correlate strongly with the degree of injury and time of return to sports activity[35]. It is also important to palpate the entire length of the fibula and both malleoli to rule out an associated bony or ligamentous injury[36].

A number of provocative stress tests have been described. The "squeeze test" is performed by compressing the tibia and fibula above the midpoint of the calf; this is positive if it induces pain at the level of the syndesmosis[37]. Although commonly used, studies have shown that the squeeze test is not reliable enough to confirm the diagnosis[25]. A far more reliable test is the "external rotation test"[25,30,33]. The patient sits with the knee flexed to 90° and the foot held in a neutral position. The foot is gently externally rotated. If this causes pain over the anterolateral ankle, proximal to the joint line, the test is considered positive. The "external rotation test" has been shown to have the best inter-observer reliability and sensitivity. A functional "stabilization test" has also been described. It is mainly used in athletes[26,38]. Athletic

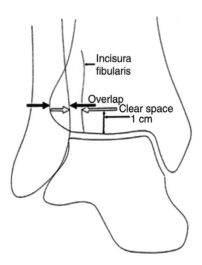

Figure 11.8 The tibiofibular clear space and overlap, which are used for detecting syndesmotic injury.

tape is tightly applied circumferentially above the ankle joint. If toe raises, walking, or jumping are less painful upon taping the test is considered positive.

Standing anteroposterior (AP), lateral, and mortise radiographs of the ankle should always be obtained. In patients who have proximal leg tenderness, additional AP and lateral views of the entire fibula should be obtained to rule out a Maisonneuve injury. It is important remember that up to 50% of all syndesmotic injuries may present with a bony avulsion of the distal anterior or posterior tibia. In chronic injuries, calcification of the syndesmosis, or even a synostosis, may be seen[39].

Three major radiological criteria define an unstable syndesmosis on radiographs (Figure 11.8).

1. **The medial clear space** is normally less than 4 mm, and is the space between the medial malleolus and medial border of the talus, 1 cm below the joint line. An increase in this space signifies an associated deltoid ligament injury[29,31,39]. Bonnin suggested that it is variable and should be used with caution[40].
2. **The tibiofibular clear space** is regarded as the most accurate parameter and is defined as the distance between the lateral cortex of the tibia and the medial cortex of the fibula, 1 cm above the joint line. In a cadaveric study, specimens without a syndesmotic injury consistently displayed a clear space of less than 6 mm[30]. A further cadaveric study noted sex-specific differences with a clear space of less than 5.2 mm in female patients and 6.5 mm in male patients[41].
3. **The tibiofibular overlap** is the overlap of the posterior tibia on fibula at the level of the incisura. It can be calculated either as an absolute amount or percentage of fibular width. Cadaveric studies have shown that tibiofibular overlap should be more than 6 mm, or 42% of the fibular width[30]. In sex-specific cadaveric studies the overlap should be greater than 2.1 mm in female and 5.7 mm in male patients, or 24% of the fibular width[41]. Although these numbers are widely accepted, it is important to remember that a radiograph of the uninjured ankle is instrumental in defining what is normal for a specific patient.

If a syndesmosis injury remains a concern, despite normal radiographs, external-rotation stress radiographs may help. While many advocate their use, the reliability of stress radiographs has been questioned. This stems from a study by Xenos who showed that there was only slight widening of the mortise when an external-rotation torque was applied to an ankle, despite sectioning all of the ligaments[34]. Negative-stress radiographs have also been obtained in patients who subsequently had an arthroscopically confirmed syndesmosis injury[42]. Therefore additional imaging studies in the form of a CT scan or MRI may be required to establish the diagnosis.

Ebraheim demonstrated in a cadaver model the superiority of CT scanning over plain radiographs. The CT shows fibular shift, rotation, shortening, and bony avulsions[43]. Routine radiographs did not show small 1 or 2 mm diastases, whereas all were detected on CT. Routine radiographs even failed to diagnose a syndesmotic injury in 50% of patients who had 3 mm diastases. It is important to evaluate the fibular rotation and tibiofibular distance at exactly the same level, if bilateral scans are obtained, to avoid misdiagnosis. An MRI gives the most detail about the integrity of the ligamentous complex and has become the standard of care in evaluating athletes suspected of having a syndesmosis injury. This stems from studies conducted by Takao who found the sensitivity, specificity, and accuracy of an MRI in identifying a syndesmotic injury to be 100%, 93.1%, and 96.2% for a tear of the AITFL and 100%, 100%, and 100% for a tear of the PITFL[44]. The sensitivity (90%) and specificity (95%) in identifying a chronic syndesmosis injury are also high[39]. Although both CT and MRI give the clinician a significant amount of information, it is important to remember that the images are non-weightbearing or unstressed. If subtle instability exists, an injury can still be missed. Lui showed that ankle arthroscopy was more sensitive than intra-operative stress radiographs in detecting syndesmotic injury[45]. Some have even advocated routine ankle arthroscopy with this in mind, especially in view of the fact that multiple studies have shown significant functional improvement with arthroscopy[29–31].

Numerous classification systems have been described for ankle syndesmosis injuries, but none clearly define the degree of injury, provide a clear therapeutic algorithm, or predict prognosis. Treatment decisions should thus be based on the patient's signs and symptoms, their level of activity, injury severity on imaging, and whether the injury is acute, subacute, or chronic.

Sprains without diastasis or instability can be managed non-operatively. The first phase is directed at protecting the ankle and limiting pain with RICE and anti-inflammatory medication. It has been also recommended that the ankle should be immobilized with a protective boot or brace, with weightbearing status determined by the patient's symptoms. The second phase begins when the acute pain has subsided and involves joint mobilization, strengthening, and neuromuscular training. In the third phase, the athlete progresses to an advanced proprioception-training program with sports-specific drills. Overall, the results of non-operative management show good to excellent results ranging from 86 to 100%[29–31].

Those with instability but no diastasis on stress testing have also been treated successfully non-operatively[29]. These patients need to be managed with a non-weightbearing cast for at least four weeks. Obtaining a repeat weightbearing radiograph is recommended at two weeks in order to confirm that reduction is maintained. After the initial four weeks, progressive weight bearing in a protective boot or walking cast may be started so that the patient is fully weight bearing at eight weeks post injury. Some authors have recommended that high-performance athletes with this degree of injury should be treated more aggressively with surgery[32]. However, this approach has yet to be justified by the literature. Ultimately, it is important to inform the patient that the recovery from syndesmosis injuries is much longer than that from a lateral ankle ligament injury, with several studies illustrating a doubling of the amount of time before being able to return to full, unrestricted activity[29,32].

Patients with frank diastasis of the syndesmosis require operative treatment, and extreme care needs to be taken to accurately reduce the fibula within the incisura. Traditionally it was recommended that the ankle needed to be held in dorsiflexion at the time of fixation, to ensure that the widest part of the talus is within the ankle mortise during fixation to avoid over-tightening of the joint. This was challenged by Tornetta who demonstrated that it is anatomic reduction of the fibula into the sigmoid notch that is the most important factor in successful syndesmosis fixation[46]. Fixation should be performed though an open lateral incision, exposing the incisura and ensuring an anatomic reduction prior to fixation. If an anatomic reduction is not possible a medial arthrotomy, to address medial pathology, should be undertaken. Historically the syndesmosis has been fixed rigidly with screws. McBryde determined that the screws should be placed 2.0 cm proximal to the tibiotalar joint, as this provides better stability than placing the screws more proximally[47]. Even with good quality intra-operative fluoroscopic imaging, postoperative CT scans have demonstrated that malreduction of the syndesmosis occurs in up to 24% of cases[39], although it has been shown that the malreduced fibula usually self-reduces anatomically after screw removal[48]. The number of screws, their size, and number of cortices fixed continues to be debated. Screws are kept in place for a minimum of six to eight weeks, while some investigators recommend that they are not removed for three months. Where the screws are left in situ, breakage and osteolysis around the screw is likely, although the patients have been shown to do well[49–50].

Bioabsorbable screws have also increased in popularity, as they do not need to be removed and provide excellent stability. An additional advantage is that although the length of time the screws take to dissolve remains unknown, if the fibula is malreduced it may reduce as the screws dissolve. The clinical results of bioabsorbable screws appear to be equivalent to those of metal screws. The main drawback is that they may create a local inflammatory reaction, which can manifest as a sterile abscess or cyst[51].

Semi-rigid fixation with polyester/polyethylene sutures secured with buttons tensioned across the syndesmosis have the theoretical advantage of maintaining movement (Figure 11.9). Thornes compared these with syndesmosis screw fixation and found that the semi-rigid fixation was at least as good as screws[52]. Seitz found a suture to be comparable to a

Peroneal Tendon Injuries

Lateral ankle sprains are the most common traumatic injury of the ankle, and other causes of lateral ankle pain are frequently overlooked. Once considered to be rare, peroneal tendon injuries in athletes have been recognized as a common cause of non-resolving pain after a "typical" ankle sprain[57]. Thus a high index of suspicion is required.

The peroneal musculature makes up the entire lateral compartment of the leg. At the level of the ankle, the tendon of the peroneus brevis (PB) lies against the retromalleolar groove of the distal fibula. The peroneus longus (PL) tendon lies behind that of the PB, compressing it in the groove. At this level both tendons are contained within a shared fibro-osseous tunnel, the fibular groove, which is deepened by a cartilaginous ridge. The tunnel is completed posteriorly and laterally by the superior peroneal retinaculum (SPR). The muscle belly of PB is more distal than that of PL, and can overstuff the tunnel and in turn predispose to injury[57]. Additional differences in the anatomy of the groove may also predispose some individuals to peroneal instability. Edwards noted that a fibular sulcus, or groove, was present in 82% of individuals, the bone was flat in 11%, and in 7% it was convex[58]. Ozbag found that 68% had a concave fibular groove, whereas the remaining specimens had a flat or convex area on the distal fibula[59].

Both tendons pass distal to the fibula and turn toward the peroneal tubercle, where the common tendon sheath bifurcates and passes under the inferior peroneal retinaculum. The PL then enters a second tunnel under the cuboid where the os peroneum, a sesamoid bone present in 10 to 20% of individuals, is located[60]. The PL ultimately inserts into the plantar aspect of the base of the first metatarsal and medial cuneiform. The PB courses over the calcaneofibular ligament, above the peroneal tubercle, and inserts into the base of the fifth metatarsal. Both tendons are relatively weak ankle plantar flexors, but do contribute significantly to hindfoot eversion[57,61]. The PL also plantar flexes the first ray. The PB is the strongest abductor of the forefoot. Both work together to dynamically stabilize the lateral ankle ligament complex.

An accessory muscle, the peroneus quartus (PQ), is present in 13 to 22% of the population[62]. It most commonly originates from the PB and inserts distally on the peroneal tubercle of the calcaneus. The

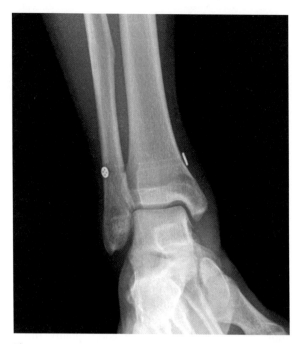

Figure 11.9 Suture endobutton syndesmotic fixation.

4.5 mm screw fixed across four cortices[53]. The semi-rigid suture technique is also associated with a shorter rehabilitation, faster return to work, and lack of complications[29,54]. In contrast, a cadaveric biomechanical study reported the failure of the suture to maintain adequate syndesmotic reduction when compared with a metallic screw, particularly with rotational forces[55].

The salvage procedure of choice for arthritis, secondary to chronic instability of the syndesmosis, is syndesmotic arthrodesis, which has been shown to produce good long-term pain relief.

In addition to chronic instability and arthritis, the most commonly cited complication following a syndesmotic injury is heterotopic ossification[26,31,39]. The presence of pain with heterotopic ossification is inconsistent[26,31,39]. Hopkinson and colleagues described nine cases of heterotopic ossification all of which were asymptomatic[26]. On the other hand, McMaster and Scranton found radiographic evidence of tibiofibular synostosis in several patients who had persistent pain three to 11 months after injury[26]. Veltri and colleagues reported two cases of symptomatic tibiofibular synostosis in collegiate and professional football players. Both returned to full activity after resection[56]. In general, it is accepted that when a painful synostosis occurs, it should be resected and sealed with bone wax to prevent recurrence.

presence of the PQ has been associated with peroneal tears, instability, and stenosing tenosynovitis by virtue of its bulk in the restricted space under the SPR[60,63]. Unfortunately, even with MRI scanning the diagnosis can be difficult to make as the accessory tendon can appear similar to a split in the PL[57].

Traditionally patients with inflamed and painful peroneal tendons are said to be suffering with "peroneal tendinitis." However, when surgical specimens of the peroneal tendon are examined histologically, very few inflammatory cells are present[64]. Instead, a much more degenerative pattern is seen, where the collagen matrix is organized in a random fashion with numerous fibroblasts[64]. Therefore the condition is better described as a "tendinosis," a description that also applies to the tendo Achillis. An acute inflammatory process of the well-vascularized tenosynovium can result in an effusion within the peroneal sheath[64]. Stenosing tenosynovitis of the peroneal tendons has been described in chronic cases, in which thickening of the tendon sheath constricts the tendons. This usually occurs in one of three areas, namely the retromalleolar sulcus, the peroneal tubercle, or the cuboid tunnel.

Typical symptoms of peroneal tendon pathology include weakness, pain, and swelling along the lateral aspect of the ankle, particularly posterior to the lateral malleolus. Pain is exacerbated by passive plantar flexion and inversion of the ankle, or by active, resisted dorsiflexion and eversion of the foot. The actual strength of the peroneal musculature is usually good, despite the pain. Circumduction of the foot and ankle is important at the time of examination as it may provoke subluxation or dislocation of the tendons. The presence of such instability alters the treatment[61,63]. A tight gastrocnemius–soleus complex, with increased calcaneal varus, should also be noted, as the presence of significant varus can ultimately result in re-injury if it is not corrected.

Radiographic examination is usually normal, and is only necessary to exclude other sources of pain and to assess the foot alignment. Rarely an acute avulsed flake of bone may be seen from the lateral tip of the fibula, where the SPR has been avulsed, and the tendons consequently dislocated. Another rare abnormality is a proximally migrated fractured os peroneum with a PL tear[65]. Tenography has been described, but is rarely used with the advent of MRI and USS. An MRI scan demonstrates fluid within the tendon sheath, although it is important to bear in mind that with the alteration in direction of the peroneal tendons at the inframalleolar region, and the flat morphology of the PB, false positive findings of tendinosis or split tears may be seen on MRI scanning as a result of the "magic angle phenomenon"[66]. A USS is more operator dependent, but can be helpful in reaching a diagnosis, as well as guiding diagnostic or therapeutic injections. It is generally recommended that injections are kept to a minimum to avoid soft-tissue atrophy and tendon rupture. One of the biggest advantages of US is the ability to dynamically assess the tendons in cases of suspected peroneal subluxation or dislocation[67–68].

The recommended non-operative management of acute peroneal tenosynovitis is RICE. Use of NSAIDs and a period of immobilization using a cast, boot, or orthosis for four to six weeks can be helpful. After symptoms subside, the patient should be mobilized as soon as possible with a course of physical therapy concentrating on proprioception, flexibility, and strengthening. Taping of the ankle or the use of an ankle brace during vigorous activity can be tried. It is extremely rare for tenosynovitis to progress to the point where surgery is required. If surgery is necessary, a tenosynovectomy and resection of any impinging bony prominences is undertaken. This, along with the correction of any associated biomechanical disorder, such as hindfoot varus, usually gives excellent results[62].

In cadaver studies, PB tears are found in 11 to 37% of specimens[69–70]. Although PL tears are less common, when they do occur they are associated with a varus hindfoot[71]. The varus position increases the force on the tendons and the peroneal tubercle. The tubercle in turn hypertrophies, further damaging the tendons. PB and PL tears usually take the form of longitudinal splits, although complete ruptures do occur leading to weakness and functional ankle instability.

Acute peroneal tears (Figure 11.10) are often the result of a sporting injury. The mechanism is usually subluxation of the PB over the posterolateral edge of the fibula as a result of injury to the SPR. Repetitive compression of the PB by the PL against the posterior fibula in the fibular groove may also cause a tear of the PB. Other contributing factors include tenosynovitis, distal insertion of the peroneus brevis muscle belly, and the presence of a PQ[72]. These last two factors lead to overcrowding of the fibular groove and predispose to tendon subluxation or dislocation.

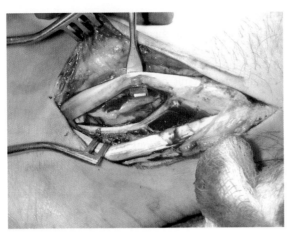

Figure 11.10 Intraoperative photograph illustrating a split tear in the peroneus brevis tendon as it courses around the distal fibula within the retromalleolar groove.

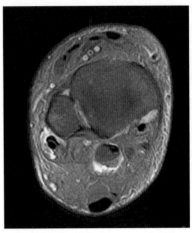

Figure 11.11 MRI demonstrating significant peroneal tendon instability with disruption of the superior peroneal retinaculum and complete dislocation of the peroneal tendons.

It is thought that flat or convex fibular groove morphology predisposes to tendon instability[57,61,63].

Conservative management is as described above for tenosynovitis, with the possible addition of an orthosis with lateral posting of the hind- and forefoot. If non-operative treatment fails, operative treatment may be needed. Krause and Brodsky described a simple classification system to help guide the surgical treatment of PB tears. This can also be applied to PL tears[73]. After an extensive tenosynovectomy and debridement, the remaining tendon is graded based on the amount of tendon still remaining. In grade 1 tears, 50% or more of the tendon is in continuity and viable after debridement. This 50% can be repaired with tubularization. In grade 2 tears less than 50% of the tendon remains viable after debridement. The abnormal tendon is excised and the stumps are tenodesed to the intact, uninvolved peroneal tendon, both proximally and distally.

Subluxation and dislocation of the peroneal tendons from the retromalleolar groove to the lateral aspect of the fibula (Figure 11.11) can cause lateral ankle pain, clicking, and instability. Frequently these injuries are misdiagnosed acutely as a routine ankle sprain. Acute peroneal tendon dislocations most commonly result from a sudden, forceful, passive dorsiflexion of an everted foot with a sudden, strong contraction of the peroneal muscles[74]. However, this injury has also been described with the foot held inverted[75]. This vigorous contraction causes the superior peroneal retinaculum to strip off the fibula at its periosteal attachment. The peroneals

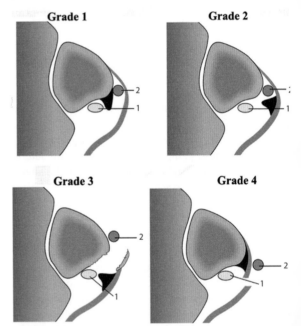

Figure 11.12 The Eckert and Davis classification of peroneal subluxation, with Oden's modification (Grade 4). 1 is the PB and 2 the PL.
(After Oden R. R. Tendon injuries around the ankle resulting from skiing. *Clin Orthop Relat Res*, 1987; 216: 63–9)

subsequently dislocate anteriorly. With chronic, recurrent dislocation, the patient presents with a snapping sensation over the distal fibula, which is usually painful.

Eckert and Davis (Figure 11.12) described three types of injury patterns[76]. In grade 1, the retinaculum and its attachment to the periosteum are stripped from the distal fibula. The peroneal tendons dislocate

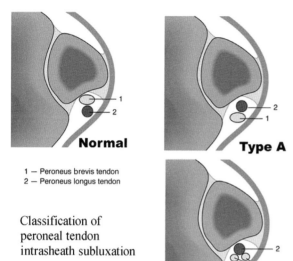

Normal

1 — Peroneus brevis tendon
2 — Peroneus longus tendon

Classification of
peroneal tendon
intrasheath subluxation

Type A

Type B

Figure 11.13 Raikin's classification of intrasheath peroneal tendon subluxation. 1 is the PB and 2 the PL.
(After Raikin et al., Intrasheath subluxion of the peroneal tendons. *J Bone Joint Surg Am.* 2008; 90: 992–9)

anteriorly into the pouch formed between the lateral border of the fibula and the periosteum/retinaculum. In grade 2 injuries, the fibrocartilagenous ridge is stripped, remaining attached to the retinaculum/periosteum. In a grade 3 injury the periosteum avulses where the cartilaginous rim attaches, giving a characteristic radiological appearance. In 1987, Oden described a grade 4 injury where the peroneal tendons dislocate through a tear in the peroneal retinaculum[74].

Intrasheath peroneal tendon subluxation (Figure 11.13) was described by Raikin and includes two subtypes. Type A is a true subluxation where the PL and PB flip over each other, reversing their positions within the retromalleolar tunnel. Type B occurs when the PL subluxes through a longitudinal split tear in the PB, again while remaining within the retromalleolar space. In both types, painful clicking occurs with activity or on clinical examination while the ankle is circumducted through a dorsiflexed, everted position. Intrasheath subluxation is best diagnosed with dynamic US[68].

The role of non-operative treatment of peroneal dislocations remains controversial. Numerous studies have been published describing various non-operative treatments ranging from short-leg, non-weightbearing casts, to simple, soft-compression dressings[57,62].

The results of non-operative treatment are disappointing and therefore surgical treatment is recommended, as it yields excellent long-term results[57,62]. For acute injuries without avulsed bony fragments, the commonest technique is repair of the superficial peroneal retinaculum, with or without deepening of the fibular groove. When the injury includes an avulsed rim of cortical bone from the insertion of the superficial peroneal retinaculum (grade 3), the fragment should be openly reduced and internally fixed. Unlike the acute injury, symptomatic, chronic dislocations must be treated surgically. Numerous procedures have been described[57,61–64,68], although the basis is usually reattachment of the retinaculum, with or without deepening of the groove. The peroneal tendons should also be repaired, according to the principles outlined above.

There are varying causes of plantar lateral foot pain. One of these is "painful os peroneum syndrome," which is often shortened to POPS. The os peroneum is a sesamoid bone, which is found in the PL tendon in 5 to 14% of individuals. The os articulates with the cuboid and calcaneus as the PL runs under the lateral border of the foot in the "cuboid tunnel." Acutely POPS can result from an acute os peroneum fracture or diastasis of a multipartite os peroneum, which lies within the substance of the PL tendon. Chronically an os peroneum fracture or diastasis of a multipartite os peroneum can create significant callus formation, which can ultimately result in a stenosing tenosynovitis of the PL within the cuboid tunnel. In addition, a partial or complete rupture of the PL tendon can also occur proximal or distal to the os peroneum, resulting in discontinuity. Clinically the patient presents with tenderness over the PL as it passes under the lateral border of the foot in the cuboid tunnel. This tenderness may be provoked by a single-stance heel rise, varus inversion stress, and resisted plantar flexion of the first ray. Standard weightbearing radiographs may show the os peroneum, which may be multipartite, fractured, or displaced proximally or distally in the case of PL rupture. Imaging the asymptomatic, contralateral foot may help in making a diagnosis. An MRI scan can also provide additional information if the diagnosis is still suspected in the setting of normal radiographs or if a rupture is apparent. A course of non-operative treatment in the absence of rupture should be attempted and includes a period of rest, non-steroidal anti-inflammatory medication, immobilization, and restricted weight bearing for two to six weeks. Once the pain subsides, a course of physical therapy can be considered. If non-operative treatment fails, the PL is ruptured, or the os peroneum is fractured with significant diastasis, surgery may be indicated. Surgery may consist of excision of the os peroneum or repair of the tendon, although reports in the literature are scarce and just of isolated case reports.

Anterior Ankle Impingement Syndrome

Many athletes complain of chronic anterior ankle pain as a result of the development of osteophytes on the anterior border of the tibial plafond and the talar neck. This was historically referred to as "footballer's ankle" as a result of its frequent occurrence in professional soccer players in Europe[77–78]. The problem has subsequently been described in a multitude of other athletes[79] and the condition is now referred to as anterior ankle impingement syndrome[80–81]. The incidence has been reported to be 45% in soccer players and 59% in dancers[64].

Mechanical factors were once believed to play an essential role in the formation of these osteophytes through repeated capsuloligamentous traction in a hyperplantarflexed foot[82–83]. Bone formation was considered to be a response to intermittent stress, through Wolff's law of bone remodeling[79]. Nevertheless, it is now known that the anterior ankle capsule attaches to the tibia 6 mm proximal to the joint line and 3 mm from the cartilage border on the talar side[79]. The difference between capsular attachment and the origin of the bony spurs makes it unlikely that traction plays a role in the development of osteophytes. It is now thought that the osteophytes may result from localized degenerative arthritis[84]. Anterior talar subluxation as a result of instability is significantly correlated with medial ankle osteophyte formation[85] and anterior bony impingement[83]. Interestingly, it has become evident that the pain most often results as a result of the synovium being caught between the talus and the ankle mortise, and not necessarily from impaction of the osteophytes[86]. When the synovial tissue is examined after resection, it reveals changes consistent with chronic inflammation and fibrosis[79]. The osteophytes, which initially develop at the non-weightbearing anterior cartilage rim of the distal tibia, merely facilitate the impingement[82].

Patients with anterior ankle impingement are typically young athletes. The diagnosis is largely clinical

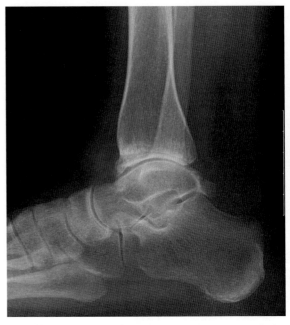

Figure 11.14 Anterior ankle impingement. Note the rim osteophytes emanating from the distal tibial plafond and talar neck. The remainder of the joint remains unaffected, which differentiates this from ankle joint osteoarthritis.

with anteromedial or anterolateral ankle pain, swelling, and limited dorsiflexion. Symptoms are exacerbated by any activity requiring ankle dorsiflexion, including walking up stairs, jumping, running, and squatting. Localized tenderness of the anterior ankle joint is evident and bony prominences may be palpable, with the hallmark finding being limited, and often painful, dorsiflexion of the ankle. Provocation of pain by hyperdorsiflexion of the ankle joint is typical. It is important to differentiate between anteromedial and anterolateral impingement. Anterolateral impingement is frequently caused by Bassett's ligament[28], which is the inferior fascicle of the anterior inferior tibiofibular ligament of the ankle syndesmosis. When hypertrophied, Bassett's ligament has the potential to impinge on the lateral talar dome and lead to osteochondral damage[28,79]. A similar picture can occur medially, with impingement of either a capsular or deltoid ligament tear.

Standard weightbearing AP, lateral, and mortise radiographs should always be obtained to evaluate the anterior tibial plafond and talar neck. A suggestive physical examination in the presence of osteophytes (Figure 11.14) confirms the diagnosis. Nevertheless the radiographs may be completely normal, or in the early stages there may be a mild periosteal reaction of the anterior tibia[79]. Additionally anteromedial osteophytes are not always visible and may require additional radiographic views. A cadaver study has shown that anteromedial osteophytes up to 7.3 mm in size can remain undetected as a result of superimposition of the prominence of the anterolateral border of the distal tibia on the lateral portion of the talar neck/body[87]. An oblique radiograph with the foot plantar flexed and the beam tilted 45° in the craniocaudal direction with the leg held in 30° of external rotation can detect these osteophytes[79,88–89]. The sensitivity of lateral radiographs for anterior tibial and talar osteophytes is 40 and 32% respectively, with a specificity of 70 and 82%[48]. When lateral radiographs are combined with an oblique anteromedial radiograph, the sensitivity increases to 85% for tibial and 73% for talar osteophytes[48,79]. The radiographic appearances of anterior impingement are similar to those of osteoarthritis of the ankle joint, but the important distinction between patients with anterior impingement and primary osteoarthritis is the lack of involvement in the remainder of the joint.

Scranton and McDermott classified the changes seen on standard radiographs into four grades.

- Grade I: an anterior tibial spur less than 3 mm.
- Grade II: a tibial spur greater than 3 mm, with no talar reaction.
- Grade III: a tibial spur greater than 3 mm, with a talar neck osteophyte.
- Grade IV: evidence of degenerative ankle arthritis[79,82].

A variant of this is the "divot sign"[90] seen in high-performance soccer players. Lateral radiographs show a divot, rather than an osteophyte, on the anterior talar neck. These athletes have the same symptoms, but tend to have no or little loss of ankle dorsiflexion.

A CT scan may be helpful, especially when x-rays are negative. This also allows further characterization of the impingement lesion if surgical intervention is being considered. The osteophytes have in the past been referred to as "kissing" osteophytes but, interestingly, a retrospective CT study by Beberian illustrated that the lesions are, in fact, not "kissing" at all[91]. Axial CT images were used to determine both tibial and talar osteophyte location by referencing them to the midline of the talar dome. 95% confidence intervals demonstrated that the talar lesion actually lies medial to the midline, while the tibial lesion lies lateral to the midline, and they typically do not overlap each other. This study suggested that the anterior tibiotalar osteophytes are consistent in their location, and further supports the thought that the pain originates from the soft tissues, rather than from any true bony impingement.

Anterior ankle impingement syndrome should initially be treated conservatively, with RICE, oral non-steroidal anti-inflammatory medication, and some form of immobilization with an AFO. The orthosis can range anywhere from a lace-up ankle brace, to a rigid CAM boot, to a non-weightbearing or weightbearing cast. The decision as to which to use depends on the severity of the patient's symptoms. The duration of immobilization ranges from two to six weeks. If pain persists an intra-articular corticosteroid injection can be considered. Physical therapy has no role in treating this condition[79].

If non-operative management fails, surgical intervention is considered. For bony lesions, the traditional approach is through an open ankle arthrotomy and cheilectomy of the distal tibial plafond and talar neck using either a chisel or osteotome[79]. Different surgical approaches have been described including a direct anterior or a dual "mini" anteriomedial and anterolateral approach. Whichever approach is used it is important to completely resect the osteophytes. McMurray reported on a series of surgically treated patients all of whom returned to professional soccer[77]. Numerous subsequent studies have also reported excellent results[79], although open surgery can be complicated by cutaneous nerve entrapment, long extensor tendon injury, and wound dehiscence or breakdown[92]. Arthroscopic surgery has now been adopted by many, and gives similarly good results to open surgery in terms of pain relief, both in the short and long term. However, arthroscopy has its own risks and limitations, including inadequate visualization leading to incomplete resection, iatrogenic cartilage injury, and superficial peroneal or saphenous nerve injury[79]. Scranton and McDermott published the only study that compared open and arthroscopic resection and showed that patients treated arthroscopically recovered in approximately half the time, with return to athletic activity one month faster[82].

A combined arthroscopic and open procedure is worth considering[48,79,86,93]. Through a small anteromedial or anterolateral incision a small instrument is introduced to resect the bone under arthroscopic guidance. This minimizes the soft-tissue dissection, decreasing the risk of wound complications, while allowing resection of the anterior osteophyte without creating the bony debris seen in a purely arthroscopic approach. The combined technique can also help resect larger osteophytes.

Patients with anterior ankle impingement and chronic instability also benefit from surgical intervention if conservative treatment fails. Cannon described the surgical treatment of 13 athletes with combined lateral instability and a painful block to dorsiflexion[94]. In this study the anterior osteophytes were debrided arthroscopically and a Brøstrom–Gould open stabilization procedure was performed. At a mean follow-up of 12 months, all 13 patients were found to have a mechanically and functionally stable ankle with an improvement in ankle dorsiflexion of 12°. All but one experienced improvement in their subjective and functional outcome scores, which suggests that combined, simultaneous ankle stabilization and anterior decompression should be considered in these patients.

Although most patients do very well following anterior decompression, some patients do go on to develop worsened pain after surgery[48,79,83]. Patients with extensive anterior arthritis, as shown by large osteophytes and narrowing of the anterior joint space, have less predictable results from surgery. Increased pain occurs in these patients as a result of their improved motion postoperatively, which in turn allows for increased contact of the arthritic joint surfaces with subsequent inflammation of the surrounding synovium. For this reason, it is extremely important to make an accurate diagnosis, so that one can be judicious when offering these patients surgery.

Posterior Ankle Impingement Syndrome

Posterior ankle pain with the ankle in plantar flexion, and pain provoked by rapid hyperplantarflexion of the ankle, is not infrequently seen. It is often seen in the ballet dancer where plantar flexion has been reported to reach 100°, as compared to the normal of up to 50°[95–96]. The patient complains of pain when performing certain active movements, such as in the relevé or en pointe positions. The pain can be severely debilitating in the athlete, but is rarely a significant issue in the non-athlete. It can be caused by overuse or a single traumatic event, with cases resultant on overuse having a better prognosis[93,96]. There are two

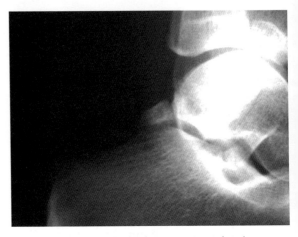

Figure 11.15 An os trigonum lying posterior to the talus.

principal pathologies associated with posterior ankle impingement: bony pathology related to the lateral process of the talus – an os trigonum or Stieda's process – and entrapment of the flexor hallucis longus (FHL) tendon.

Between the ages of 8 and 11 years, a secondary ossification center forms posterior to the lateral process of the talus. In 15% of individuals the ossification center remains separate to the talus and forms the "os trigonum" (Figure 11.15), in the other 85% it fuses to the talus[97]. The resultant posterolateral process of the talus can be long and prominent; in which case it is referred to as a "Stieda's" or "trigonal" process[96–97]. Both the os trigonum and Stieda's process can cause posterior impingement. A differential diagnosis of an os trigonum is a fracture of the lateral process of the talus, also known as a "Shepherd's fracture." A Shepherd's fracture, or an injury to the synchondrosis between the os trigonum and the talus, causes posterior impingement symptoms.

The soft tissue structures of importance in the posterior ankle include the capsule of the ankle and subtalar joints, the ligaments of the posterior ankle and FHL. The FHL tendon runs in a fibro-osseous tunnel between the posteromedial and posterolateral processes of the talus, where it is predisposed to stenotic lesions and the development of tenosynovitis[87,93]. It is important to note that some individuals have a low-lying FHL muscle belly, which can become entrapped at the entrance of the fibro-osseous tunnel during motion, causing pain. In general, the posterior aspect of the ankle does not accommodate the soft tissues well, which in turn makes them prone to impingement.

Regardless of whether the impingement is bony or soft tissue, patients usually complain of pain and swelling posterior to the ankle. Posterolateral impingement is the most common, although it is important to bear in mind that posteromedial impingement has been described[93,97].

Bony and FHL pathology may coexist, or be seen individually. Differentiating the two can be difficult. A useful clinical sign is reproducible pain with rapid, forced, passive plantar flexion of the ankle, which is only seen with posterior impingement, as opposed to FHL entrapment[93]. A rotational moment in maximal plantar flexion will cause the posterior talar process/ os trigonum to impinge between the tibia and calcaneus, producing additional discomfort[97]. Dorsiflexion of the great toe with the foot and ankle held fully plantar flexed may induce pain from the FHL, although it may also, less commonly, induce os trigonum pain[97]. Flexor hallucis longus discomfort is frequently associated with palpable crepitus felt along the tendon, although this is often difficult to assess given the deep anatomic location of the FHL. Additionally, the point of maximum tenderness in posterior impingement is usually posterolateral, whereas it is usually posteromedial in FHL pathology.

An injection of local anesthetic, with or without corticosteroid, into the posterior ankle can be very helpful both from a diagnostic and therapeutic perspective, but should be done under US guidance, in order to avoid inadvertently injuring the neurovascular bundle. The forced plantar flexion test is repeated after local anesthesia, and if symptoms are no longer present, then the diagnosis is clear[97].

Diagnostic studies should start with a lateral weightbearing radiograph of the ankle. This may show an os trigonum or Stieda's process, but often the posterolateral process is superimposed on the posteromedial process[93]. A lateral radiograph with the foot in 25° of external rotation may show the lateral process.[93,96,97]. Additionally a lateral radiograph with the ankle fully plantar flexed may show impingement of the os trigonum or Stieda's process between the posterior tibia and calcaneus. If doubt remains a CT can be obtained to delineate the bony anatomy. An MRI scan may also be helpful where the impingement is suspected to be primarily soft tissue in nature. It easily detects subtle details that can differentiate, for example, between ankle synovitis and FHL tenosynovitis (Figure 11.16).

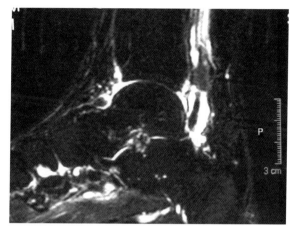

Figure 11.16 Flexor hallucis longus tendonitis and tenosynovitis. An MRI can be extremely valuable in determining the cause of posterior ankle impingement as it is not uncommon for an athlete to have both a symptomatic os trigonum and FHL tendon pathology.

Non-operative management, depending on the severity of the patient's presenting symptoms, can consist of RICE, oral anti-inflammatory medication, injections, and, in more extreme cases, a CAM boot or short leg cast. In high-performance athletes and dancers, many surgeons use injections under US guidance to return the patient to competition. Although, before giving the injection, it is recommended that an MRI scan is obtained to exclude other causes of the pain. Physical therapy has shown inconsistent results as the underlying cause of the pain is primarily due to mechanical factors[87,93,95–97].

If non-operative management fails to improve the patient's symptoms after six weeks, surgical intervention can be considered. The open surgical approach, either posteromedial or posterolateral, can be used. The posterolateral approach is used most commonly, but a posteromedial approach should be considered if one needs to address pathology of the FHL tendon and sheath during the same procedure. Hamilton reported good or excellent results in 75% of dancers undergoing such surgery through a mixture of medial and lateral incisions. Twenty-six operations were performed for a mixture of FHL and bony pathologies; nine for isolated FHL pathology; and six for bony impingement syndrome[98]. In the athlete, open debridement has generally favorable outcomes with most investigators reporting around 70 to 80% good or excellent results[99–100].

Posterior ankle arthroscopy has been popularized in recent years, although it can present a significant challenge to the surgeon due to the limited space and the surrounding neurovascular structures. Posterior ankle arthroscopy allows the os trigonum and Stieda's process to be excised, as well as allowing decompression of the FHL tendon sheath. The posterior ankle joint is also accessible for the treatment of osteochondral lesions and loose bodies. Some report that they are able to access lesions even better arthroscopically than by the traditional open approach[101], with a low rate of complications[102–104]. Wound infection rates range from 0 to 5%. Sural nerve injury rates of up to 8% have been reported, although they are usually transient neurapraxias. The proposed benefit of arthroscopic over an open excision is the shorter recovery time, which may be attributable to the early mobilization after arthroscopic surgery.

Turf Toe

Many different injuries of the hallux can lead to significant pain and disability if left undiagnosed or inadequately treated, but a first MTPJ capsulo-ligamentous injury or "turf toe" is extremely disabling to the athlete[105]. After it was described by Bowers and Martin in 1976, turf toe has received a lot of attention due to its increasing prevalence, in particular in American footballers as opposed to soccer players[106]. The initial study described an average of 5.4 turf toe injuries per season in football players at the University of West Virginia, but Rodeo in 1990 found that 45% of players in the National Football League had experienced such an injury, with 83% of those occurring on artificial turf[107]. Nigg and Segesser demonstrated that these MTPJ injuries had a propensity to occur on artificial turf because of the enhanced friction that is inherent in the playing surface[108]. The surface has since mostly been exonerated, with the propensity to injury being related to the more flexible cleat, or stud, designs used on these surfaces. Although this injury classically occurs in football players, turf toe injuries can occur in any sport, on any surface, and can lead to chronic problems including loss of push-off strength, persistent pain, progressive deformity, and joint degeneration if not treated appropriately[109–110].

Like many other joints in the foot, the first MTPJ has little inherent bony stability. This results in a moving center of rotation during motion, such that Kelikian described the MTPJ as having a dynamic acetabulum[109,111]. Most of the stability comes from

the surrounding capsuloligamentous–sesamoid complex, which is a confluence of multiple different structures, including the medial and lateral collateral ligaments and the medial and lateral metatarso-sesamoid suspensory ligaments. The plantar plate is a separate fibrous structure that courses from a weaker proximal attachment to the metatarsal neck through the joint capsule to a firm attachment on the proximal phalanx. The tendons of the FHB run along the plantar aspect of the hallux, split, and encompass the sesamoids just before they insert into the base of the proximal phalanx. The abductor and adductor hallucis tendons also insert on the medial and lateral aspects of the hallux MTPJ capsule. It is important to differentiate a plantar plate from a sesamoid injury, which can be challenging as a result of their proximity.

During the normal gait cycle, the hallux typically supports twice the load taken by the lesser toes, withstanding forces that reach up to 60% of body weight[112]. The peak forces approach two to three times body weight with jogging and running, and eight times body weight with a running jump[108]. The typical mechanism of most turf toe injuries is through an axial load to a foot that is held in a fixed equinus position with the first MTPJ in hyperextension[109–110]. Unrestricted hyperextension disrupts the plantar plate complex. The joint surface of the proximal phalanx and the dorsal and plantar articular cartilage of the metatarsal head may also be damaged[105,110].

The diagnosis acutely requires a high index of suspicion. Pain with weight bearing may be the only symptom, as ecchymosis and swelling are not always apparent on initial presentation. It is imperative, when examining the first MTPJ, to do so with careful palpation to localize tenderness and discriminate between the many structures found in this region. The presence of instability, as well as the range of motion of the first MTPJ in all planes, should be assessed and compared with the contralateral side. Varus and valgus stress can be placed on the joint to determine the integrity of the collateral ligaments. Decreased resistance to dorsiflexion suggests a plantar plate injury[111]. The drawer test, similar to the Lachman test of the knee, provides important information about the integrity of the plantar plate and must be conducted whenever a plantar plate injury is suspected[109–110]. Any increase in translation or softening of the end point, relative to the contralateral side,

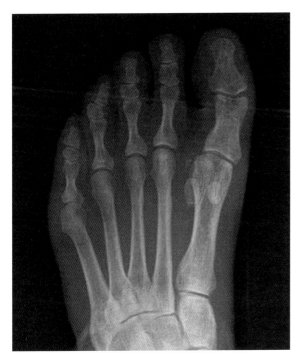

Figure 11.17 Turf toe. Note the proximal migration of the sesamoids, avulsion fracture, and MTPJ incongruity.

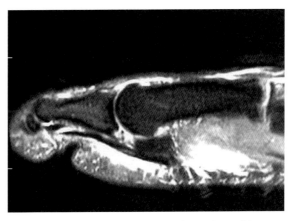

Figure 11.18 MRI scan showing a complete avulsion of the plantar plate.

indicates an injury of the plantar capsulo-ligamentous complex.

A clinical classification system has been described to help guide treatment[105,110].

- **Grade 1** is a mild injury with stretching of the plantar capsulo-ligamentous structures without any evidence of tear. The patient has minimal pain with localized tenderness at the plantar aspect of the MTPJ, minimal swelling, and little to no ecchymosis.

- **Grade 2** is a partial tear of the plantar plate and clinically differs from a grade 1 injury with diffuse ecchymosis, swelling, and tenderness across the plantar structures. Range of motion is significantly limited by pain.

- **Grade 3** injuries have a complete tear of the plantar plate. There is severe tenderness, marked swelling, and pain, especially on movement. In these patients an underlying osteochondral injury and other associated medial/lateral injuries as well should be considered. A drawer test is clearly positive.

Following a thorough physical examination, standard radiographs, including weightbearing AP, lateral,

oblique of the foot, and sesamoid views, should be obtained. Obtaining contralateral radiographic views for comparison can be very helpful in detecting subtle injuries. Standard radiographs are usually normal, although Prieskorn has reported that patients with a complete rupture of the plantar plate tend to have proximal migration of the sesamoids (Figure 11.17)[105,113]. Rodeo described a forced dorsiflexion lateral radiograph of the MTPJ[107]. He noted that with passive hyperextension of the first MTPJ the sesamoids normally migrate distally, but with a plantar plate injury they paradoxically migrate proximally[110]. The distance from the base of the proximal phalanx to the distal pole of either sesamoid should be less than 3 mm of the sesamoid position on the contralateral foot. If a bipartite sesamoid is present, the normal distance should be less than 10 mm for the tibial sesamoid and 13 mm for the fibular sesamoid. Measurements greater than this suggest plantar plate disruption 99.7% of the time[110–111]. A small fleck of bone from the insertion site of the plantar plate may also be seen. Although multiple imaging modalities can play a role in its diagnosis, MRI has become the standard of care, as it identifies the soft tissue injuries as well as articular damage (Figure 11.18)[114]. It is debatable whether an MRI should be obtained for grade 1 injuries, but well accepted that grade 2 and 3 injuries require an MRI scan to guide treatment and indicate prognosis.

For all grades of injury, RICE should be instituted in addition to an anti-inflammatory medication to help alleviate pain. Unlike other injuries of the foot and ankle, corticosteroid injections are not advised as

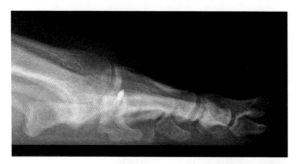

Figure 11.19 The plantar plate can be repaired. Here a suture anchor was used to reattach it to the proximal phalanx.

they can cause the plantar plate to attenuate further and even rupture completely.

With a grade 1 injury, return to competition with little or no loss of playing time is the norm[109]. Following such an injury the toe may benefit from being taped into slight plantar flexion to restrict the potential for further injury, as well as providing added stability. Additionally the athlete should use a stiff-soled shoe with a carbon fiber insert in an effort to reduce the amount of motion seen at the joint during the push-off phase of gait.

A grade 2 injury generally results in at least a two-week absence from sports and may need to be immobilized, or at the very least protected, as a result of discomfort[109]. This can be accomplished either with a CAM walker boot or postoperative shoe. Return to play is dictated by the patent's symptoms.

A grade 3 injury may require anywhere from eight weeks to six months of treatment before symptoms begin to improve[109]. A longer period of immobilization in a CAM walker usually suffices but, for the most severe injuries, a short leg weightbearing cast with a toe spica may be required. Although return to competition is again dictated by patient symptoms, the patient should be able to achieve 50 to 60° of painless passive dorsiflexion at the first MTPJ prior to being allowed to return to sport[111]. Fortunately, surgical treatment is rarely necessary as most turf toe injuries do well if the MTPJ is adequately immobilized for an appropriate length of time. If significant instability is still present despite the above, repair of the avulsed plantar plate can be undertaken using a suture anchor or drill hole through the metatarsal (Figure 11.19). Postoperatively, the patient limits weight bearing on

the forefoot for four to six weeks, and uses a rigid-soled shoe on their return to sport.

Chronic instability requiring late reconstruction of a turf toe injury may be necessary in the athlete who was improperly treated or who continues to perform in the face of injury. As a result of unrestrained dorsiflexion, secondary disorders can occur such as longitudinal tears of the FHL tendon or hallux rigidus with significant joint degeneration[105,109]. Other sequelae include a progressive hallux valgus or varus and a cock-up toe with an interphalangeal joint flexion contracture. In these situations, surgical reconstruction is more difficult because of scarring of the soft tissues. The sequelae of turf toe injuries occur after conservative treatment and, less commonly, after surgical treatment, with the most common problems being joint stiffness and pain[115].

Key Points
Ankle Ligaments
- Acute injuries are treated non-operatively in the majority of cases, excepting the occasional elite athlete with instability to clinical testing.
- Chronically the patient with mechanical, as opposed to functional, instability is more likely to benefit from operative treatment.
- Surgical repairs are broadly of two types – anatomical repair or tenodesis.
- Both types of repair have high success rates.
- Correction of heel varus should be considered.

Syndesmosis
- A high index of suspicion for a "high ankle sprain" is important.
- Radiological diagnosis may be difficult, and CT, MRI, or even ankle arthroscopy may be required.
- Sprains without diastasis or instability can be managed non-operatively.
- Patients with frank diastasis of the syndesmosis require operative treatment.
- Fixation may be with screws or suture techniques.

Peroneal Tendons
- Peroneal tendon pathology is not uncommon in the sporting population.

- The principal pathologies are tears of the brevis tendon and tendon dislocation associated with superficial peroneal retinaculum injury.
- Both injuries often require surgical treatment.
- Peroneal tendon tears can either be repaired with tubularization if <50% is involved, or tenodesis of the longus to the brevis if >50% is involved.
- Dislocation is treated with repair of the retinaculum +/– deepening of the groove.
- Correction of heel varus should be considered.

Anterior Ankle Impingement

- Patients present with anterior pain, swelling, and a block to dorsiflexion.
- Surgery is associated with excellent results, whatever technique is used.
- If anterior impingement is associated with instability, both the instability and impingement should be addressed with surgery.

Posterior Ankle Impingement/FHL Entrapment

- Patients present with posterior ankle pain, which is often reproduced on forced plantar flexion.
- There are two common pathologies, posterior impingement from an os trigonum or Stieda's process, and FHL entrapment. Often both are present simultaneously.
- Surgery is associated with 75% good or excellent results, whatever technique is used.
- Arthroscopic techniques are associated with a shorter recovery.

First Metatarsophalangeal Joint

- Patients present with pain and swelling of the first MTPJ following a dorsiflexion injury.
- Radiographs and MRI are the imaging modalities of choice.
- Most acute injuries are treated non-operatively.

References

1. Colville M. Surgical treatment of the unstable ankle. *J Am Acad Orthop Surg.* 1998; 6:368–77.

2. DiGiovanni BF, Partal G, Baumhauer J. Acute ankle injury and chronic lateral instability in the athlete. *Clin. Sports Med.* 2004; 23:1–19.

3. Ajis A, Mafulli N. Conservative management of chronic ankle instability. *Foot Ankle Clin N Am.* 2006; 11:531–7.

4. Kelikian H, Kelikian AS. *Disorders of the Ankle.* (Philadelphia, PA: W.B. Saunders, 1985).

5. Hubbard T, Wikstrom E. Ankle sprain: pathophysiology, predisposing factors, and management strategies. *Journal of Sports Medicine.* 2010; 1:115–22.

6. Ferran NA, Maffulli N. Epidemiology of sprains of the lateral ankle ligament complex. *Foot Ankle Clin.* 2006; 11:659–62.

7. Hertel J. Functional anatomy, pathomechanics, and pathophysiology of lateral ankle instability. *J Athl Train.* 2002; 37:364–75.

8. Brostrom L. Sprained ankles: anatomic lesions on recent sprains. *Acta Chir Scand.* 1964; 128:483–95.

9. Krips R, de Vries J, van Dijk CN. Ankle instability. *Foot Ankle Clin N Am.* 2006; 11:311–29.

10. Frost HM, Hanson CA. Technique for testing the drawer sign in the ankle. *Clin Orthop Relat Res.* 1977; 123:49–51.

11. Griffith J, Brockwell J. Diagnosis and imaging of ankle instability. *Foot Ankle Clin N Am.* 2006; 11: 475–96.

12. Mafulli N, Ferran N. Management of acute and chronic ankle instability. *J Am Acad Orthop Surg.* 2008; 16: 608–15.

13. Malliaropoulos N, Papacostas E, Papalada A, Maffulli N. Acute lateral ankle sprains in track and field athletes: an expanded classification. *Foot Ankle Clin.* 2006; 11:497–507.

14. Ardèvol J, Bolíbar I, Belda V, Argilaga S. Treatment of complete rupture of the lateral ligaments of the ankle: a randomized clinical trial comparing cast immobilization with functional treatment. *Knee Surg Sports Traumatol Arthrosc.* 2002; 10(6):371–7.

15. Kerkhoffs GM, Rowe BH, Assendelft WJ, Kelly K, Struijs PA, van Dijk CN. Immobilisation and functional treatment for acute lateral ankle ligament injuries in adults. *Cochrane Database Syst Rev.* 2002.

16. Kerkhoffs GM, Struijs PA, Marti RK, Blankevoort L, Assendelft WJ, van Dijk CN. Functional treatments for acute ruptures of the lateral ankle ligament: a systematic review. *Acta Orthop Scand.* 2003; 74(1):69–77.

17. Broström L. Sprained ankles: Surgical treatment of "chronic"

ligament ruptures. *Acta Chir Scand.* 1966; 132:551–65.

18. Gould N, Seligson D, Gassman J. Early and late repair of lateral ligament of the ankle. *Foot Ankle.* 1980; 1:84–9.

19. Chrisman OD, Snook GA. Reconstruction of lateral ligament tears of the ankle: An experimental study and clinical evaluation of seven patients treated by a new modification of the Elmslie procedure. *J Bone Joint Surg Am.* 1969; 51:904–12.

20. Evans DL. Recurrent instability of the ankle: a method of surgical treatment. *Proc R Soc Med.* 1953; 46:343–4.

21. Watson-Jones R. Recurrent forward dislocation of the ankle joint. *J Bone Joint Surg Br.* 1952; 134:519.

22. Miller AG, Raikin SM, Ahmad J. Near-anatomic allograft tenodesis of chronic lateral ankle instability. *Foot Ankle Int.* 2013; 34(11):1501–7.

23. Sammarco VJ. Complications of lateral ankle ligament reconstruction. *Clin Orthop.* 2001; 391:123–32.

24. Rasmussen O. Stability of the ankle joint: analysis of the function and traumatology of the ankle ligaments. *Acta Orthop Scand.* 1985; 211:1–75.

25. Boytim MJ, Fischer DA, Neumann L. Syndesmotic ankle sprains. *Am J Sports Med.* 1991; 19(3):294–8.

26. Rammelt S, Zwipp H, Grass R. Injuries to the distal tibiofibular syndesmosis: an evidence-based approach to acute and chronic lesions. *Foot Ankle Clin.* 2008; 13(4):611–33

27. Sarrafian SK. *Anatomy of the Foot and Ankle: Descriptive, Topographic, Functional.* (Philadelphia, PA: JB Lippincott, 1983).

28. Bassett FH, Gates HS, Billys JB, Morris HB, Nikolaou PK. Talar

impingement by the anteroinferior tibiofibular ligament: a cause of chronic pain in the ankle after inversion sprain. *J Bone Joint Surg.* 1990; 72A:55–9.

29. Clanton T, Paul P. Syndesmosis injuries in athletes. *Foot Ankle Clin N Am.* 2002; 7:529–49.

30. Espinosa N, Smerek JP, Myerson MS. Acute and chronic syndesmosis injuries: pathomechanisms, diagnosis and management. *Foot Ankle Clin.* 2006; 11(3):639–57.

31. Pena F, Coetzee JC. Ankle syndesmosis injuries. *Foot Ankle Clin N Am.* 2006; 11:35–50.

32. Mak MF, Gartner L, Pearce CJ. Management of syndesmosis injuries in the elite athlete. *Foot Ankle Clin.* 2013; 18(2):195–214.

33. Ogilvie-Harris D, Reed S, Hedman T. Disruption of the ankle syndesmosis: biomechanical study of the ligamentous restraints. *Arthroscopy.* 1994; 10:558–60.

34. Xenos J, Hopkinson W, Mulligan M, Olson E, Popovic N. The tibiofibular syndesmosis: evaluation of the ligamentous structures, methods of fixation, and radiographic assessment. *J Bone Joint Surg.* 1995; 77A:847–56.

35. Nussbaum ED, Hosea TM, Sieler SD. Prospective evaluation of syndesmotic ankle sprains without diastasis. *Am J Sports Med.* 2001; 29(1):31–5.

36. Taweel NR, Raikin SM, Karanjia HN, Ahmad J. The proximal fibula should be examined in all patients with ankle injury: a case series of missed Maisonneuve fractures. *J Emerg Med.* 2013; 44(2):251–5.

37. Hopkinson WJ, St. Pierre P, Ryan JB. Syndesmosis sprains of the ankle. *Foot Ankle.* 1990; 10:325–30.

38. Wolf BR, Amendola A. Syndesmosis injuries in the athlete: when and how to operate.

Curr Opin Orthop. 2002; 31:151–4.

39. Mosier-LaClair S, Pike H, Pomeroy G. Syndesmosis injuries: acute, chronic, new techniques for failed management. *Foot Ankle Clin.* 2002; 7(3):551–65.

40. Bonnin J. *Injuries to the Ankle.* (London: W. Heinemann Medical Books Ltd, 1950).

41. Ostrum RF, De Meo P, Subramanian R. A critical analysis of the anterior-posterior radiographic anatomy of the ankle syndesmosis. *Foot Ankle Int.* 1995; 16(3):128–31.

42. Ogilvie-Harris DJ, Reed SC. Disruption of the ankle syndesmosis: diagnosis and treatment by arthroscopic surgery. *Arthroscopy.* 1994; 10:561–8.

43. Ebraheim NA, Lu J, Yang H. Radiographic and CT evaluation of tibiofibular syndesmotic diastasis: a cadaver study. *Foot Ankle Int.* 1997; 18:693–8.

44. Takao M, Ochi M, Oae K. Diagnosis of a tear of the tibiofibular syndesmosis. The role of arthroscopy of the ankle. *J Bone Joint Surg Br.* 2003; 85:324–9.

45. Lui TH, Ip K, Chow HT. Comparison of radiologic and arthroscopic diagnoses of distal tibiofibular syndesmosis disruption in acute ankle fracture. *Arthroscopy.* 2005; 21(11):1370.

46. Tornetta P, Spoo JE, Reynolds FA. Overtightening of the ankle syndesmosis: is it really possible? *J Bone Joint Surg Am.* 2001; 83:489–92.

47. McBryde A, Chiasson B, Wilhelm A. Syndesmotic screw placement: a biomechanical analysis. *Foot Ankle Int.* 1997; 18:262–6.

48. Tol JL, Verhagen RA, Krips R. The anterior ankle impingement syndrome: diagnostic value of oblique radiographs. *Foot Ankle Int.* 2004; 25(2):63–8.

49. Song DJ, Lanzi JT, Groth AT, et al. The effect of syndesmosis screw

removal on the reduction of the distal tibiofibular joint: a prospective radiographic study. *Foot Ankle Int.* 2014; 35(6):543–8.

50. Stuart K, Panchbhavi VK. The fate of syndesmotic screws. *Foot Ankle Int.* 2011; 32(5):S519–25.

51. Ahmad J, Raikin SM, Pour AE, Haytmanek C. Bioabsorbable screw fixation of the syndesmosis in unstable ankle injuries. *Foot Ankle Int.* 2009; 30(2):99–105.

52. Thornes B, Walsh A, Hislop M. Suture-endobutton fixation of ankle tibiofibular diastasis: a cadaveric study. *Foot Ankle Int.* 2003; 24:142–6.

53. Seitz WH, Bachner EJ, Abram LJ. Repair of the tibiofibular syndesmosis with a flexible implant. *J Orthop Trauma.* 1991; 5(1):78–82.

54. Thornes B, Shannon F, Guiney AM, Hession P, Masterson E. Suture-button syndesmosis fixation: accelerated rehabilitation and improved outcomes. *Clin Orthop Relat Res.* 2005; 431:207–12.

55. Thornes B, Shannon F, Guiney AM. Suture-button syndesmosis fixation: accelerated rehabilitation and improved outcomes. *Clin Orthop Relat Res.* 2005; 431:207–12.

56. Veltri DM, Pagnani MJ, O'Brien SJ, Warren RF, Ryan MD, Barnes NP. Symptomatic ossification of the tibiofibular syndesmosis in professional football players: a sequela of the syndesmotic ankle sprain. *Foot Ankle Int.* 1995; 16(5):285–90.

57. Cerrato RA, Myerson MS. Peroneal tendon tears, surgical management and its complications. *Foot Ankle Clin.* 2009; 14(2):299–312.

58. Edwards ME. The relation of the peroneal tendons to the fibula, calcaneus, and cuboideum. *Am J Anat.* 1928; 42:213–53.

59. Ozbag D, Gumusalam Y, Uzel M. Morphometrical features of the human malleolar groove. *Foot Ankle Int.* 2008; 29:77–81.

60. Sobel M, Pavlov H, Geppert MJ. Painful os peroneum syndrome: a spectrum of conditions responsible for plantar lateral foot pain. *Foot Ankle Int.* 1994; 15:112–24.

61. Rosenfeld P. Acute and chronic peroneal tendon dislocations. *Foot Ankle Clin N Am.* 2007; 12:643–57.

62. Molloy R, Tisdel C. Failed treatment of peroneal tendon injuries. *Foot Ankle Clin N Am.* 2003; 8:115–29.

63. Ferran NA, Maffulli N, Oliva F. Management of recurrent subluxation of the peroneal tendons. *Foot Ankle Clin N Am.* 2006; 11:465–74.

64. *Mann's Surgery of the Foot and Ankle*, 9th edn. (Elsevier Health Sciences, 2014).

65. Peacock KC, Resnick EJ, Thoder JJ. Fracture of the os peroneum with rupture of the peroneus longus tendon. A case report and review of the literature. *Clin Orthop Relat Res.* 1986; 202:223–6.

66. Wang XT, Rosenberg ZS, Mechlin MB, Schweitzer ME. Normal variants and diseases of the peroneal tendons and superior peroneal retinaculum: MR imaging features. *Radiographics.* 2005; 25(3):587–602.

67. Neustadter J, Raikin SM, Nazarian LN. Dynamic sonographic evaluation of peroneal tendon subluxation. *AJR Am J Roentgenol.* 2004; 183(4):985–8.

68. Raikin SM, Elias I, Nazarian LN. Intrasheath subluxation of the peroneal tendons. *J Bone Joint Surg Am.* 2008; 90(5):992–9.

69. Sobel M, Bohne WH, Levy, ME. Longitudinal attrition of the peroneal brevis tendon in the fibular groove: an anatomic study. *Foot Ankle.* 1991; 11:124–8.

70. Sobel M, DiCarlo EF, Bohne WH, Collins L. Longitudinal splitting of the peroneus brevis tendon: an anatomic and histologic study of cadaver material. *Foot Ankle.* 1991; 12:165–70.

71. Vienne P, Schoniger R, Helmy N. Hindfoot instability in cavovarus deformity: static and dynamic balancing. *Foot Ankle Int.* 2007; 28:96–102.

72. Sobel M, Geppert MJ, Olson EJ. The dynamics of peroneus brevis tendon splits: a proposed mechanism, technique of diagnosis, and classification of injury. *Foot Ankle.* 1992; 13:413–22.

73. Krause JO, Brodsky JW. Peroneus brevis tendon tears: pathophysiology, surgical reconstruction, and clinical results. *Foot Ankle Int.* 1998; 19:271–9.

74. Oden RR. Tendon injuries about the ankle resulting from skiing. *Clin Orthop Relat Res.* 1987; 216:63–9.

75. Safran MR, O'Malley MR, Fu FH. Peroneal tendon subluxation in athletes: new exam technique, case reports, and review. *Med Sci Sports Exerc.* 1999; 31:S487–92.

76. Eckert WR, Davis EA Jr. Acute rupture of the peroneal retinaculum. *J Bone Joint Surg Am.* 1976; 58:670–2.

77. McMurray TP. Footballer's ankle. *J Bone Joint Surg.* 1950; 32:68–9.

78. Morris LH. Report of cases of athlete's ankle. *J Bone Joint Surg.* 1943; 25:220.

79. Tol J, van Dijk CN. Anterior ankle impingement. *Foot Ankle Clin N Am.* 2006; 11:297–310.

80. Biedert R. Anterior ankle pain in sports medicine: etiology and indications for arthroscopy. *Arch Orthop Trauma Surg.* 1991; 110(6):293–7.

81. Ferkel RD, Fasulo GJ. Arthroscopic treatment of ankle injuries. *Orthop Clin North Am.* 1994; 25(1):17–32.

82. Scranton PE, McDermott JE. Anterior tibiotalar spurs: a

comparison of open versus arthroscopic debridement. *Foot Ankle*. 1992; 13(3):125–9.

83. Tol JL, van Dijk CN. Etiology of the anterior ankle impingement syndrome: a descriptive anatomical study. *Foot Ankle Int*. 2004; 25(6):382–6.

84. Hawkins RB. Arthroscopic treatment of sports-related anterior osteophytes in the ankle. *Foot Ankle*. 1988; 9(2):87–90.

85. Watson A. Ankle instability and impingement. *Foot Ankle Clin N Am*. 2007; 12: 177–95.

86. Tol JL, Verheyen CP, van Dijk CN. Arthroscopic treatment of anterior impingement in the ankle. *J Bone Joint Surg Br*. 2001; 83(1):9–13.

87. van Dijk CN, Tol JL, Verheyen CC. A prospective study of prognostic factors concerning the outcome of arthroscopic surgery for anterior ankle impingement. *Am J Sports Med*. 1997; 25:737–45.

88. Ray RG, Gusman DN, Christensen JC. Anatomical variation of the tibial plafond: the anteromedial tibial notch. *J Foot Ankle Surg*. 1994; 33(4):419–26.

89. van Dijk CN, Wessel RN, Tol JL. Oblique radiograph for the detection of bone spurs in anterior ankle impingement. *Skeletal Radiol*. 2002; 31(4):214–21.

90. Raikin SM, Cooke PH. The divot sign: a new observation in anterior impingement of the ankle. *Foot Ankle Int*. 1999; 20(8):532.

91. Berberian WS, Hecht PJ, Wapner KL, DiVerniero R. Morphology of tibiotalar osteophytes in anterior ankle impingement. *Foot Ankle Int*. 2001; 22(4):313–7.

92. Cutsuries AM, Saltrick KR, Wagner J. Arthroscopic arthroplasty of the ankle joint. *Clin Podiatr Med Surg*. 1994; 11(3):449–67.

93. van Dijk CN. Anterior and posterior ankle impingement.

Foot Ankle Clin N Am. 2006; 11:663–83.

94. Cannon LB, Hackney RG. Anterior tibiotalar impingement associated with chronic ankle instability. *J Foot Ankle Surg*. 2000; 39(6):383–6.

95. Hamilton WG, Hamilton LH, Marshall P. A profile of the musculoskeletal characteristics of elite professional ballet dancers. *Am J Sports Med*. 1992; 20:267–73.

96. Roche AJ, Calder JD, Lloyd Williams R. Posterior ankle impingement in dancers and athletes. *Foot Ankle Clin*. 2013; 18(2):301–18.

97. Chao W. Os trigonum. *Foot Ankle Clin N Am*. 2004; 9:787–96.

98. Hamilton WG, Geppert MJ, Thompson FM. Pain in the posterior aspect of the ankle in dancers. Differential diagnosis and operative treatment. *J Bone Joint Surg Am*. 1996; 78:1491–500.

99. Abramowitz Y, Wollstein R, Barzilay Y. Outcome of resection of a symptomatic os trigonum. *J Bone Joint Surg Am*. 2003; 85:1051–7.

100. Leutloff D, Perka C. Posterior ankle impingement syndrome in dancers: a short-term follow-up after operative treatment. *Foot Ankle Surg*. 2002; 8:33–9.

101. Lee JC, Calder JD, Healy JC. Posterior impingement syndromes of the ankle. *Semin Musculoskelet Radiol*. 2008; 12:154–69.

102 Galla M, Lobenhoffer P. Technique and results of arthroscopic treatment of posterior ankle impingement. *Foot Ankle Surg*. 2011; 17:79–84.

103. Guo QW, Hu YL, Jiao C. Open versus endoscopic excision of a symptomatic os trigonum: a comparative study of 41 cases. *Arthroscopy*. 2010; 26:384–90.

104 Scholten PE, Sierevelt IN, Van Dijk CN. Hindfoot endoscopy for posterior ankle impingement.

J Bone Joint Surg Am. 2008; 90:2665–72.

105. Coker TP, Arnold JA, Weber DL. Traumatic lesions of the metatarsophalangeal joint of the great toe in athletes. *J Ark Med Soc*. 1978; 74(8):309–17.

106. Bowers KD, Martin RB. Turf-toe: a shoe-surface related football injury. *Med Sci Sports*. 1976; 8(2):81–3.

107. Rodeo SA, O'Brien S, Warren RF. Turf-toe: an analysis of metatarsophalangeal joint sprains in professional football players. *Am J Sports Med*. 1990; 18(3):280–5.

108. Nigg BM. *Biomechanics of Running Shoes*. (Champaign, IL: Human Kinetics Publishers, 1986).

109. Maskill J, Bohay D, Anderson J. First ray injuries. *Foot Ankle Clin N Am*. 2006; 11:143–63.

110. McCormick J, Anderson R. The great toe: failed turf toe, chronic turf toe, and complicated. *Foot Ankle Clin N Am*. 2009; 14:135–50.

111. Watson TS, Anderson RB, Davis WH. Periarticular injuries to the hallux metatarsophalangeal joint in athletes. *Foot Ankle Clin*. 2000; 5(3):687–713.

112. Stokes AF, Hutton WC, Scott JR. Forces under the hallux valgus foot before and after surgery. *Clin Orthop Rel Res*. 1979; 142:64–72.

113. Prieskorn D, Graves SC, Smith RA. Morphometric analysis of the plantar plate apparatus of the first metatarsophalangeal joint. *Foot Ankle*. 1993; 14(4):204–7.

114. Tewes DP, Fischer DA, Fritts HM. MRI findings of acute turf toe. A case report and review of anatomy. *Clin Orthop Relat Res*. 1994; 304:200–3.

115. Clanton TO, Butler JE, Eggert A. Injuries to the metatarsophalangeal joints in athletes. *Foot Ankle*. 1986; 7(3):162–76.

Chapter

12

Ankle Arthroscopy

Ian G. Winson and Stephen W. Parsons

Introduction

Arthroscopic surgery of the ankle and hindfoot is increasingly popular. Arthroscopy for visualization of joints was reported in cadavers in 1931, this included the ankle[1].

The advantage of arthroscopic surgery is in having a technique that can assist with both diagnosis and treatment of pathologies in the ankle and hindfoot, while minimizing the collateral damage to the soft tissue envelope. The aim is to reduce the morbidity associated with the soft tissue stripping, allowing early discharge from hospital, faster rehabilitation, improved healing, and fewer complications. Classically, arthroscopy is used for intra-articular pathologies, although its versatility has led to a more recent increase in its use for tendon and ligament abnormalities.

Initial Assessment

Arthroscopy is a surgical tool. It is only employed after meticulous assessment, both clinically and radiologically.

The aim of clinical assessment is to establish a diagnosis, its functional impact, to record the patient's comorbidities, and to counsel the patient as to the expected outcome of the arthroscopic intervention. Clinical assessment uses the systematic interview technique and features of examination outlined in Table 12.1.

Radiological examination should include a weightbearing AP view of the ankle, with an additional mortise view if deemed necessary; a weightbearing lateral view of the whole foot and ankle; a dorsoplantar weightbearing view of the foot; and an oblique view of the foot. Additional views may be of assistance, for example a limb alignment view for assessment of deformity, and an ankle anteromedial oblique impingement view is helpful for medial bony impingement from talar neck osteophytes.

Computed tomography scanning is useful to evaluate deformity, the presence of occult arthritis, tarsal coalitions, and occult fractures. The use of SPECT-CT scanning may be helpful in better localizing pathology. Magnetic resonance imaging can provide useful additional information regarding the soft tissue envelope, particularly the ligaments and tendons, but also the presence of bone edema, infection, and avascular necrosis (AVN). Ultrasound is a valuable dynamic tool, particularly in the assessment of pathology and trauma in tendons and ligaments. Image-guided joint injections of local anesthetic and contrast medium also help in localization.

Table 12.1 The core elements of history and examination

History	
Symptoms	Soreness, stiffness, swelling, stability, shape
Function	Mobility, work, activities of daily living, sport
Examination	
Shape	Coronal–sagittal
Swelling	Soft tissue–bony
Gait	Velocity: stride; length: cadence
Stance tests	Ski stance dorsiflexion, double stance heel raise, single stance heel raise, weightbearing supination, heel rock
Tenderness	
Range of movement	Active–passive
Compensatory movements	
Stress tests	
Neurology	
Vascularity	

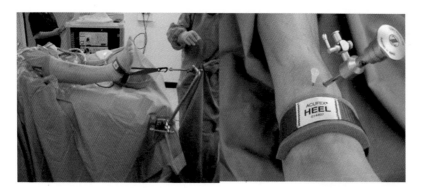

Figure 12.1 Shows the position to allow traction, with the knee slightly bent and the initial access achieved with a hypodermic needle. A 4.0 mm arthroscope is inserted in the anteromedial portal.

Ankle Arthroscopy

A variety of techniques of positioning and joint distraction are available. The authors prefer a simple set up, with the patient placed supine in a marginal head-down position. An ipsilateral bolster under the buttock is used to correct external rotation and align the ankle in a neutral position. The lower leg is placed on a thick cushion, flexing the knee to approximately 20°. Traction, if required, can be applied through an ankle strap, attached to a fixed arm at the end of the table (Figure 12.1). The traction is increased and decreased not by any complex mechanism, but by elevating or depressing the end of the table. The standard 30°, 4.0 mm arthroscope is the workhorse, but narrower diameters (2.7 mm "Panvision") are preferable for smaller and tighter ankles, as well as for children. A reliable and stable fluid-management system with a relatively low-pressure setting is employed. A camera system should allow an adjustment of aperture and of focus. It should be routine to record pictures or videos.

An initial "examination under anesthetic" should be recorded. This should include stability in the sagittal and coronal planes. Three portals are used regularly (Figure 12.2):

- the anteromedial, which is medial to the tibialis anterior
- the medial midline, between the tibialis anterior and extensor hallucis longus
- the anterolateral, which is just lateral to the extensor digitorum longus.

The level of the ankle joint is usually determined with a small hypodermic needle. The tibialis anterior, the extensor digitorum longus, and the lateral branch or trunk of the superficial peroneal nerve are marked if possible. A technique for identifying the superficial

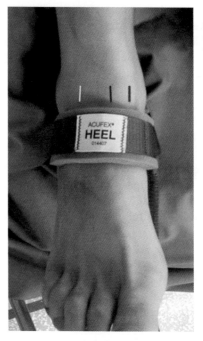

Figure 12.2 The commonly used anterior portals for ankle arthroscopy. Red: anteromedial; mauve: medial midline; yellow: anterolateral.

peroneal nerve in thinner patients is to hold the fourth toe plantar flexed and invert the foot. The nerve can usually be seen and felt subcutaneously. It is important to note that the structures can shift horizontally when traction is applied.

The anteromedial and anterolateral portals are the most commonly used. The medial portal is established first, with a skin incision being made with a knife followed by deep dissection to the joint with fine scissors. A blunt trocar within the arthroscope sheath is then used to establish access, before introducing the arthroscope into the anterior recess of the ankle. While traction allows easy initial access to the joint, it is often necessary to release the traction before undertaking surgery in the anterior recesses of the

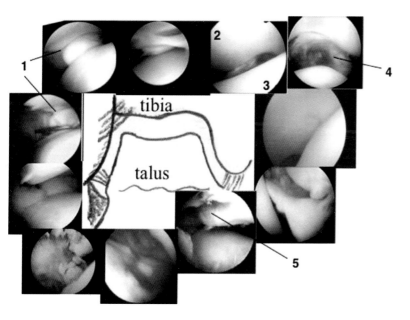

Figure 12.3 The systematic review of the ankle joint. 1: tibiofibular syndesmosis; 2: tibial plafond; 3: talar dome; 4: posteromedial recess; 5: anterior margin of the tibia.

ankle, as the ligament distraction increases soft tissue tension and thereby increases the risk of neurovascular injury. If the anteromedial portal is established first, the light can be used to transilluminate the lateral superficial structures and reduce the risk of damage to the superficial peroneal nerve. Once the two portals are established the initial view may be limited by fat, synovitis, or scarring within the anterior gutter. This can be removed using a 3.5 power-assisted shaver with suction. Care should be taken to keep the resection device facing backward into the joint to prevent iatrogenic damage to the anterior neurovascular bundle. Once the anterior gutter is cleared, a systematic review of the ankle can be performed (Figure 12.3).

Systematic review of the joint starts on the opposite side of the joint to the primary portal. Thus we work from the anterior inferior tibiofibular ligament visualizing the tibiofibular syndesmosis, the articular surfaces of the lateral sides of the talus and the tibia, the posterior recess of the inferior tibiofibular joint, the posterior inferior tibiofibular ligament, and the posterior transverse intermalleolar ligament. This leads you across to the posteromedial corner. As one returns anteriorly, the superior part of the medial gutter can be inspected with the medial surfaces of the joint. Once you have returned to the anterior recess the traction can be temporarily removed and the deeper part of the medial gutter and the deltoid ligament can be visualized. The anterior recess can be

further inspected – particularly the talar neck. This brings you back to the lateral gutter allowing you to view the anterior talofibular ligament. At this point it is important to check the stability of the inferior tibiofibular joint with the traction off. At all stages, the joint surfaces of both the tibia and talus should be carefully reviewed.

Posterior Ankle Arthroscopy

Approaches to the posterior ankle joint and posterior subtalar joint can be performed with the patient in the prone position[2] or the lateral position. No distraction is required. Posteromedial and posterolateral portals can be used adjacent to either side of the tendo Achillis, at the level of the tip of the fibula. It is necessary to take care to avoid damage to the sural nerve laterally and the posterior tibial nerve medially during portal placement.

Alternative portal placements may be helpful. If the patient is in the lateral position the ankle can be instrumented or visualized through two posterolateral incisions – one close to the peroneal tendons and one close to the tendo Achillis. The arthroscope is introduced into the lateral portal. A soft tissue resector is then introduced medially (Figure 12.4). The resector is tapped against the arthroscope and then, when localized, the resector is used to clear a space in the fat. As a pocket is created the visualization improves and the FHL tendon comes into view. It is critical to

223

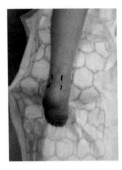
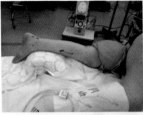
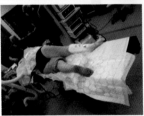

Bad side down showing ankle and subtalar portals

Figure 12.4 The set up for posterior ankle and subtalar arthroscopy. The "bad" leg is down. The ankle (superior) and subtalar portals are marked.

Table 12.2 The soft tissue pathologies seen during ankle arthroscopy

Soft tissue and synovial pathology	
Infection	
Inflammation:	inflammatory arthropathy, crystal arthropathy, hemophilia
Neoplasia:	pigmented villonodular synovitis, synovial osteochondromatosis
Degenerative:	post-traumatic, degenerative
Trauma:	fibrosis, ligament injuries, scarring, impingement

Soft Tissue Pathology

The pathologies affecting the synovium and soft tissues are numerous and are outlined in Table 12.2. A common indication for arthroscopy is persistent anterior ankle pain, with or without instability, following an ankle "sprain." The patient usually presents with anterolateral pain, from synovitis, fibrosis, or scarring, which impinges on ankle dorsiflexion[3]. The impingement is from a mass of fibrotic tissue, which builds up in the anterolateral ankle and resembles the meniscus of the knee – a "meniscoid lesion" (Figure 12.6a). Arthroscopic resection is easily undertaken with a soft tissue shaver. Such surgery has a 90% rate of success with purely soft tissue lesions[4–5], but the success rate is lower if there is articular surface damage or arthrosis. It is important to also assess the syndesmosis[6], and deltoid ligament. Impingement lesions can also occur anteromedially or posteriorly. On occasions the inferior margin of the anterior inferior tibiofibular ligament can impinge on the lateral talar dome – in this case it is known as Bassett's ligament (Figure 12.6b). Arthroscopic resection of the prominent ligament is effective[7].

Bony Pathology

Anterior bony impingement of the ankle is a common indication for arthroscopy. The usual sites are an anterolateral tibial or a medial talar neck osteophyte. Osteophytes also occur on the anterior edges, as well as the tips, of the medial and lateral malleoli. They may also be seen on the lateral shoulder of the neck of the talus. Removal of an anterior tibial osteophyte is performed using a 3.5 mm barrel burr, introduced through the anterolateral portal. The normal tibia

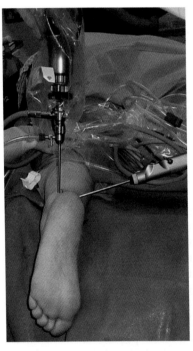

Figure 12.5 The arthroscope is introduced toward the second toe. The shaver is introduced medially, and located initially by tapping it against the arthroscope.

remain lateral to the FHL tendon, until adequate visualization is obtained – this avoids inadvertent damage to the posterior tibial artery and nerve (Figure 12.5). Once the posterior ankle capsule and fat are removed, the transverse tibiofibular and talofibular ligaments, the posterior ankle joint, and the subtalar joint can be viewed.

(a)

(b)

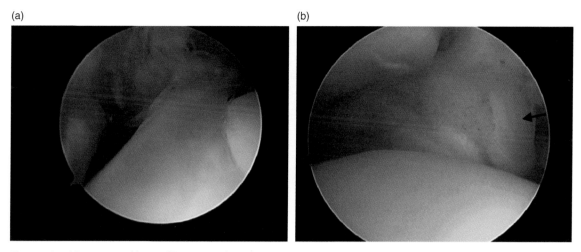

Figure 12.6 (a) A meniscoid lesion. (b) A Bassett's ligament (arrow) that was impinging on the talar dome.

above the osteophytic shelf is identified and the osteophyte is resected to a level flush with the anterior face of the tibia. Adequate resection is also marked when the articular cartilage returns to normal. Repeated dorsiflexion of the ankle helps identify adequate clearance of the impingement. The areas that are easily missed include the extreme anterolateral corner of the tibia, and the front of the medial malleolus. Results suggest 90% of patients are improved following surgery, although this is reduced to 50% if the joint space is narrowed on preoperative radiographs[8–9].

It has also been shown that ossicles that are symptomatic and enhance on MRI scanning respond well to arthroscopic excision[10].

As well as anterior impingement, posterior ankle impingement syndrome is increasingly recognized in ballet dancers and athletes. The typical history is of posterior, or posteromedial, ankle pain worsened by plantar flexion. Posterior ankle impingement is thought to arise from osseous impingement between the posterior process of the talus, or an os trigonum, and the tibia. Secondary inflammation may occur in the mobile ankle, leading to mechanical entrapment of the FHL tendon. This typically occurs as the FHL runs posterior to the talus, between the medial and lateral talar tubercles. In about 7% of the population an os trigonum lying just posterior to the lateral tubercle, which is the more prominent of the two tubercles, is present. In some individuals the lateral tubercle is long, in which case it is called a Stieda's process. The os trigonum or Stieda's process can be excised with a posterior ankle arthroscopy (Figure 12.7),

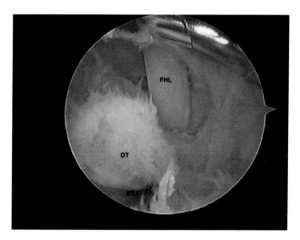

Figure 12.7 The space posterior to the ankle is cleared of fat, staying lateral to the FHL. An os trigonum (OT) and the subtalar joint (STJ) are also shown.

and provides 80% good or excellent results at two to five years' follow-up[11].

Joint Surface Pathology

Joint surface lesions include chondral lesions, osteochondral lesions, cysts, and arthritis. All of these lesions produce persistent deep-seated pain, catching, locking, and instability, with swelling from the associated synovitis. Following ankle injury these deep symptoms are differentiated from soft tissue pain or impingement, which tend to cause anterior joint line pain.

Even if the MRI does not show an articular surface lesion, arthroscopy may well reveal joint laxity,

225

(a)
(b)

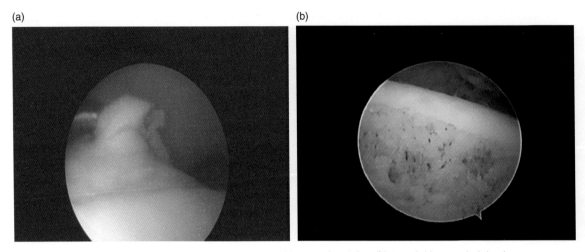

Figure 12.8 (**a**) A large talar dome flap will always have exposed bone underneath it. (**b**) A medial lesion, which has been debrided and microfractured.

ligament damage, synovitis, fibrosis, a meniscoid lesion, chondral damage[12], and loose bodies. Tibial and talar osteophytes may be identified and treated.

The Berndt and Hardy radiological classification of osteochondral lesions of the talar dome has been updated to an MRI classification, as only about 50% of osteochondral defects are visible on plain radiographs. The MRI classification is[13]:

- Stage I: Articular cartilage injury only
- Stage IIA: Cartilage injury with bony fracture and edema
- Stage IIB: Stage IIA without bony edema
- Stage III: Detached but undisplaced bony fragment
- Stage IV: Detached and displaced fragment
- Stage V: Subchondral cyst formation

Lesions of the lateral talar dome are said to be superficial with chondral flaps (Figure 12.8a). Posteromedial lesions are said to be typically deeper and associated with osteochondral cysts. There is a range of treatments including microfracture, osteochondral grafting, chondrocyte implantation, and even the implantation of particulated juvenile articular cartilage. Microfracture, with the creation of holes in the subchondral plate 3 to 4 mm apart (Figure 12.8b) to stimulate the bone marrow to produce fibrocartilaginous cover, has been reported as giving good results in 80 to 85% of lesions that are less than 15 mm in diameter. However, poorer outcomes, with less than 50% good results, are seen in cystic lesions[14], and lesions larger than 15 mm[15]. There is evidence that bone grafting can produce comparable results to

microfracture. Early weight bearing following microfracture gives equal results to non-weightbearing[16].

Success has been reported with repeat arthroscopic surgery[17–18], when the first arthroscopic operation fails. Nevertheless, in treating larger cystic lesions and those cases where microfracture has failed, a variety of techniques can be used. Cylindrical osteochondral autografting, or mosaicplasty, has been reported as having 87% excellent or good results[19], although concerns remain about the knee, from which the graft is often harvested. Osteochondral allografts have also been reported to give satisfactory results.

An alternative is autologous chondrocyte implantation (ACI), which can be embedded within a matrix (MACI). This is a two-stage procedure. In the first stage, the chondrocytes are harvested. They are then cultured. The cultured chondrocytes are then reintroduced, either embedded in a matrix (MACI), or not (ACI). The results of these techniques appear comparable. A meta-analysis of ACI in the talus showed an overall clinical success rate of 89.9%[20].

Isolated lesions of the distal tibia are much rarer than talar lesions; nevertheless, the success rate of arthroscopic treatment appears to be similar to that for talar dome lesions[21].

Arthritis

Ankle arthroscopy can be used in two ways for the treatment of ankle arthritis: firstly, to debride the joint; and, secondly, to fuse the joint. The value of arthroscopic debridement of the arthritic ankle is open to debate. Although the removal of flaps and loose bodies can be of assistance with mechanical symptoms, it should be noted that 90% of patients without joint space narrowing have good or excellent results after excision of the anterior tibial osteophyte, whereas only 50% of patients with joint space narrowing on preoperative weightbearing radiographs had good or excellent results. Furthermore pain relief at two years after surgery was significantly improved in the pure anterior impingement group, but not the group with joint space narrowing[9]. Care should also be taken in those cases where the joint is clearly starting to sublux in the sagittal plane. In those patients with end-stage arthritis the role of arthroscopic surgery lies with arthroscopic ankle arthrodesis.

Postoperative Management

Postoperatively we use a bulky compression bandage for two to three days. The patient is advised to elevate the ankle for ten days postoperatively, until the soft tissues have settled. During this time, the ankle is mobilized regularly and iced to reduce any swelling. Weight bearing will depend on the complexity of the surgery, but is best guided by the patient's level of discomfort.

It is reasonable to warn patients of a greater level of pain and discomfort following an ankle arthroscopy than a knee arthroscopy. A prudent approach is to warn the patients that they may require four to six weeks to recover, for example the average return to dance was at seven weeks in a small group of elite dancers[22]. Nevertheless the time from surgery to maximum recovery is usually three to six months.

Complications

The treatment of lesions that are not amenable to conservative arthroscopic treatment, such as end-stage arthritis or large osteochondral cystic lesions, can lead to failure. Persisting symptoms may also occur as a result of the incomplete removal of bone or soft tissue pathologies. Patients with extensive soft tissue scarring or undergoing repeat arthroscopy are at a greater risk of complications in general. Care must be taken not to traumatize the portals by excessive, repeated introduction of instrumentation.

More specifically:

- Damage to the superficial nerves can occur both as a result of poor portal placement and from inside out, if care is not taken with the resectors when debriding the anterior or posterior gutter.
- Aneurysms of the dorsalis pedis artery have been reported.

- Bleeding is uncommon, but hemarthrosis, leading to pain and infection, can occur if considerable resection has been performed and the leg has not been elevated and rested postoperatively.
- Superficial infections in the portals are rare, and deep infection is rarer.

Arthroscopic Ankle Arthrodesis

Ankle arthritis is most commonly post-traumatic (70%), with primary arthritis being rare (<10%)[23]. There are numerous other causes (Table 12.3). It is now clear that the pain and disability arising from end-stage ankle arthritis can be as severe as that experienced by patients with hip or knee arthritis[24]. Arthroscopic ankle arthrodesis gives good pain relief, stability, correction of deformity, and postoperative function, with a low rate of complications and morbidity in these severely disabled patients[25–31].

Table 12.3 Causes of ankle arthritis

Post-traumatic

Ankle fracture
Pilon fracture
Talar fracture
Avascular necrosis
Osteochondral fractures

Inflammatory

Sero-positive
Sero-negative
Crystal
Hemophilia

Neuropathic

Diabetes
HMSN (CMT)
Peripheral neuropathies

Deformity

Chronic ligament instability
Pes cavovarus
Pes planovalgus
Physeal arrest

Infective

Septic arthritis
Osteomyelitis, chronic

Tumors

Pigmented villonodular synovitis (PVNS)
Chondrocalcinosis
Intraosseous

Clinical assessment should record the severity of the pain and the limitations to function imposed by the arthritis. On examination, limp, soft tissue, bony swelling, and limitation of movement should be noted. It is important to consider the limb alignment in the coronal, sagittal, and axial planes. It is also important to differentiate between deformity arising from the ankle and that deriving from the foot, for example heel varus and the plantar flexed first ray in cavovarus. Vascular and neurological status should also be noted.

The basic imaging of the arthritic ankle is with plain weightbearing x-rays. These may be supplemented by image-guided injections of local anesthetic into the ankle joint to confirm the source of the pain. The injection should be with contrast, to ensure that there is no connection to the subtalar joint. CT scanning may be used to help define complex deformities and assess the degree of arthritis in other joints. MRI scanning has a role in the rarer diagnoses, such as infection and avascular necrosis.

Advantages of Arthroscopic Technique

Compared to open ankle arthrodeses, there is lower perioperative morbidity, less blood loss, fewer reported postoperative complications, a shorter hospital stay, a quicker rehabilitation and decreased time to union, and a reduction in cost[32–33].

Planning and Risk Factors

The specific planning and risk factors are outlined in Table 12.4. The reduced size of the incisions and the reduction in soft tissue dissection allow arthroscopic fusion to be undertaken in a diabetic and even in patients with peripheral vascular disease. Great caution should be taken with patients who hold unreasonable expectations and those who may be uncooperative with the postoperative management. Cigarette smokers should also be counseled to cease, as they have higher delayed and non-union rates[34].

In planning surgery, the knee and foot should be considered. Severe deformity of the knee from arthritic change should be corrected first. Similarly, if significant foot deformity, such as planovalgus or pes cavus, is present, additional corrective foot surgery may well need incorporating in the surgical plan. Distal arthritis also needs consideration, as the presence of radiological and particularly symptomatic subtalar and midtarsal arthritis may require simultaneous fusions or, alternatively, the use of ankle arthroplasty as opposed to arthrodesis.

Table 12.4 Considerations in arthroscopic ankle arthrodesis

Acceptable indications
Skin and soft tissues:
Poor quality skin, scarring, and grafts
Deformity:
Varus, valgus, equinus
Modified management
General conditions:
Diabetes, peripheral vascular disease, peripheral neuropathy
Bone:
Osteoporosis, avascular necrosis, treated infection
Adjacent joints:
Pes cavus, planovalgus, subtalar arthritis, midfoot arthritis
Contraindications
Patient factors:
Smoking, unreasonable expectation, poorly compliant patient

Local conditions such as avascular necrosis (AVN) may be apparent on MRI. Avascular necrosis does not preclude arthroscopic ankle arthrodesis, indeed the tibia is an ideal vascularized bone graft. Nevertheless, the strength of the fixation and the postoperative protected weightbearing regime will need to be increased.

Operative Procedure
Patient Positioning

The patient is positioned as for an ankle arthroscopy – supine, with a bolster under the ipsilateral buttock, the lower leg supported on a cushion, with intermittent soft tissue ankle distraction performed using an ankle sling, adjusted by movements of the table end. The patient is placed in a slightly head-down position. In the operating theater, room should be made for an image intensifier on the ipsilateral side, with the x-ray monitor alongside, so that the surgeon has a clear view when inserting the screws.

Procedure

The portal placements are the same as those described for standard ankle arthroscopy. Anterior osteophytes,

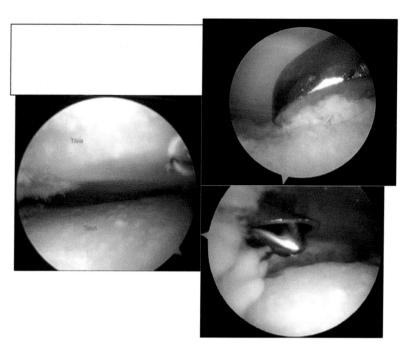

Figure 12.9 Preparation of the talar dome and the tibia for arthrodesis must penetrate the subchondral bone. A variety of instruments, both power and hand held, can be used to achieve this.

synovitis, and scar tissue are removed using power shavers. A visual assessment is then performed of the congruity of the joint, with particular reference to those areas of the joints that have been eroded by the arthritic process. Decortication is usually undertaken using a 4.5 barrel burr, using continuous-flow irrigation to remove the debris. Curettes can be of assistance with cystic lesions, and curved or reversed osteotomes be helpful in decortication of the posterior talus (Figure 12.9).

In a varus ankle, it is common to see significant cartilage and bony erosion on the medial side of the tibia, with anterior subluxation of the talus and large anterolateral tibial and talar osteophytes. This may be combined with erosion of the medial malleolus, and osteophytes in the medial gutter of the talus, at the tip of the medial malleolus, and on the anterior aspect of the lateral malleolus. In the valgus ankle the erosions are lateral.

Decortication usually begins anteriorly on the talar dome, and proceeds posteriorly. Talar and tibial preparation can be alternated to create space and allow easier posterior access. The medial gutter should be decorticated, to add mobility to the joint. Similarly, in cases of significant deformity, the lateral gutter is decorticated, combined with the removal of the gutter osteophytes. It is usual to be able to

decorticate fully to the posterior capsule, allowing the talus to be positioned correctly and anatomically below the tibia. The tip of the lateral malleolus may be removed to prevent impingement, if necessary.

In pes cavovarus the hindfoot may be varus with a pronation deformity in the mid- and forefoot. Correcting the forefoot flat to the floor will drive the hindfoot further into varus. When a tibiotalar arthrodesis is performed for such a deformity then the varus at the ankle is corrected in the coronal plane, anterior subluxation corrected in the sagittal plane, and internal rotation of the talus on the tibia corrected in the axial plane. However, the primary foot deformity remains hindfoot varus and forefoot pronation. These may well require correction by a lateral displacement os calcis osteotomy, and a dorsiflexion osteotomy of the first ray. If this deformity is associated with neurological conditions causing muscle imbalance, rebalancing may be required with transfer of the peroneus longus to brevis. If tibialis anterior muscle weakness is significant occasionally a tibialis posterior tendon transfer to the dorsum of the foot as part of a Bridle procedure is needed. A Bridle procedure consists of a tibialis posterior tendon transfer through the interosseous membrane to the dorsum of the foot with a dual anastomosis to the tendon of the tibialis anterior and the peroneus longus tendon, which is rerouted in front of the lateral malleolus.

Feet with planovalgus deformity can develop a valgus tilt in the ankle, which is sometimes associated with arthrosis. There are three radiological patterns of ankle disease associated with the flat foot.

1. An arthritic pattern, without tilt or deformity, above a planovalgus foot.
2. Ankle arthritis with a valgus tilt, above a planovalgus foot.
3. A valgus-tilted ankle without significant arthritic disease.

All three can be treated by arthroscopic ankle arthrodesis, should this prove to be necessary. Additional treatment for the planovalgus foot will depend on the severity of the deformity, and the mobility of the subtalar and transverse tarsal joints. In some patients, the deformity is acceptable if the foot is comfortable and the joints are mobile. For these patients correction of the planovalgus foot is often deemed unnecessary. If the flat foot produces significant symptoms it should be corrected according to its pathology.

In some conditions, a plantaris deformity of the forefoot may accompany an arthritic ankle. Some correction for the combined deformity can be made in the arthrodesis of the ankle, but severe plantaris deformity requires corrective osteotomy or arthrodesis of the midfoot, to correct the foot to plantargrade, which reduces loading under the forefoot.

Fixation

With the ankle deformity corrected, fixation is with two or three 6.5 mm cannulated screws inserted under x-ray control, from the medial tibia laterally into the talus. These screws are usually placed parallel; the more proximal screw is positioned anterolaterally and the more distal screw more posteromedially (Figure 12.10). Careful use of the image intensifier is necessary to avoid screw penetration into the subtalar joint, in particular by the posteromedial screw. The positioning of the foot should be the same as for open arthrodesis. It should be plantargrade, with the heel in 5° of valgus, the forefoot square to the ground and neutral to 10° of external rotation in the axial plane.

Postoperative Management

The authors' preference is to rest the lower leg below the knee in a splint or backslab, elevating the leg

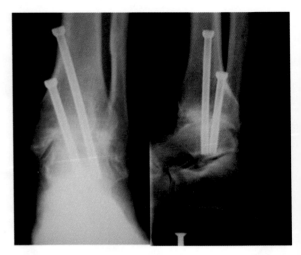

Figure 12.10 Screw fixation position for a fusion has to emphasize rigidity over attempts at parallel placement for compression.

overnight in hospital. At two weeks, when the wounds have healed, the patient is transitioned to either a below-knee walking cast or proprietary boot, increasing weight bearing as pain allows[35]. The patient is encouraged to progressively build up their walking distance over the subsequent weeks. If at three months the patient is capable of unprotected weight bearing, is non-tender on examination, and x-rays show satisfactory progress toward union, the patient is weaned from the boot. Varying amounts of swelling, weakness, and discomfort will be experienced, and so it is prudent to warn the patients before surgery to expect these symptoms, particularly in the first six months postoperatively. Improvement continues for at least 12 months after surgery, nevertheless the severe, disabling pain experienced preoperatively is normally starting to resolve by three months.

Outcomes

Union rates are 95% to 98%. High union rates depend, to some degree, on identifying the risk factors associated with delayed or non-union, particularly smoking, diabetes, peripheral neuropathy, and peripheral vascular disease.

Managing Complications
Infection

Infection is rare. Superficial infections may respond well to simple antibiotics, but deep infection can compromise union of the arthrodesis and may not be eradicated without removal of particularly cannulated screws and overdrilling of the tracks. A regime where the screws are removed, the ankle is immobilized while treating with antibiotics for six weeks, followed by simple replacement of the screws at a later date, is viable.

Nerve Injury

Nerve injury is infrequent, but patches of numbness can occur, usually in the distribution of the branches of the superficial peroneal nerve, as with standard ankle arthroscopy.

Malalignment

Malalignment of the arthrodesis at the tibiotalar joint is avoided by scrupulous surgical technique, in particular decortication of the gutters, removal of osteophytes, and careful imaging during fixation.

It is important to predict malposition from factors outside the ankle, including the knee, tibia, and foot. Preoperative planning should predict such malalignment and whether the arthrodesis can be modified to compensate. If the deformity cannot be corrected through the ankle fusion, extra-articular surgery may be required. If obvious residual deformity of the ankle is seen postoperatively it is best corrected early, while extra-ankle deformity is probably best dealt with once solid union has been achieved.

Subtalar Arthritis

It is recognized that 20 years after ankle arthrodesis radiological arthritis in the ipsilateral foot is accelerated, compared to the non-fused side[36]. It is not always symptomatic, and may not need surgical treatment. It is not entirely clear if this subtalar arthritis is the result of the arthrodesis, preexists the ankle fusion, or both[37]. It is therefore prudent to carefully assess the subtalar joint prior to ankle fusion. Both scans and targeted injections of local anesthetic will help determine whether symptomatic subtalar arthritis is present. Moderate to severe subtalar arthritis will require either simultaneous subtalar arthrodesis or the use of an alternative technique, such as subtalar arthrodesis combined with ankle replacement. Patients with minor, asymptomatic subtalar degenerative change can pose a greater challenge to decision making. One option is to undertake the ankle arthrodesis and only to treat the subtalar joint if it becomes symptomatic.

Impingement

When correcting deformity, or in the presence of exuberant osteophytes, impingement, particularly of the malleoli against the talus or calcaneum, may prevent proper apposition of the decorticated joint surfaces. It is therefore important to remove osteophytes, and if necessary to shorten the fibula or rarely the medial malleolus. Particular areas to concentrate on are the anteromedial talar neck, the tip of the lateral malleolus, and the anterior edge of the lateral malleolus. Similar impingement lesions can be seen at the back of the ankle. It is therefore important to remove the posterior osteophytes or fibrosed capsule during decortication, to allow correct positioning of the talus underneath the tibia. After fusion, if further impingement occurs this can be dealt with surgery targeted to the affected area.

Non-Union

Non-unions are rare, and in treating them it is important to identify correctable, systemic risk factors that might have been overlooked, such as smoking, obesity[38], poorly controlled diabetes, and vascular impairment. Vitamin D deficiency may also be an issue.

Technical causes for non-union, such as impingement, need to be excluded, and therefore multiaxial imaging is important in the assessment. It is also important to consider and exclude low-grade infection.

Non-union resulting from an arthroscopic ankle arthrodesis does not inevitably mean that revision arthrodesis needs to be an open procedure. It is entirely feasible, with the aid of image intensification, to identify the pseudarthrosis and to arthroscopically repeat the decortication. Meticulous care must once again be taken to remove any impingement lesions, to fully decorticate the gutters, and to shorten the malleoli, so that good bony apposition is achieved. At least one side of the proposed arthrodesis must have a good blood supply. If dead or infected bone is present on both sides of the arthrodesis, then an open technique may well be required. Bone graft for osteoinductive purposes can be inserted through arthroscopic portals. Fixation needs to be stable. Postoperatively, weight bearing can be introduced with care as pain allows. Immobilization should be continued until union is established clinically and radiologically, which may take six months or more. CT scanning should be employed if there is doubt.

When undertaking a revision arthrodesis, if there is evidence of significant degenerative change distal to the ankle, in particular of the subtalar joint, it may be prudent to include this joint in the fusion.

Key Points

Ankle Arthroscopy

- Arthroscopic surgery allows diagnosis and treatment of pathology with minimal soft tissue damage.
- Anteromedial, medial midline, and anterolateral portals provide safe anterior access.
- Posterior ankle arthroscopy portals require careful technique to avoid neurological injury: in particular staying lateral to the FHL tendon.
- Arthroscopic resection has a 90% rate of success for soft tissue lesions causing anterior impingement.
- Bony anterior ankle impingement can be treated successfully in 90% of patients, although if there is preoperative joint space narrowing the success rate falls to 50%.
- Arthroscopic microfracture is more successful for osteochondral lesions less than 15 mm.

Arthroscopic Arthrodesis

- Open and arthroscopic ankle arthrodesis is highly successful treatment for end-stage ankle arthritis with low morbidity, low complications, and early mobilization.
- Arthroscopic ankle arthrodesis is appropriate for both normally aligned and deformed joints.
- Arthroscopic ankle arthrodesis has a lower perioperative morbidity, less blood loss, fewer reported postoperative complications, shorter hospital stay, quicker rehabilitation, decreased time to union, and a reduction in cost compared to open techniques.
- Arthroscopic arthrodesis is particularly helpful for patients with a poor soft tissue envelope and can be used, with caution, for patients with peripheral vascular disease and neuropathies.
- Deformities proximal to the ankle should be corrected before arthrodesis, and foot deformities planned for secondary correction after union.
- Fixation is by two or three parallel screws from medial tibia to talus.
- Weight bearing can commence at two weeks. Standard immobilization time is three months.

References

1. Burman MS. Arthroscopy or the direct visualisation of joints: an experimental cadaver study. *J Bone Joint Surg*. 1931; 13:669.

2. van Dijk CN, van Bergen CJ. Advancements in ankle arthroscopy. *J Am Acad Orthop Surg*. 2008; 16(11):635–46.

3. Molloy S, Solan MC, Bendall SP. Synovial impingement in the ankle. a new physical sign. *J Bone Joint Surg Br*. 2003; 85(3):330–3.

4. Baums MH, Kahl E, Schultz W, Klinger HM. Clinical outcome of the arthroscopic management of sports-related "anterior ankle pain": a prospective study. *Knee Surg Sports Traumatol Arthrosc*. 2006; 14(5):482–6.

5. Urgüden M, Söyüncü Y, Ozdemir H, Sekban H, Akyildiz FF, Aydin

AT. Arthroscopic treatment of anterolateral soft tissue impingement of the ankle: evaluation of factors affecting outcome. *Arthroscopy*. 2005; 21(3):317–22.

6. Lui TH, Ip K, Chow HT. Comparison of radiologic and arthroscopic diagnoses of distal tibio-fibular syndesmosis disruption in acute ankle ankle fracture. *Arthroscopy*. 2005; 21(11):1370.

7. Bassett FH 3rd, Gates HS 3rd, Billys JB, Morris HB, Nikolaou PK. Talar impingement by the anteroinferior tibiofibular ligament. A cause of chronic pain in the ankle after inversion sprain. *J Bone Joint Surg Am*. 1990; 72(1):55–9.

8. Ogilvie-Harris DJ, Mahomed N, Demazière anterior impingement

of the ankle treated by arthroscopic removal of bony spurs. *J Bone Joint Surg Br*. 1993; 75(3):437–40.

9. van Dijk CN, Tol JL, Verheyen CC. A prospective study of prognostic factors concerning the outcome of arthroscopic surgery for anterior ankle impingement. *Am J Sports Med*. 1997; 25:737–45.

10. Han SH, Choi WJ, Kim S, Kim SJ, Lee JW. Ossicles associated with chronic pain around the malleoli of the ankle. *J Bone Joint Surg Br*. 2008; 90(8):1049–54.

11. Van Dijk NC. Anterior and posterior ankle impingement. *Foot Ankle Clin*. 2006; 11(3):663–83.

12. Rolf CG, Barclay C, Riyami M, George J. The importance of early arthroscopy in athletes with

painful cartilage lesions of the ankle: a prospective study of 61 consecutive cases. *J Orthop Surg Res.* 2006; 1:4.

13. Hepple S, Winson IG, Glew D. Osteochondral lesions of the talus: a revised classification. *Foot Ankle Int.* 1999; 20(12):789–93.

14. Robinson DE. Winson IG, Harries WJ, Kelly AJ. Arthroscopic treatment of osteochondral lesions of the talus. *J Bone Joint Surg Br.* 2003; 85(7):989–93.

15. Chuckpaiwong B, Berkson EM, Theodore GH. Microfracture for osteochondral lesions of the ankle: outcome analysis and outcome predictors of 105 cases. *Arthroscopy.* 2008; 24(1):106–12.

16. Lee DH, Lee KB, Jung ST, Seon JK, Kim MS, Sung IH. Comparison of early versus delayed weightbearing outcomes after microfracture for small to midsized osteochondral lesions of the talus. *Am J Sports Med.* 2012; 40(9):2023–8.

17. Schuman L, Struijs PA, van Dijk CN. Arthroscopic treatment for osteochondral defects of the talus. Results at follow-up at 2 to 11 years. *J Bone Joint Surg Br.* 2002; 84(3):364–8.

18. Savva N, Jabur M, Davies M, Saxby T. Osteochondral lesions of the talus: results of repeat arthroscopic debridement. *Foot Ankle Int.* 2007; 28(6):669–73.

19. Zengerink M, Struijs PA, Tol JL, van Dijk CN. Treatment of osteochondral lesions of the talus: a systematic review. *Knee Surg Sports Traumatol Arthrosc.* 2010; 18(2):238–46.

20. Niemeyer P, Salzmann G, Schmal H, Mayr H, Südkamp NP. Autologous chondrocyte implantation for the treatment of chondral and osteochondral defects of the talus: a meta-analysis of available evidence.

21. Mologne TS, Ferkel RD. Arthroscopic treatment of osteochondral lesions of the distal tibia. *Foot Ankle Int.* 2007; 28(8):865–72.

22. Nihal A, Rose DJ, Trepman E. Arthroscopic treatment of anterior ankle impingement syndrome in dancers. *Foot Ankle Int.* 2005; 26(11):908–12.

23. Saltzman CL, Salamon ML, Blanchard GM, et al. Epidemiology of ankle arthritis: report of a consecutive series of 639 patients from a tertiary orthopaedic center. *Iowa Orthop J.* 2005; 25:44–6.

24. Glazebrook M, Daniels T, Younger A, et al. Comparison of health-related quality of life between patients with end-stage ankle and hip arthrosis. *J Bone Joint Surg Am.* 2008; 90(3):499–505.

25. Townshend D, Di Silvestro M, Krause F, et al. Arthroscopic versus open ankle arthrodesis: a multicenter comparative case series. *J Bone Joint Surg Am.* 2013; 95(2):98–102.

26. Gougoulias NE, Agathangelidis FG, Parsons SW. Arthroscopic ankle arthrodesis. *Foot Ankle Int.* 2007; 28(6):695–706.

27. Dannawi Z, Nawabi DH, Patel A, Leong JJ, Moore DJ. Arthroscopic ankle arthrodesis: are results reproducible irrespective of pre-operative deformity? *Foot Ankle Surg.* 2011; 17(4):294–9.

28. Winson IG, Robinson DE, Allen PE. Arthroscopic ankle arthrodesis. *J Bone Joint Surg Br.* 2005; 87(3):343–7.

29. Rippstein P, Kumar B, Muller M. Ankle arthrodesis using the arthroscopic technique.

Oper Orthop Traumatol. 2005; 17(4–5):442–56.

30. Mazur JM, Schwartz E, Simon SR. Ankle arthrodesis: long-term follow-up with gait analysis. *J Bone Joint Surg Am.* 1979; 61:964–75.

31. Ferkel RD, Hewitt M. Long-term results of arthroscopic ankle arthrodesis. *Foot Ankle Int.* 2005; 26(4):275–80.

32. Peterson KS, Lee MS, Buddecke DE. Arthroscopic versus open ankle arthrodesis: a retrospective cost analysis. *J Foot Ankle Surg.* 2010; 49(3):242–7.

33. Nielsen KK, Linde F, Jensen NC. The outcome of arthroscopic and open surgery ankle arthrodesis: a comparative retrospective study on 107 patients. *Foot Ankle Surgery.* 2008; 14(3):153–7.

34. Cobb TK, Gabrielsen TA, Campbell DC 2nd, et al. Cigarette smoking and nonunion after ankle arthrodesis. *Foot Ankle.* 1994; 15:64–7.

35. Cannon LB, Brown J, Cooke PH. Early weight bearing is safe following arthroscopic ankle arthrodesis. *Foot Ankle Surgery* 2004; 10(3):135–9.

36. Coester LM, Saltzman CL, Leupold J, et al. Long-term results following ankle arthrodesis for post-traumatic arthritis. *J Bone Joint Surg Am.* 2001; 83-A:219–28.

37. Sheridan BD, Robinson DE, Hubble MJW, Winson IG. Ankle arthrodesis and its relationship to ipsilateral arthritis of the hind- and mid-foot. *J Bone Joint Surg Br.* 2006; 88(2):206–7.

38. Collman DR, Kaas MH, Schuberth JM. Arthroscopic ankle arthrodesis: factors influencing union in 39 consecutive patients. *Foot Ankle Int.* 2006; 27(12):1079–85.

Chapter 13

Foot Arthroscopy and Tendonoscopy

Stephen W. Parsons and Ian G. Winson

Introduction

Following the successful introduction of diagnostic and operative arthroscopy in the ankle, the techniques have been extended to the joints and tendons of the foot. In this chapter we describe these newer techniques, and their applications to conditions such as tarsal coalitions.

Subtalar Joint Arthroscopy

Diagnostic arthroscopy and arthroscopic surgery of the subtalar joint is a recent development, one of the earliest reports of subtalar arthroscopy was as recent as 1985. There are a number of reasons that this technique has not reached the same levels of popularity as arthroscopy of the ankle joint. The subtalar joint is a complex structure, into which it is relatively difficult to introduce an arthroscope. It is composed of a large posterior facet, which has close congruence. The posterior facet is separated from the middle and anterior facets by the sinus tarsi, which contains blood vessels, nerves, fat, and the talocalcaneal ligaments. Visualization and intervention can be challenging. On the other hand subtalar arthroscopy is a low-risk procedure and, with appropriate training, practice, and care, effective surgery can be undertaken[1].

Pathologies

There is a wide variety of pathological and traumatic processes that can affect the subtalar joint (Box 13.1). Although similar to the ankle joint, there are some pathologies that are specific to the subtalar joint, in particular talocalcaneal and calcaneonavicular coalitions.

Clinical Assessment

As with the ankle joint, there are good clinical indications for arthroscopic surgery (Box 13.2). Clinical examination is similar to that of the ankle, with the emphasis on assessment of subtalar movement, weightbearing supination and pronation, and non-weightbearing passive movement. Direct palpation may show specific areas of tenderness, such as over the lateral process, the sinus tarsi, or the anterior process of the os calcis. It is important to try to differentiate between joint-related pain and pain from the peroneal or posterior tibial tendons.

Radiological

Whereas the standard weightbearing foot and ankle series and the non-weightbearing oblique foot remain

---

Box 13.1 The variety of subtalar pathologies

Chondral lesions
Osteochondral lesions
Osteophytes
Adhesions – arthrofibrosis or synovitis
Loose bodies
Fracture fragments – lateral or anterior process
Os trigonum syndrome
Posterior impingement
Coalitions
Arthrosis

Box 13.2 Indications for subtalar arthroscopy

Excision of osteophytes
Lysis of adhesions – arthrofibrosis or synovitis
Removal of loose bodies
Excision of fracture fragments
Excision of os trigonum
Excision of posterior impingement
FHL transfer for tendo Achillis ruptures
Excision of calcaneonavicular coalitions
Excision of talocalcaneal coalitions
Arthrodesis

extremely useful, the Harris and Broden's views are little used, and have been replaced by the use of CT, MRI, and US scanning. Image intensifier guided local anesthetic injections, particularly when undertaken with an arthrogram, can again be extremely helpful in confirming that clinical symptoms arise from the identified pathology.

Techniques

There are two main approaches to subtalar arthroscopy – posterior and sinus tarsi.

Posterior Arthroscopy

The posterior approaches to the subtalar joint are similar to the posterior approach to the ankle joint. The only difference is that the portals can be placed lower using the tip of the distal fibula as the reference level. Fluoroscopy can be helpful.

Sinus Tarsi Approach

Positioning

The patient is positioned at 45° or in the "saggy" lateral, half way between supine and lateral. The exact angle is determined by the rotational mobility of the hip. This position is adjusted, so that the foot can be moved between the vertical and lateral position. The leg is supported by a firm, well-padded cushion, allowing the foot to hang free and inverted off the end of the cushion. The surgeon stands at the patient's heel, and the camera screen is placed opposite, next to the patient's head. The x-ray monitor is then placed alongside the arthroscopy stack, and the C-arm beside that, so that it can be brought in at 90° to the limb if fluoroscopy is required.

The patient is prepared and draped in the standard manner, with a pouch to collect fluid. If an arthrodesis is planned, the patient should have primary draping above the knee, so that the correct limb alignment can be confirmed visually.

Portals

The standard incisions are known as the anterolateral and the accessory anterolateral "sinus tarsi" portals. The anterolateral portal is situated immediately above the calcaneum at the angle of Gissane, beneath the lateral process of the talus, approximately 1 cm distal and 2 cm anterior to the tip of the fibula. The

accessory anterolateral portal is positioned approximately 1.5 cm more distal, and 0.5 cm more dorsal. Each portal is checked before incision, by using a hypodermic needle to ensure the sinus tarsi is entered. Radiology can be used if in doubt. It is important to recognize that there is the potential for damage to both branches of the sural nerve and the lateral branch of the superficial peroneal nerve. Therefore the skin is incised with a knife and then round-ended scissors are used to separate the deep tissues until the sinus tarsi is entered. The separation is undertaken in the long axis of the foot. The scissors can then be rotated 90° and opened to spread the portals. Accessory portals can be established more posteriorly. These accessory posterior portals include the posterolateral portal from posterior ankle arthroscopy, and an accessory posterolateral portal, just posterior to the peroneal tendons. The accessory posterolateral portal does have a higher risk of damage to the sural nerve (Figure 13.1).

Standard Arthroscopic Tour

The arthroscope is inserted into the anterolateral portal and instruments into the accessory anterolateral portal. Initially the view may be obscured by the fat of the sinus tarsi. A 3.5 mm soft tissue resector is used to excise the fat adjacent to the arthroscope. Care is taken to leave the talocalcaneal ligaments undamaged. The initial area prepared is the anterior margin of the posterior facet of the subtalar joint, this is then extended into the lateral gutter, between the joint and the peroneal tendons. Swapping portals assists in visualization of the lateral gutter. Thus the anterolateral edge of the posterior facet is identified, and the foot gently moved to show the subtalar movement. Any osteophytes can then be removed using a small burr. A blunt periosteal elevator is then inserted into the joint, to open it for inspection. If chondral or osteochondral injuries are identified, the accessory posterolateral portal may be necessary to distract the joint, to allow debridement.

The tour then proceeds distally; any excess fat, synovitis, inflammatory tissue, or scarring is identified and removed. It is usually possible to bypass the talocalcaneal ligaments, leaving them intact to identify the middle facet, but they are removed for arthrodesis. The arthroscope is returned to the anterolateral portal and the resector to the accessory anterolateral portal allowing inspection of the anterior process of the

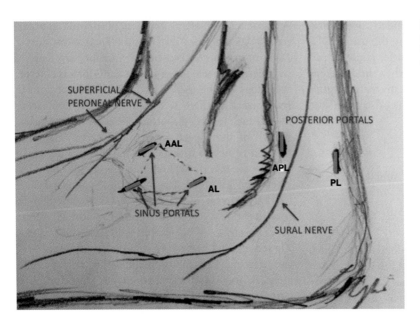

Figure 13.1 Portals for access to the subtalar joint. AL: anterolateral; AAL: accessory anterolateral; PL: posterolateral; APL: antero-posterolateral.

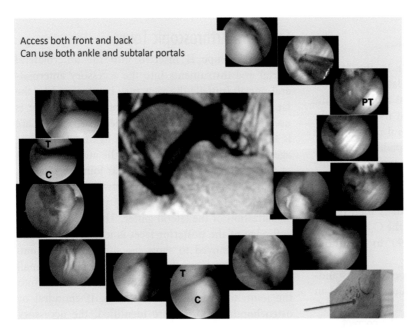

Figure 13.2 Tour of the subtalar joint. PT: peroneal tendons; T: talus; C: calcaneus

calcaneum, the bifurcate ligament, the spring ligament, and the anterior facet of the subtalar joint. The head of the talus can be followed into the talonavicular joint, although soft tissue will need to be resected to clearly visualize the joint. It is possible to track along the anterior process of the calcaneum to identify the calcaneocuboid joint, and the quadrilateral point between the calcaneum, cuboid, navicular, and talus.

This allows identification and treatment of osteophytes, loose bodies, un-united fractures, coalitions, and soft tissue pathologies (Figure 13.2).

Postoperatively, the wounds are closed with sutures or glue and adhesive tape. A wool and crepe compression bandage is applied for 48 hours. It is important to avoid hematoma and therefore intraoperative diathermy is used and postoperative

(a)

(b)

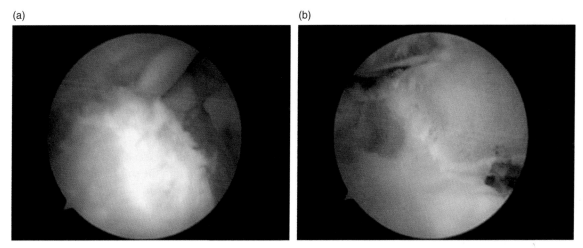

Figure 13.3 Calcaneonavicular coalition: initial view (**a**) and at partial resection (**b**).

elevation of the foot emphasized. The patient is advised to mobilize the foot and ankle, weight bearing as pain permits, in the ten days following surgery, and is then referred for progressive mobilization, guided by a physiotherapist.

Tarsal Coalitions

Tarsal coalitions may present in adolescence or adulthood. The history is of increasing, activity-related pain, stiffness, and recurrent instability. Tarsal coalitions are defined as either complete or incomplete. Complete tarsal coalitions have continuity of bony bridging, whereas a mixture of fibrous and cartilaginous tissue fills incomplete coalitions. The two most common tarsal coalitions are the calcaneonavicular and talocalcaneal. Both of these coalitions are amenable to arthroscopic resection.

Examination usually identifies a restriction of subtalar movement. Careful investigation is mandatory, with a full set of x-rays and either MRI or CT scanning. CT scanning, including 3D reconstruction, is particularly useful in defining talocalcaneal coalitions[2].

Resection of coalitions is usually considered when the symptoms are not improved with orthoses and rest in a cast. Extensive degenerative changes or a large talocalcaneal coalition are better treated by a subtalar or a triple arthrodesis. Preoperative valgus deformity will not improve following resection of the coalition, and may have to be separately addressed by calcaneal osteotomy, or even an arthroereisis implant.

Calcaneonavicular Coalition

A calcaneonavicular coalition bridges the gap from the anterior process of the calcaneum, across the quadrilateral point, to the lateral side of the navicular. It may be complete or incomplete. The coalition replaces the calcaneonavicular band of the bifurcate ligament. The rigidity of the coalition stiffens the movement of the hindfoot joint complex.

Resection can be undertaken arthroscopically[3], through two sinus tarsi portals. The patient is positioned as for a subtalar arthroscopy. An anterolateral portal is established. A second accessory anterolateral portal is made slightly distal to the standard portal, over the calcaneonavicular coalition. The excision is performed with a 3.5 mm shaver and barrel burr. Adequacy of removal is assessed by direct vision (Figure 13.3) and by fluoroscopy. The excision must be wide and complete, and allow the restoration of hindfoot movement. This will help prevent re-calcification and recurrent formation of the coalition. The patient is mobilized early post-surgery.

Good results from arthroscopic resection of calcaneonavicular coalitions have been reported, with few complications[4–5]. The reported complications include hematoma formation, scar pain, infection, and damage to the branches of the sural or superficial peroneal nerves. Despite not using interposition grafting with fat or muscle, recurrent calcification or bony bridging is rare if the excision is adequate. Pain and stiffness can occur if there is established degenerative change in the talonavicular or subtalar joints, which has not been identified preoperatively.

237

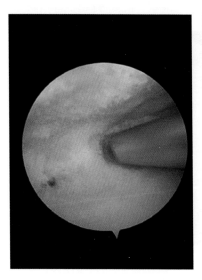

Figure 13.4
Talocalcaneal coalition – during resection.

Talocalcaneal Coalitions

Talocalcaneal coalitions once again may be complete or incomplete. Preoperative imaging is essential to determine the position, type, and extent of the coalition. Different shapes and extents of coalition can be identified on CT scanning, particularly with 3D reconstructions. The coalitions usually involve the middle facet, and may extend to a greater or lesser degree into the posterior facet. One particular type involves only the posterior medial aspect of the posterior facet and can require both sinus tarsi and posterior approaches for arthroscopic excision.

Smaller talocalcaneal coalitions, which are predominantly restricted to the middle facet with only limited extension into the posterior facet, are amenable to removal through a sinus tarsi approach (Figure 13.4). The positioning and portals are as for subtalar arthroscopy. Image intensification may be of assistance in guiding resection. The first step is to identify the limits of the coalition. Its extent into the posterior facet is noted, but also its extent into the anterior facet. Resections are undertaken using a combination of a 3.5 mm soft tissue resector and a 3.5 mm barrel burr. Care is required in the resection at the proximal end of the posterior facet, particularly where the FHL tendon is visualized, as this is in close proximity to the neurovascular bundle. Following adequate excision of the coalition, increased movements of the subtalar joint should be observed. The talocalcaneal ligaments can be released to enhance movement and correct deformity.

When the coalition extends to the posteromedial aspect of the posterior facet, but is still sufficiently small to be resected, a combination of approaches can be used. The patient is positioned 45° prone, which permits both the sinus tarsi approach and the posterior approach to remove a peripheral coalition while preserving the joint surface and medial soft tissues. Wounds are closed in the standard manner.

General complications are similar to those listed for calcaneonavicular resections. In addition, over-aggressive resection into the soft tissues medial to the posterior facet can result in damage to the posterior tibial nerve. Poor selection of too extensive a tarsal coalition produces a large raw area of bony surface at the end of the procedure, which may lead to reformation of the coalition, or even the formation of a painful pseudarthrosis.

Studies have shown arthroscopic resection of talocalcaneal coalitions to be a feasible and effective technique[6].

Posterior Subtalar Arthroscopy

Posterior subtalar arthroscopy can be used for excision of posteromedial talocalcaneal coalitions, which are a rare variant. The posterior approach can also be used to harvest the FHL for transfer in the salvage of late diagnosed tendo Achillis rupture in patients with poor quality soft tissues, or significant medical comorbidities. The patient is placed prone and the standard posteromedial and posterolateral portals are used.

Arthroscopic Subtalar Arthrodesis

In circumstances where the subtalar or transverse tarsal joints are degenerative and non-operative management of the pain has failed, the operation of choice is arthrodesis. Subtalar and hindfoot arthrodeses are also the mainstay of treatment for fixed deformity or deformity with degeneration.

Improvements in the internal fixation techniques used to stabilize the arthrodesis have resulted in improvements in the rates of union. Nevertheless there can be problems with the quality of the soft tissue envelope. This can be worsened by severe deformity where correction of the foot shape can lead to post-operative tension in the soft tissues on the concave side of the deformity. The tension can lead to wound breakdown, which can be complicated by infection, painful scar formation, and nerve dysfunction.

(a)

(b)

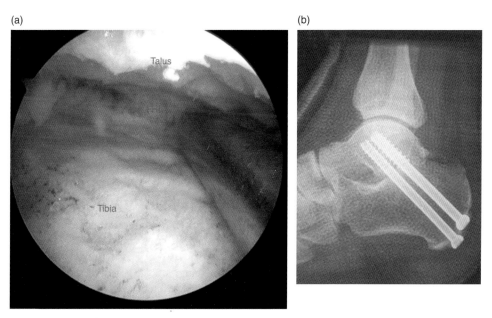

Figure 13.5 The subtalar joint prepared (**a**) for introduction of screws (**b**).

As arthroscopic ankle arthrodesis became established as an effective surgical technique, with high union rates and reduced complications, it was inevitable that subtalar arthroscopy would be considered and utilized for subtalar arthrodesis. The indications for arthroscopic subtalar arthrodesis are in situ fusion, or where correction of the rotational or angulatory deformities can be corrected by soft tissue releases and decortication alone. It is not indicated if there is a requirement for major bony excision or if there is significant bone loss requiring structural bone grafting, for example in the elevation of the talus after depressed calcaneal fractures. Similarly, if there are large cavities, which require extensive bone grafting, an arthroscopic technique should not be used.

There are a number of published reports of case series reviewing in situ arthroscopic subtalar arthrodeses, performed through a posterior approach[7-9], with usually an accessory sinus tarsi portal. Fusion rates are reported as being high, over 90%, but series numbers are low. We prefer the sinus tarsi approach for subtalar arthrodesis[10]. Using this approach, not only the posterior facet but the middle and anterior facets can be prepared, allowing a full decortication of the joint and therefore a greater correction of any rotary or angulatory deformity.

The patient is positioned as for subtalar arthroscopy, in the 45° semi-lateral, supine position. The standard sinus tarsi portals are created. The contents of the sinus tarsi, including the ligaments, can be removed for clear visualization and mobilization of the joint. A 4.5 mm soft tissue resector can be utilized for this purpose. Decortication is usually undertaken with a 4.5 mm barrel burr, starting at the anterior aspect of the posterior facet, and proceeding from the lateral side, posteriorly and medially. Once the medial side of the facet is reached, the decortication is completed from posterior to anterior, along the medial edge, with careful attention being made to identify the flexor hallucis longus tendon, which is an important landmark for the adjacent posterior neurovascular bundle. During decortication, prominent osteophytes and other pathologies, such as lateral process non-unions, may require removal. Similarly, tarsal coalitions may need to be removed from the middle facet, or from the medial side of the posterior facet. Once decortication of the posterior facet is complete, the middle and anterior facets are also decorticated. Care must be taken to avoid entering the talonavicular joint. Decortication allows considerable mobility, which allows the correction of deformity.

Apposition of the raw surfaces can be checked arthroscopically, and with fluoroscopy (Figure 13.5). Fixation is usually undertaken with one or two 6.5 mm cannulated titanium screws, inserted from the

239

calcaneal tuberosity into the body and neck of the talus under radiological control. It is important to visually assess the alignment of the limb after the insertion of the cannulated guide wires to ensure correct heel alignment and rotation of the foot. Screws should have a short enough thread to allow compression.

Postoperatively the lower leg is immobilized in a backslab. The patient is advised to elevate the limb for the majority of the time for the first two weeks, to reduce swelling and the risk of a hematoma. At two weeks a below-knee cast is applied. Weight bearing is then permitted with the use of crutches. It is reasonable to utilize a removable boot, which can be removed to allow non-weightbearing active mobilization of the remaining joints. At 12 weeks following surgery, providing the patient can fully bear weight, with no pain on stressing the joint and x-rays showing no joint line lucency, the boot may be progressively discarded and rehabilitation continued.

Outcomes and Complications

Union rates of 97% have been achieved in the two authors' separate practices[11], and good results have been reported by others[12–15]. Complications specific to arthroscopic subtalar arthrodesis include poor healing of sinus tarsi portal wounds, and heel pain from the screw insertion scars on the heel, or from prominent metalwork. To avoid the latter, care should be taken to countersink the heads of the screws. Infection is uncommon but if deep infection occurs, cannulated screws may need to be removed, the tracks debrided and extensively washed out. The screws can then be replaced with either solid screws or external fixation if the union is not sound.

Midtarsal Joints

Pathologies

The talonavicular and calcaneocuboid joints can be affected by arthritis, osteochondral lesions, osteophyte formation, coalitions, and midfoot fractures. Arthroscopic techniques are particularly useful for the removal of coalitions (see above), for the removal of loose bodies, un-united fractures, and for arthrodesis.

Arthroscopic Technique

To access the transverse tarsal joints the portals are modified, with the anterolateral sinus tarsi portal

being inserted just anterior to the angle of Gissane, 5 mm distal to the standard portal, and the second portal more distal and dorsal on the lateral side of the foot. This portal is positioned to lie approximately halfway along the line of the talonavicular joint, when imaged on the lateral foot x-ray. If the anterior process of the calcaneum is the source of pathology, for example a non-united fracture, then the portals are those described for the calcaneonavicular coalition resection.

Triple and Double Arthrodeses

The indications for both double and triple arthrodesis are significant pain or deformity arising from the hindfoot joints. These are clearly defined by radiology, multiplanar imaging, and, if required, image-guided injections of local anesthetic. A triple arthrodesis is normally indicated when all three joints are degenerative, or require decortication for correction of deformity. A double arthrodesis, defined here as talonavicular and subtalar joints, can be undertaken for patients with deformity that can be corrected without mobilizing a pristine calcaneocuboid joint.

Two or three portals may be utilized[16]. The standard sinus tarsi portal at the angle of Gissane, the second portal at the quadrilateral point, and a third dorsolateral talonavicular portal if necessary. The posterior facet of the subtalar joint is decorticated first. The posterior subtalar facet preparation is extended through the middle and anterior subtalar facets, following the head of the talus, into the talonavicular joint. Decortication of the talonavicular joint starts inferiorly and laterally, and progresses dorsally and medially. The calcaneocuboid joint is identified, if uncertain, with the aid of fluoroscopy, and decortication is then completed from dorsal to plantar, and usually medially to laterally. Decortication must be sufficient to allow mobilization of the joints to a corrected position if there is deformity. If the foot position cannot be corrected an open procedure should be undertaken.

Fixation of the subtalar joint is performed as previously described. The talonavicular fixation uses a 5 mm headed, partially threaded titanium compression screw from the navicular tuberosity to the head and neck of the talus, with one or two further compression screws passed dorsally from the navicular into the talus (Figure 13.6). Preoperative marking of the dorsalis pedis pulse is useful, and staying to the

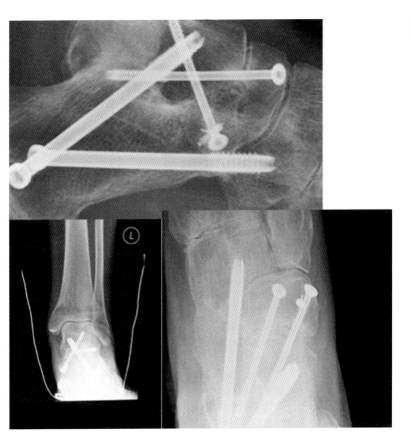

Figure 13.6 Radiographs following arthroscopic triple fusion.

medial side of the extensor hallucis longus tendon will also help avoid the artery. The calcaneocuboid joint may be fixed by passing a screw from the posterior calcaneum through to the cuboid, or using compression screws from the cuboid into the calcaneum. It is critical during surgery to expose the lower limb from the knee, to check alignment of the hindfoot in all three planes, compared to the knee and the axis of the tibia.

Talonavicular Arthrodesis

For patients in whom degenerative change is localized to the talonavicular joint, an isolated talonavicular arthrodesis may well be considered. If there is no significant bone loss arthroscopic talonavicular arthrodesis can be considered, particularly if the soft tissue envelope is poor.

A sinus tarsi approach can be used, as described for the triple and double arthrodesis, although the portals are positioned to ease access to the talonavicular joint. The sinus tarsi portals are positioned more distally and the dorsolateral talonavicular portal can be used so that decortication can be undertaken from lateral to medial. An accessory dorsomedial portal, medial to extensor hallucis longus, can be considered, particularly if dorsal osteophytes need to be removed. The dorsolateral and dorsomedial portals both risk damaging the adjacent neurological structures, and care must be taken with portal placement[17-18]. Fixation is as described above.

Tips

It is important to resect the soft tissues around the talonavicular joint and the calcaneonavicular component of the bifurcate ligament, to allow adequate visualization. Fluoroscopy can be extremely helpful, particularly during the learning curve. It helps in positioning the portals and the instruments, to ensure that decortication is complete. Optimum alignment of the hindfoot is vital to achieve the best results. Thus it is worth undertaking a trial reduction and fixation, secured with guide wires, to assess whether the talonavicular or subtalar joint is best positioned and secured first to allow optimum hindfoot position.

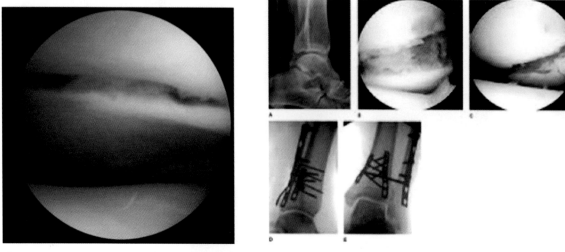

Figure 13.7 Intraoperative views of a posterior malleolar fracture, which has been openly reduced and internally fixed.

Postoperative Management

This is as for the triple fusion, although non-weightbearing is prolonged to six, as opposed to two, weeks.

Outcomes and Complications

Arthroscopic double[19] and triple arthrodesis is feasible[20-21], although it has to be borne in mind that major hindfoot fusions are salvage procedures, not reconstructions, and although marked improvement of symptoms and correction of deformity are achieved, there is often postoperative discomfort. Any muscular imbalance present, for example secondary to neurological disease, should be corrected with a tendon transfer. Complications are similar to those outlined for subtalar arthrodesis. Non-unions can be a problem in the talonavicular joint, as with open surgery, but in our arthroscopic series these have been associated with poor case selection, rather than failure of technique.

Ankle and Hindfoot Arthroscopy for Trauma

Arthroscopy of the ankle and subtalar joints can be used as a supplement to open surgical approaches to assess the degree of joint surface damage and confirm the adequacy of reduction. This is true in ankle fractures where the syndesmosis or the posterior malleolus has been displaced (Figure 13.7).

Subtalar arthroscopy in conjunction with the percutaneous treatment of calcaneal fractures may also prove a good technique, as it minimizes the soft tissue damage (Figure 13.8). Both the posterior facet of the subtalar joint and the angle of Gissane are visualized arthroscopically. Although often thought of as being at the more difficult end of arthroscopic techniques, the presence of fracture lines and displacement means that it is surprisingly easy to gain access to the joint. Care must be taken to avoid compartment syndrome by allowing the portals to be relatively "leaky." It may be that this form of direct visualization will prove to be more accurate than the use of intraoperative CT scanning.

Arthroscopy of the First Metatarsophalangeal Joint

Arthroscopy of the first metatarsophalangeal joint is used for conditions causing pain, not deformity. These are usually associated with acute or chronic injury or early hallux rigidus. Plain radiographs may show no abnormality but dorsal osteophytes may be seen. Ultrasound and MRI scanning can be used to detect osteochondral lesions, degeneration, and intra-articular meniscoid lesions.

Surgical Technique

Appropriate anesthesia is provided by a nerve block sufficiently proximally to provide muscle relaxation,

(a)

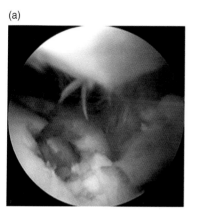

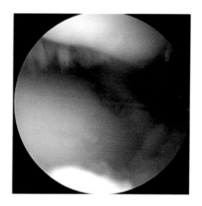

Figure 13.8 Intraoperative views of the subtalar joint, before and after reduction (**a**). The fracture was fixed percutaneously (**b**).

(b)

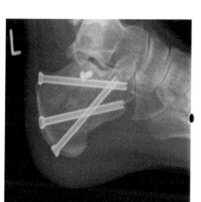

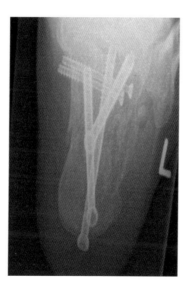

or a general anesthetic. This is to allow distraction of the joint, which can either be achieved by manual distraction or a Chinese finger trap. The adjustability of manual traction allows easier visualization of the extra-articular areas of the joint.

The joint is pre-inflated with up to 5 ml of normal saline. A 2.7 mm arthroscope can be introduced through either a dorsolateral or dorsomedial portal (Figure 13.9). These are approximately 5 mm either side of the extensor hallucis longus tendon and a couple of millimeters proximal to the joint line so that natural curve of the joint line can be entered, aiming slightly distally. The arthroscope is usually introduced into the lateral portal as this is easiest. Once the lateral portal is established the second portal is made using a needle followed by a knife and spreading an artery clip.

An additional portal can be made on the medial side of the joint to visualize the inferior part of the joint just above and distal to the medial sesamoid. This portal must be placed above the sesamoid articulation with the first metatarsal head, to avoid the digital nerve. Although smaller arthroscopes make it easier to access the joint, visualization is more difficult. The 2.9 mm resectors and burrs are also useful.

Therapeutically we find first metatarsophalangeal joint arthroscopy useful for the resection of meniscoid lesions and dorsal osteophytes. Osteochondral lesions (Figure 13.10) can be debrided and microfractured. The published results show a low level of complications and high levels of patient satisfaction.

243

Postoperatively, light dressings are used to permit gentle early movement with heel weight bearing in a wedge shoe. Physiotherapy can be used to maximize the range of movement.

Tendo Achillis

Introduction

The use of arthroscopic techniques in the treatment of the tendo Achillis remains controversial, but is certainly feasible and as such worthy of consideration and further study. There are three pathologies that potentially can be treated by arthroscopic techniques.

Insertional Tendonopathy with Haglund's Deformity

Perhaps best established is the use of arthroscopic techniques to debride a Haglund's deformity of the

posterosuperior aspect of the calcaneal tuberosity and excise the pretendinous bursa.

History and Examination

The patient presents with pain at the insertion of the tendo Achillis, with persistent swelling. Most patients will have tried non-operative treatment, which should include protracted periods of rest, anti-inflammatory medication, icing, and shoe modification. Physiotherapy can help but stretching exercises are usually ineffective. The physical findings are of swelling and local tenderness at the insertion of the tendo Achillis.

Preoperative Investigation

A standing lateral radiograph of the foot and ankle may show an increased pitch of the calcaneum and prominence of the posterior superior part of the calcaneal tuberosity, which can look relatively osteopenic. The presence of calcification in the tendon insertion should be noted, as if extensive it is a relative contraindication to the use of an arthroscopic technique, and open excision of the "enthesophyte" with detachment of the tendon will be needed.

Surgical Technique

The patient can be positioned prone using a portal on either side of the tendon. An alternative, the "bad side down position," allows general anesthesia without intubation and paralysis. This commits the surgeon to using two medial portals. These will need to be separated to improve triangulation and means one is working away from, rather than back toward, oneself. This approach can also be utilized for more proximal tendon pathology. The proximal portal is 3 to 4 cm and the distal portal 1 to 2 cm above the posterior

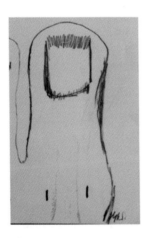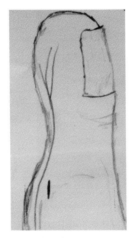

Figure 13.9 The three portals for first MTPJ arthroscopy. Two dorsal and one plantar-medial.

(a)

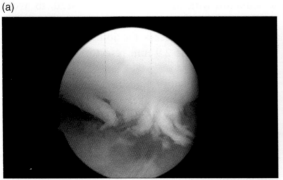

(b)

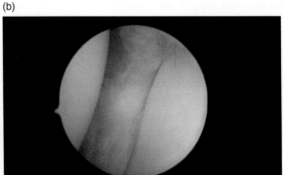

Figure 13.10 Arthroscopic view of an osteochondral lesion (**a**) in an otherwise normal (**b**) first MTPJ.

process. Prior to establishing the portals, the bursa anterior to the tendon is inflated with 5 ml of normal saline. We use a 4.5 mm arthroscope with 3.5 mm and 4.5 mm power instruments. Although one is effectively instrumenting a "virtual" space anterior to the tendo Achillis, the advantage of using the larger instruments is that they act as their own retractors. The arthroscope is introduced through the distal portal into the bursa. A soft tissue resector is then introduced through the proximal portal and is tapped against the arthroscope to identify its tip. Careful initial resection of the retrocalcaneal bursa and fat pad allows the development of a working space anterior to the tendon. The Haglund's deformity is visualized and a burr used to resect bone until no contact occurs between it and the insertion of the tendon through a full range of movement. Care must be taken to ensure that the bone on both the lateral and medial sides is resected clear of the tendon (Figure 13.11).

Postoperatively the patient is mobilized with partial weight bearing on crutches as comfort allows. In the early stages prior to wound healing and removal of sutures it is important that the patient rests and only undertakes gentle stretching exercises. Protected weight bearing is maintained for six weeks with no impact activity for three months.

Although the published results are limited, our experience is favorable. Cadaveric studies have shown that you can resect sufficient bone arthroscopically to reduce the pressure between bone and tendon.

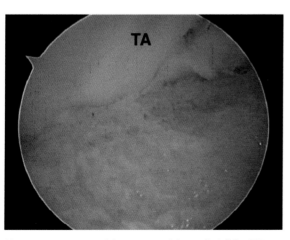

Figure 13.11 A view of the insertion of the tendo Achillis (TA) as it inserts into the calcaneum, after resection of the Haglund's deformity.

Midsubstance Tendinopathy of TA and Plantaris Syndrome

Surgery for Achilles tendinosis should be considered when the non-operative options have failed. The mechanism by which surgery works is poorly understood, with the possible exception of "plantaris syndrome." It is recognized that the plantaris is stiffer and stronger than the TA and inflammation between the two tendons can make them adhere, leading to a localized tendinopathy[22]. Broadly there is no difference between open surgery and arthroscopic surgery; the only advantage of arthroscopic over open techniques lies in their relatively low complication rate.

Preoperative Assessment

The usual presentation is tendo Achillis pain persisting despite conservative treatment with rest, anti-inflammatory medication, and physiotherapy. In plantaris syndrome the pain is localized to the medial side of the TA. On examination, the common findings are localized tenderness in the midsubstance of the tendon often associated with variable localized swelling. Occasionally when paratendinitis is present crepitus will be felt. It is common for the calf muscle complex to be tight producing reduced ankle dorsiflexion.

Investigations

Both MRI and US scanning can be used to image the tendon. Ultrasound is dynamic, making it possible to see whether the tendon is fixed by the thickening of the paratenon and to demonstrate whether the plantaris tendon is adherent to it. Ultrasound also allows visualization of the neovascularization of the tendon. A disadvantage of US scanning is the operator dependence.

Surgical Technique

The patient is positioned and anesthetized as for insertional tendinitis. We prefer to use a 4.5 mm arthroscope and large instruments. In the "bad side down position" two medial portals are established. The proximal portal is 5 to 7 cm above the posterior process of the calcaneum, with the second portal 3 to 5 cm distal to this. Prior to making the portal, the space between the tendon and skin is inflated with up to 20 ml of saline. It is sometimes possible to inject the saline within the paratenon, but care should be taken not to inject into the tendon itself.

The arthroscope is introduced into the space between the skin and tendon through the inferior portal. A soft tissue resector is then introduced through the proximal portal and the "tapping the arthroscope" technique is used to feel for the tip. Careful initial resection of soft tissue allows a working space to be developed. The paratenon can usually be identified lying on the tendon and, if present, the plantaris is seen medially. The paratenon can be stripped off the tendon with a soft tissue resector. If the plantaris is clearly stuck to the main tendon it can be simply sacrificed and resected. If the TA is significantly degenerate then it is possible to simply tease the tendon fibers apart, akin to the recognized open and closed techniques, to split the tendon longitudinally, effectively decompressing it. Once the tendon is lying freely, the wounds are simply closed with sutures and dressing applied.

The postoperative regime is as described above, although there is a greater emphasis on TA stretching exercises, particularly eccentrically.

Arthroscopic Flexor Hallucis Longus Transfer: Surgical Technique

One of the established open techniques for patients presenting with either a missed TA rupture or a re-rupture is an FHL tendon transfer. A particularly difficult therapeutic problem occurs in the older patient when the skin is of poor quality. The FHL transfer can be achieved arthroscopically, preserving the soft tissue envelope and reducing the risk of wound complications.

The patient is placed prone and standard posteromedial and posterolateral portals for subtalar arthroscopy are employed. The FHL tendon is identified and traced distally to the sustentaculum tali. The tendon is divided with arthroscopic scissors and brought back through the posteromedial portal. A whipstitch is then placed into the tendon. Through this portal, or through a more distal medial accessory portal over the calcaneum, a medial drill hole is made into the tuberosity of the calcaneum. The whipstitched suture tail is then passed from medial to lateral using a guide wire with a needle eye, and the stump of the FHL is then pulled into the drill hole. The foot is placed in equinus, and the FHL tendon is tensioned before the stump is then secured with a biotenodesis screw.

Postoperatively the patient is placed in an equinus backslab for two weeks. This is changed at two weeks to an adjustable walking boot. The patient is allowed to weight bear with the foot in at least 20° of equinus with gradually increasing load as pain allows. Over a six- to eight-week period the foot is gradually brought up to neutral. Once the foot is plantigrade the boot can be removed and the patient is encouraged to start non-weightbearing active ankle movements. The walking boot is used for weightbearing activity for a minimum of six weeks.

We believe that this technique has the same advantages as open surgery while limiting the risks of soft tissue complications. Our results have been encouraging.

Peroneal Tendons

The use of arthroscopic techniques in the treatment of peroneal tendon pathology is well established. Compared to open techniques they do not necessitate dividing the retinaculum and allow early movement. Patients typically present with pain along the line of the tendons and clicking. There is often a history of trauma. Examination shows tenderness, swelling, clicking, and snapping of the tendons. Peroneal tendon disease is often part of a cavovarus foot.

Preoperative investigation includes the use of both MRI and US scanning. We prefer to use US as it is dynamic and identifies abnormal tendon movement or subluxation. It is recognized that the tendons can partially or completely sublux over the lateral border of the lateral malleolus, or internally within the sheath, including through longitudinal splits in the other tendon. They can also be affected by bony prominences and scarring of the peroneal tunnel following trauma.

Surgical Technique

The patient is positioned in the classic lateral position or in the lazy lateral, with a large sandbag under the buttock. It is important that the foot is freely mobile. Once the patient has been prepared and draped, then the peroneal tunnel can be pre-inflated with up to 10 ml of normal saline. A 2.7 mm arthroscope with a 30° offset is used with soft tissue resectors and burrs up to 3.5 mm in diameter. Up to three portals are used, one just above the peroneal tuberosity, one at the level of the lateral malleolus, and one 3 to 4 cm proximal to the tip of the lateral malleolus. It is easiest to establish the distal portal first, visualizing the tendons from their anterior surface. The peroneus brevis lies anterior to the longus. The portal at the tip of the fibula is created by placing a needle into the peroneal tendon sheath under direct vision. A small stab incision, which is broadened by blunt dissection, is developed into a portal. The proximal portal is created in a similar manner if required.

It is possible to see and treat a variety of pathologies including post-traumatic or inflammatory synovitis, tendon tears, intrasheath subluxation of the tendons, and tethering of a tendon by a thickened vincula. In these cases it is usually possible to debride or release the tendon. With longitudinal splits, commonly of the brevis tendon, it is possible to select the smaller redundant part of the tendon and resect it. Open surgery should be considered if there is any doubt about the nature of the tear, or which is the larger or more stable segment. Similarly if the tear involves more than 50% of the tendon it maybe necessary to undertake open surgery with a tenodesis of the brevis and longus (see Chapter 11). Arthroscopic resection usually starts in the axilla of the tear and involves working along the tear until resection is complete. It is also possible to remove post-traumatic fibular exostoses and deepen the retromalleolar fibular groove in which the tendons run. Retinacular repair for true peroneal tendon instability is difficult to perform arthroscopically, but may become feasible with improvements in technology in the future.

The postoperative regime is similar for all pathologies, with weight bearing, as comfort allows, on crutches for at least two weeks, until the wounds are healed. Mobilization is then commenced.

The results of are good, with a low incidence of primary complications[23]. Effectively the portals are on an intraneural line, although the superficial peroneal nerve is at risk proximally and the sural nerve distally.

Posterior Tibial Tendon

The two major indications for tendonoscopy of the posterior tibial tendon are postfracture scarring with tethering of the tendon, and persistent inflammatory tenosynovitis. In the presence of tenosynovitis it is important to ensure that there is no progressive planovalgus deformity of the foot, as this requires reconstructive surgery. Arthroscopic surgery is only appropriate for Johnson and Strom stage I tibialis posterior tendon disease. In a more experimental form tendonoscopy has been used to guide resection of the tibialis posterior tendon at the time of reconstructive surgery, when the tendon is not exposed, for example during a triple fusion. It remains to be seen whether this is an acceptable form of treatment, or even necessary.

Surgical Technique

The patient is positioned either with a large sandbag under the contralateral side or in the "bad side down" lateral. The use of the 2.7 mm arthroscope and smaller soft tissue resectors and burrs is most satisfactory. The tendon sheath is pre-inflated with 5 to 10 ml of saline. Three portals along the line of the tendon are used, two distal to the tip of the medial malleolus and one proximal. The proximal portal is placed at a point close to the entry of the tibialis posterior into its tunnel – this is usually at a point not more than 5 cm above the tip of the medial malleolus. The distal portals are just distal to the tip of the medial malleolus at a point 2 to 3 cm short of the navicular tuberosity. It is easiest to start distally and work proximally, using the technique used for the peroneal tendons to create the more proximal portals.

Unlike the peroneal tendons it is entirely reasonable to release the tendon sheath and with synovitis a full synovectomy can be performed. Bone can be taken from behind the medial malleolus to free the tendon. The tendon should be lying freely and moving freely at the end of the procedure.

The postoperative regime is as for peroneal tendonoscopy. Again at the present reports of clinical results are limited but low complication results and satisfactory functional outcomes have been observed. Posterior tibial tendonoscopy has been shown to be effective both diagnostically and therapeutically[24–25].

Key Points
Subtalar Arthroscopy

- There are two main approaches to subtalar arthroscopy – posterior and sinus tarsi.
- The technique's indications have been expanded successfully to treat talocalcaneal coalitions, talonavicular coalitions, and to fuse the subtalar joint.

- Double and triple arthrodeses of the hindfoot can also be undertaken arthroscopically.

Tendonoscopy

- The tendo Achillis, peroneal, tibialis posterior, and FHL tendons are the principal tendons amenable to tendonoscopy in the foot and ankle.

- Arthroscopic surgery is the same as open surgery, but with reduced soft tissue damage.

- Stage I tibialis posterior tendon disease can be debrided arthroscopically.

- Plantaris syndrome and Achilles tendonosis have been successfully treated with arthroscopic surgery.

References

1. Ahn JH, Lee SK, Kim KJ, Kim YI, Choy WS. Subtalar arthroscopic procedures for the treatment of subtalar pathologic conditions: 115 consecutive cases. *Orthopedics*. 2009; 32(12):891.

2. Rozansky A, Varley E, Moor M, Wenger DR, Mubarak SJ. A radiologic classification of talocalcaneal coalitions based on 3D reconstruction. *J Child Orthop*. 2010; 4(2):129–35.

3. Lui TH. Arthroscopic resection of the calcaneonavicular coalition or the "too long" anterior process of the calcaneus. *Arthroscopy*. 2006; 22:903.

4. Singh AK, Parsons SW. Arthroscopic resection of calcaneonavicular coalition/ malunion via a modified sinus tarsi approach: an early case series. *Foot Ankle Surg*. 2012; 18:266–9.

5. Knörr J. Accadbled F, Abid A, et al. Arthroscopic treatment of calcaneonavicular coalition in children. *Orthop Traumatol Surg Res*. 2011; 97:565–8.

6. Jagodzinski NA, Hughes A, Davis NP, Butler M, Winson IG, Parsons SW. Arthroscopic resection of talocalcaneal coalitions: a bicentre case series of a new technique. *Foot Ankle Surg*. 2013; 19(2):125–30.

7. Carro LP, Golanó P, Vega J. Arthroscopic subtalar arthrodesis: the posterior approach in the prone position. *Arthroscopy*. 2007; 23(4):445.

8. Amendola A, Lee KB, Saltzman CL, Suh JS. Technique and early experience with posterior arthroscopic subtalar arthrodesis. *Foot Ankle Int*. 2007; 28(3):298–302.

9. Beimers L, de Leeuw PA, van Dijk CN. A 3-portal approach for arthroscopic subtalar arthrodesis. *Knee Surg Sports Traumatol Arthrosc*. 2009; 17(7):830–4.

10. Tasto JP. Arthroscopic subtalar arthrodesis. *Tech Foot Ankle Surg*. 2003; 2:122–8.

11. Jeavons L, Butler M, Shyam M, Parsons W. Arthroscopic subtalar fusion: results of a series of 33 isolated subtalar arthrodeses *J Bone Joint Surg Br*. 2012; 94-B Suppl XX1:139.

12. Scranton P. Comparison of open isolated subtalar arthrodesis with autogenous bone graft versus outpatient arthroscopic subtalar arthrodesis using injectable bone morphogenic protein-enhanced graft. *Foot Ankle Int*. 1999; 20(3):162–5.

13. Stroud CC. Arthroscopic arthrodesis of the ankle, subtalar, and first metatarsophalangeal joint. *Foot Ankle Clin N Am*. 2002; 7:135–46.

14. El Shazly O, Nassar W, El Badrawy A. Arthroscopic subtalar fusion for post traumatic subtalar arthritis. *Arthroscopy*. 2009; 25(7):783–7. Epub 2009 Mar 17.

15. Lee KB, Park CH, Seon JK, Kim MS. Arthroscopic subtalar arthrodesis using a posterior 2-portal approach in the prone position. *Arthroscopy*. 2010; 26(2):230–8.

16. Hughes AM, Gosling O, McKenzie J, Amirfeyz R, Winson IG. Arthroscopic triple fusion joint preparation using two lateral portals: a cadaveric study to evaluate efficacy and safety. *Foot Ankle Surg*. 2014; 20:135–9.

17. Hammond AW, Phisitkul P, Femino J, Amendola A. Arthroscopic debridement of the talonavicular joint using dorsomedial and dorsolateral portals: a cadaveric study of safety and access. *Arthroscopy*. 2011; 27(2):228–34.

18. Lui TH, Chan LK. Safety and efficacy of talonavicular arthroscopy and arthroscopic triple arthrodesis. A cadaveric study. *Knee Surg Sports Traumatol Arthrosc*. 2010; 18(5):607–11.

19. Oloff L, Schulhofer SD, Fanton G, Dillingham M. Arthroscopy of the calcaneocuboid and talonavicular joints. *J Foot Ankle Surg*. 1996; 35(2):101–8.

20. Jagodzinski NA, Parsons AMJ, Parsons SW. Arthroscopic triple and modified double hindfoot arthrodesis. *Foot Ankle Surg*. 2015; 21(2):97–102.

21. Lui TH. Arthroscopic triple arthrodesis in patients with Müller–Weiss disease. *Foot Ankle Surg*. 2009; 15(3):119–22.

22. Pearce CJ, Carmichael J, Calder JD. Achilles tendinoscopy and plantaris tendon release and division in the treatment of non-insertional Achilles tendinopathy.

Foot Ankle Surg. 2012; 18(2):124–7.

23. Kennedy JG, van Dijk PA, Murawski CD, et al. Functional outcomes after peroneal tendoscopy in the treatment of peroneal tendon disorders. *Knee Surg Sports Traumatol Arthrosc.* 2016; 24(4):1148–54.

24. Gianakos AL, Ross KA, Hannon CP, Duke GL, Prado MP, Kennedy JG. Functional outcomes of tibialis posterior tendoscopy with comparison to magnetic resonance imaging. *Foot Ankle Int.* 2015; 36(7):812–19.

25. Khazen G, Khazen C. Tendoscopy in stage I posterior tibial tendon dysfunction. *Foot Ankle Clin.* 2012; 17(3):399–406.

Heel Pain

Matthew C. Solan, Andrew Carne, and Mark S. Davies

Introduction

Heel pain is widely perceived as a minor ailment that will get better by itself. This is not always true and both plantar fasciitis and tendo Achillis (TA) problems are prevalent, affecting millions of people each year. Most sufferers will improve with a combination of time and proper stretching regimens. Nevertheless a proportion of patients suffer with resistant symptoms that can be difficult to manage and require operative treatment.

Heel pain is classified as either posterior or plantar[1]. Posterior heel pain is usually from the TA. Tendinopathy of TA is associated with sport and is an increasingly common complaint as people continue to exercise into older age[2]. Plantar heel pain is most commonly caused by plantar fasciitis. In the United States over 1 million people seek help for this pain every year[3]. The majority of cases never reach the secondary care sector. This chapter aims to outline the treatment of these two causes of heel pain.

General Management of Heel Pain

Clinical History

Pain, especially with the first steps in the morning or after a period of rest, is the main symptom. Most patients report that the pain improves after an initial period of painful stiffness, but that after prolonged standing (plantar fasciitis) or after exercise (TA) the symptoms return. Inability to walk long distances and reduced exercise and sports participation are also common complaints.

There may be no distinct injury preceding the symptoms, but there is frequently an alteration in activity levels, new sports shoes, increase in body weight, including pregnancy, or alteration in working patterns requiring longer periods of standing. In chronic cases the nature of the pain and its radiation is important. Plantar heel pain radiating to the arch of the foot may indicate disease in the more distal plantar fascia but, especially if associated with tingling or numbness, can indicate a neurological cause.

The duration of symptoms should be noted as so many cases run a self-limiting course and little active intervention is needed for uncomplicated cases of recent onset. Conversely chronic cases, particularly when proper first-line treatments have been tried and failed, need more help. There is increasing awareness of the association between adverse biomechanics, particularly isolated gastrocnemius tightness, and heel pain. Specific enquiry regarding symptoms of other conditions associated with gastrocnemius tightness should be part of the history. Conditions associated with gastrocnemius tightness include posteromedial pain and swelling from the tibialis posterior tendon with an acquired flat foot, previous medial gastrocnemius calf muscle tear (tennis leg), forefoot overload, hallux valgus, difficulty wearing flat shoes, and calf cramps.

Examination

In moderate or severe cases the patient limps into the clinic. In chronic cases in non-athletes there is a strong association with raised body mass index. Planovalgus foot posture is more common than "normal," reflecting the association of heel pain with calf contracture, but a cavus foot with increased calcaneal pitch may also be associated with plantar fascia pain. Similarly forefoot ground clearance may be reduced and Silfverskiöld's test should be performed once the patient is seated to confirm and quantify the gastrocnemius contracture. Pulses and sensation are checked. If symptoms suggest an atypical cause for the pain then full lumbar spine and neurological assessment is needed, particularly looking for signs of lumbar radiculopathy. Tarsal tunnel syndrome is very rare, but a Tinel's test over the tibial nerve, lying just behind the medial malleolus, should still be recorded. The calcaneal squeeze test where the heel is squeezed between the thenar eminences of both hands is often weakly positive in long-standing cases of plantar fasciitis, but if the heel is very tender this may indicate a calcaneal stress fracture.

Local examination of the plantar fascia is conveniently performed with the patient sitting on a high couch with their legs dangling over the side, facing the examiner who is seated in a lower chair. In plantar fasciitis tenderness is usually maximal at the medial calcaneal tuberosity on the plantar aspect of the foot. Posterior tenderness may seem "plantar" when it is in fact from insertional Achilles tendinopathy. Central plantar tenderness may indicate traumatic or iatrogenic fat pad atrophy as a result of steroid injections or, rarely, a bursa. It is important to palpate along the non-insertional plantar fascia as it extends into the medial longitudinal arch, because tenderness or lumps in this part of the plantar fascia may merit different treatment strategies. Plantar fibromata are best managed with relief orthotics because the rate of complications after attempted excision is devastatingly high. Midfoot arthrosis occasionally presents as plantar arch pain.

The TA and its insertion may be examined with the clinician and patient sitting as described above, but it is also convenient to ask the patient to kneel on a chair (as one would to perform Simmonds' test for an TA rupture). This affords a better view of the heel and allows accurate palpation of the tendon from the musculo-tendinous junction to the insertion.

It is important to distinguish between disease of the main body (non-insertional) and insertional part of the TA, as the treatment of the two areas differs. Tendinopathy of the main body of the tendon is associated with tenderness and swelling, which may be discrete or involve a long section of the tendon. Tenderness and swelling that remains in the same location when the ankle is put through a full range of dorsiflexion and plantar flexion is due to inflammation of the paratenon rather than the tendon itself. Paratendinitis is relatively uncommon. This clinical sign is sometimes known as the Royal London Hospital test. Other soft tissue swellings may present around the TA and may be benign or very rarely malignant.

The insertion of the TA is relatively complex in anatomical terms (Figure 14.1). Pathology here may be seen in the retrocalcaneal bursa, superficial bursa, bursal projection, or the insertion of the TA itself. It is in fact usually a combination of these structures, but if tenderness is marked to the medial or lateral sides of the tendon then retrocalcaneal bursitis most likely predominates. Distinct midline tenderness is more indicative of calcific tendinopathy. A sports person will occasionally present with tenderness at the widest reaches of the tendon's expansion due to a small avulsion injury.

Classification

After clinical and radiological assessment it should be possible to accurately classify the nature of the

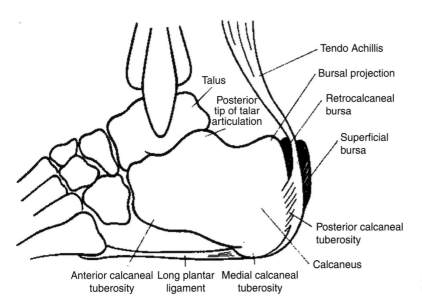

Figure 14.1 Posterior heel anatomy. (From Stephens, with permission)

251

Table 14.1 Guildford classification of heel pain

1. Posterior heel pain

    a. Tendinopathy of the main body of the tendo Achillis
    b. Insertional tendinopathy

2. Plantar heel pain

    a. Plantar fasciopathy of the calcaneal insertion
    b. Atypical fasciopathy (distal/fibroma)

Table 14.2 A suggested pathway for management of heel pain. The figures represent the percentage of patients who might be expected to recover at each step

1. Less than three months	Home stretches	80%
2. More than three months	Physio eccentric stretches	80%
3. More than six months	Heel pain clinic Biomechanics Images	80%

problem (Table 14.1). As in all fields of medicine, a precise diagnosis allows targeted treatment and should lead to improved results.

Logistics

The self-limiting nature of the symptoms in the majority of cases, and the need for the prudent use of healthcare resources, means that it is appropriate to triage patients presenting with heel pain. The protocol outlined in Table 14.2 is practical, rather than scientific, but in the authors' opinion steers a sensible path between masterful inactivity and overinvestigation. Using this protocol only 4% of those patients who seek medical attention will ever require assessment in secondary care. The majority of the discussion below will focus on this group.

Less Than Three Months of Symptoms

Patients presenting to primary care with heel pain of relatively recent onset can reasonably be expected to improve with simple "home stretches," time, and activity modification. Stretches should focus in the calf muscle. Lowering the heel over the edge of a step is a simple stretch that patients can easily understand.

A gel heel cushion can be helpful for plantar heel pain. It is important that the patient understands that it is necessary to perform the stretches regularly. Failure to improve should prompt referral for physiotherapy.

More Than Three Months of Symptoms

If symptoms persist then physiotherapy is indicated, and very likely to help. Formal calf stretching programs are widely considered to be the best first-line treatment for both plantar fasciitis and non-insertional achilles tendinopathy[11,22]. The TA even recovers its normal structure after eccentric stretching[4]. With plantar fasciitis there are further benefits from stretches targeting the fascia itself[5-6]. We believe that treatments in primary care should focus upon, and be restricted to, these stretches. There is little or no evidence for acupuncture, orthoses, or steroid injection.

More Than Six Months of Symptoms

Optimum management of stubborn cases of both plantar fascia pain and disorders of the TA requires a thorough clinical assessment and appropriate radiological investigation. Many patients have suffered for years while trying to relieve their symptoms. Multiple interventions have usually been tried without success. Our heel pain clinic is devoted to the investigation and treatment of these recalcitrant plantar fascia and TA problems. Patients are assessed and most commonly investigated by US scan, with color-Doppler capability. A critical part of the clinical examination is assessment of the calf muscle tension. There is a strong association between isolated tightness of the gastrocnemius and complaints of plantar fasciitis or TA pain. We believe that local treatments for heel pain are much less likely to be of benefit in the face of the adverse biomechanics consequent upon gastrocnemius tightness. Initial emphasis is therefore placed upon correcting this. Physiotherapy treatment is prescribed, but a proportion of cases are subsequently offered surgical gastrocnemius lengthening (Figure 14.2).

After clinical and US assessment, patients can be divided into groups on the basis of their biomechanical profile and the exact nature of their tendinopathy or fasciopathy. Treatment can be tailored accordingly.

Those who do not exhibit tight gastrocnemius, or remain symptomatic after gastrocnemius release, are candidates for local therapy (Table 14.3).

Table 14.3 Local treatments for heel pain

Plantar fasciopathy	
Insertional	ESWT
Non-insertional	ESWT or injection prolotherapy
Tendo Achillis (main body)	
Neovascularity on USS	Injection prolotherapy
No neovascularity	ESWT
Tendo Achillis (insertion)	
Retrocalcaneal bursitis	USS-guided cortisone injection
Tendinopathy	ESWT or injection prolotherapy

ESWT: extra-corporeal shockwave therapy; USS: ultrasound scanning.

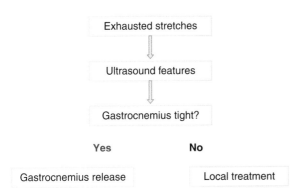

Figure 14.2 Gastrocnemius shortening is a malign influence and sometimes requires operative correction.

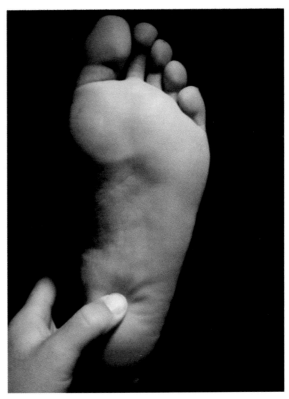

Figure 14.3 Tenderness at the medial calcaneal tuberosity.

Plantar Fasciopathy

Heel pain is common[7–8]. Pain, especially after a period of rest or with the first steps of the morning, is characteristic. Other complaints include difficulty standing for long periods, reduced ability to walk long distances, and an inability to play sport or run. Plantar heel pain is most commonly caused by plantar "fasciitis." This term implies acute inflammation and is therefore something of a misnomer. We prefer the term plantar fasciopathy, which is consistent with the current nomenclature used for disorders of the TA.

Examination

Patients with recalcitrant plantar fasciopathy are nearly always either sedentary and overweight, often with a very high body mass index, or, conversely, very athletic.

An assessment of the overall foot shape, when standing, is important. There is a strong association between planovalgus foot posture, gastrocnemius contracture, and heel pain. Hallux valgus or hallux rigidus impair the function of the medial column of the foot and should be noted. Careful examination of the whole plantar fascia is imperative. The site of maximal tenderness is most commonly at the medial calcaneal tuberosity (Figure 14.3). Any tenderness more distally in the fascia is particularly relevant. Pulses and sensation should be documented, paying particular attention to the presence of altered sensation or a positive Tinel's sign behind the medial malleolus, as this raises the possibility of a diagnosis of tarsal tunnel syndrome. The calcaneum is squeezed between the examiner's two hands; tenderness may indicate a calcaneal stress fracture, but the squeeze is often mildly tender in patients who have had plantar fascia pain for months or years. Calcaneal stress fracture is commoner in running athletes who have increased their training or in older female patients.

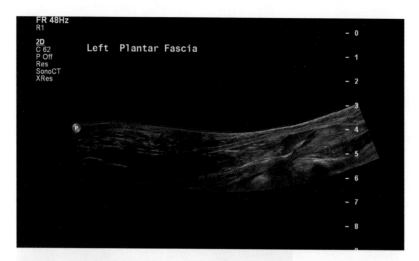

Figure 14.4 Ultrasound scan of plantar fascia.

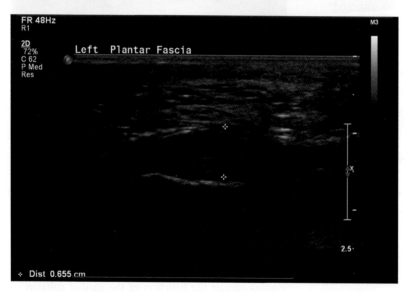

Figure 14.5 Thickening of the calcaneal insertion of the plantar fascia.

Imaging

Plantar fasciopathy is not routinely imaged and treatment is started empirically. Recalcitrant cases benefit from investigation when first-line treatments have failed. A plain lateral weightbearing radiograph of the foot and ankle allows assessment of foot shape and may show: a healing calcaneal stress fracture; erosions to suggest inflammatory arthropathy; and a plantar heel spur, which confuses both the patient and many practitioners – as it can be absent in the presence of disease, or present in the absence of disease!

We use USS as our primary imaging modality for all recalcitrant cases (Figure 14.4). Experience with this has led to an improved ability to distinguish between plantar fasciopathy affecting the insertion of the fascia at the os calcis, and patients with "atypical" findings.

A cohort of patients was followed prospectively with USS, and the scans were reviewed noting the characteristics of their plantar fascia disease.

This study included 125 feet, in 120 patients[9]. Sixty-six percent had only "typical insertional" pathology on USS (Figure 14.5). The remaining 34% had "atypical distal fascia disease" or a combination of insertional and distal disease. Patients with distal disease had either distal thickening or, occasionally, discrete fibromata.

The proportion of atypical, non-insertional disease was higher than expected and indicates that USS is valuable both for determining location and characterizing the nature of pathology in the plantar fascia. Atypical cases are harder to treat and so the information is useful when counseling patients and deciding about management options.

We advocate the classification of plantar heel problems into insertional fasciopathy or non-insertional fasciopathy. This mirrors the current classification of Achilles tendinopathy, and it is important to remember that the treatment of insertional disease is more predictable than that of non-insertional fasciopathy.

Empirical treatment is not adequate for recalcitrant cases of plantar fasciopathy and we advocate USS to confirm the clinical picture and classify the pathology.

Treatment

There are many different treatments that are used for plantar fasciopathy. The evidence for most is weak[7–8]. Formal calf stretching with additional stretches for the plantar fascia is the best first-line treatment[5–6]. The mechanism by which these stretches help is not well established[10]. Calf contracture is associated with a variety of clinical problems in the foot and ankle[11–12]. There is also laboratory evidence that increased plantar fascia strain is seen with increased calf muscle tension[13]. Many patients who have already "had physiotherapy" or "done stretches" have, on close questioning, either not performed the stretches properly or, more commonly, have not been sufficiently diligent with the program. Even after months or years of symptoms we advocate further intensive stretching efforts, including plantar fascia stretches and gastrocnemius-specific calf stretches. Night splints are a useful adjunct to the stretching program but may not be well tolerated.

For many years steroid injections have been used to alleviate pain from plantar fasciitis. Currently many orthopedic foot and ankle surgeons recommend that this is done under image guidance. The imaging modality can be fluoroscopy, sometimes under anesthetic as a day-case procedure, or alternatively under US guidance as an outpatient. Anecdotal experience is that this is a satisfactory treatment. However, a recent published randomized controlled trial showed no benefit of steroid over placebo after one month[14]. It is important to remember that cortisone injections are not free from side effects – thinning of the plantar fat pad and rupture of the plantar fascia can be particularly difficult to treat as there is

no answer to the chronic pain that both these problems can cause.

Extra-corporeal shockwave therapy (ESWT) is a non-invasive treatment that administers pulsed, radial waves of energy that penetrate body tissues. Originally it was used to break up kidney stones. Lower energy ESWT has been used to treat calcific tendinitis of the shoulder, tennis elbow, plantar fasciitis, and both insertional and non-insertional tendinopathy of TA. There have been several modifications of the technology and this has led to confusion within the literature regarding the effectiveness of ESWT in treating musculoskeletal complaints.

The few well-designed studies that do exist have shown that radial ESWT is effective in the management of tendinopathy of TA and plantar fasciitis[15–17].

The UK's National Institute for Care and Health Excellence (NICE) has reviewed the available evidence for the use of shockwave therapy in plantar fasciitis and tendinopathy of TA. Their recommendation is that further high-quality research is needed.

Our experience has been favorable when using ESWT for the treatment of plantar fasciopathy affecting the insertion of the fascia onto the calcaneum. However, in the face of persistent biomechanical imbalance – contracture of the gastrocnemius – there is a much lower success rate. Patients who have gastrocnemius shortening are likely to fail to improve with ESWT, and yet the same patients are greatly improved after surgical gastrocnemius release. For this reason we advocate that gastrocnemius contracture that persists in spite of three months of proper stretching, ideally supervised by specialist physiotherapists, is treated surgically before considering the use of ESWT.

Non-insertional or atypical plantar fasciopathy is difficult to manage. ESWT does help a proportion of cases, usually when the USS demonstrates a short segment of fusiform swelling. More widespread abnormalities or discrete fibromata are probably best served with the provision of a relief orthotic.

What about the patient for whom all this still proves ineffective? Firstly, it is important to reconsider the diagnosis. There are very rare distal entrapment syndromes of the tibial nerve or its plantar branches[18]. More proximally an accessory soleus muscle may be responsible for plantar heel pain, which is usually exercise related, by exerting a mass effect upon the neurovascular bundle. Tarsometatarsal arthritis can also masquerade as arch pain with plantar tenderness located over the main body of the plantar fascia in the midfoot.

If the plantar fascia does still seem to be the cause of the pain then Topaz (radiofrequency needle ablation) treatment can be considered, and may be performed under tibial nerve block or general anesthesia. There are few published series[19] and although sometimes beneficial the results in our experience are unpredictable.

When all conservative measures fail, surgical release of the plantar fascia has traditionally been performed, sometimes in combination with release of the first branch of the lateral plantar nerve[20]. Success rates as high as 90% have been reported in the literature[20-21], but there are risks of plantar fascia rupture, plantar nerve injury, wound complications, and lateral column pain. In one study of 47 heels undergoing a plantar fascia release only 48% of patients were satisfied[22]. In light of the uncertain results and significant complications surgical plantar fasciotomy is not a treatment that we recommend.

Tendinopathy of Tendo Achillis

Posterior heel pain not arising from the TA is rare. Tendo Achillis pain was classified by Clain and Baxter as being either from the insertional or from the non-insertional portion of the tendon[23]. This division is helpful clinically as the management of the two different tendinopathies is very different.

Non-insertional TA pathology is much commoner than the insertional variety. As with tendinopathies elsewhere (knee, shoulder, elbow, and hip) there is degeneration within the substance of the tendon, thickening of the paratenon, and sometimes both. Modern research emphasizes that the changes seen in cases of tendinopathy are attributable to a "failed healing response," rather than an acute inflammatory process.

Terminology

Maffulli proposed a logical system (Table 14.4) for describing TA pathologies. This reduced the use of the many terms that have confused the literature. The triad of pain, swelling, and impaired function is best referred to as tendinopathy of TA[24]. The pathology seen in chronic tendinopathy is of necrosis and mucoid degeneration. There is no inflammatory response and granulation tissue is rarely seen histologically. Thus the term tendinitis should be abandoned[25].

Table 14.4 Terminology of tendo Achillis pain

Clinical

1. Tendinopathy – pain, swelling, and impaired function
2. Paratenonopathy – affects the paratenon clinically
3. Pantendinopathy – affects both tendon and paratenon clinically

Histological

1. Tendinosis – mucoid degeneration and collagen disorganization
2. Paratenonitis – hyperemia and inflammatory cells; fibrosis and thickening; more common in younger patients

Demographics

Although tendinopathy of TA is known to be common, reliable epidemiological data are not available[26]. The association with sports and athletic training suggests that overuse is the principal cause. Age also plays a role. Young athletes have a lower incidence of TA pain than older individuals participating in the same sport. Tendo Achillis pain is also seen in sedentary individuals[39]. Older athletes have a higher prevalence of insertional tendinopathy than their younger counterparts[27]. Symptomatic non-insertional tendinopathy is four times more prevalent than symptomatic insertional tendinopathy.

Examination

Overpronation of the foot with excessive heel valgus, a low medial longitudinal arch, and forefoot varus causes secondary TA injury[28]. Patients with a plano-valgus foot posture also invariably have an adaptive shortening of the gastrocnemius, demonstrable by Silfverskiöld's test. This test must be performed with the forefoot held in a position to ensure reduction of the talonavicular joint. If the talonavicular joint is not reduced then false negative findings occur, as the heel escapes into valgus, masking the gastrocnemius contracture by shortening the distance between the knee and heel[29].

Anatomy

The TA inserts onto the middle third of the posterior surface of the os calcis. Insertion into the bone comprises zones of transitional tissues: tendon, fibrocartilage, mineralized fibrocartilage, and, finally, bone. This arrangement is considered to afford a means of force dissipation. Immediately proximal to the insertion the tendon is closely related to the bone and the bone's surface is covered by fibrocartilage. The retrocalcaneal bursa lies in the potential space between the tendon and calcaneus. It is normally small. Between the distal TA and the skin there is another bursa called the superficial bursa (Figure 14.1).

Insertional Tendinopathy

A large postero-superior margin of the calcaneal tuberosity is called the bursal projection, or Haglund's deformity[30-31]. This bony protuberance can impinge against the anterior surface of the tendon and give rise to retrocalcaneal bursitis or degenerative changes in the tendon itself. A separate pathology is seen where calcification arises within the central portion of the tendon. A spur (enthesophyte) may be seen arising from the middle third of the calcaneus on a lateral radiograph.

If the insertion of the tendon is tendinopathic, or there is an enthesophyte then tenderness is maximal in the center of the insertion. In cases where there is swelling, most commonly just anterior to the lateral edge of the tendon, and the maximal tenderness is not midline, then inflammation within the retrocalcaneal bursa is the likely cause. Retrocalcaneal bursitis is well demonstrated on MRI or US scan.

It is important to recognize that many patients with insertional TA pain have a mixture of pathologies, although one may predominate.

Non-Insertional Tendinopathy

In non-insertional tendinopathy, the main body of the TA is thickened and tender a few centimeters proximal to the insertion of the tendon into the calcaneum (Figure 14.6). The focal area of tendinosis will move proximal to distal as the ankle, and by implication the tendon, is put through a range of movement from dorsiflexion to plantar flexion. In the rare cases of true paratendinopathy the tenderness does not move with movement of the ankle, as the paratenon does not move. This is known as the "Royal London test."

Imaging

Routine standing plain x-rays allow assessment of the overall foot shape. A lateral weightbearing view of the foot and ankle may show posterior enthesophytes,

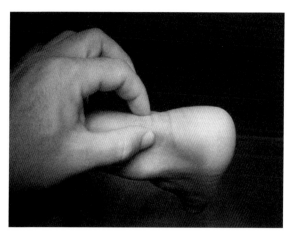

Figure 14.6 Non-insertional TA palpation.

a prominent calcaneal tuberosity, and an increased calcaneal pitch.

It is worth remembering that calcification at the insertion of the TA is easily missed on an MRI scan. A plain radiograph is much more revealing, and radiographs should be obtained before obtaining MRI scans, which are expensive. If operative resection is considered, then a CT scan helps to define the medial–lateral extent of the enthesophyte, which is useful for planning.

Anteroposterior weightbearing views of both feet, and an oblique view to supplement the weightbearing lateral film, are useful when assessing the degree of planovalgus deformity (dorsolateral peritalar subluxation). With cavus posture a weightbearing AP and mortise views of the ankle should also be obtained.

In tendinopathy of TA our initial choice of imaging is USS, which provides useful information about the tendon, insertion, and bursae[32]. Although there is no permanent image that the treating surgeon can later refer to, this is less important if the surgeon and radiologist are present together at the time of the scan. The advantages of USS include a dynamic assessment with Doppler capability (Figure 14.7) to determine the extent of neovascularity. Ultrasound scanning also provides the option of proceeding directly to injection treatment.

Treatment of Non-Insertional Tendinopathy

Accurate assessment to identify the source of the pain guides treatment. Non-operative treatment is preferred initially. Stretching regimens for non-insertional tendinopathy are extremely effective, with

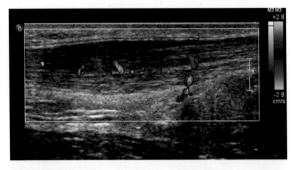

Figure 14.7 Neovascularity of the main body of the tendo Achillis.

up to 90% of patients responding when the stretches are performed properly[33]. Achieving this level of compliance is not easy. If the hamstrings are tight with a large popliteal angle then stretches of this muscle group should be added to the regimen[34].

Steroid injection is avoided for non-insertional tendinopathy because of the risk of tendon rupture. Cases of non-insertional tendinopathy associated with neovascularization. and hypervascularity on the anterior surface of the tendon respond well to sclerosant injection treatment, sometimes called injection prolotherapy. However, the amount of evidence in the literature to support this and, for that matter, other injection treatments is limited[35–36]. Another option is the use of a high-volume injection to non-operatively strip the anterior paratenon away from the tendon, again disrupting the neovascular infiltration[37].

Injection prolotherapy or high-volume injection is less useful in cases where there is no notable neovascularity on Doppler USS. In these cases we recommend ESWT. Stretching exercises are continued throughout the course of therapy.

If symptoms are not improved with these modalities then surgical debridement of the tendon is offered. Such is the success of the less invasive modalities that this is not performed as frequently now as it was a decade ago. If the tendinopathy is severe and resistant to all these treatments then excision of the tendon and reconstruction using FHL is a good salvage procedure[38–39]. We advise excising the native TA, as its retention can cause residual pain.

Treatment of Insertional Tendinopathy

Insertional tendinopathy is more difficult to treat non-operatively and stretches often exacerbate symptoms, rather than reducing symptoms. The results of

stretching programs in cases of insertional tendinopathy show that only one-third of patients respond[33]. Shockwave therapy for calcific tendinopathy is very painful and poorly tolerated. Once there is a moderate or large enthesophyte then the efficacy of shockwave therapy is poor. Retrocalcaneal bursitis improves with targeted injection of steroid but recurrence is frequent. Steroid injection into the superficial bursa is not recommended, because of the risk of skin atrophy at a potentially sensitive site. Recalcitrant cases do well with surgery but the recovery period is lengthy[1].

Retrocalcaneal endoscopy and debridement is good for dealing with retrocalcaneal bursitis and bony prominence of the tuberosity, but does not address the insertional spur or tendinopathy of the distal tendon. An open procedure through a para-median incision to remove the "Haglund" and bursitis affords a better opportunity to debride the tendon, but still does not address the enthesophyte. A midline posterior approach through the tendon allows the enthesophyte to be removed as well as the bursa and posterior prominence of the tuberosity, but there is a risk of inadvertent tendon detachment and this dictates a slower rehabilitation[1]. Suture anchors and newer devices for reattachment of the TA allow greater confidence in reattaching the tendon and so formal deliberate detachment for aggressive debridement of bone and tendon does not always require FHL transfer to reconstruct the tendon. Closing wedge osteotomy of the os calcis is reported to improve pain. There is currently no consensus on the best form of operative treatment for insertional tendinopathy of TA.

Gastrocnemius Lengthening for Recalcitrant Heel Pain

DiGiovanni, in what might be considered a landmark paper[11], noted plantar fascia and TA pathologies are among the conditions that are associated with isolated gastrocnemius contracture. The best published evidence for the association between plantar fasciopathy and contracture of the gastrocnemius is the recent paper by Patel et al.[40]. They prospectively reviewed 254 patients with plantar fasciopathy. They stratified the groups into acute and chronic, choosing nine months as the cut-off. Eighty-three percent of patients had reduced ankle dorsiflexion. Fifty-seven percent had an isolated contracture of the gastrocnemius, 26% had a contracture of the whole gastrocnemius–soleus complex, and 17% had no limit of dorsiflexion.

The authors concluded that limited ankle dorsiflexion is strongly associated with plantar fasciopathy.

Where surgery is considered for the treatment of a calf contracture it is essential that the chosen technique is appropriate to the type of contracture. Silfverskiöld's test[41] will allow the surgeon to determine whether the contracture is in both the gastrocnemius and the soleus, or confined to the gastrocnemius portion of the triceps surae.

Cadaver studies have shown that the degree by which forefoot pressures increase is similar whether contracture is from the whole triceps or just the gastrocnemius[42]. Surgical release of the TA is associated with a risk of weakness due to overlengthening. There is also a lengthy rehabilitation period. For these reasons, when Silfverskiöld's test confirms that the contracture is confined to the gastrocnemius, release of just the gastrocnemius portion of the calf may be preferred[42].

Gastrocnemius Lengthening Surgery

The pioneering work on gastrocnemius release was carried out by Vulpius and Stoffel[43], Silfverskiöld[41], and Strayer[44]. Classification of the anatomic level of the gastrocnemius–soleus complex where the release is performed (Figure 14.8) is helpful in understanding the surgical options[45]. We recommend the proximal medial gastrocnemius release described by Barouk. If the contracture is severe then the more powerful

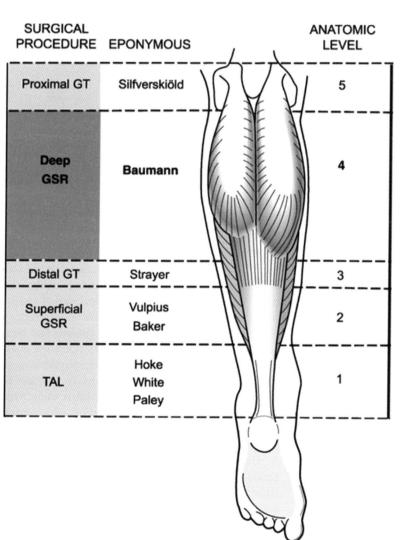

Figure 14.8 Levels of surgical lengthening.

SURGICAL PROCEDURE	EPONYMOUS	ANATOMIC LEVEL
Proximal GT	Silfverskiöld	5
Deep GSR	Baumann	4
Distal GT	Strayer	3
Superficial GSR	Vulpius Baker	2
TAL	Hoke White Paley	1

Strayer release is preferred even though recovery is longer and requires cast or boot immobilization. There are currently no reliable methods for measuring the degree of gastrocnemius tightness.

Strayer described a release of the gastrocnemius at the insertion onto the TA (level three)[44]. He allowed the gastrocnemius to retract and reattached the muscle more proximally. This places the sural nerve at risk. The sural nerve can be superficial, deep, or closely applied to the fascia at the level of a Strayer release[46]. After surgery the patient is immobilized in a cast or boot for a period of at least two weeks[47–48]. This is another disadvantage of a surgical release at this level. There is an overall 6% complication rate of the Strayer release, with 5% of patients complaining of poor wound cosmesis, and 3% of patients of nerve damage.

The Strayer release has also been described as an endoscopic procedure[49]. The sural nerve remains at risk[49], with neurapraxia reported in three of 18 patients in one series[50]. The aponeurosis at this level is a thick structure and there are reports of difficulties using the shaver to release it completely. In a cadaver study half of the specimens were not fully released[49].

Level four is the ideal level to perform an isolated release of the gastrocnemius. The lengthening is restricted to the tight gastrocnemius aponeurosis. There is no damage to either the insertion or the origin of the muscle, and the risk of neurological complication is extremely low. Barouk[51] reported a simple and safe level four gastrocnemius release (Figure 14.9). As the medial head has been found to be the source of most of the gastrocnemius tightness[52–53], release of the aponeurosis of the medial head in isolation is sufficient. This procedure is safe and in adults can be performed under local anesthetic and sedation. Postoperatively patients mobilize immediately without a protective plaster. The wound heals very well with none of the complications seen with the Strayer release[54–55].

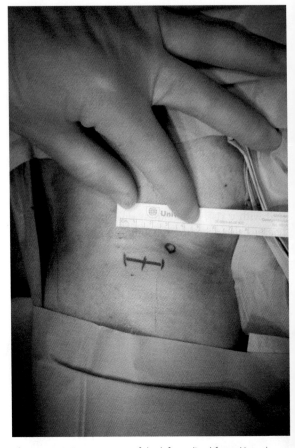

Figure 14.9 Posterior view of the left popliteal fossa. Note the central incision.

Results of Gastrocnemius Lengthening
Plantar Foot Pain

Maskil et al. reported on surgical release of the gastrocnemius at the musculotendinous junction[56] for a cohort of patients all of whom had "foot pain with no structural abnormality." Thirty-eight patients were followed up with good results. As well as "plantar fasciitis" (n = 25) there were cases of "metatarsalgia"

and "arch pain." It is not clear whether the diagnoses were purely clinical or whether the plantar fasciitis was confirmed with imaging. Abbassian et al.[57] reported the results of proximal medial gastrocnemius release in a cohort of patients with refractory plantar fasciitis. Before surgery the patients had been treated with at least one year of non-operative treatment. Treatment included orthoses, physiotherapy, and, in some cases, steroid injections. In addition to their previous physiotherapy, all patients underwent at least a further three-month period of eccentric stretching, as popularized by Alfredson[58], under the supervision of a specialist physiotherapist.

Unlike patients in previous studies, all of these patients had a radiological as well as a clinical diagnosis of plantar fasciitis. Imaging included radioisotope bone scan, MRI, or USS.

At an average of 24 months (range of 8 to 36 months) after surgery, 17 of the 21 heels (81%) reported total or significant pain relief. Fifteen patients (88%) would recommend this operation to a friend. There were no major complications. One minor wound complication occurred, which resolved without intervention.

Gastrocnemius Lengthening for Tendinopathy of TA

The literature regarding gastrocnemius lengthening for the treatment of TA pain is even more limited than that for plantar fasciopathy. There is a published case report of tendinopathy of TA, which was treated by gastrocnemius lengthening[59] producing a good result. A small series of patients who were treated by midcalf lengthening also enjoyed good results[60].

Gurdezi et al. reviewed eleven patients (five female, six male) who had a total of fifteen proximal medial head of gastrocnemius releases. Four patients required further surgery (one release of the lateral head; three tendon debridements, one of which required a supplementary FHL transfer). Despite these additional procedures, the patient group reported that the gastrocnemius surgery was helpful.

The improvement in ankle dorsiflexion was maintained at one year and there was no subjective or objective muscle weakness.

Key Points

- Recalcitrant heel pain does not receive the attention it deserves.
- Proper management requires clinical and radiological assessment.
- Ultrasound has an important role in the diagnosis and treatment of both TA and plantar fasciopathy.
- Accurate diagnosis guides treatment.
- Local treatments are less effective in the presence of adverse biomechanical features, most notably shortening of the gastrocnemius.
- Gastrocnemius tightness should be addressed, surgically if necessary, before considering local treatment of the heel.
- No advanced treatments should be instituted until first-line stretches have been properly performed for six months.
- Frequently, insufficient compliance is a cause of failure of stretching to resolve symptoms.

References

1. Solan M, Davies M. Management of insertional tendinopathy of the Achilles tendon. *Foot Ankle Clin.* 2007; 12(4):597–615.

2. Jarvinen TA, Kannus P, Maffulli N, Khan KM. Achilles tendon disorders: etiology and epidemiology. *Foot Ankle Clin.* 2005; 10(2):255–66.

3. Riddle DL, Schappert SM. Volume of ambulatory care visits and patterns of care for patients diagnosed with plantar fasciitis: a national study of medical doctors. *Foot Ankle Int.* 2004; 25(5):303–10.

4. Ohberg L, Lorentzon R, Alfredson H. Eccentric training in patients with chronic Achilles tendinosis: normalised tendon structure and decreased thickness at follow up. *Br J Sports Med.* 2004; 38(1):8–11.

5. DiGiovanni BF, Nawoczenski DA, Lintal ME, et al. Tissue-specific plantar fascia-stretching exercise

enhances outcomes in patients with chronic heel pain. A prospective, randomized study. *J Bone Joint Surg.* 2003; 85-A(7):1270–7.

6. Digiovanni BF, Nawoczenski DA, Malay DP, et al. Plantar fascia-specific stretching exercise improves outcomes in patients with chronic plantar fasciitis. a prospective clinical trial with two-year follow-up. *J Bone Joint Surg.* 2006; 88(8):1775–81.

7. Crawford F. Plantar heel pain and fasciitis. *Clin Evid.* 2003; 10:1431–43.

8. Hennessy MS, Molloy AP, Sturdee SW. Noninsertional Achilles tendinopathy. *Foot Ankle Clin.* 2007; 12(4):617–41.

9. Ieong E, Afolayan J, Carne A, Solan M. Ultrasound scanning for recalcitrant plantar fasciopathy. Basis of a new classification. *Skeletal Radiol.* 2013; 42(3):393–8.

10. Knobloch K, Kraemer R, Lichtenberg A, et al. Achilles tendon and paratendon microcirculation in midportion and insertional tendinopathy in athletes. *Am J Sports Med.* 2006; 34(1):92–7.

11. DiGiovanni CW, Kuo R, Tejwani N, et al. Isolated gastrocnemius tightness. *J Bone Joint Surg.* 2002; 84-A(6):962–70.

12. DiGiovanni CW, Langer P. The role of isolated gastrocnemius and combined Achilles contractures in the flatfoot. *Foot Ankle Clin.* 2007; 12(2):363–79.

13. Carlson RE, Fleming LL, Hutton WC. The biomechanical relationship between the tendoachilles, plantar fascia and metatarsophalangeal joint dorsiflexion angle. *Foot Ankle Int.* 2000; 21(1):18–25.

14. McMillan AM, Landorf KB, Gilheany MF, Bird AR, Morrow AD, Menz HB. Ultrasound guided

corticosteroid injection for plantar fasciitis: randomised controlled trial. *BMJ*. 2012; 344:e3260.

15. Gerdesmeyer L, Frey C, Vester J, et al. Radial extracorporeal shock wave therapy is safe and effective in the treatment of chronic recalcitrant plantar fasciitis: results of a confirmatory randomized placebo-controlled multicenter study. *Am J Sports Med*. 2008; 36(11):2100–9.

16. Rompe JD, Furia J, Maffulli N. Eccentric loading compared with shock wave treatment for chronic insertional Achilles tendinopathy. A randomized, controlled trial. *J Bone Joint Surg*. 2008; 90(1):52–61.

17. Rompe JD, Furia J, Maffulli N. Eccentric loading versus eccentric loading plus shock-wave treatment for midportion Achilles tendinopathy: a randomized controlled trial. *Am J Sports Med*. 2009; 37(3):463–70.

18. Donovan A, Rosenberg ZS, Cavalcanti CF. MR imaging of entrapment neuropathies of the lower extremity. Part 2. The knee, leg, ankle, and foot. *Radiographics*. 2010; 30(4):1001–19.

19. Weil L, Jr, Glover JP, Weil LS, Sr. A new minimally invasive technique for treating plantar fasciosis using bipolar radiofrequency: a prospective analysis. *Foot Ankle Spec*. 2008; 1(1):13–18.

20. Sinnaeve F, Vandeputte G. Clinical outcome of surgical intervention for recalcitrant infero-medial heel pain. *Acta Orthop Belg*. 2008; 74(4):483–8.

21. Sammarco GJ, Helfrey RB. Surgical treatment of recalcitrant plantar fasciitis. *Foot Ankle Int*. 1996; 17(9):520–6.

22. Davies MS, Weiss GA, Saxby TS. Plantar fasciitis: how successful is surgical intervention? *Foot Ankle Int*. 1999; 20(12):803–7.

23. Clain MR, Baxter DE. Achilles tendinitis. *Foot Ankle*. 1992; 13(8):482–7.

24. Maffulli N, Khan KM, Puddu G. Overuse tendon conditions: time to change a confusing terminology. *Arthroscopy*. 1998; 14(8):840–3.

25. Khan KM, Cook JL, Kannus P, Maffulli N, Bonar SF. Time to abandon the "tendinitis" myth. *BMJ*. 2002; 324(7338):626–7.

26. Maffulli N, Wong J, Almekinders LC. Types and epidemiology of tendinopathy. *Clin Sports Med*. 2003; 22(4):675–92.

27. Schepsis AA, Jones H, Haas AL. Achilles tendon disorders in athletes. *Am J Sports Med*. 2002; 30(2):287–305.

28. James SL, Bates BT, Osternig LR. Injuries to runners. *Am J Sports Med*. 1978; 6(2):40–50.

29. Silfverskiöld N. Uber die subkutane totale Achillessehnenruptur and deren Behandlung. *Acta Chir Scand*. 1941; 84:393.

30. Keener BJ, Sizensky JA. The anatomy of the calcaneus and surrounding structures. *Foot Ankle Clin*. 2005; 10(3):413–24.

31. Stephens MM. Haglund's deformity and retrocalcaneal bursitis. *Orthop Clin North Am*. 1994; 25(1):41–6.

32. Bleakney RR, White LM. Imaging of the Achilles tendon. *Foot Ankle Clin*. 2005; 10(2):239–54.

33. Fahlstrom M, Jonsson P, Lorentzon R, Alfredson H. Chronic Achilles tendon pain treated with eccentric calf-muscle training. *Knee Surg Sports Traumatol Arthrosc*. 2003; 11(5):327–33.

34. Harty J, Soffe K, O'Toole G, Stephens MM. The role of hamstring tightness in plantar fasciitis. *Foot Ankle Int*. 2005; 26(12):1089–92.

35. Gross CE, Hsu AR, Chahal J, Holmes GB, Jr. Injectable treatments for noninsertional

Achilles tendinosis: a systematic review. *Foot Ankle Int*. 2013; 34(5):619–28.

36. Yelland MJ, Sweeting KR, Lyftogt JA, Ng SK, Scuffham PA, Evans KA. Prolotherapy injections and eccentric loading exercises for painful Achilles tendinosis: a randomised trial. *B J Sports Med*. 2011; 45(5):421–8.

37. Chan O, O'Dowd D, Padhiar N, et al. High volume image guided injections in chronic Achilles tendinopathy. *Disabil Rehabil*. 2008; 30(20–22):1697–708.

38. Den Hartog BD. Flexor hallucis longus transfer for chronic Achilles tendonosis. *Foot Ankle Int*. 2003; 24(3):233–7.

39. Martin RL, Manning CM, Carcia CR, Conti SF. An outcome study of chronic Achilles tendinosis after excision of the Achilles tendon and flexor hallucis longus tendon transfer. *Foot Ankle Int*. 2005; 26(9):691–7.

40. Patel A, DiGiovanni B. Association between plantar fasciitis and isolated contracture of the gastrocnemius. *Foot Ankle Int*. 2011; 32(1):5–8.

41. Silfverskiöld N. Reduction of the uncrossed two-joint muscles of the leg to one joint muscles in spastic conditions. *Acta Chir Scandinavica*. 1923–1924; 56:315–30.

42. Aronow MS, Diaz-Doran V, Sullivan RJ, Adams DJ. The effect of triceps surae contracture force on plantar foot pressure distribution. *Foot Ankle Int*. 2006; 27(1):43–52.

43. Vulpius O, Stoffel A. *Tenotmie der end schnen der mm. gastrocnemius et soleus mittels rutschenlassens nach vulpius. Orthopadishe Operationslehre*. (Stuttgart: Verlag von Ferdinand Enke, 1913).

44. Strayer LM, Jr. Recession of the gastrocnemius; an operation to relieve spastic contracture of the calf muscles. *J Bone Joint Surg Am*. 1950; 32-A(3):671–6.

45. Herzenberg JE, Lamm BM, Corwin C, Sekel J. Isolated recession of the gastrocnemius muscle: the Baumann procedure. *Foot Ankle Int.* 2007; 28(11):1154–9.

46. Pinney SJ, Sangeorzan BJ, Hansen ST, Jr. Surgical anatomy of the gastrocnemius recession (Strayer procedure). *Foot Ankle Int.* 2004; 25(4):247–50.

47. Pinney SJ, Hansen ST Jr., Sangeorzan BJ. The effect on ankle dorsiflexion of gastrocnemius recession. *Foot Ankle Int.* 2002; 23(1):26–9.

48. Rush SM, Ford LA, Hamilton GA. Morbidity associated with high gastrocnemius recession: retrospective review of 126 cases. *J Foot Ankle Surg.* 2006; 45(3):156–60.

49. Tashjian RZ, Appel AJ, Banerjee R, DiGiovanni CW. Endoscopic gastrocnemius recession: evaluation in a cadaver model. *Foot Ankle Int.* 2003; 24(8):607–13.

50. Saxena A, Widtfeldt A. Endoscopic gastrocnemius recession: preliminary report on 18 cases. *J Foot Ankle Surg.* 2004; 43(5):302–6.

51. Barouk LS, Barouk P, Toulec E. Resulltats de la liberation proximale des gastrocnemiens. *Etude Prospective Symposium "Brieveté des Gastrocnemiens," Journées de Printemps SFMCP-AFCP.* (Toulouse: Med.Chir.Pied 2006) pp. 151–6.

52. Barouk P. Comparaison de deux types de liberation proximale des gastrocnemeiens medial et lateral, versus gastrocnemien medial isole. *Med Chir Pied.* 2006; 22:156.

53. Hamilton PD, Brown M, Ferguson N, Adebibe M, Maggs J, Solan M. Surgical anatomy of the proximal release of the gastrocnemius: a cadaveric study. *Foot Ankle Int.* 2009; 30(12):1202–6.

54. Barouk LS, Barouk P. *Brièveté des gastrocnémiens. Compte rendu du symposium n°3, Journées de Printemps SFMCP-AFCP; 2006;* (Toulouse: Maître Orthopedique, 2006) p. 22–8.

55. Kohls-Gatzoulis JA, Solan M. Results of proximal medial gastrocnemius release. *J Bone Joint Surg Br.* 2009; 91-B(Supp II):361.

56. Maskill JD, Bohay DR, Anderson JG. Gastrocnemius recession to treat isolated foot pain. *Foot Ankle Int.* 2010; 31(1):19–23.

57. Abbassian A, Kohls-Gatzoulis J, Solan MC. Proximal medial gastrocnemius release in the treatment of recalcitrant plantar fasciitis. *Foot Ankle Int.* 2012; 33(1):14–19.

.58. Alfredson H, Pietila T, Jonsson P, Lorentzon R. Heavy-load eccentric calf muscle training for the treatment of chronic Achilles tendinosis. *Am J Sports Med.* 1998; 26(3):360–6.

59. Gentchos CE, Bohay DR, Anderson JG. Gastrocnemius recession as treatment for refractory Achilles tendinopathy: a case report. *Foot Ankle Int.* 2008; 29(6):620–3.

60. Kiewiet NJ, Holthusen SM, Bohay DR, Anderson JG. Gastrocnemius recession for chronic noninsertional Achilles tendinopathy. *Foot Ankle Int.* 2013; 34(4):481–5.

Chapter 15

Disorders of the Tendo Achillis

Andrew J. Roche and James D. F. Calder

Introduction

Clinicians frequently encounter patients with a painful tendo Achillis (TA). They present with pain, swelling, and reduced function.

Anatomy

The TA is the thickest and strongest tendon in the body. The gastrocnemius–soleus complex is a tri-articular muscle; it crosses the knee, ankle, and subtalar joints. It is innervated by the posterior tibial nerve. The medial and lateral heads of gastrocnemius originate, respectively, from the posterior aspect of the medial and lateral femoral condyles. The soleus muscle has a complex origin from the posterior aspect of the tibia, fibula, and interosseous membrane. The two muscles coalesce to form the TA.

The Tendo Achillis

The TA varies in length, but averages 15 cm in adults (11–26 cm). At the proximal end it can measure up to 8 cm wide, narrowing to its thinnest cross-section in the midportion (1.5–2.5 cm). It then widens to around 4 cm above the insertion, from where it gradually widens and flattens as it reaches the calcaneal insertion. At the posterior calcaneus midpoint it measures 2 to 4.8 cm in width.

The TA is composed of cellular and extracellular matrix. The cellular component is primarily fibroblasts, which make up around 20% of the volume. The extracellular matrix accounts for around 80% and is mainly type I collagen, with lesser quantities of type III and IV. Collagen makes up over 70% of the extracellular matrix, with the remainder being proteoglycan-rich ground substance to stabilize the collagen fibrils, and elastin allowing the network of collagen to stretch and recoil.

The collagen fibrils are wrapped in a thin endotenon, which in turn is enveloped by epitenon. The paratenon, or peritendineum, is a thin layer of areolar connective tissue around the epitenon, which further protects and stabilizes the tendon.

The collagen fibers of the tendon are not vertical but orientated in a spiral manner. As the fibers descend from the musculotendinous junction they spiral through 90° and come to lie in the configuration shown in Figure 15.1. The degree of fiber rotation depends at which level the gastrocnemius and soleus muscles fuse to form the tendon – a more distal fusion resulting in more rotation. A rotational fiber pattern allows tendon elongation and recoil during locomotion, with efficient energy storage and dissipation. It also ensures less fiber buckling when the tendon is lax and less deformation under stress, which increases overall tendon strength.

The blood supply to the TA is poor and worsens with age. The tendon is supplied by two arteries – the posterior tibial and peroneal. There are three vascular territories. The midsection is supplied by the peroneal artery, and the proximal and distal sections are supplied by the posterior tibial artery[2].

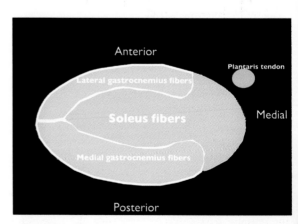

Figure 15.1 Cross-section of the tendo Achillis 1 cm above the calcaneum. (Fascicles of the adult human tendo Achillis, adapted from Szaro et al.[1]).

The vascularity of the midsection, 2 to 7 cm from the calcaneal insertion, is poorest, with blood entering through the anterior surface. The proximal third of the tendon receives vessels via the muscle bellies. The distal third receives its supply at the level of the insertion and the supply travels proximally. The midsection is the site most commonly affected by tendinopathy.

The paratenon is vascular although vessels may not be uniformly distributed throughout its length.

The tendon and paratenon are innervated by the same nerves as the musculature, with small branches from the cutaneous nerves, particularly the sural nerve.

The Tendo Achillis Insertion

The posterior calcaneal tuberosity is divided into three facets. The upper and middle facets are separated by a shallow groove, the middle and lower facets by a rough ridge. The upper facet lies anterior to the retrocalcaneal bursa. The TA inserts onto the middle and lower facets, and is confluent with the plantar fascia[3].

The superficial calcaneal bursa lies superficial to the TA between the tendon and the skin. Deep to the tendon is the retrocalcaneal bursa. The superior facet of the calcaneal tuberosity forms the anterior wall of the retrocalcaneal bursa and the tendon lies posteriorly. Periosteal fibrocartilage overlies the tuberosity anteriorly. Sesamoid fibrocartilage overlies the tendon posteriorly. On the inner surface of the fibrocartilage is a synovial membrane, it is mainly smooth on the posterior TA surface but richly layered with vascular folds on the anterior aspect.

Kager's triangle is often described on imaging and is bounded inferiorly by the superomedial calcaneum, anteromedially by the flexor hallucis longus (FHL) tendon, and posteriorly by the TA (Figure 15.2). It contains Kager's fat pad. Three parts of the fat pad have been identified:

The TA-associated part is encapsulated by the paratenon and held to the TA. The FHL-associated part lies anteriorly and within the FHL tendon sheath. Between these two parts is the retrocalcaneal bursal wedge.

Kager's fat pad minimizes pressure changes within the retrocalcaneal bursa as the wedge of fat displaces into the retrocalcaneal space on plantar flexion of the foot. It has an excursion of 10 to 12 mm, on

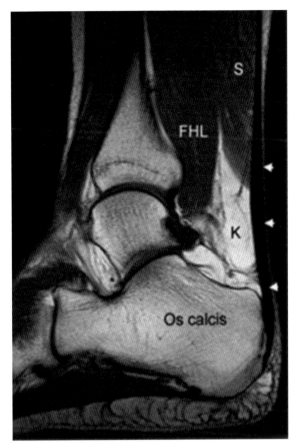

Figure 15.2 The MRI appearance of Kager's triangle, containing Kager's fat pad. S: soleus; FHL: flexor hallucis longus; K: Kager's fat pad. The three arrows delineate the tendo Achillis.
(Picture courtesy of Dr. J. Healey, Chelsea and Westminster Hospital, UK)

loadbearing dorsiflexion/plantar flexion. The fat pad also protects the tortuous vascular supply to the TA in its TA-associated part.

The Plantaris Tendon

The plantaris tendon is present in approximately 93% of individuals. It arises laterally in the knee from the linea aspera and oblique popliteal ligament. It then runs between the gastrocnemius and soleus muscles. It passes obliquely, coming to lie medial to the TA, inserting on the posterior calcaneus. In 3% of individuals there is a variable insertion, 1 to 16 cm above the calcaneus, into the TA or calf complex itself[4]. The role of the plantaris in tendinopathy of TA is being increasingly recognized and may explain the reason why symptoms can be more severe on the medial side of the TA.

Nomenclature of Tendo Achillis Disorders

There are a number of different descriptions of TA disorders. The term "tendinitis" of the TA has been recognized distinctly as having "insertional" and "non-insertional" components. Authors have since suggested abandoning the term "tendinitis" and replacing it with "tendinopathy," as histologically there is no inflammatory change[5]; there is in fact an incomplete healing response to repeated micro-injury or overuse. This also helps to distinguish between "paratendinopathy" and "tendinopathy." *Paratendinopathy* is inflammation or degeneration of the paratenon, which surrounds the tendo Achillis.

The terminology for TA disorders has developed incorporating location, symptoms, clinical findings, and histology. The following conditions are included in the "non-insertional disorders":

- midportion tendinopathy of tendo Achillis
- acute paratendinopathy (also called paratendinitis)
- chronic paratendinopathy.

Many incorrectly use the term "insertional tendinopathy" to describe any disorder located around the TA insertion. It is important to appreciate other distinct causes of pain around the TA insertion, which may coexist and make diagnosis difficult. The following conditions are included under insertional disorders:

- insertional tendinopathy of tendo Achillis
- retrocalcaneal bursitis
- superficial calcaneal bursitis.

Epidemiology

The incidence of tendinopathy of TA is rising, largely as a result of mass participation in recreational activities with increasingly demanding training regimens. Fifty-five to 65% of tendinopathy of TA is midportion tendinopathy, insertional disorders are about 25%, with 3% ruptures, and 8% myotendinous pain[6].

The sports most associated with TA disorders are middle- and long-distance running, with up to 10% of runners affected[7].

Normal aging can affect the tendon in a similar fashion as a result of overuse. A cadaveric study demonstrated that 34% of previously healthy individuals have evidence of tendinopathic change[8].

There is a correlation between tendinopathy and chronic disease, such as diabetes mellitus, obesity, hypertension, hypercholesterolemia, and mixed hyperlipidemia[9].

Etiology

Genetics

Tendinopathy of TA is multifactorial but research into the genetic susceptibilities to tendinopathy has revealed links to a variety of factors. Collagen forms 80% of the dry mass of tendons and genetic polymorphisms within the genes for collagen types 1, 2, and 12 have been linked with tendinopathy of TA and rupture. For example, individuals carrying a single nuclear polymorphism, the TT genotype of the GDF5-rs143383 variant, have twice the risk of tendinopathy compared with non-carriers[10]. Homeostasis and remodeling of the extracellular matrix is controlled in part by matrix metalloprotease (MMP) enzymes, tissue inhibitors of MMPs (TIMPs), and growth factors such as transforming growth factor β (tgf-β). Imbalances in the remodeling of the extracellular matrix can lead to collagen disturbances and tendinopathic change. Genotypes of these enzymes and growth factors have been linked to tendinopathy of AT and rupture. The deleterious effect of quinolone antibiotics (ciprofloxacin) is also mediated by MMPs and TIMPs.

The major cell type in the tendon is the tenocyte. Damaged tenocytes are removed by apoptosis. However, repetitive loading can cause excessive tenocyte apoptosis such that the tenocytes are unable to maintain the extracellular matrix and the tendon does not heal normally. The apoptosis signaling cascade has been implicated in the development of tendinopathic changes[11], and in turn this pathway has genetic polymorphisms that are linked to tendinopathy of TA.

Epigenetics, the effect of external or environmental factors on genetic expression, is also an area that is being increasingly recognized as important, as aging and exercise regimes can modulate the expression of genetic material. This may help to explain why some individuals develop musculoskeletal conditions, while others do not.

Insertional Tendinopathy of Tendo Achillis

Predisposing factors to insertional tendinopathy of TA include increasing age, seronegative inflammatory arthropathy, corticosteroids, diabetes mellitus, hypertension, obesity, gout, hyperostotic conditions, hyperlipidemias, and medications such as quinolone antibiotics.

There are extrinsic and intrinsic etiological factors in insertional tendinopathy of AT.

Extrinsic Factors

Increased, repetitive loading, which is common in runners[7] and athletes in "springing" sports, such as badminton, causes insertional disease. New training regimens can also trigger stress-related structural change. Increased hindfoot eversion, reduced ankle dorsiflexion speed, and knee flexion during running are associated with tendinopathic change[12].

Coronal plane malalignment of the knee, ankle, and particularly the subtalar joint predisposes to insertional disorders. Both varus and valgus malalignment may cause the tendon to shorten. Malalignment also causes atypical stress, which can initiate a sequence of repetitive microtears and tendinopathic changes. Thus shoes with uneven wear can contribute to disease as a result of excessive subtalar joint movement. Poor shock absorption and uneven surfaces may also be contributors.

Sagittal malalignment and calcaneal pitch can influence the interface between the tendon and calcaneum producing a bursal inflammatory response, rather than degenerative change.

Intrinsic Factors

There are four principal pathologies of the TA insertion: Haglund's deformity; enthesophytes; the retrocalcaneal bursa; and degeneration of the tendon itself.

1. Prominence of the posterosuperior calcaneum, originally described by Haglund, is associated with local attritional wear of the TA insertion causing pain, swelling, and tenderness. The so-called "Haglund's deformity" probably also contributes to retrocalcaneal bursitis.

2. The anterior surface of the TA insertion is often more affected than the posterior surface in insertional tendinopathy, despite the posterior surface undergoing a higher strain on dorsiflexion[13]. Insertional spurs, or enthesophytes, form by endochondral ossification of the enthesis fibrocartilage on the anterior, stress-shielded aspect of the TA[14]. Thus the precise role loading has to play is complex. Enthesophytes do not appear to need preceding

microtears or inflammatory change to initiate them.

3. The retrocalcaneal bursa is lined with synovium and fibrocartilage. These layers are apposed during ankle dorsiflexion and the tendon is compressed against the calcaneum. Synovial fold hypertrophy, calcification of the sesamoid fibrocartilage, and cellular degeneration with bursal debris have been demonstrated in the retrocalcaneal bursa[14]. This may be the cause of retrocalcaneal bursitis.

4. The poor tendon blood supply seen in normal entheses reduces further with age. Thus midsubstance tendinopathy may exacerbate insertional tendinopathy.

Non-Insertional Tendinopathy of Tendo Achillis

Extrinsic Factors

As with insertional tendinopathy of TA, shoes have been linked to non-insertional tendinopathy. The shoes may cause slight varus or valgus of the heel and therefore change the direction of pull of the TA, adversely affecting the tendon.

Positioning of the foot while running can lead to tendinopathy. Hyperpronation of the hindfoot, in particular, is related to the development of tendinopathy of AT. As with insertional tendinopathy, an increase in activity can adversely affect the TA. Similarly, environmental factors such as changes in the surface or surface orientation can influence ankle biomechanics and the resultant strain force on the tendon itself.

Intrinsic Factors

The tendon itself is predisposed to tendinopathic change by virtue of its shape. As described above the collagen fibers spiral through 90° so the medial fibers proximally lie posteriorly distally. This produces areas of high stress, which could be a factor in ischemic change in the tendon.

Neovascularization on US scanning of the tendinopathic TA has been the focus of recent study[15]. The evidence is somewhat conflicting and confusing. It is assumed that normal tendons exhibit no vascular flow on color Doppler US, whereas tendinopathic tendons exhibit increased flow[16].

Increased vascularity is thought to be a physiological, adaptive response to increased load, although it may be a direct reaction to hypoxia secondary to reduced vascularity and degeneration. Alfredson has correlated pain with histological tendinopathic change, showing that neovascularization at the site of pain correlates with biopsies of tendinopathic material[17]. On the other hand intratendinous flow does not increase, in fact it may decrease, with repetitive loading[18].

Plantaris Tendon

The plantaris tendon is closely related to the medial aspect of the tendo Achillis. It is stiffer than the TA and acts as a weak hindfoot invertor. The soleus muscle forms the medial fibers of the TA and is an ankle plantar flexor. The differing action and stiffness of plantaris and the medial TA can produce differing excursions of the two tendons during gait. This is proposed as a cause of TA pain, especially in patients complaining of medial symptoms.

Presentation

History

The history of insertional and non-insertional disease differs. Pertinent features for both conditions include whether the onset was associated with an increase in activity, alteration in shoes, and the presence of a generalized inflammatory arthropathy or systemic disease.

Non-Insertional Tendinopathy of Tendo Achillis

The patient with non-insertional tendinopathy often describes the gradual onset of pain, but may also remember an isolated incident. Symptoms may have been present for years. In more severe cases, patients complain of pain even with the activities of daily living. Typically there is stiffness in the morning and after periods of sitting. Night pain can be a feature. There is often variable swelling and tenderness of the tendon.

Paratendinitis

The history is usually more acute with a rapid onset of symptoms, which include diffuse swelling and pain around the tendon, sometimes associated with erythematous change. The pain is usually in the middle third of the tendon and can be more prominent medially.

Insertional Tendinopathy of Tendo Achillis

The main feature is pain located at the insertion of the TA. Affected populations include the younger athlete in running and jumping sports, who has often started a new regimen, and the sedentary older individual who presents with a more chronic picture, and may or may not describe progressive planovalgus foot deformity. The posterior heel pain is sharp and exacerbated by rubbing shoes, with increased pain on start-up.

Retrocalcaneal Bursitis

Retrocalcaneal pain is worse on walking or running. The pain is "to the side" or "in front" of the tendon insertion. The pain is exacerbated by activity or new shoes. Use of NSAIDs often dramatically improves the symptoms.

Superficial Calcaneal Bursitis

Often affecting women, the symptoms include an inability to wear shoes with firm uppers.

Examination

For both insertional and non-insertional disorders the general alignment is important, as planovalgus and cavovarus can predispose to heel pain. The patient should be observed standing and walking. The presence of calf wasting should be noted.

In paratendinitis the tendon is exquisitely tender and swollen with crepitus being felt on movement. In both insertional and non-insertional tendinopathy the affected area is tender, firm, and swollen. There is usually a discrete, fusiform swelling of the tendon in non-insertional tendinopathy, although occasionally the tendon may be diffusely involved (Figure 15.3). A posterior prominence at the insertion is seen in insertional tendinopathy (Figure 15.4). With retrocalcaneal bursitis the skin is typically warm and erythematous with the swelling and tenderness localized just anterior and to the sides of the tendon. The range of motion in dorsiflexion is often limited, although plantar flexion strength is usually normal.

Investigations

Plain Radiographs

The role of plain radiographs is limited in non-insertional tendinopathy, although calcification of the tendon is occasionally seen. However, in the investigation of "heel pain," or insertional tendinopathy,

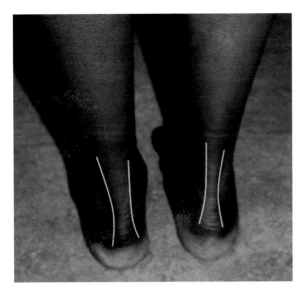

Figure 15.3 The clinical appearance of a thickened, diffuse non-insertional tendinopathy of tendo Achillis on the left side.

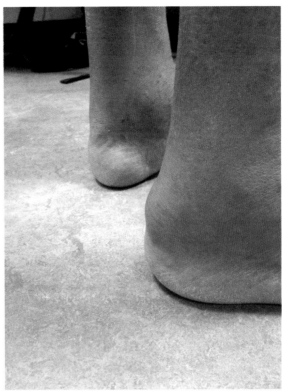

Figure 15.4 The clinical appearance of an insertional tendinopathy of tendo Achillis with posterior prominence on the right side.

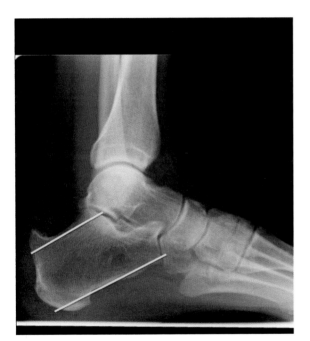

Figure 15.5 A large posterosuperior prominence of the calcaneum, demarcated by Pavlov's parallel pitch lines.

plain radiographs, specifically a weightbearing lateral view, are much more useful. The three major features to note are:

1. posterosuperior prominences (Haglund's deformity[19], various authors have measured the posterosuperior prominence on radiographs – one such example is the method by Pavlov[20], see Figure 15.5)
2. ossification of the insertion of the tendon (enthesophytes, see Figure 15.6)
3. swelling in Kager's fat pad, anterior to the usually well-demarcated tendo Achillis.

Ultrasound Scanning

Ultrasound is useful both diagnostically and therapeutically in tendo Achillis disease. It is operator dependent, but can also be used to guide injection therapies.

In the prone position, patients are assessed with a linear high-frequency probe (7–18 MHz) examining in the transverse and longitudinal planes. The use of color Doppler shows neovascularization. The normal tendon exhibits an echogenic pattern of parallel, fibrillar lines in the longitudinal plane, and a round or oval shape in the transverse plane (Figures 15.7 and 15.8).

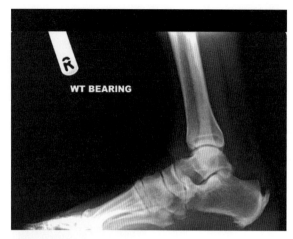

Figure 15.6 Enthesophytes at the distal insertion of the tendo Achillis.

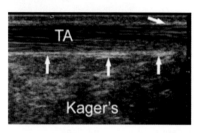

Figure 15.7
A normal tendo Achillis in the longitudinal plane. TA: tendo Achillis; top right arrow indicates the paratenon.
(Picture courtesy of Dr. J. Healey, Chelsea and Westminster Hospital, London, UK)

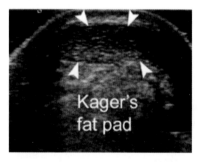

Figure 15.8
A normal tendo Achillis in the transverse plane. Arrows point to the tendon.
(Picture courtesy of Dr. J. Healey, Chelsea and Westminster Hospital, London, UK)

Ultrasound of non-insertional tendinopathy of TA shows diffuse or fusiform thickening with hypo- or hyperechogenic lesions within the tendon. The Doppler is used to show neovascularity[16–17].

Non-insertional tendinopathy of TA may be indistinguishable clinically from paratendinitis, but in paratendinitis the US shows a normal tendon with a circumferential hypoechogenic halo, which may be hypervascular on power Doppler. Contrast-enhanced MRI has probably superseded US for the diagnosis of isolated acute paratendinitis.

In insertional disorders partial tears may be demonstrated, usually on the ventral surface with expansion of the tendon in the AP dimension. There is heterogeneous loss of reflectivity and the normal fibrillar pattern. Enthesophytes and a Haglund's deformity are also visualized.

The retrocalcaneal and subcutaneous calcaneal bursae are not demonstrable by ultrasonography in healthy people. Abnormal bursae are usually well defined, although US is poorly sensitive but highly specific in making the diagnosis of retrocalcaneal bursitis compared to MRI. In a true bursitis increased blood flow can be seen on color or power Doppler.

Magnetic Resonance Imaging

The normal MRI scan of the TA shows a low signal, homogeneous structure on T1 and T2 weighted images (Figure 15.2). Standard sequences include T1-weighted and fluid-sensitive sequences such as short-tau inversion recovery (STIR) and fat-suppressed T2, or intermediate (proton) density weighted sequences in the axial and sagittal planes.

The sensitivity of MRI scanning in detecting TA abnormalities is 94% with a specificity of 81% and positive predictive value of 90%[21]. The tendinopathic TA on MRI appears with a variable amount of ill-defined longitudinal high signal, with fusiform expansion of the tendon on the sagittal images. Enhancement of the paratenon is best visualized with gadolinium contrast. Presence of a calcaneal prominence, especially with bone edema, is of significance (Figure 15.9).

Magnetic Resonance Imaging or Ultrasound?

Ultrasound shows neovascularization and images the tendon dynamically. It also has a therapeutic role with injection therapies. MRI may be more useful to detect multiple lesions (Figure 15.9). Sagittal MRI is the optimal tool to diagnose a significant retrocalcaneal bursitis, especially when coupled with insertional pathology, although US shows vascularization in cases with insertional tendinopathy. Both modalities clearly demonstrate tendon thickening and partial tears.

Treatment

The treatment of tendinopathy of TA is multimodal. The requirements of the low-demand patient with multiple comorbidities differ from those of the elite athlete. Treatment also depends on the area of pathology. Pathologies can coexist, for example in non-insertional

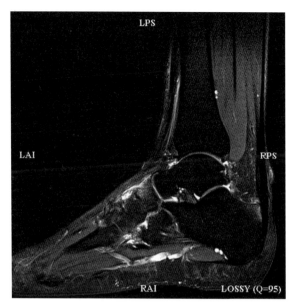

Figure 15.9 Sagittal MRI showing edematous changes in the posterosuperior calcaneum, an inflamed retrocalcaneal bursa, and tendinopathic change with inflammatory change in the posterior paratenon.

disorders an acute paratendinitis can coexist with a tendinopathy. There is no one strategy for either insertional or non-insertional disorders and therefore complicated treatment algorithms have been avoided.

Non-Insertional Tendinopathy of Tendo Achillis

Non-Surgical Treatment

Non-Steroidal Anti-Inflammatory Drugs (NSAIDs)

NSAIDs have been shown to have a modest effect on symptoms from three trials reported in the Cochrane Review[22], but a randomized study found no benefit over placebo[23]. Additionally, the scientific basis for their use in chronic tendinopathy is questionable in view of the histological absence of inflammatory cells in the tendinopathic tissue. Thus their short-term benefit is likely to be due to their analgesic effect. There are some studies that highlight the possible detrimental effects of NSAIDs. Celecoxib inhibits tenocyte migration and proliferation[24] and NSAIDs increase leukotriene B, which may contribute to the development of tendinopathy of TA[25].

Eccentric Exercises

Eccentric exercises are supported by multiple studies. Nevertheless, the therapeutic effect of eccentric exercises is poorly understood. Öhberg showed that they lead to normalization of the tendon structure and reduction in the neovascularization seen on US[26]. Rees demonstrated increased stretching of the tendon with eccentric, when compared to concentric, exercises[27]. Alfredson, in a randomized study, reported 82% of individuals returning to normal activities at 12 weeks with eccentric, as opposed to 36% with concentric, stretches[28]. Many now use a 12-week regimen as the gold-standard therapy for treating non-insertional tendinopathy; however, shorter, six-week regimens have been described with reasonable results[29]. Clinical trials comparing different eccentric protocols are lacking and thus it remains to be seen whether a shorter regimen is as effective as a 12-week regimen.

Shockwave Therapy

In trials, extra-corporeal shockwave therapy (ESWT), typically low energy, has given rise to conflicting results, although recent randomized trials have demonstrated improvement when ESWT is combined with eccentric exercises, when compared to eccentric exercises alone[30]. A non-randomized case-control study of patients failing to improve following at least three non-operative treatments, for a minimum of six months, found improved visual analogue scores at 12 months in the ESWT group[31].

The mechanism of action of ESWT is not absolutely clear, but ESWT causes cavitation of the tendon with interstitial and extracellular disruption leading to a healing response[32]. At the cellular level, ESWT promotes cell growth and collagen synthesis in cultured human tenocytes. It is suggested that this increases the efficacy of tendon repair after injury[33]. Changes in TGF-β1 and IGF-1 expression and decrease in some interleukins and MMPs have been demonstrated in rat and human cultured tenocytes[34].

Extra-corporeal shockwave therapy also causes selective dysfunction of sensory unmyelinated nerve fibers and changes in the dorsal root ganglia. It appears to have a role in treatment if other conservative measures have failed, as it is safe and inexpensive.

Corticosteroids

Corticosteroid injections are reported to reduce pain and swelling, and improve the US appearance of the TA. This may be through their vasoconstrictive effects[35]. Corticosteroid injections may have some

271

early benefit but later complications are reported including tendon rupture[36] and the risks appear to outweigh the benefits.

Nitric Oxide

A randomized double-blind, placebo-controlled study demonstrated impressive improvement in symptoms from glyceryl trinitrate (GTN) patches applied over the tendon. A follow-up study showed the benefit was maintained in the GTN compared to the control group[37]. Doubts have been raised as to the blinding of this study, as the GTN group required significantly more paracetamol to treat headaches. A subsequent randomized study demonstrated no additional benefit for GTN patches[38]. More worryingly, increased nitric oxide levels have also been implicated in the development of degenerative conditions, including tendinopathy[39]. It has been suggested therefore that GTN may in fact be detrimental to the underlying pathological process.

Injection Therapies

Dry needling and autologous blood injections are said to provide cellular and humoral mediators, which promote the healing of tendinopathy. Good results are reported in the treatment of medial epicondylitis of the elbow and patellar tendinopathy, although no good quality studies have reported benefit in tendinopathy of TA.

Platelet rich plasma (PRP) is widely used in orthopedic practice; however, recent publications have failed to demonstrate significant improvement using PRP to treat tendinopathy of TA[40]. A meta-analysis concluded that while there may be benefit in using PRP to increase the healing strength in tendo Achillis repair following acute rupture, there was no evidence to support the use of PRP in the treatment of tendinopathy of TA[41].

High-volume injections with limited follow-up have demonstrated reduced pain and improved function following high-volume injection (10 ml bupivacaine and 40 ml normal saline) anterior to the tendo Achillis[42]. However, they also injected 25 mg hydrocortisone, which has been shown to provide early symptomatic improvement, but is associated with a higher rate of later complications. It should be noted that there were no control groups, and the results were early, at 30 weeks follow-up. It is proposed that the mechanical effect of the volume of fluid causes damage to the neovessels and neural ingrowth.

Intratendinous hyperosmolar dextrose (prolotherapy) has been used since the 1940s and is thought to produce a local inflammatory response and increase in tendon strength. Evidence to support prolotherapy is lacking. A pilot study by Maxwell et al. demonstrated that ultrasonographically guided injection of 25% dextrose led to a reduction in TA pain both at rest and during exercise[43].

Aprotinin is a potent MMP inhibitor and some studies demonstrated its success in treating tendinopathy of TA; however, it was withdrawn in May 2008 due to severe complications in its use during open heart surgery.

Sclerosants have been used to reduce neovascularization in the tendinopathic tendon. Early reports using polidocanol injected under Doppler US guidance into the abnormal vessels on the ventral aspect of the TA led to significant improvements in pain and function[44]. This was a small study with limited follow-up and has not been reproduced at other institutions.

Finally, electrocautery has been used to destroy the neovascularization, with one study reporting good results in a series of 11 patients followed up for six months[45].

Other Non-Surgical Modalities

No significant benefits have been shown for kinesiotape, deep frictional massage, or dorsiflexion night splints. Therapeutic US reduces the swelling in the acute inflammatory phase of soft tissue disorders and may enhance tendon healing. It has been demonstrated that therapeutic US is beneficial in the treatment of tennis elbow and calcific tendinopathy of the shoulder, but systematic reviews and meta-analyses have failed to demonstrate any benefit over placebo for tendinopathy[46].

Surgical Treatment
Open Surgery

Surgical treatment is classically an open release of adhesions with or without resection of the paratenon through a longitudinal posteromedial incision. Macroscopic areas of tendinopathy are excised through a central longitudinal tenotomy (Figure 15.10) and multiple further tenotomies are made in the surrounding tissue to initiate vascular ingrowth and a healing response.

Even after extensive debridement there is usually enough tendon to achieve side-to-side closure of the

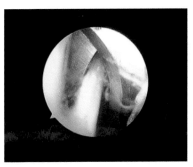

Figure 15.11
The endoscopic view of the plantaris tendon being transected.

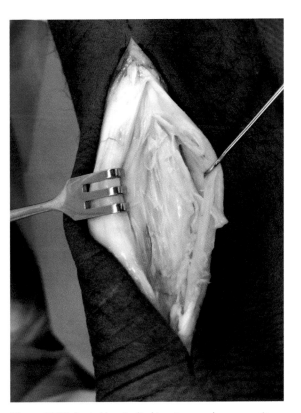

Figure 15.10 Central longitudinal tenotomy and macroscopic tendo Achillis degeneration.

tenotomy. However, if more than 50% of the tendon has been debrided augmentation is recommended – small defects may be covered with a turn-down flap of the plantaris tendon, but larger defects may require tendon transfer with peroneus brevis, flexor digitorum longus, or flexor hallucis longus (FHL)[47]. The FHL is the most commonly used. Success rates reported for open surgery vary widely but are generally said to be greater than 75%[48]. Nelen reported on surgery in 146 tendo Achillis cases with 18 months of symptoms. He detailed an 86% success rate in isolated paratendinopathy, a 73% success in tendinosis, and those requiring augmentation with a turn-down flap had an 87% success rate[49].

Complications are not uncommon and Paavola, in a large series of 432 consecutive patients, reported an overall complication rate of 11% and reoperation rate of 3%. This included 3% wound necrosis, 2.5% superficial infection, and 1% sural nerve injury[50].

Minimally Invasive Surgery

Minimally invasive techniques may reduce the risks associated with open surgery. Maffulli et al. reported

the results of multiple percutaneous tenotomies performed under local anesthetic. Good or excellent results were seen in 37 of 48 patients at a minimum follow-up of 22 months[51].

Stripping of the paratenon from the tendinopathic TA is thought to remove the neovascularization and denervate the diseased area of tendon. Steenstra reported good results in 16 of 20 patients treated using an endoscopic technique[52].

The Role and Treatment of the Plantaris Tendon

The plantaris tendon is stiffer and stronger than the TA and tethering of the plantaris tendon to the medial aspect of the TA may initiate an inflammatory response and localized tendinopathy, which leads to localized pain and swelling along the medial border of the TA – known as "plantaris syndrome." Stripping the plantaris in such patients has given good outcomes with both mini-incision and endoscopic techniques (Figure 15.11). A significant reduction in pain with improved function was reported in 11 patients, at two years follow-up, using an endoscopic technique[53]. At open surgical debridement the plantaris can be released and resected above the area of tendinopathy (Figures 15.12 and 15.13).

Gastrocnemius Lengthening

Ankle dorsiflexion of 10° with the knee extended is required in the terminal stance phase for normal gait. Furthermore, as a result of the different contributions from the gastrocnemius and soleus, the stress in the TA is non-uniform. This produces abnormal concentrations of load, which can result in localized damage to the fibers. Duthan et al. studied 14 patients who underwent a gastrocnemius lengthening (Strayer) and found that 79% were able to return to their previous sporting activities at two years follow-up[54]. More recently, proximal release of the medial gastrocnemius aponeurosis for both insertional and non-insertional tendinopathy of TA has shown promising

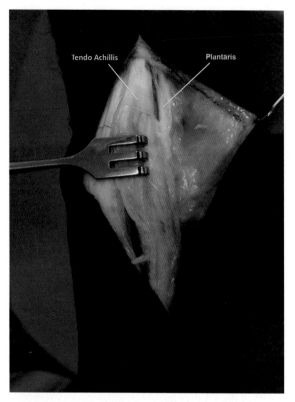

Figure 15.12 The plantaris tendon adherent to the tendo Achillis.

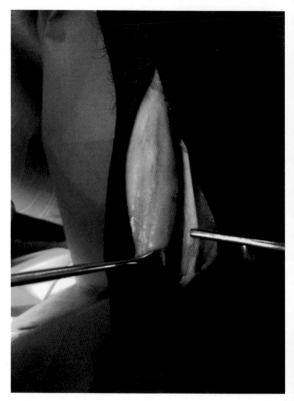

Figure 15.13 The plantaris tendon released from the tendo Achillis ready for resection.

results in patients with a tight gastrocnemius complex, as assessed by the Silfverskiöld test[55].

Insertional Tendinopathy of Tendo Achillis

Non-Surgical Treatment

Immobilization and Stretching

There is no definitive evidence to support immobilization in isolation for any form of insertional tendinopathy, and prolonged immobilization should be avoided. Despite this immobilization is frequently used in the acute setting to control exacerbations of symptoms. Following immobilization a treatment plan is required that should involve the gradual integration of loadbearing activity and monitored physical therapy, including a stretching regime.

A study of patients with retrocalcaneal pain treated with initial immobilization for six to eight weeks, followed by stretching, showed that after six months' treatment 88% of patients were satisfied. Diabetes, previous steroid injections, Haglund's deformity, and smoking were associated with poorer results. It is difficult to ascertain whether it was the immobilization or stretching that contributed most to the success of the regime[56].

Orthoses

A heel lift may alleviate pressure and potentially reduce symptoms.

Eccentric Full Range of Motion Activity

The 12-week eccentric exercise program described by Alfredson has been used with considerable success in non-insertional disorders, with good outcomes in 80 to 90%[28]. A recent systematic review[57] has shown that a successful outcome following eccentric loading exercise is less likely in insertional disorders, with success rates of around 30% reported. These poorer results in insertional disease may be because by dorsiflexing the ankle under load the retrocalcaneal bursa is compressed against the tendinopathic fibers of the anterior aspect of the TA.

Eccentric Floor-Level Activity

To determine if the effect of ankle dorsiflexion was detrimental in the full motion eccentric program, the activities were modified by Jonsson. Ankle dorsiflexion was eliminated by using floor-level exercises only. Interestingly they found improved outcomes in 67%, compared to 32% for the original activities[58]. Although not supported by further evidence as yet, this regimen is promising.

Extra-Corporeal Shockwave Therapy

The number of impulses and their energy are important parameters for ESWT. ESWT can be of high or low energy. As it is believed that high-energy ESWT is too damaging for use in tendinopathy, low-energy therapy (<0.2 mJ/mm^2) over three or four sessions is usually used. The number of impulses emitted per treatment is usually in the 1500 to 2500 range.

Rasmussen reported, in a double-blind RCT with sham and genuine ESWT, improvements in the AOFAS score from 70 to 88 in the intervention arm and 74 to 81 in the sham arm (p = 0.05)[59]. This study included both insertional and non-insertional tendinopathy. Furia reported good or excellent results in 83% of ESWT patients, compared to 40% of traditionally treated patients. Although a significant difference was found, with strict inclusion criteria of insertional tendinopathy only and a standardized ESWT procedure in a large cohort, the control arm group's treatment was variable and not clearly stratified[60]. A recent systematic review suggests promising results for ESWT at a minimum of three months' follow-up, although this study did not differentiate results according to whether the disease was insertional or non-insertional[61].

The use of ESWT is increasing and the development of cheaper, smaller machines is likely to accelerate the use of ESWT.

Injections

There is a variety of injection modalities; in reviewing these it is important to note that the studies are largely uncontrolled. Corticosteroid use in retrocalcaneal bursitis has been used in isolated cases; however, the volume of evidence is lacking and risk of tendon rupture probably explains its relatively infrequent use.

Prolotherapy essentially irritates the tendon to stimulate a healing response through release of pro-inflammatory mediators. Hyperosmolar dextrose solution is commonly used, often with local anesthetic. Widely quoted is the study by Ryan who treated 22 patients with a median of five (range 1–13) injections (1 ml lignocaine, 1 ml 50% dextrose) given once every three to eight weeks. The VAS significantly reduced over 28 months. Satisfaction scales were not used[62].

Sclerosing agents are used to reduce the neovascularization and innervation. Only one study using polidocanol for insertional disease is available. In this study 11 patients with up to five repeated injections showed an improved VAS after eight months with a 73% satisfaction rate[63].

Platelet-rich plasma has been used in insertional tendinopathy following failed non-invasive conservative treatments. There is limited objective data. Monto treated 30 patients (eight insertional tendinopathy, 22 non-insertional) with a single injection of PRP. The results seem impressive with average AOFAS scores increasing from 34 to 88 at 24 months; however, two of the eight insertional tendinopathies were classed as treatment failures, and required subsequent surgery[64].

Radiofrequency Coblation

A single study of 47 cases was reported using a technique where 20 separate stab incisions are made over the tendon insertion, and treatment with a radiofrequency probe inserted into each incision is undertaken. There was a 6.4% tendon rupture rate and a 15% re-operation rate, with no functional outcome data[65].

Surgical Treatment
Endoscopic Surgery

Calcaneoplasty with removal of the posterosuperior prominence of the calcaneum and retrocalcaneal bursal debridement can be undertaken open or endoscopically. The endoscopic technique has minimal morbidity and allows a rapid return to activity. The patients are selected after the failure of non-operative treatment. The patient is positioned prone, with portals placed anterior to the tendon on the medial and lateral sides. Surgery has a good or excellent outcome in 75 to 95% of cases (Figure 15.14); however, complications such as early rupture of the tendon have been reported[66].

Calcaneal osteotomy for retrocalcaneal bursitis

The increasing popularity of endoscopic treatments means osteotomies are less frequently undertaken. Zadek[67] described an osteotomy which excises a

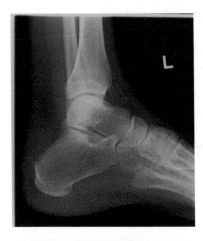

Figure 15.14 Postoperative lateral radiograph demonstrating resection of the prominence (preoperative x-rays are shown in Figure 15.5).

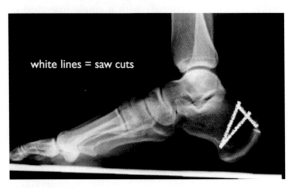

white lines = saw cuts

Figure 15.15 Preoperative lateral radiograph demonstrating the osteotomy lines.
(Picture courtesy of Mr. Sunil Dhar, Nottingham, UK)

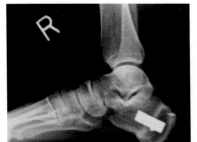

Figure 15.16 Postoperative lateral radiograph with fixation using a two-hole plate. (Picture courtesy of Mr. Sunil Dhar, Nottingham, UK)

dorsomedial wedge from the calcaneal tuberosity. The wedge is then closed, this reduces the prominence and decompresses the retrocalcaneal bursa and the tendon insertion (Figures 15.15 and 15.16).

Open Surgery on the Tendon Insertion

Open, as opposed to endoscopic, surgery can be used in cases of simple excision of a Haglund's deformity.

However, in cases where the tendon is degenerate and requires reconstruction, or the presence of an enthesophyte, open techniques are required. It is necessary to consider:

1. Debridement of the degenerate insertion
2. Decompression and debridement of bursal tissue
3. Resection of the Haglund's deformity or enthesophyte
4. Reattachment of the tendon insertion
5. Augmentation of the Achilles with a tendon transfer.

Caution should be exercised in patients whose skin is "at risk." This includes smokers, diabetics, and those with peripheral vascular disease.

Which Incision?

Numerous incisions are advocated, including longitudinal tendon splitting, medial, lateral, and Cincinnati, or transverse. The medial and lateral incisions can be extended with a transverse incision at the lower level of the insertion forming a "hockey stick." We prefer a medial incision, with a lateral hockey stick extension if required.

Reattachment

In surgery to excise a TA enthesophyte it is necessary to, at least partially, detach the TA. Biomechanical and clinical data suggest that 50% of the insertion can be safely debrided, without formal reattachment, while maintaining a minimal postoperative risk of detachment[68]. Reattachment using bone anchors (Figures 15.17 and 15.18) or transosseous sutures may be required for larger detachments of the tendon.

It is important to ensure the anchors are spaced symmetrically with equal tension on the insertion. Recent mechanical data suggest single- or double-row repairs are equivalent in peak load to failure[69], although anatomically the footprint of the insertion is better restored with a double-row technique. With accurate reattachment of the tendon normal plantar flexion should be maintained and Nunley achieved 96% satisfaction with good function at seven years' follow-up[70].

Reconstruction

If the tendon is degenerate at its point of insertion to the calcaneum it may be necessary to reconstruct it. Wagner compared V–Y advancement to simple debridement, and showed no functional difference

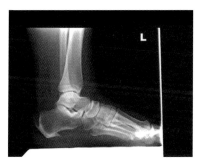

Figure 15.17
Lateral radiograph before excision of TA enthesophytes using osseous anchors to reattach the tendon insertion.

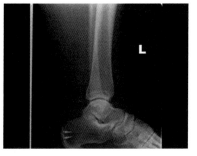

Figure 15.18
Lateral radiograph after excision of TA enthesophytes using osseous anchors to reattach the tendon insertion.

between the two groups; however, those requiring advancements had more extensive disease. The V–Y advancement was undertaken at the musculotendinous junction in the mid-calf and bridges insertional defects of more than 2 cm[72].

The commonest tendon used to augment the TA is the FHL, other options include autografts, and patella-bone or quadriceps-bone grafts, but these all have their own risks. Peroneus brevis and FDL tendon transfers have also been described. Harvesting the peroneus brevis can leave the ankle unstable and prone to invert. The FDL is about 50% weaker than the FHL and rerouting the tendon brings it across the posterior tibial nerve. Thus the FHL is ideal as it is in phase, is anatomically adjacent, has good vascularity with its low-lying muscle belly, and is the second strongest plantar flexor of the ankle. The FHL tendon can either be harvested through the one posterior incision, sectioning it as it passes into the foot behind the talus or, alternatively, a second incision in the foot can be utilized. The two-incision technique allows a 3 to 10 cm longer tendon to be harvested[71].

A recent systematic review reports 20% minor and 3.1% major complications[57]. Wound infection rates vary between 0 and 15% but many series report on a mixture of insertional and non-insertional

reconstructions[73]. The largest study reviewed 432 patients and found 4.7% of the insertional group had wound complications of which one was significant[50]. No particular approach is more prone to wound breakdown and rarely are there any serious consequences. Re-ruptures are reported but are usually secondary to a further injury.

Van Dijk quotes an 89% overall satisfaction rate[57], with other studies reporting satisfaction rates between 82 and 97% with significant improvements in functional scores[48,70]. There is no evidence to suggest any one technique is superior to another, but there are few comparative studies.

Summary

These conditions affect a huge spectrum of patients from the older diabetic patient to the young elite long-distance runner. The treatments offered may therefore differ widely. However, the majority of patients with non-insertional tendinopathy will respond to non-surgical management, activity modification, and supervised therapy. Injection therapy, such as high-volume injections around the tendon, and shockwave therapy certainly have a role and treatment can often be coupled with other modalities.

Surgery is effective in resistant cases and, depending on the surgeon's preference, minimally invasive techniques may reduce the risks of complications. The "plantaris effect" should be considered when pain and swelling are isolated to the medial border of the tendo Achillis. Satisfactory outcome following surgery may be expected in about 85% of patients.

It is important to appreciate that insertional disorders can encompass a number of distinct pathologies and as a result differing therapies can be instituted. Supervised injection therapies are evolving and shockwave therapy is low risk, but is probably less effective in insertional than in non-insertional disease. Retrocalcaneal bursa injections are successful but must be used with caution with a tendinopathic tendon. The endoscopic surgical excision of calcaneal prominences or bursae has good evidence to support its use; however, the procedure can be technically challenging, although it can be performed carefully under direct radiography. Open surgery for insertional tendinopathy should be considered after all other treatment modalities fail, with >80% of patients likely to gain significant benefit.

Key Points

Non-Insertional Tendinopathy

- Non-insertional tendinopathy is twice as common as insertional.
- Thirty percent of patients may not be sports active, although running is the predominant association.
- Correcting hindfoot malalignment is important.
- The plantaris may cause medial midportion TA pain.
- Physiotherapy does not just mean "eccentric" loading, although eccentric stretches are the mainstay of non-operative treatment.
- Extra-corporeal shockwave therapy has results comparable to loading activities.
- Open surgery gives greater than 75% good results.

Insertional Tendinopathy

- Loading exercises and ESWT are less successful in insertional disorders.
- Correcting hindfoot malalignment is important.
- Injection therapies must be image guided and used with caution if tendinopathy is present.
- Retrocalcaneal bursitis can be treated successfully with local anesthetic/steroid injection.
- Endoscopic calcaneoplasty/bursal resection is an effective procedure for resection of bony prominence of the calcaneum and retrocalcaneal bursitis.
- Open surgery is needed to excise the TA enthesophyte.
- Reattachment/augmentation of the tendon may be necessary if more than 50% of the TA is detached.
- Open surgery gives greater that 80% good results.

References

1. Szaro P, Witkowski G, Smigielski R, Krajewski P, Ciszek B. Fascicles of the adult human Achilles tendon: an anatomical study. *Ann Anat.* 2009; 191(6):586–93.
2. Chen TM, Rozen WM, Pan W-R, Ashton MW, Richardson MD, Taylor GI. The arterial anatomy of the Achilles tendon: anatomical study and clinical implications. *Clin Anat.* 2009; 22(3):377–85.
3. Lohrer H, Arentz S, Nauck T, Dorn-Lange NV, Konerding MA. The Achilles tendon insertion is crescent-shaped: an in vitro anatomic investigation. *Clin Orthop Relat Res.* 2008; 466(9):2230–7.
4. van Sterkenburg MN, Kerkhoffs GM, Kleipool RP, Niek van Dijk C. The plantaris tendon and a potential role in mid-portion Achilles tendinopathy: an observational anatomical study. *J Anat.* 2011; 218(3):336–41.
5. Maffulli N, Khan KM, Puddu G. Overuse tendon conditions: time to change a confusing terminology. *Arthroscopy.* 1998; 14(8):840–3.
6. Kvist M. Achilles tendon injuries in athletes. *Ann Chirurg Gynae.* 1991; 80(2):188–201.
7. Lysholm J, Wiklander J. Injuries in runners. *Am J Sports Med.* 1987; 15(2):168–71.
8. Kannus P, Jozsa L. Histopathological changes preceding spontaneous rupture of a tendon. A controlled study of 891 patients. *J Bone Joint Surg Am.* 1991; 73(10):1507.
9. Holmes GB, Lin J. Etiologic factors associated with symptomatic Achilles tendinopathy. *Foot Ankle Int.* 2006; 27(11):952–9.
10. Ribbans WJ, Collins M. Pathology of the tendo Achillis: do our genes contribute? *Bone Joint J.* 2013; 95-B(3):305–13.
11. Nell EM, van der Merwe L, Cook J, Handley CJ, Collins M, September AV. The apoptosis pathway and the genetic predisposition to Achilles tendinopathy. *J Orthop Res.* 2012; 30(11):1719–24.
12. Munteanu SE, Barton CJ. Lower limb biomechanics during running in individuals with Achilles tendinopathy: a systematic review. *J Foot Ankle Res.* 2011; 4:15.
13. Lyman J, Weinhold PS, Almekinders LC. Strain behavior of the distal Achilles tendon: Implications for insertional Achilles tendinopathy. *Am J Sports Med.* 2004; 32(2):457–61.
14. Rufai A, Ralphs JR, Benjamin M. Structure and histopathology of the insertional region of the human Achilles tendon. *J Orthop Res.* 1995; 13(4):585–93.
15. Yang X, Coleman DP, Pugh ND, Nokes LD. The volume of the neovascularity and its clinical implications in Achilles tendinopathy. *Ultrasound Med Biol.* 2012; 38(11):1887–95.
16. Öhberg L, Lorentzon R, Alfredson H. Neovascularisation in Achilles tendons with painful tendinosis but not in normal tendons: an ultrasonographic investigation. *Knee Surg Sports Traumatol Arthrosc.* 2001; 9(4):233–8.
17. Alfredson H, Ohberg L, Forsgren S. Is vasculo-neural ingrowth the cause of pain in chronic Achilles tendinosis? An investigation using

ultrasonography and colour Doppler, immunohistochemistry, and diagnostic injections. *Knee Surg Sports Traumatol Arthrosc.* 2003; 11(5):334–8.

18. Boesen AP, Boesen MI, Torp-Pedersen S, et al. Associations between abnormal ultrasound color Doppler measures and tendon pain symptoms in badminton players during a season: A prospective cohort study. *Am J Sports Med.* 2012; 40(3):548–55.

19. Haglund P. Beitrag zur klinik der achillessehne. *Zeitschr Orthop Chir.* 1928; 49:49–58.

20. Pavlov H, Heneghan MA, Hersh A, Goldman AB, Vigorita V. The Haglund syndrome: initial and differential diagnosis. *Radiology.* 1982; 144(1):83–8.

21. Leung JL, Griffith JF. Sonography of chronic Achilles tendinopathy: a case–control study. *J Clin Ultrasound.* 2008; 36(1):27–32.

22. McLauchlan GJ, Handoll HH. Interventions for treating acute and chronic achilles tendinitis. *Cochrane Database Syst Rev.* 2001; 2(2):CD000232.

23. Aström M, Westlin N. No effect of piroxicam on Achilles tendinopathy. A randomized study of 70 patients. *Acta Orthop Scand.* 1992; 63(6):631–4.

24. Tsai WC, Hsu CC, Chou SW, Chung CY, Chen J, Pang JH. Effects of celecoxib on migration, proliferation and collagen expression of tendon cells. *Connect Tissue Res.* 2007; 48(1):46–51.

25. Li Z, Yang G, Khan M, Stone D, Woo SL, Wang JH. Inflammatory response of human tendon fibroblasts to cyclic mechanical stretching. *Am J Sports Med.* 2004; 32(2):435–40.

26. Öhberg L, Lorentzon R, Alfredson H. Eccentric training in patients with chronic Achilles tendinosis: normalised tendon structure and

decreased thickness at follow up. *Br J Sports Med.* 2004, 38(1):8–11.

27. Rees JD, Lichtwark GA, Wolman RL, Wilson AM. The mechanism for efficacy of eccentric loading in Achilles tendon injury; an in vivo study in humans. *Rheumatol.* 2008; 47(10):1493–7.

28. Alfredson H, Pietilä T, Jonsson P, Lorentzon R. Heavy-load eccentric calf muscle training for the treatment of chronic Achilles tendinosis. *Am J Sports Med.* 1998; 26(3):360–6.

29. Verrall G, Schofield S, Brustad T. Chronic Achilles tendinopathy treated with eccentric stretching program. *Foot Ankle Int.* 2011; 32(9):843–9.

30. Rompe JD, Furia J, Maffulli N. Eccentric loading versus eccentric loading plus shock-wave treatment for midportion Achilles tendinopathy: a randomized controlled trial. *Am J Sports Med.* 2009; 37(3):463–70.

31. Furia JP. High-energy extracorporeal shock wave therapy as a treatment for chronic noninsertional Achilles tendinopathy. *Am J Sports Med.* 2008; 36(3):502–8.

32. Ogden JA, Tóth-Kischkat A, Schultheiss R. Principles of shock wave therapy. *Clin Orthop Relat Res.* 2001; 387:8–17.

33. Vetrano M, d'Alessandro F, Torrisi MR, Ferretti A, Vulpiani MC, Visco V. Extracorporeal shock wave therapy promotes cell proliferation and collagen synthesis of primary cultured human tenocytes. *Knee Surg Sports Traumatol Arthrosc.* 2011; 19(12):2159–68.

34. Han SH, Lee JW, Guyton GP, Parks BG, Courneya J-P, Schon LC. Effect of extracorporeal shock wave therapy on cultured tenocytes. *Foot Ankle Int.* 2009; 30(2):93–8.

35. Suzuki T, Nakamura Y, Moriya T, Sasano H. Effects of steroid

hormones on vascular functions. *Microsc Res Tech.* 2003; 60(1):76–84.

36. Smith AG, Kosygan K, Williams H, Newman RJ. Common extensor tendon rupture following corticosteroid injection for lateral tendinosis of the elbow. *Br J Sports Med.* 1999; 33(6):423–5.

37. Paoloni JA, Appleyard RC, Nelson J, Murrell GA. Topical glyceryl trinitrate application in the treatment of chronic supraspinatus tendinopathy: a randomized, double-blinded, placebo-controlled clinical trial. *Am J Sports Med.* 2005; 33(6):806–13.

38. Kane TP, Ismail M, Calder JD. Topical glyceryl trinitrate and non-insertional Achilles tendinopathy. A clinical and cellular investigation. *Am J Sports Med.* 2008; 36(6):1160–3.

39. Calder JD, Buttery L, Revell PA, Pearse M, Polak JM. Apoptosis: a significant cause of bone cell death in osteonecrosis of the femoral head. *J Bone Joint Surg Br.* 2004; 86(8):1209–13.

40. de Jonge S, de Vos RJ, Weir A, et al. One-year follow-up of platelet-rich plasma treatment in chronic Achilles tendinopathy: a double-blind randomized placebo-controlled trial. *Am J Sports Med.* 2011; 39(8):1623–9.

41. Sadoghi P, Rosso C, Valderrabano V, Leithner A, Vavken P. The role of platelets in the treatment of Achilles tendon injuries. *J Orthop Res.* 2013; 31(1):111–18.

42. Chan O, O'Dowd D, Padhiar N, et al. High volume image guided injections in chronic Achilles tendinopathy. *Disabil Rehabil.* 2008; 30(20–22):1697–708.

43. Maxwell NJ, Ryan MB, Taunton JE, Gillies JH, Wong AD. Sonographically guided intratendinous injection of hyperosmolar dextrose to treat chronic tendinosis of the Achilles tendon: a pilot study.

Am J Roentgenol. 2007; 189(4): W215–20.

44. Willberg L, Sunding K, Ohberg L, Forssblad M, Fahlström M, Alfredson H. Sclerosing injections to treat midportion Achilles tendinosis: a randomised controlled study evaluating two different concentrations of polidocanol. *Knee Surg Sports Traumatol Arthrosc.* 2008; 16(9):859–64.

45. Balasubramaniam P, Prathap K. The effect of injection of hydrocortisone into rabbit calcaneal tendons. *J Bone Joint Surg Br.* 1972; 54(4):729–34.

46. Robertson VJ, Baker KG. A review of therapeutic ultrasound: effectiveness studies. *Phys Ther.* 2001; 81(7):1339–50.

47. Den Hartog BD. Flexor hallucis longus transfer for chronic Achilles tendonosis. *Foot Ankle Int.* 2003; 24(3):233–7.

48. Paavola M, Kannus P, Orava S, Pasanen M, Järvinen M. Surgical treatment for chronic Achilles tendinopathy: a prospective seven month follow up study. *Br J Sports Med.* 2002; 36(3):178–82.

49. Nelen G, Martens M, Burssens A. Surgical treatment of chronic Achilles tendinitis. *Am J Sports Med.* 1989; 17(6):754–9.

50. Paavola M, Orava S, Leppilahti J, Kannus P, Järvinen M. Chronic Achilles tendon overuse injury: complications after surgical treatment, an analysis of 432 consecutive patients. *Am J Sports Med.* 2000; 28(1):77–82.

51. Maffulli N, Testa V, Capasso G, Bifulco G, Binfield PM. Results of percutaneous longitudinal tenotomy for Achilles tendinopathy in middle- and long-distance runners. *Am J Sports Med.* 1997; 25(6):835–40.

52. Steenstra F, van Dijk CN. Achilles tendoscopy. *Foot Ankle Clin.* 2006; 11(2):429–38.

53. Pearce CJ, Carmichael J, Calder JD. Achilles tendinoscopy and plantaris tendon release and division in the treatment of non-insertional Achilles tendinopathy. *Foot Ankle Surg.* 2012; 18(2):124–7.

54. Duthon VB, Lübbeke A, Duc SR, Stern R, Assal M. Noninsertional Achilles tendinopathy treated with gastrocnemius lengthening. *Foot Ankle Int.* 2011; 32(4):375–9.

55. Gurdezi S, Kohls-Gatzoulis J, Solan MC. Results of proximal medial gastrocnemius release for Achilles tendinopathy. *Foot Ankle Int.* 2013; 34(10):1364–9.

56. Johnson MD, Alvarez RG. Nonoperative management of retrocalcaneal pain with AFO and stretching regimen. *Foot Ankle Int.* 2012; 33(7):571–81.

57. Wiegerinck JI, Kerkhoffs GM, van Sterkenburg MN, Sierevelt IN, van Dijk CN. Treatment for insertional Achilles tendinopathy: a systematic review. *Knee Surg Sports Traumatol Arthrosc.* 2013; 21(6):1345–55.

58. Jonsson P, Alfredson H, Sunding K, Fahlström M, Cook J. New regimen for eccentric calf-muscle training in patients with chronic insertional Achilles tendinopathy: results of a pilot study. *Br J Sports Med.* 2008; 42(9):746–9.

59. Rasmussen S, Christensen M, Mathiesen I, Simonson O. Shockwave therapy for chronic Achilles tendinopathy: a double-blind, randomized clinical trial of efficacy. *Acta Orthop* 2008; 79(2):249–56.

60. Furia JP. High-energy extracorporeal shock wave therapy as a treatment for insertional Achilles tendinopathy. *Am J Sports Med.* 2006; 34(5):733–40.

61. Al-Abbad H, Simon JV. The effectiveness of extracorporeal shock wave therapy on chronic Achilles tendinopathy: a systematic review. *Foot Ankle Int.* 2013; 34(1):33–41.

62. Ryan M, Wong A, Taunton J. Favorable outcomes after sonographically guided intratendinous injection of hyperosmolar dextrose for chronic insertional and midportion Achilles tendinosis. *AJR Am J Roentgenol.* 2010; 194(4):1047–53.

63. Öhberg L, Alfredson H. Sclerosing therapy in chronic Achilles tendon insertional pain-results of a pilot study. *Knee Surg Sports Traumatol Arthrosc.* 2003; 11(5):339–43.

64. Monto RR. Platelet rich plasma treatment for chronic Achilles tendinosis. *Foot Ankle Int.* 2012; 33(5):379–85.

65. Shibuya N, Thorud JC, Humphers JM, Devall JM, Jupiter DC. Is percutaneous radiofrequency coblation for treatment of Achilles tendinosis safe and effective? *J Foot Ankle Surg.* 2012; 51(6):767–71.

66. Ortmann FW, McBryde AM. Endoscopic bony and soft-tissue decompression of the retrocalcaneal space for the treatment of Haglund deformity and retrocalcaneal bursitis. *Foot Ankle Int.* 2007; 28(2):149.

67. Zadek I. An operation for the cure of achillobursitis. *Am J Surg.* 1939; 43(2):542–6.

68. Calder JD, Saxby TS. Surgical treatment of insertional Achilles tendinosis. *Foot Ankle Int.* 2003; 24(2):119–21.

69. Pilson H, Brown P, Stitzel J, Scott A. Single-row versus double-row repair of the distal Achilles tendon: a biomechanical comparison. *J Foot Ankle Surg.* 2012; 51(6):762–6.

70. Nunley JA, Ruskin G, Horst F. Long-term clinical outcomes

following the central incision technique for insertional Achilles tendinopathy. *Foot Ankle Int.* 2011; 32(9):850–5.

71. Tashjian RZ, Hur J, Sullivan RJ, Campbell JT, Digiovanni CW. Flexor hallucis longus transfer for repair of chronic Achilles tendinopathy. *Foot Ankle Int.* 2003; 24(9):673–6.

72. Wagner E, Gould JS, Kneidel M, Fleisig GS, Fowler R. Technique and results of Achilles tendon detachment and reconstruction for insertional Achilles tendinosis. *Foot Ankle Int.* 2006; 27(9):677–84.

73. DeVries JG, Summerhays B, Guehlstorf DW. Surgical correction of Haglund's triad using complete detachment and reattachment of the Achilles tendon. *J Foot Ankle Surg.* 2009; 48(4):447–51.

Chapter 16

Rupture of the Tendo Achillis

Rebecca Kearney and Matthew Costa

Introduction

As the triceps surae descends toward the heel it enters a broad aponeurosis. From the musculotendinous junction, the tendon gradually becomes rounded, approximately 4 cm above the calcaneus, where the tendon fibers spiral laterally through 90°. The tendo Achillis (TA) connects the triceps surae distally to the middle one-third of the posterior surface of the calcaneus. This enables the forces produced by the triceps surae to be transmitted to the hindfoot[1].

Macroscopically the TA is composed of multiple fibers, which in turn are composed of fibrils; this structure enables the tendon to resist high tensile forces with minimal loss of energy and deformation (Figure 16.1). However, when considering mechanisms of injury and rehabilitation it is also important to consider that tendons are viscoelastic tissues. As such they display decreased stress with time under constant deformation (stress relaxation) and increased deformation with time under constant load (creep). Finally, the tension generated across the tendon is also dependent on the type of muscle contraction, eccentric loads producing the highest, followed by concentric, and finally isometric muscle contractions[2–5].

Epidemiology and Etiology

The TA is the most commonly ruptured tendon in the human body and the incidence is rising[6–7]. European figures show approximately 18 per 100 000 people per year sustain the injury[8]. The pattern of incidence displays a bimodal distribution according to age, with the first peak consisting of men aged 30 to 40 years and the second women aged 60 to 80 years[7–8].

From Figure 16.1 one would expect all TA ruptures, "macroscopic failures," to occur during forced and unexpected dorsiflexion of the ankle, for example in a fall or road traffic accident. Nevertheless, both of the cohorts outlined above most commonly sustain

TA ruptures below the threshold of macro-failure[9]. The explanation for this is widely accepted to be that ruptures occur on a background of preexisting abnormalities in the tendon resultant on tendinopathy[10].

People with tendinopathy can be symptomatic, experiencing pain on loading activities, or asymptomatic. In either case the tendon displays characteristic features of tendinopathy on a cellular level, these include decreased cellularity, abnormal matrix organization, neovascularization, and increased type III collagen[11]. These features occur as a result of an imbalance between the protective/regenerative functions within the tendon; MMPs are thought to have a key role but the exact mechanisms are not fully understood[11]. These changes in the tendon structure predispose to TA rupture.

While both the younger and older groups of patients sustain tendon ruptures on a background of tendinopathy, they have contrasting mechanisms of injury. The "typical" injury of a 30- to 40-year-old male is during participation in sport, and occurs during eccentric loading of the tendon, such as sprint starts, landing from a jump, and lunging – actions typical in football and racquet sports[7]. In contrast the "typical" injury for a 60- to 80-year-old female occurs during normal daily activities, such as climbing stairs[7]. With an aging population it is this second cohort that is largely responsible for the rising incidence[7].

Classification

Acute Musculotendinous Junction Rupture

Ruptures of the TA that occur in the region of the aponeurosis are classified as musculotendinous junction ruptures. As the name suggests, these injuries involve both the tendon and the muscle. Consequently, ruptures at this level may not have the characteristic palpable gap, but may have increased

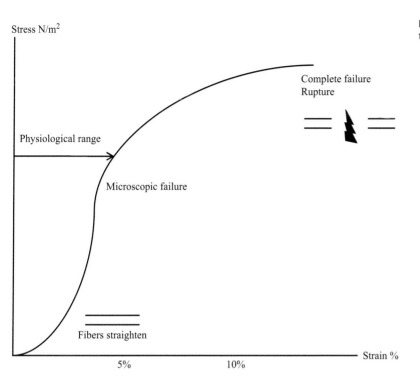

Figure 16.1 The stress–strain curve of tendon.

Stress N/m²

Complete failure
Rupture

Physiological range

Microscopic failure

Fibers straighten

5%   10%   Strain %

bruising and severe pain due to the muscle involvement[12].

Acute Midsubstance Rupture

Midsubstance TA ruptures are defined as those occurring approximately 2 to 6 cm above the tendon insertion, at the point where the tendon is most rounded and the tendon fibers spiral through 90°. In contrast to musculotendinous junction ruptures, midsubstance ruptures are characterized acutely by a defined palpable gap[13].

Acute Insertional Rupture

Insertional TA ruptures occur in the distal 2 cm of the tendon and involve the attachment to the os calcis. Insertional injuries may be more difficult to diagnose, as the palpable gap noted in midsubstance injuries is far less obvious. However, in the acute situation, the patient can usually localize the pain to the distal 2 cm of the tendon.

Chronic Rupture

There is a lack of consensus as to the exact time frame during which a ruptured TA is considered "chronic,"

although any presentation after the first two weeks is more difficult to diagnose[14]. The patient will usually describe an eccentric loading injury followed by pain and a limp, so the history can be more informative than the clinical findings. Rarely, the patient cannot recall an exact event.

Presentation

Acute Rupture

The patient typically presents with a sudden pain in the area of the TA[13]. The most common comment made by the patient during the subjective history is a feeling that they have been "kicked in the back of the leg"[13]. During the objective assessment physical findings include a positive "calf-squeeze test," decreased ankle plantar flexion strength, presence of a palpable gap, and increased ankle dorsiflexion on dorsiflexion of the ankle by the examiner[13]. The only published guidelines on this topic have been produced by the American Academy of Orthopaedic Surgeons (AAOS) who concluded that based on current literature there was strong evidence to support a diagnosis of a midsubstance TA rupture based on two of these four physical findings.

Chronic

The diagnosis of chronic rupture of the TA is more complicated than that of acute ruptures[14]. Firstly, the patient often does not present with pain and the clinical findings are more subtle. In contrast to the presentations of an acute rupture, this group of patients is more likely to report reduced power during activities that require greater "push-off" strength, for example walking upstairs or climbing a ladder. They may also report instability of the ankle, altered walking patterns, or a lack of balance.

A TA rupture that is not treated acutely will often "heal" with scar tissue filling the gap, therefore a palpable gap is rarely felt. Nevertheless on occasion palpation may identify a change in tissue consistency at the site of rupture. Additional physical findings will be largely due to the functional length of the healed tendon: commonly increased passive dorsiflexion, decreased plantar flexion power, and plantar flexion fatigue on repeated activity[14].

Investigations

For acute TA ruptures, the diagnosis is usually clinical, although US may be used to identify the exact location of the rupture or in cases where the diagnosis is uncertain. The routine use of US, MRI, or radiographs in the diagnosis of TA ruptures is not supported by the current literature[13]. Imaging in the diagnosis of chronic TA ruptures can provide confirmation, where uncertainty exists[14].

Dynamic US assessment has been suggested to be of value as a selection tool for which treatment pathways patients should be directed toward[15]. Such studies have used this assessment to determine if retracted torn tendon ends can be approximated on plantar flexion. However, the literature on this topic is not definitive, consequently dynamic US is not routine practice for most centers, as shown in a recent UK survey of current practice[16].

Non-Operative Treatment

Non-operative management options fall into three categories: plaster cast immobilization, combined plaster cast and functional bracing, or functional bracing alone[16]. There is no consensus in the literature regarding an exact protocol for these categories, so the following discussion is based on a recent survey of UK practice carried out by the British Orthopaedic Foot and Ankle Society[16].

Plaster cast immobilization involves an initial plaster cast applied in the "gravity equinus" position; this is the position that the foot naturally adopts when unsupported. Full equinus is avoided as this may lead to stiffness and gait abnormalities[17]. Once in plaster the patient is often advised not to bear weight; in fact the equinus position of the cast precludes normal weight bearing. Over a period of approximately two months, as the tendon heals, the position of the plaster cast is changed at two-week intervals until the foot is plantigrade. Patients gradually begin to introduce weight bearing. After two months the cast is removed and the patient is clinically evaluated for any signs that the tendon is not in continuity. As long as the TA heals in continuity the patient is referred for physiotherapy.

Plaster-cast immobilization combined with functional rehabilitation involves the same initial plaster-cast treatment; however, after approximately one month the cast is exchanged for a functional weight-bearing brace. The functional weightbearing brace often mimics the more traditional serial casting, with return of the foot to plantigrade, but using heel raise inserts inside the brace so that the foot plate of the brace is flat to the floor, despite the ankle being plantar flexed. There are two basic designs of brace: rigid rocker bottom style (Figure 16.2) or the more flexible carbon-fiber dorsal brace[18] (Figure 16.3). The flexible brace generally allows a greater range of movement than the more rigid designs. This increased, but controlled, movement has been suggested as being beneficial to tendon healing. Obviously increased flexibility must be weighed up against the possible complications of the tendon healing in a lengthened position or tendon re-rupture[18].

Functional bracing alone involves the immediate use of the brace, with either heel inserts or fixing the brace in plantar flexion and allowing immediate weight bearing. As with the two methods described above, the brace is worn for approximately two months, with the ankle gradually being moved to plantigrade, with the removal of heel inserts or adjustment of the brace settings.

This range of protocols exemplifies the complexity of this early rehabilitative intervention. For this reason synthesis of the literature comparing different rehabilitation protocols is a challenge[19]. Saleh et al. in 1992[20] were the first authors to publish a randomized

(a)

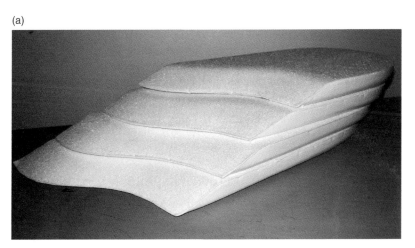

Figure 16.2 A rocker bottom style brace, for the treatment of tendo Achillis rupture. The wedges (**a**) are fitted into the boot (**b**), which is completed with an anterior shell. The wedges are then sequentially removed, bringing the foot to neutral.

(b)

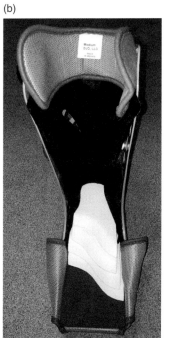

(c)

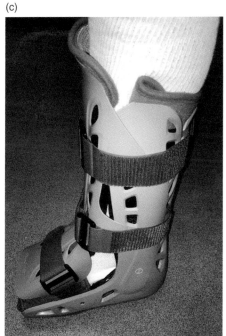

controlled trial (RCT) comparing different conservative management protocols. However, the trials in this area have been small, with no definitive conclusions, as outlined in the AAOS guidelines[13].

Surgical Treatment

Acute Musculotendinous Junction Rupture

As a result of the anatomy of the musculotendinous junction, there is a consensus that operative management is unnecessary – it is very difficult to achieve an adequate surgical repair when the muscle, which does not satisfactorily hold sutures, is involved[12].

Acute Midsubstance Rupture

Surgical management can be broadly divided into open or percutaneous techniques, with or without augmentation[8].

Open longitudinal repair involves an incision just medial to the TA, to avoid the sural nerve, and provides a clear view of the retracted tendon, which is sutured end to end[8]. Percutaneous repair techniques

285

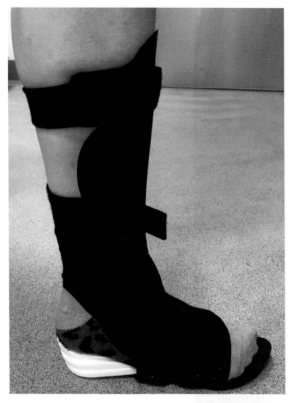

Figure 16.3 An alternative to the rocker bottom boot, a flexible dorsal brace that is worn with heel wedges, as shown in Figure 16.2a.

vary, but generally involve several small incisions on either side of the tendon rupture, with sutures then being blindly passed through the tendon ends, as first described by Ma and Griffith[21].

The first RCT to compare open with percutaneous techniques was published by Schroeder et al. in 1997[22], followed by three further RCTs in 2001, 2008, and 2009[23–25]. The main advantage of the percutaneous method is reduced infection and wound complication rates. However, this proposed advantage needs to be weighed against the risks, which include an increase in sural nerve injury[8]. With regard to functional outcomes, the literature remains inconclusive; nevertheless, the trend is toward percutaneous or "mini-open" surgical repair with transverse rather than longitudinal incisions.

The question as to whether to augment the repair remains. Autogenous options include primary augmentation with tendon transfer from the plantaris, peroneus, gracilis, flexor hallucis longus, flexor digitorum longus, free-grafts with hamstrings, or a gastrocnemius fascial turndown flap[14]. However, these all share the problem of donor-site morbidity. Synthetic grafts have therefore been suggested as an alternative, including polyester tape, Marlex® mesh, and carbon fiber, but as with all synthetic grafts there is always the risk of an immune response[28]. The most recent Cochrane Review identified only two RCTs[26–27], consequently augmentation has not been adopted in routine practice.

Acute Insertional Rupture

Surgical repair of these injuries is complicated by the fact that there is very little, if any, tendon distal to the rupture. While the proximal end of the tendon can usually be brought down to the heel using a standard tendon suture technique, the distal end is seldom amenable to this approach, and transosseous sutures or bone anchors are usually required to achieve satisfactory distal fixation. An alternative is to use the flexor hallucis longus either through a bone tunnel or attached to the bone with anchors, if the fixation is tenuous or the TA has retracted.

Chronic Rupture

There is no consensus as to when a TA rupture becomes chronic, although four weeks is often quoted. Pragmatically, if the gap is difficult to bridge alternative strategies to simple end-to-end suture will need to be considered. Kuwada classified ruptures according to the gap found at the time of surgery, recommending different operative techniques based on the size of the defect. However, as there is no evidence to suggest that such a classification system improves outcome, it is largely accepted that management should be on a case-by-case basis, with the technique used depending on surgical preference, clinical examination, and patient factors[14].

Following the decision to operate on a chronic rupture, the technique is liable to be open, rather than percutaneous, as it is necessary to mobilize the tendon ends to approximate them as closely as possible, or to introduce bridging material into the gap. After a year or so a neotendon often forms, which can closely resemble the normal tendon, although on close examination it will be noted to be homogeneous, without the fibrillar structure of the normal TA. Simple end-to-end repairs are often not possible, and therefore chronic tendon repairs frequently require augmentation. Local tissue, local tendons, and allografts can be used to reconstruct the tendon. The FHL tendon is convenient. It lies anterior to the TA, is the second strongest plantar flexor of the foot, after the gastrocnemius–soleus, and it works in phase with the triceps surae. The FHL can be harvested short, behind the ankle, or long, in the foot, depending on the length of graft required. There may be weakness of flexion of the interphalangeal joint of the great toe, although this is well tolerated. Transfer of the FHL has become the workhorse for reconstructing the late-presenting TA rupture in many surgical practices.

Physiotherapy

Following the removal of the brace or cast immobilization, patients are usually referred to physiotherapy[16]. There is no agreed physiotherapy protocol[16]. Therefore therapy is usually based upon the degree of healing, with loading activity increasing as the tendon matures and remodels.

Remodeling is thought to occur from approximately two to twelve months. The scar tissue is initially very stiff and relatively vulnerable to tensile loads and excessive stretching[29–30]. Therefore the early stages of rehabilitation concentrate on high-repetition, low-impact muscle training, using for example static bike work. Loading activities have been shown to stimulate fibroblast activity and type III collagen maturation[31–32] so it is important, even in the early stages after immobilization, that loading activities are initiated in a controlled and progressive manner. As the tendon healing progresses the tensile strength of the tendon increases, and the focus turns to gait rehabilitation and range of movement exercises.

Once the patient has regained a normal gait cycle and a good range of movement, the rehabilitation can progress to introduce loadbearing strengthening exercises that are focused predominantly on the disuse atrophy of the calf muscles. Strengthening exercises should aim to gradually increase the load through the tendon, first beginning with isometric and concentric exercises, before progressing to eccentric and finally plyometric/high-impact exercises such as sprinting, hopping, and jumping[16]. Although there is no consensus on the exact rehabilitation protocol, there is a consensus in the literature that any protocol should initially restrict impact activities and gradually introduce increasing load through the healing tendon.

Once a patient has completed a rehabilitation program of gradually increasing loads and more

demanding high-impact exercises they may want to consult on the issue of reintroduction to sport. A TA rupture does not preclude anyone returning to any specific sporting activity; however, the literature suggests that return to pre-injury sporting levels is unlikely as a result of weakness of plantar flexion. Furthermore, the risks of sustaining a re-rupture should be fully explained to include the risk profiles of different sporting activities, given the mechanism of injury associated with this condition. Once a decision to return to sports has been made, a physiotherapist will guide a patient through a program of sport-specific exercises. Patients can then progress from sport-specific exercises in a controlled rehabilitation environment to participating in full training activities, as appropriate. Finally, there is the transition to participating in sports on a competitive level, which again should be introduced gradually.

Complications and Outcome

Historically, re-rupture is the major concern following both operative and non-operative management of TA rupture. However, the more recent literature has investigated functional recovery of the patient through either patient-reported or objective functional outcome measurements[33].

Re-rupture at the musculotendinous junction is rare. This is thought to be because the blood supply, and therefore the healing process, is better than that in the midsubstance of the tendon.

A recent review[8] published data on complication rates among operatively and non-operatively managed midsubstance TA ruptures. This suggested a 5% incidence of re-rupture among those managed with surgery, as opposed to 12% in those managed non-operatively. However, these results are confounded to some degree by the rehabilitation protocols; patients having surgical repair traditionally also have accelerated rehabilitation regimes, which may per se reduce the incidence of re-rupture.

The other major concern following a TA rupture is the risk of deep vein thrombosis (DVT) and pulmonary embolism (PE). This is an area of great contention, with variation in incidence varying hugely. An incidence of symptomatic DVT of 0.43% and symptomatic PE of 0.34% was reported in 2011[34]. Incidences of DVT up to 34% have been reported using color Doppler, although of this 34%, 84% were below the knee. The issue as to whether to use chemoprophylaxis for thromboembolism is similarly controversial. Surprisingly the only RCT in this area found that the use of dalteparin did not affect the incidence of DVT[35].

Complications other than re-rupture and DVT/PE are common. When the authors of the Cochrane Review evaluated all complications, except re-rupture, they found an incidence of 29% complications among surgically managed patients and 8% in non-operatively managed patients. These complications were mainly scar adhesion, infection, wound healing problems, and sural nerve injury.

Therefore it is clear that when considering whether a patient with a TA rupture should be treated operatively, or non-operatively, the overall risk profile of complications in each patient needs careful balancing. The risk of re-rupture needs to be weighed against the risk of, the mainly soft tissue, complications of surgery.

Chronic Rupture Complications

Due to the range of presentations of this patient group, extrapolating case study and case series data of complication profiles is problematic. Although the incidence of specific complications is less clear, the nature of complications reported is the same as for acute midsubstance presentations.

Functional Recovery Following a Rupture

The literature indicates that patients have long-term functional deficits following TA rupture[17]. These have been assessed using physical measures such as single leg heel raises, calf muscle strength testing, and gait analysis[36]. Examples in the literature using gait analysis show a decrease in forefoot pressures of around 33%, with a concomitant increase of 40% in heel pressures six months after injury[17]. Further examples measuring calf circumference and calf muscle strength one year after injury have shown a decrease of 1.4 cm in calf circumference and a loss of 20% plantar flexion compared to the unaffected limb[39].

Functional recovery can also be assessed using patient-reported outcome measures. The first such measure was introduced in 1994 by the American Orthopaedic Foot and Ankle Society (AOFAS) who published the design and development of a rating system for ankle hindfoot pathologies. A recent review in this area has subsequently identified a

further 16 such measures published in the literature[36]. Of these only one measure, the Achilles Tendon Rupture Score (ATRS), has been developed using recognized methodology for outcome measure development, as opposed to expert opinion alone. The ATRS is a series of ten questions asking patients to score their limitations/symptoms from 0 to 10. The questions range from "Are you limited due to decreased strength in the calf/Achilles tendon/foot?" to "Are you limited in performing hard physical labour?"

Discussion Points

This chapter has outlined the management options following a TA rupture. With regard to the most common midsubstance injuries, there are three key decisions to be made:

- whether to operate or not
- if operating, which operation to perform – open or minimally invasive?
- the choice of rehabilitation protocol.

In 1981, the first RCT comparing operative with non-operative treatment was published. This was followed by a long line of RCTs addressing the same question, which have been collated and meta-analyzed by a Cochrane Review group[8]. Although the authors of this Review have presented pooled results, with particular regard to the incidence of complications, the choice of operative or non-operative management is confounded by differences in the choice of early rehabilitation. The results are therefore difficult to interpret in the context of the increasing use of early weight bearing and accelerated mobilization in recently published operative versus non-operative studies in 2008, 2010, and 2011[37-40].

Although associated with a lower risk of re-rupture in the current literature, patients undergoing operative treatment have a higher incidence of other complications, mostly associated with wound healing. Proponents of percutaneous repair argue that the evidence would clearly favor operative management if open repairs were excluded. However, this presumes that the rate of re-rupture is the same in percutaneous repair and open repair, and also ignores the residual confounding associated with the choice of early rehabilitation. Conversely, proponents of open repair point out that sural nerve injuries occur more commonly in percutaneous repair. Therefore despite the relatively large number of trials in this area, there is still debate regarding the best form of surgery, even when the decision has been made to operate.

Regarding rehabilitation method, it has been shown among patients who have had operative management that early weight bearing, functional brace protocols result in lower re-rupture rates than those reported in the Cochrane Review, i.e., lower than plaster-cast treatment. This is to the extent that the AAOS guidelines state that early weight bearing is best practice[13]. However, among non-operatively managed patients the literature is confined to only two RCTs, published in 1992[20] and 2002[41]. These suggested that there was a reduced re-rupture rate of 2.4% in the functional bracing group, compared with 12.2% in the casting group. This level of re-rupture rate combined with an already low risk profile of other complications may then indicate that surgery is redundant. However, given the small numbers and limited quality of these studies the results are far from conclusive, but certainly indicative of an area for further research.

Thus there are several interacting factors to consider when a patient presents with a rupture of their TA including the location of the rupture, the time since the event, whether to operate or not, and what type of operation or rehabilitation to use. There is considerable uncertainty in the field that upcoming and ongoing registered clinical trials will address. In the meantime, surgeons can only present the options, including associated risk profiles and likely functional outcomes, and allow their patients to make an informed decision regarding their management.

Key Points

- The incidence of TA rupture is approximately 18 per 100 000 and is increasing in the Western world.
- TA rupture is associated with underlying tendinopathy, even in younger patients.
- Clinical tests are usually sufficient to make the diagnosis in acute presentations.
- Dynamic US is the optimal imaging technique in cases of uncertainty and in late presentations.
- Patients choosing surgery have a lower rate of re-rupture but higher risk of wound-healing complications, although the evidence base is confounded by the choice of early rehabilitation.
- Early weight bearing in a functional brace is recommended following operative repair, but the optimal rehabilitation strategy following non-operative management is still to be determined.

References

1. Standring S. *Gray's Anatomy*. 39th edn. (London: Elsevier, Churchill Livingstone; 2005).

2. Evans NA, Stanish WD. The basic science of tendon injuries. *Curr Orthop.* 2000; 14(6):403–12.

3. Maganaris CN, Narici MV, Maffulli N. Biomechanics of the Achilles tendon. *Disabil Rehabil.* 2008; 30(20–22):1542–7.

4. Wang JH, Iosifidis MI, Fu FH. Biomechanical basis for tendinopathy. *Clin Orthop Rel Res.* 2006; 464:320–32.

5. Fenwick SA, Hazleman BL, Riley GP. The vasculature and its role in the damaged and healing tendon. *Arthritis Res.* 2002; 4(4):252–60.

6. Leppilahti J, Puranen J, Orava S. Incidence of Achilles tendon rupture. *Acta Orthop Scand.* 1996; 67(3):277–9.

7. Houshian S, Tscherning T, Riegels-Nielsen P. The epidemiology of Achilles tendon rupture in a Danish county. *Injury.* 1998; 29(9):651–4.

8. Jones MP, Khan RJ, Carey Smith RL. Surgical interventions for treating acute Achilles tendon rupture: key findings from a recent Cochrane review. *J Bone Joint Surg Am.* 2012; 94(12):e88.

9. Maffulli N. Rupture of the Achilles tendon. *J Bone Joint Surg Am.* 1999; 81(7):1019–36.

10. Tallon C, Maffulli N, Ewen SW. Ruptured Achilles tendons are significantly more degenerated than tendinopathic tendons. *Med Sci Sports Exerc.* 2001; 33(12):1983–90.

11. Riley G. Tendinopathy: from basic science to treatment. *Nat Clin Pract Rheumatol.* 2008; 4(2):82–9.

12. Ahmad J, Repka M, Raikin SM. Treatment of myotendinous Achilles ruptures. *Foot Ankle Int.* 2013; 34(8):1074–8.

13. AAOS. The diagnosis and treatment of acute Achilles tendon rupture: guideline and evidence report [Online]. (www.aaos.org/research/guidelines/atrguideline.pdf). First edn 2009.

14. Maffulli N, Ajis A. Management of chronic ruptures of the Achilles tendon. *J Bone Joint Surg Am.* 2008; 90(6):1348–60.

15. Hutchison AM, Topliss C, Beard D, Evans RM, Williams P. The treatment of a rupture of the Achilles tendon using a dedicated management programme. *Bone Joint J.* 2015; 97-B(4):510-5.

16. Kearney RS, Parsons N, Underwood M, Costa ML. Achilles tendon rupture rehabilitation: a mixed methods

investigation of current practice among orthopaedic surgeons in the United Kingdom. *Bone Joint Res.* 2015; 4(4):65–9.

17. Costa ML, Kay D, Donell ST. Gait abnormalities following rupture of the tendo Achillis: a pedobarographic assessment. *J Bone Joint Surg Br.* 2005; 87(8):1085–8.

18. Kearney RS, Lamb SE, Achten J, Parsons NR, Costa ML. In-shoe plantar pressures within ankle-foot orthoses: implications for the management of Achilles tendon ruptures. *Am J Sports Med.* 2011; 39(12):2679–85

19. Kearney RS, McGuinness KR, Achten J, Costa ML. A systematic review of early rehabilitation methods following a rupture of the Achilles tendon. *Physiotherapy.* 2012; 98(1):24–32.

20. Saleh M, Marshall PD, Senior R, MacFarlane A. The Sheffield splint for controlled early mobilisation after rupture of the calcaneal tendon. A prospective, randomised comparison with plaster treatment. *J Bone Joint Surg Br.* 1992; 74(2):206–9.

21. Ma GW, Griffith TG. Percutaneous repair of acute closed ruptured Achilles tendon: a new technique. *Clin Orthop Relat Res.* 1977;128:247–55.

22. Schroeder L, Lehmann M, Steinbrueck. Treatment of acute Achilles tendon ruptures: open vs. percutaneous repair vs. conservative treatment. *Orth Trans.* 1997; 21:1228.

23. Lim J, Dalal R, Waseem M. Percutaneous vs. open repair of the ruptured Achilles tendon: a prospective randomized controlled study. *Foot Ankle Int.* 2001; 22(7):559–68.

24. Gigante A, Moschini A, Verdenelli A, Del Torto M, Ulisse S, de Palma L. Open versus percutaneous repair in the treatment of acute Achilles tendon rupture: a randomized prospective study. *Knee Surg Sports Traumatol Arthrosc.* 2008; 16(2):204–9.

25. Aktas S, Kocaoglu B. Open versus minimal invasive repair with Achillon device. *Foot Ankle Int.* 2009; 30(5):391–7.

26. Pajala A, Kangas J, Siira P, Ohtonen P, Leppilahti J. Augmented compared with nonaugmented surgical repair of a fresh total Achilles tendon rupture. A prospective randomized study. *J Bone Joint Surg Am.* 2009; 91(5):1092–100.

27. Aktas S, Kocaoglu B, Nalbantoglu U, Seyhan M, Guven O. End-to-end versus augmented repair in the treatment of acute Achilles tendon ruptures. *J Foot Ankle Surg.* 2007; 46(5):336–40.

28. Kearney RS, Costa ML. Collagen-matrix allograft augmentation of bilateral rupture of the achilles tendon. *Foot Ankle Int.* 2010; 31(6):556–9.

29. Sharma P, Maffulli N. Tendon injury and tendinopathy: healing and repair. *J Bone Joint Surg Am.* 2005; 87(1):187–202.

30. Woo SL, Hildebrand K, Watanabe N, Fenwick JA, Papageorgiou CD, Wang JH. Tissue engineering of ligament and tendon healing. *Clin Orthop Rel Res.* 1999; 457(367 Suppl):S312–2S3.

31. Enwemeka CS. Functional loading augments the initial tensile strength and energy absorption capacity of regenerating rabbit Achilles tendons. *Am J Phys Med Rehabil.* 1992; 71(1):31–8.

32. Enwemeka CS, Spielholz NI, Nelson AJ. The effect of early functional activities on experimentally tenotomized Achilles tendons in rats. *Am J Phys Med Rehabil.* 1988; 67(6):264–9.

33. Kearney RS, Costa ML. Current concepts in the rehabilitation of an acute rupture of the tendo Achillis. *J Bone Joint Surg Br.* 2012; 94(1):28–31.

34. Patel A, Ogawa B, Charlton T, Thordarson D. Incidence of deep vein thrombosis and pulmonary embolism after Achilles tendon rupture. *Clin Orthop Relat Res.* 2012; 470(1):270–4.

35. Lapidus LJ, Rosfors S, Ponzer S, et al. Prolonged thromboprophylaxis with dalteparin after surgical treatment of Achilles tendon rupture: a randomized, placebo-controlled study. *J Orthop Trauma.* 2007; 21(1):52–7.

36. Kearney R, Achten J, Plant C, Lamb S. A systematic review of patient reported outcome measures used to assess Achilles tendon rupture management: what's being used and should we be using it? *Br J Sports Med.* 2012; 46(16):1102–9.

37. Nistor L. Surgical and non-surgical treatment of Achilles tendon rupture. A prospective randomized study. *J Bone Joint Surg Am.* 1981; 63(3):394–9.

38. Metz R, Verleisdonk E-JMM, van der Heijden GJMG, et al. Acute Achilles tendon rupture: minimally invasive surgery versus nonoperative treatment with immediate full weightbearing – a randomized controlled trial. *Am J Sports Med.* 2008; 36(9):1688–94.

39. Willits K, Amendola A, Bryant D, et al. Operative versus nonoperative treatment of acute Achilles tendon ruptures: a multicenter randomized trial using accelerated functional rehabilitation. *J Bone Joint Surg Am.* 2010; 92(17):2767–75.

40. Kearney RS, Achten J, Parsons NR, Costa ML. The comprehensive cohort model in a pilot trial in orthopaedic trauma. *BMC Med Res Methodol.* 2011; 11(1):39.

41. Petersen OF, Nielsen MB, Jensen KH, Solgaard S. Randomized comparison of CAM walker and light-weight plaster cast in the treatment of first-time Achilles tendon rupture. *Ugeskr Laeger.* 2002; 164(33):3852–5.

Benign Tumors of the Foot and Ankle

Lee Parker, Nicholas Cullen, Panagiotis D. Gikas, Paul O'Donnell, and Dishan Singh

Introduction

The foot and ankle are relatively common sites for tumors. The lack of muscle coverage in this region results in a tendency toward early presentation[1]. Foot and ankle tumors are more likely to be benign than malignant: one large series from a general foot and ankle clinic reported that 16% of all tumors were malignant[2]. Even in a tertiary referral center, we have found that most tumors of the foot and ankle are benign. Osteochondroma is the commonest benign bone lesion and xanthomatous and giant cell-rich tumors are the most frequently encountered benign soft tissue lesions[3].

Benign and malignant tumors in the foot and ankle can be clinically indistinguishable and therefore there is a risk of incomplete surgical excision if the preoperative planning is poor[4]. If there is a suspicion of a malignant bone or soft tissue tumor from the history, examination, and basic imaging, then prompt referral to a regional musculoskeletal tumor service is advised, so that appropriate imaging, biopsy, and staging can be performed and, once accurate diagnosis had been obtained, definitive management[5].

This chapter focuses on the commonly encountered benign foot and ankle tumors and their management.

Clinical Evaluation

Tumors in the foot and ankle can be difficult to accurately diagnose clinically. In one series only 58 out of 101 tumors in the foot were accurately diagnosed prior to surgery[6]. A thorough patient history and clinical examination are important and can help guide imaging. A malignant tumor may be painless and very small, thus these features should never be used alone to distinguish between benign and malignant lesions.

Often the patient will present early with a painless mass that interferes with footwear or walking. If there

is a history of pain, the timing, duration, severity, and response to analgesia are important. Osteoid osteomas classically present with nocturnal pain, relieved by NSAIDs.

Although foot and ankle tumors tend to be primary in origin, it is important to determine whether there has been previous exposure to ionizing radiation or chemicals, both of which predispose to development of a soft tissue sarcoma. As tumors grow, pressure effects on nerves may lead to numbness. Tendon subluxation, tendon rupture, and loss of joint motion are also occasional presentations. A family history may reveal a familial tendency to tumors, such as multiple hereditary exostoses.

Trauma and infection, especially after foreign travel, should be considered in the differential diagnosis. Rarely, tumors develop as the result of chronic infection.

The site, size, and consistency of the tumor should be recorded. Fluctuance, transillumination, and a smooth defined surface suggest a ganglion, which may move with tendon motion. Any tethering, either deeply or to skin, should be noted. The examination of a foot or ankle tumor should also include an assessment of joint, tendon, and neurovascular function.

Imaging

Weightbearing AP and lateral radiographs with an oblique view are obtained[7] for both osseous and non-osseous lesions. Tumor location can be an important predictor of the histological type, for example chondroblastomas have a tendency to be epiphyseal/subarticular. The radiolucency or radio-opacity of an osseous lesion is noted. Osseous lesions can be described in terms of their "zone of transition." This defines the interface between normal and abnormal bone. A lesion with a narrow zone of transition often shows "geographic" bone destruction and in many circumstances is benign. When the transition between normal and abnormal bone is less obvious or "wide," the growth rate is likely to be greater, which indicates a more aggressive, possibly malignant, bone tumor[8]. It is also necessary to establish what effect the osseous lesion is having on the bone: is there erosion or "scalloping" of the endosteum, or pathological fracture? Analyze what the bone is doing in response to the lesion: is there periosteal new bone formation? If there is a geographic lesion with surrounding sclerosis as the only major host-bone reaction, the lesion is more likely to be slow growing and benign. Calcification in the soft tissues may be observed on x-rays of soft tissue lesions; extra-osseous extension (and most bone lesions) should be further evaluated with MRI scanning.

Ultrasound is the investigation of choice for differentiating solid from cystic soft tissue tumors. It also shows the vascularity of masses and is particularly useful for superficial lesions. It is ideal for investigating suspected lipomas, hemangiomas, and nerve sheath tumors. It showed a sensitivity of 94.1% and a specificity of 99.7% in identifying malignant, superficial musculoskeletal tumors in a large case series[9]. Ultrasound is a dynamic investigation and allows an appreciation of the tumor relationship to the surrounding tendons and nerves. It can also guide the aspiration of simple ganglia.

Deep and solid soft tissue lesions should be further evaluated with MRI scanning, which gives useful information about the presence or absence of marrow infiltration, multifocal tumors, for example "skip" lesions in osteosarcoma, and the extent of the "reactive zone" around the tumor. The extent of this reactive zone is especially useful in planning resection margins and identifying very "active" tumors, such as osteoid osteomas.

Computed tomography scanning remains an alternative cross-sectional imaging technique, which provides greater osseous detail, but less tissue-specific information, and less accurate evaluation of extra-osseous extent and neurovascular involvement. It is occasionally needed for local tumor staging if there are contraindications to MRI. CT angiography can also help reveal vascular encasement by a tumor.

Technetium bone scanning assesses bone turnover and blood supply, and can be useful for osteoid osteomas and bone metastases. SPECT-CT can add further anatomic detail, which is typically lacking in standard SPECT.

Anatomical Factors

The foot and ankle are unique in having a great number of articular surfaces, which serve as barriers to tumor extension. The epiphyses, however, are relatively thin with multiple vascular channels through which tumor extension into the soft tissues is possible. Within the forefoot, fascial compartments between the rays provide a relative barrier to tumor extension, although the lack of thick soft tissue coverage means bone tumors can easily spread into the soft tissues[10].

Biopsy

Most tumors in bone and soft tissue require confirmation of histological diagnosis prior to surgery, and in our unit the vast majority undergo imaging-guided needle biopsy. On the relatively infrequent occasions when imaging appearances are diagnostic, excision biopsy will be performed and is sufficient treatment for benign or low-grade malignant lesions, aiming to remove the tumor and its reactive zone, avoiding potential tumor seeding to uninvolved tissue. However, poorly planned and executed biopsy may complicate subsequent limb-salvage surgery and therefore it is recommended that biopsy be performed in the tumor center, or the excision by the surgeon ultimately tasked with resecting and managing the tumor[11].

The approach to a potentially malignant lesion requires meticulous planning at a multidisciplinary musculoskeletal tumor center. The planning involves a tumor surgeon, musculoskeletal radiologist, pathologist, and oncologist.

Tumor Staging

Staging provides the basis for further surgical and oncological management. Staging is determined by the clinical, radiological, and histological features. For benign tumors of bone and soft tissue the staging system is[12]:

Stage 1	A latent lesion or a lesion with a tendency to spontaneously heal
Stage 2	An active lesion showing a tendency to continued growth with less mature histological appearance
Stage 3	A locally aggressive, histologically immature lesion with progressive growth, not confined by the usual anatomical barriers such as growth plates

Surgical Margins

Surgical margins are defined as follows[13]:

Intralesional	The lesion is removed with its margin passing through the reactive tumor zone
Marginal	The lesion is removed with the resection margin passing just outside the reactive zone with the possibility of leaving microscopic tumor deposits behind
Wide	The lesion with a surrounding cuff of normal tissue is removed without breaching the reactive zone
Radical	The lesion and its entire anatomical compartment is removed

The planned choice of margin depends on:

- the staging of the tumor
- its location
- whether or not it involves neurovascular structures or joint surfaces
- the anticipated functional deficit after tumor removal.

For soft tissue benign stage 1 and 2 lesions, a wide excision is ideal, providing this will not affect functional outcome, in which case marginal excision may be acceptable. For benign stage 3 lesions, a wide surgical margin is obligatory. If there is extensive involvement of a single metatarsal or toe, a ray amputation may be preferred[10].

Benign Soft Tissue Tumors of the Foot and Ankle

Fibrous Tumors

Plantar Fibromas and Fibromatosis

These lesions are superficial fibroblastic proliferations – other common examples are Dupuytren's and Peyronie's disease. The fibromatoses include isolated plantar fibroma, juvenile aponeurotic fibroma, and deep (desmoid-type) fibromatosis[14]. Characteristically occurring along the medial border of the plantar fascia, either singly or multiply, they can be debilitating and painful due to their location under the medial longitudinal arch (Figure 17.1). They often become noticeable in adolescence, grow to 2 to 3 cm and then become indolent. Calcification within a more dorsally located fibroma is suggestive of a juvenile aponeurotic fibroma[15]. Desmoid-type fibromatosis can also occur in the foot and may be larger and more aggressive, with infiltration into the dermis, between the web-spaces and neurovascular structures.

(a)

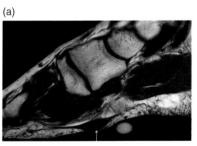

(b)

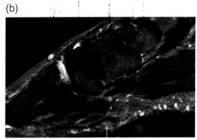

(c)

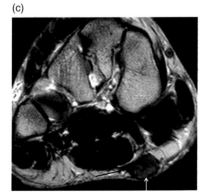

Figure 17.1 Plantar fibroma, M/31y. (a) Sagittal T1 and (b) STIR MRI of right foot. Small, elliptical mass arising from the plantar fascia at TMT joint level (white arrows). The mass is hypointense on fluid-sensitive sequences, in keeping with its fibrous content. (c) Coronal T2 MRI: lobular hypointense fibroma (white arrow) arises from the central band of the fascia (black arrow).

In those lesions that demonstrate rapid growth, a soft tissue sarcoma is the differential diagnosis and so the lesion should always be biopsied.

The mainstay of treatment of plantar fibromas should be non-operative with footwear modification, offloading insoles, and patient reassurance. There are isolated reports of success with intralesional steroid injections[16].

Surgery should be reserved for painful lesions unresponsive to orthotic management or, occasionally, when there is evidence of neurovascular infiltration by aggressive fibromatosis. Wide excision of the fibromatosis and its adjacent fascia is recommended, paying close attention so that the skin incision is situated away from the loadbearing area of the foot[17]. Despite this, attempted surgical resection may be incomplete, leading to rapid local recurrence with additional scarring and pain. Dermofasciectomy with skin grafting has been performed for recurrent plantar fibromatosis, particularly when there is skin infiltration, but painful neuroma formation seems to be more disabling than the original fibromatosis[18].

Vascular Tumors

Glomus tumor

These rare tumors arise from a neuroarterial structure called the "glomus body," which is thought to be responsible for thermoregulatory control, particularly in the digits[19]. They present as bright-red to bluish masses, and can occur beneath the nail. They are usually too small to palpate but are very painful, and especially tender to cold and direct pressure[20]. Radiographs may demonstrate a distal phalangeal bone erosion, but MRI is the investigation of choice. MRI shows a well circumscribed mass with a low signal on T1- and a high signal on T2-weighted images[21]. Treatment is by excision, occasionally necessitating subungual resection. Subungual melanoma should always be considered and the lesion should always be sent for histological analysis.

Hemangioma

Many adult hemangiomas are more accurately classified as "malformations," rather than neoplasms. The malformations arise from congenitally dysplastic vessels, often unappreciated at birth, which slowly enlarge and can cause pain and limb overgrowth and do not regress. The malformations may be high flow (arteriovenous malformations and fistulae) or low flow (venous, lymphatic, capillary)[22].

Infantile hemangioma is a separate entity presenting in the first few weeks of life as a slowly enlarging benign vascular tumor, which then regresses.

These tumors can occur anywhere in the body, but are rare in the foot and ankle. In one review of 83 soft tissue tumors of the foot, only one hemangioma was found[23]. They can be associated with gigantism of the limb and equinus deformities of the ankle if they are intramuscular[24].

Multiple hemangiomata should alert one to the possibility of an accompanying syndrome (Klippel–Trenaunay, Sturge–Weber, Maffucci, Proteus). Plain x-rays may show a soft tissue mass with multiple phleboliths. Ultrasound demonstrates low or no flow on Doppler, with tumor compressibility useful to help differentiate from sarcomas. On MRI, hyperintense vascular channels interspersed between the solid soft tissue matrix are seen on T2-weighted images, with fluid–fluid levels in areas of static blood and signal voids due to phleboliths[25].

Hemangiomata in isolation do not usually require surgical excision and are best managed with compression hosiery and camouflage make-up of the skin for cosmesis. The infiltrative nature of hemangiomata means they are difficult to separate from normal tissue, often prompting sacrifice of uninvolved tissue and risking incomplete excision. The literature is made up of case reports of successful resection of hemangiomata in the foot[26–27]. If surgical excision is contemplated for a large hemangioma, preoperative embolization may be required in high flow-lesions. Ethanol sclerotherapy has been used with some success to reduce pain and induce lesion involution in symptomatic malformations. Sclerotherapy would be advocated over surgery in most cases[28].

Neural Tumors

Neurilemmoma and Neurofibroma

Neurilemmomas are also known as schwannomas. They are benign tumors of the peripheral nerve sheath. The lesions are usually solitary, well-encapsulated, and situated on the surface of the nerve. In contrast, a neurofibroma is a spindle cell tumor, which is more permeative and less easy to separate from the surrounding normal nerve fibers. It can be solitary or multiple in association with neurofibromatosis[29]. Neurilemmoma in the foot is rare. In one series of 303 neurilemmomas, none were located in the foot[30].

The usual mode of presentation is of a painful nodule with a positive Tinel sign in the nerve distribution. Neural tumors affecting the tibial or plantar nerves around or distal to the tarsal tunnel can mimic plantar fasciitis. The patient presents with deep-seated heel pain without the palpable nodule or Tinel sign, and this can be easily misdiagnosed as plantar fasciitis[31].

Magnetic resonance imaging is the investigation of choice for neurilemmomas and neurofibromas. MRI can help differentiate a neurofibroma within the nerve from a neurilemmoma on the nerve surface, compressing and displacing the nerve[32]. The MRI scan may also demonstrate the target-pattern of central fibrocollagenous (Antoni A) and peripheral myxoid (Antoni B) tissue characteristic of a benign nerve sheath tumor (Figure 17.2)[33].

Neurilemmomas are well encapsulated and can usually be removed from the nerve without damaging the adjacent nerve fibers. Local recurrence and malignant transformation are rare. In contrast, the lack of a clear plane of dissection around a neurofibroma means the affected section of nerve often requires sacrificing.

Lipomatous Tumors

Although lipomas are one of the most commonly encountered benign soft tissue tumors, they are relatively rare in the foot owing to the scarcity of adipose tissue. In a large series of 67 000 tumors and other lesions of the foot, lipomas only constituted 0.24%[34].

Lipomas are subclassified depending on their morphological features and non-lipomatous elements. Thus there are conventional lipomas, fibrolipomas, angiolipomas, spindle-cell lipomas, myelolipomas, and pleomorphic lipomas. Conventional lipomas are soft, mobile, and painless and are treated by simple marginal excision[35]. Angiolipomas are frequently painful. Atypical presentations of lipoma variants include pain from tibial nerve compression within the tarsal tunnel[36].

Subcutaneous lipomas are usually easy to diagnose. Deeper intramuscular, parosteal, or intraosseous lipomas often require imaging evaluation. Plain radiography may show large lipomas as areas of relative radiolucency compared to the surrounding tissue. Calcification is present in about 11% of lipomas. Ultrasound and MRI scanning are usually diagnostic.

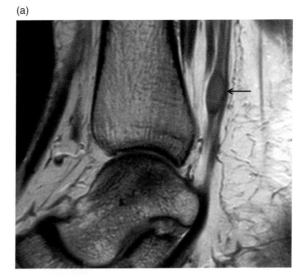

(a)

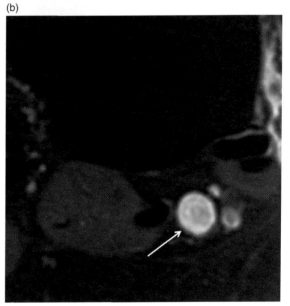

(b)

Figure 17.2 (**a**) Neurofibroma, F/38y. Sagittal PD MRI shows an elliptical intraneural mass in the tibial nerve proximal to the ankle (arrow). (**b**) Axial PD fat saturated MRI shows the mass (arrow) has a slightly eccentric relation to the nerve and a faint target sign (relatively low signal center, hyperintense periphery), suggesting a benign nerve sheath tumor.

On MRI, incomplete suppression of signal on fat-suppressed sequences, enhancing thick nodular septa, and focal non-lipomatous areas should raise the possibility of an atypical lipomatous tumor/lipoma-like well-differentiated liposarcoma, but there is overlap in the imaging of these benign and malignant fatty lesions[37].

(b)

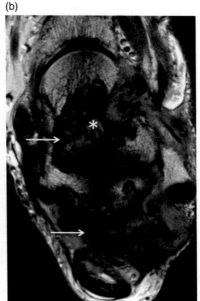

(a)

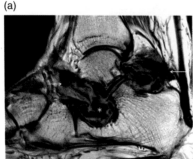

Figure 17.3 Tenosynovial giant cell tumor/pigmented villonodular synovitis, F/56y. (**a**) Sagittal and (**b**) axial proton density (PD) MRI of the left hindfoot showing a hypointense tumor in the posterior subtalar joint (arrows), anteriorly extending into the sinus tarsi. There is deep erosion of the calcaneum (*).

Synovial Tumors

Tenosynovial Giant Cell Tumor

Giant cells are found in many bone and soft tissue lesions. Tenosynovial giant cell tumor (giant cell tumor of the tendon sheath) arises in synovial spaces (joint, bursa, or tendon sheath) and is classified as either *localized* (also known as nodular tenosynovitis or giant cell tumor of the tendon sheath – localized type, GCT-LT) or *diffuse* (also known as pigmented villonodular synovitis/tenosynovitis or diffuse-type giant cell tumor – GCT-DT)[38].

Giant cell tumor of the tendon sheath typically presents with a focal, slow-growing, painless nodular swelling in the foot, adjacent to a small joint or tendon. It can produce pain as a result of compressive effects. GCT-DT develops from the synovial lining of joints and typically presents with painful or painless swelling and recurrent hemarthrosis.

Plain radiographs of GCT only rarely show soft tissue calcification adjacent to a small joint or tendon but may show bone erosion. MRI evaluation characteristically identifies a hemosiderin-laden soft tissue matrix of low signal intensity on T2-weighted images (exaggerated on T2 gradient echo (T2*) images), helping to differentiate tenosynovial GCT from other soft tissue tumors. Biopsy of both localized and diffuse GCT is advised: periarticular malignancies such as synovial, clear cell, and epithelioid sarcoma can certainly mimic localized GCT. Wide excision is the treatment of choice as intralesional resection leads to a high rate of local recurrence[39].

GCT-DT (Figure 17.3) arises from the synovial lining of joints but may be intra- or extra-articular. Joint aspiration of a brownish, hemosiderin-laden fluid is diagnostic, but imaging with plain radiography and MRI is necessary to establish whether the recurrent hemarthroses have caused joint erosions and the extent of the disease. GCT-DT can extend for long distances along tendon sheaths. Meticulous surgical planning is advised – ideally in a multidisciplinary setting since the recurrence rates with incomplete excision of the disease are high.

Although arthroscopic synovectomy is occasionally possible, the extent of disease often precludes complete excision. Therefore arthrotomy, if necessary using multiple approaches, is the treatment of choice. Radiosynovectomy with yttrium-90 has been utilized as an adjunct after subtotal surgical synovectomy in the knee. In the ankle it has resulted in severe complications, including full thickness skin necrosis, and is therefore not recommended[40].

Synovial Chondromatosis

Synovial chondromatosis is a process of chondral metaplasia within the synovium producing multiple cartilaginous bodies, which become detached and lie loose in the ankle joint. They can cause pain, locking, instability, or a palpable mass.

(a)

(b)

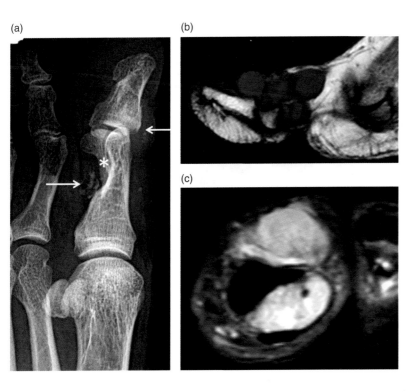

(c)

Figure 17.4 (**a**) Synovial chondromatosis in the left great toe, F/56y. Oblique radiograph shows pressure erosion of the plantar surface of the proximal phalanx distally (*) and calcified masses on the dorsal and plantar aspects of the toe, arising from the interphalangeal joint (arrows). (**b**) Sagittal T1 MRI shows a lobular hyperintense mass arising from the dorsal aspect of the interphalangeal joint. (**c**) Axial PD fat-saturated MRI shows the mass, which is homogeneously hyperintense, on both the dorsal and plantar aspects of the joint.

Plain radiographs may show multiple smooth, spherical loose bodies if they are calcified. MRI characteristically shows the loose bodies as low signal on T1-weighted images and high signal on T2-weighted images with multiple signal voids of calcification[41]. Occasionally, MRI shows a chondral mass with no significant punctate mineralization, arising from a joint or within a tendon sheath (Figure 17.4). Radiographs are useful to show mineralization in these cases.

Synovectomy and retrieval of the loose cartilaginous bodies is often required as longstanding chondromatosis can lead to osteoarthritis, necessitating arthrodesis or joint replacement. Synovial chondromatosis in the foot and ankle is rare, with only small cohorts reported in the literature. Chondrosarcomatous differentiation has been reported and it is suggested that in cases with rapid recurrence, especially with significant erosive joint destruction, repeat biopsy should be performed[42].

Miscellaneous

Ganglion

Ganglia are well-encapsulated fluid-filled lesions arising as a result of mucoid degeneration of tendon sheaths and joint capsules. Treatment is reserved for ganglia producing pressure or mechanical symptoms, as otherwise they tend to be painless. The cystic nature of the lesion should be confirmed with USS prior to intervention. At aspiration, a gelatinous clear fluid is obtained and this helps confirm the diagnosis. MRI scanning (Figure 17.5) is helpful to find the origin of the lesion and plan excision, the aspiration track being excised with the tumor. Marginal excision is the treatment of choice for symptomatic ganglia, ensuring excision of a portion of the degenerate joint capsule or tendon sheath. The patient should be warned that the recurrence rate of foot and ankle ganglia is reported as being up to 43%, which is higher than in the wrist[43].

Tendon Xanthomas

Most common in the tendo Achillis, xanthomas are pathognomic of familial hypercholesterolemia. They manifest clinically as discrete fusiform swellings within the tendon (Figure 17.6) and can be painful, but are usually painless. Xanthomas are infiltrative and difficult to dissect free from the tendon substance, necessitating reconstructive procedures rather than simple debulking. Management includes medical referral for investigation and management of hypercholesterolemia[44].

(a)

(b)

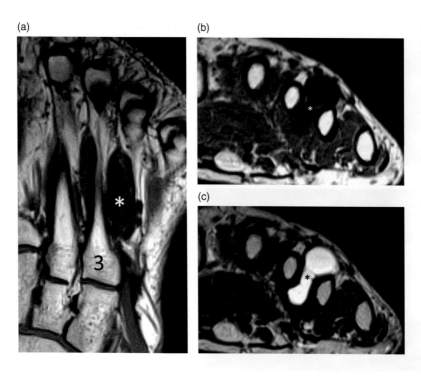

(c)

Figure 17.5 Ganglion, F/73y. (a) Coronal T1 MRI of the left forefoot shows an elongated fluid signal mass (*) adjacent to the third metatarsal (3). (b) Axial T1 and (c) T2 MRI demonstrate the ganglion (*) abutting the third and fourth metatarsals.

Infection

Infection should always be entertained in the differential diagnosis of a patient with a mass, particularly when accompanied by a history of an inoculating foreign body. Not uncommonly, bacterial infections such as tuberculosis and more indolent fungal infections such as Madura foot, particularly in patients from overseas or with a history of travel, are encountered and the relevant investigations including blood tests, imaging, and even biopsy should be undertaken[45].

Benign Bone Tumors

The surgical treatment of benign bone tumors follows the same principles as those of benign soft tissue tumors. Stage 1 and 2 lesions are most often treated with intralesional curettage. The resulting bone defects are managed with bone graft or, in the case of large voids left by giant cell tumors, polymethyl methacrylate cement. Cement augmentation not only provides structural support to the surrounding native bone, but the heat generated during polymerization also sterilizes the reactive zone. It may be appropriate to treat some stage 2 and 3 lesions with wide surgical resection. When the tumor involves the articular surfaces it is better to arthrodese the joint to prevent late local recurrence[46].

Bone-Forming Tumors
Osteochondroma

Solitary lesions rarely occur in the foot and ankle. They arise from the paraphyseal region of growing long bones. They develop as a consequence of the aberrant growth of cells from the proliferative zone of the physis, and hence appear during childhood and cease growing when the physis fuses. They characteristically have an osseous stalk directed away from the physeal plate with a thin (<2 cm) cartilage cap. The normal metaphyseal bone is said to "flow into" the osseous stalk[47]. Osteochondromas are benign, but the cartilage cap undergoes malignant transformation into a chondrosarcoma in approximately 1% of non-syndromic lesions. This presents with an increase in size and pain after physeal closure. Benign lesions can, however, cause symptoms as a result of the local mechanical irritation of tendons and nerves. Pain is an indication for excision.

Hereditary multiple exostoses or diaphyseal aclasis is an autosomal dominant disorder with a greater incidence of malignant transformation, in which the exostoses are larger and the metaphyses are widened and dysplastic. In this condition the exostoses can cause growth arrest and potentially ankle deformity, which may require corrective surgery[48].

(a)

(b)

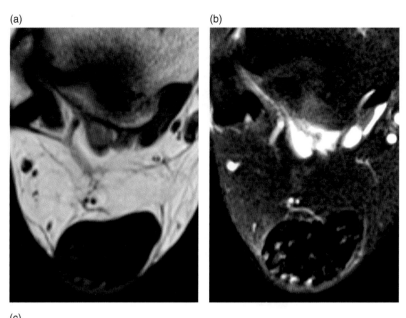

Figure 17.6 Tendon xanthoma, F/62y. (**a**) Axial T1 and (**b**) PD fat-saturated MRI showing a speckled/reticulated appearance of the tendo Achillis. Sagittal scans showed fusiform enlargement but little internal signal change. (**c**) Longitudinal ultrasound image shows a lobular area of low reflectivity, bulging the superficial aspect of the tendon (*), blending with more normal tendon fibers (arrows).

(c)

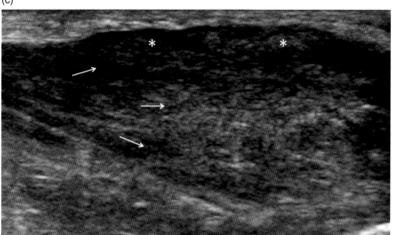

Subungual Exostosis

Subungual exostoses develop as a painful lesion on the tip of the distal phalanx (Figure 17.7). They usually present with nail deformity and pain. Treatment is with marginal excision.

Osteoid Osteoma and Osteoblastoma

Although osteoid osteomas classically present in young adults with a history of self-limiting, localized, nocturnal inflammatory pain, which is not related to activity and may be improved by NSAIDs, it is worth remembering that many cases present atypically. Osteoblastoma, although morphologically

similar, is almost always progressive and occasionally locally aggressive.

Plain radiography sometimes shows a small (<1 cm), intracortical, intramedullary, or subperiosteal nidus. The most reliable way of showing the reactive inflammatory change that surrounds the nidus is with MRI. Nevertheless on MRI scans, hindfoot osteoid osteomas may only show as edema, the nidus not being visible; in these cases CT scanning is helpful[49]. More recently SPECT-CT scanning has proved useful in diagnosing these lesions. Computed tomography is also used to guide radiofrequency ablation of these osteoid osteomas[50]. Some are not

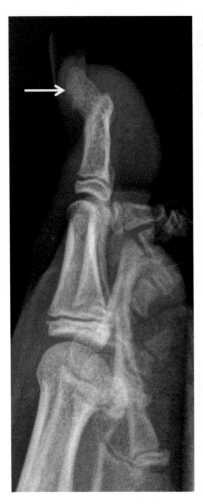

Figure 17.7
Subungual exostosis, F/15y. A large exostosis arising from the dorsal aspect of the tip of the distal phalanx of the great toe (arrow).

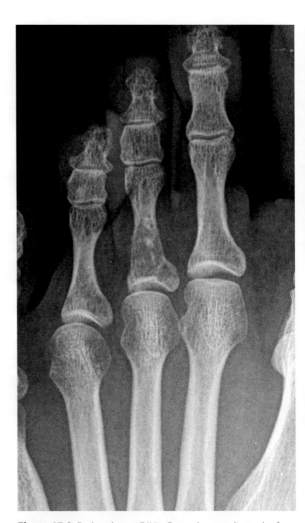

Figure 17.8 Enchondroma, F/35y. Dorsoplantar radiograph of the left foot. Lucent lesion in the proximal aspect of the proximal phalanx of the third toe, with cortical thinning and punctate matrix mineralization. No cortical breach or extra-osseous mass.

amenable to radiofrequency ablation, for example superficial lesions or those in close proximity to major neurovascular structures risk thermal damage to the skin or adjacent nerves. In these it may be necessary to attempt either en bloc resection or intra-lesional curettage making sure to completely remove the nidus.

Osteoblastoma is classically described as a larger variant (>1 cm) of an osteoid osteoma, although it also behaves differently. In contrast to osteoid osteoma, the history of nocturnal pain relieved with NSAIDs is inconsistent. They are also progressive and can be locally destructive with a tendency for recurrence. Some even undergo malignant transformation. Subperiosteal osteoblastomas can give rise to a peri-osteal reaction with a soft tissue mass, which mimics a sarcoma. They have a particular affinity for the dorsal junction of the head and neck of the talus, but they have also been known to cause pathological fracture in the smaller tubular bones of the foot. Osteoblastomas may be treated by intralesional curettage and bone grafting[51].

Cartilage-Forming Tumors
Enchondroma

Enchondromas are benign cartilage tumors arising from displaced nests of cartilage cells from the physis. They are often diagnosed incidentally on plain radiographs, where they appear as radiolucent lesions with areas of stippled, calcified chondroid matrix (Figure 17.8). They can occasionally lead to pathological fracture.

Asymptomatic lesions can simply be followed radiographically with serial x-rays. Symptomatic lesions, or lesions with a pathological fracture, are treated by intralesional curettage, bone grafting, and, if needed, internal fixation.

Differentiating radiologically between a benign enchondroma and a low-grade chondrosarcoma is difficult. Malignant transformation to a chondrosarcoma is very rare, but increasing size, length greater than 5 cm (in a long tubular bone), and deep endosteal scalloping are suggestive of low-grade chondrosarcoma[52].

Chondroblastoma

Chondroblastomas are benign, locally aggressive lesions, which characteristically form in the epiphyses of growing long bones. One large series reported that 13% of chondroblastomas occurred in the foot, mainly in the tarsal bones. There was a predilection for the posterior subchondral areas of the talus, calcaneus, and calcaneal apophysis[53]. This periarticular location can lead to pain, joint effusion, and restricted movement.

Plain radiographs shows a distinctive, geographic radiolucent lesion with a surrounding rim of sclerotic bone with occasional chondral matrix production (Figure 17.9). The differential diagnosis of a subchondral radiolucent lesion in a young patient includes infection, degenerative joint disease, rheumatoid arthritis, pseudogout, and crystal deposition diseases[54]. Biopsy is advised, even with classical appearance.

Intralesional curettage and bone grafting are the surgical treatments of choice; however, when there is subchondral involvement, primary arthrodesis of the joint may be required to adequately resect the tumor and achieve a pain-free, functional limb. Radiofrequency ablation is often a useful alternative to surgery.

Periosteal Chondroma

This benign surface cartilage tumor of tubular bones presents as a painless enlarging mass in young patients. In the foot it usually occurs in the metatarsals, with characteristic pressure erosion of the cortex on plain radiographs[55]. If asymptomatic these lesions can be observed with serial radiographs over one to two years. Symptomatic lesions are treated with intralesional curettage.

Fibrous Cortical Defect

Fibrous cortical defects, which are histologically identical to the larger non-ossifying fibromas, are usually an incidental finding on a plain radiograph of a long tubular bone. Their appearance is of a cortically based radiolucent tumor with a sclerotic margin[56]. Occasionally pathological fracture occurs, which leads to spontaneous healing; otherwise intralesional curettage is sufficient. Symptomatic lesions are treated with curettage, with or without bone grafting. However, the majority are asymptomatic and can be documented and treated non-operatively.

Fibrous Dysplasia

Fibrous dysplasia was until fairly recently thought to be a developmental condition, but is now confirmed to be a bone tumor, where trabecular bone is replaced by fibrous tissue. The bone is weakened and can deform or fracture. Reports of fibrous dysplasia of the foot are scanty.

Fibrous dysplasia is often seen as an incidental finding on plain radiographs. It is characterized by a "ground-glass" fibrous matrix. Smaller lesions require no treatment. Larger lesions occupying over one-third of the diameter of a long bone may predispose to deformity or pathological fracture and should be monitored. On occasions the lesions fracture pathologically and as the fracture heals with the same defective fibrous matrix, bone grafting and internal fixation are required.

Unicameral Bone Cyst

Unicameral bone cysts are fluid-filled lesions, which are often found incidentally on plain radiographs during adolescence. In the foot and ankle, they most frequently occur in the calcaneum. Unlike unicameral cysts elsewhere, calcaneal unicameral cysts do not spontaneously resolve and can be seen in adults. Operative treatment is recommended for symptomatic or large cysts, which occupy most of the calcaneum from the medial to the lateral wall on cross-sectional imaging. Reported treatments include aspiration and injection of methylprednisolone, injection of demineralized bone powder with autologous bone marrow, and intralesional curettage and bone grafting. There is no clear benefit of one technique over another[57–58]. Certainly if there is pathological fracture, internal fixation with bone grafting is recommended as few of these lesions heal spontaneously[59].

Intraosseous Lipoma

The differential diagnosis of a radiolucency in the calcaneum is an intraosseous lipoma, which has a

(a)

(b)

(c)

(d)

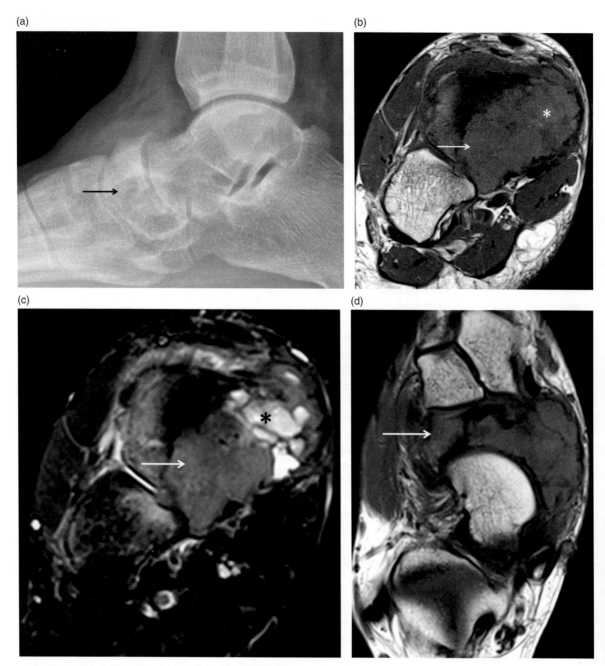

Figure.17.9 Chondroblastoma of right navicular, M/18y. (**a**) Lateral radiograph of right hindfoot shows a well-defined lucent lesion in the navicular (arrow). (**b**) Coronal T1 and (**c**) STIR MRI show an expansile mass destroying the navicular. A solid component is seen laterally (arrow) and a multilocular cystic component, suggesting secondary ABC change, medially (*) (fluid levels were seen on axial fluid sensitive images). Edema is seen in the adjacent cuboid and navicular. (**d**) Axial T1 MRI shows a tumor in the medial aspect of the navicular and edema-like hypointensity in the residual lateral aspect (arrow).

tendency to lie directly beneath the angle of Gissane. This fat-containing benign tumor is usually asymptomatic and often has a central focus of calcification, which can differentiate it from a unicameral cyst. The fat content is well shown by MRI scanning (Figure 17.10). Usually lipomas require no treatment, but if they are symptomatic they are treated like a unicameral cyst[60].

(a)

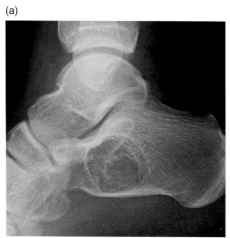

Figure 17.10 Intraosseous lipoma in right calcaneum, M/27y. (**a**) Lateral radiograph shows a lucency inferior to the angle of Gissane, with a non-aggressive, sclerotic border. (**b**) Coronal T1 and (**c**) axial T2 MRI show a mildly expansile lesion in the body of the calcaneum, with a fatty signal at the periphery (arrows) and a proteinaceous fluid signal centrally (*).

(b)   (c)

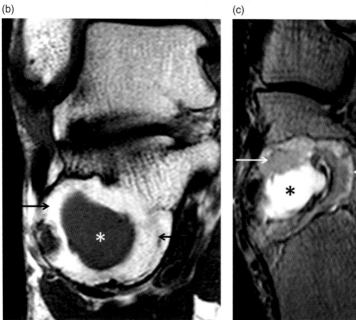

Aneurysmal Bone Cysts and Giant Cell Tumors

In the foot and ankle in young patients aneurysmal bone cysts (ABCs) and giant cell tumors (GCTs) may be confused. Classically ABCs develop in the metaphyseal region of long bones and appear radiographically as expansile, radiolucent lesions with a thin surrounding rim of cortical bone. On cross-sectional imaging ABCs are more likely to demonstrate fluid levels than GCTs (Figure 17.11). In the foot ABCs are commonest in the metatarsals, but when in the hindfoot they are most commonly seen in the calcaneus.

They have a tendency to "blow-out" the cortex and therefore present early as a painful, palpable mass.

Giant cell tumors are more likely to occur in the hindfoot, especially the talus, and radiographically are geographic, with an ill-defined non-sclerotic margin. Giant cell tumors are more locally aggressive, stage 3 benign, and present with pain and swelling (Figure 17.12). Pathological fracture into the adjacent joint is commoner with GCTs[61].

Intralesional curettage is the treatment of choice for both ABCs and GCTs. The local recurrence rate for ABCs is approximately 20%. The recurrence rate for GCTs depends upon the grade of the lesion;

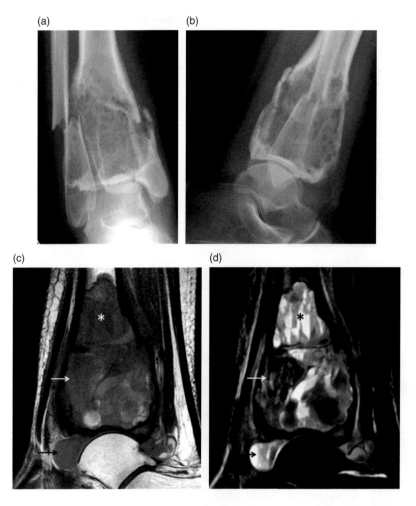

(a) (b)

(c) (d)

Figure 17.11 ABC right distal tibia, F/14y. (**a**) AP and (**b**) lateral radiograph of right distal tibia and fibula show a pathological fracture of the tibia after minor trauma. There is an expansile, lucent lesion in the distal tibia extending to the subarticular bone. There are some atypical radiographic features, raising the possibility of a sarcoma, but the diagnosis of ABC was proven on biopsy. A transverse fracture of the fibula was also noted. (**c**) Sagittal T1 and (**d**) STIR MRI of the right distal tibia. Proximally, a well-defined lesion containing multiple fluid–fluid levels is seen (*). Distally, the appearance is altered due to hemorrhage following the fracture (white arrow). A hemarthrosis is noted, in keeping with intra-articular fracture (black arrow).

those that have broken through the cortical bone are more likely to recur. In such lesions, adjuvant agents such as polymethyl methacrylate can help reduce local recurrence by thermal necrosis and providing instant subchondral support[62]. Local recurrence rates of 3 to 17% were found following curettage with adjuvant therapy[63–64]. A number of malignant tumors can contain areas of secondary ABC, therefore histological examination of the curettings is important.

Following local recurrence, treatment options include wide excision, bone grafting, and arthrodesis.

Miscellaneous

Infection, Inflammation, and Metabolic Bone Disease

It must not be forgotten that infection (Figure 17.13), inflammatory arthritis, and metabolic bone disease may mimic bone and soft tissue tumors. The differential diagnosis for soft tissue tumors includes inflammatory bursae, rheumatoid nodules, and tophaceous gout.

The differential diagnosis for benign bone lesions includes the brown tumor, which is seen in hyperparathyroidism. Infection can produce a metaphyseal radiolucent Brodie's abscess. A thorough history and examination with analysis of serum inflammatory markers, renal function, calcium, phosphate, parathyroid hormone, and uric acid should help.

Intraosseous Ganglia and Degenerative Bone Cysts

Intraosseous ganglia are occasional incidental findings on plain radiographs, usually involving the medial malleolus in foot and ankle patients. In the majority of cases they are asymptomatic and have a well-defined radiolucent appearance, in which case they can be treated expectantly. If painful they can be treated with curettage and bone grafting.

(a)

(b)

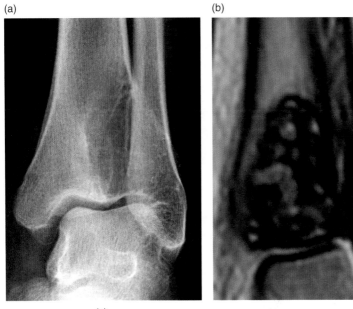

Figure 17.12 Giant cell tumor in the left distal tibia, M/18y. (**a**) AP radiograph of the left distal tibia. Eccentric subarticular tumor at the lateral aspect of the distal tibia, showing a well-defined, predominantly non-sclerotic edge (narrow zone of transition) and septation. There is a solid periosteal reaction at the medial aspect of the distal tibia. (**b**) Coronal and (**c**) axial T2 MRI show a lobular hypointense tumor, occupying the anterolateral aspect of the distal tibia. Low signal intensity reflects chronic hemorrhage.

(c)

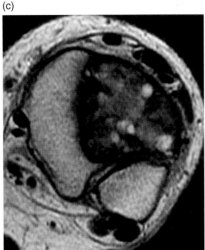

Many subchondral cysts and larger subarticular geodes are related to degenerative joint disease, and hence are seen on radiographs performed for joint pain. The cysts communicate with the joint and contain a synovial-like fluid. Their treatment is that of the degenerative joint (Figure 17.14).

Key Points

- Imaging is crucial in the diagnosis of tumors of the foot and ankle. Clinical examination alone is insufficient.
- For radiologically indeterminate lesions, biopsy planning within the scope of a musculoskeletal tumor service is required.

- Infection, metabolic bone disease, crystal deposition disease, and degenerative and inflammatory arthritis are the differential diagnoses of tumors in the foot and ankle.
- Many benign tumors are discovered incidentally and in such cases after diagnosis all that is required is reassurance and non-operative management, with adequate clinical follow-up.
- Staging is the basis of treatment. It is determined by the clinical, radiological, and histological features.
- Surgical margins are intralesional, marginal, wide, and radical.

305

(a)   (b)

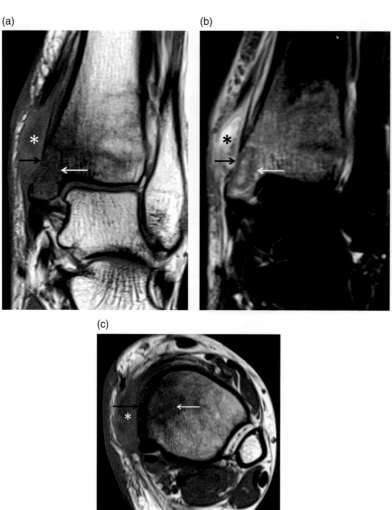

(c)

Figure 17.13 Granulomatous infection, F/25y. (a) Coronal T1, (b) STIR, and (c) axial T1 MRI show a part cystic (*), part solid mass overlying the medial malleolus, with periosteal reaction and erosion of the adjacent tibia (black arrow), and early bone abscess formation (white arrow). Marked marrow/soft tissue edema and thickening of the overlying skin also suggest infection.

(a)   (b)

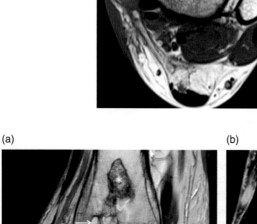

Figure 17.14 Geode/degenerative subarticular cyst in the distal tibia, M/54y. (a) Sagittal PD MRI and (b) coronal PD fat-saturated MRI of the left ankle. There is a lobular cyst in the tibial plafond (arrow), with adjacent articular surface irregularity (likely joint communication) and surrounding marrow edema. Proximal to the cyst is a demarcated area of heterogeneous, edematous fat, consistent with an infarct (*). There is advanced ankle osteoarthritis and the subtalar joint is fused.

References

1. Enneking WF. *Musculoskeletal Tumour Surgery. Volume 1.* (New York: Churchill Livingstone, 1983) pp. 719–20.

2. Hart WJ, Hemmady M, Cool WP. A review of the tumour workload presenting to a foot and ankle clinic over an eighteen month period. *J Bone Joint Surg Br.* 2005; 87-B(Suppl I):2.

3. Ozdemir HM, Yildiz C, Yilmaz C, Saqlik Y. Tumours of the foot and ankle: analysis of 196 cases. *J Foot Ankle Surg.* 1997; 36(6):403–8.

4. Temple HT, Worman DS, Mnaymneh WA. Unplanned surgical excision of tumours of the foot and ankle. *Cancer Control.* 2001; 8(3):262–8.

5. Ashwood N, Witt JD, Hallam PJ, Cobb JP. Analysis of the referral pattern to a supraregional bone and soft tissue tumor service. *Ann R Coll Surg Engl.* 2003; 85:272–6.

6. MacDonald D, Holt G, Vass K, Marsh A, Kumar CS. The differential diagnosis of foot lumps: 101 cases treated surgically in North Glasgow over 4 years. *Ann R Coll Surg Engl.* 2007; 89(3):272–5.

7. Peh WC, Gilula LA. Plain film approach to tumours and tumour-like conditions of bone. *Br J Hosp Med.* 1995; 54(11):549–57.

8. Helms CA. *Fundamentals of Skeletal Radiology*, 4th edn. (Philadelphia, PA: Elsevier-Saunders, 2014) pp. 35–6.

9. Hung EH, Griffith JF, Ng AW, Lee RK, Lau DT, Leung JC. Ultrasound of musculoskeletal soft-tissue tumors superficial to the investing fascia. *Am J Roentgenol.* 2014; 202(6): W532–40. doi: 10.2214/AJR.13.11457.

10. Coughlin MJ, Mann RA, Saltzmann CL. *Surgery of the Foot and Ankle. Vol 1*, 8th edn. (Philadelphia, PA: Mosby-Elsevier, 2007), p. 710.

11. Mankin HJ, Lange TA, Spanier SS. The hazards of biopsy in patients with primary bone and soft tissue tumours. *J Bone Joint Surg Am.* 1982; 64:1121–7.

12. Enneking WF, Spanier SS, Goodman MA. A system for the surgical staging of musculoskeletal sarcoma. *Clin Orthop Relat Res.* 1980; 153:106–20.

13. Ramachandran M. *Basic Orthopaedic Sciences. The Stanmore Guide.* (CRC Press, 2006), p. 64.

14. Enneking WF. *Musculoskeletal Tumour Surgery. Volume 1* (New York: Churchill Livingstone, 1983) pp. 747–75.

15. Keasby LE. Juvenile aponeurotic fibroma (calcifying fibroma). A distinctive tumor arising in the palms and soles of young children. *Cancer.* 1953; 6:338–46.

16. Pentland AP, Anderson TF. Plantarfibromatosis responds to intralesional steroids. *J Am Acad Dermatol.* 1985; 12(1 Pt. 2):212–14.

17. Lee TH, Wapner KL, Hecht PJ. Plantar fibromatosis: current concepts review. *J Bone Joint Surg Am.* 1993; 75A:1080–5.

18. Wapner KL, Ververelli PA, Moore JH, Hecht PJ, Becker CE, Lackman RD. Plantar fibromatosis: a review of primary and recurrent surgical treatment. *Foot Ankle Int.* 1995; 16(9):548–51.

19. Carroll RE, Berman AT. Glomus tumors of the hand. *J Bone Joint Surg.* 1972; 54A(4):691–703.

20. Rettig AC, Strickland JW. Glomus tumor of the digits. *J Hand Surg.* 1977; 2A(4):261–5.

21. Mohler DG, Lim CK, Martin B. Glomus tumour of the plantar arch: a case report with magnetic resonance imaging findings. *Foot Ankle Int.* 1997; 18(10):672–4.

22. Lowe LH, Marchant TC, Rivard DC, Scherbel AJ. Vascular malformations: classification and terminology the radiologist needs to know. *Semi Roentgenol.* 2012; 106–17.

23. Kirby EJ, Shereff ML, Lewis MM. Soft-tissue tumours and tumour-like lesions of the foot. An analysis of eighty-three cases. *J Bone Joint Surg.* 1989; 71A:621–6.

24. Nakamura T, Matsumine A, Nishiyama M, Uchida A, Sudo A. Recurrent ankle equinus deformity due to intramuscular hemiangioma of the gastrocnemius: case report. *Foot Ankle Int.* 2011; 32(9):905–7.

25. Adam A, Dixon AK, Gillard JH, Schaefer-Prokop CM. *Grainger and Allison's Diagnostic Radiology: A Textbook of Medical Imaging, Vol. 2*, 6th edn. (Churchill-Livingstone-Elsevier, 2014) pp. 1143–4.

26. Urguden M, Ozdemir H, Duygulu E, Aydin AT. Cavernous hemangioma behaving like peroneal tenosynovitis. *Foot Ankle Int.* 2000; 21(10):856–9.

27. Yetkin H, Kanatli U, Guzel VB, Poyraz A. Multiple hemangiomas of the foot: a case report. *Foot Ankle Int.* 2001; 22(2):150–2.

28. Crawford EA, Slotcavage RL, King JJ, Lackman RD, Ogilvie CM. Ethanol sclerotherapy reduces pain in symptomatic musculoskeletal hemangiomas. *Clin Orthop Relat Res.* 2009; 467(11):2955–61.

29. Love S, Louis DN, Ellison DW. *Greenfield's Neuropathology. Vol. 2*, 8th edn. (CRC Press, 2008) pp. 2049–53.

30. Das Gupta T, Brasfield R, Strong E, Hajdu S. Benign solitary schwannomas (neurilemmomas). *Cancer.* 1969; 24:355–66.

31. Marui TM, Yamamoto T, Akisue T, et al. Neurilemmoma in the foot as a cause of heel pain: a report of two cases. *Foot Ankle Int.* 2004; 25(2):107–11.

32. Cerefolini E, Landi A, DeSantis G, Maiorana A, Canossi G,

Romagnoli R. MR of benign peripheral nerve sheath tumours. *J Comput Assist Tomogr.* 1991; 15:593–7.

33. Varma DG, Moulopoulos A, Sara AS, et al. MR imaging of extracranial nerve sheath tumous. *J Comput Assist Tomogr.* 1992; 16:448–53.

34. Berlin SJ. A laboratory review of 67,000 foot tumours and lesions. *J Am Podiatr Med Assoc.* 1984; 74:341–7.

35. Kumar V, Abbas AK, Fausto N, Aster JC. *Robbins and Cotran Pathologic Basis of Disease*, 8th edn. (Saunders-Elsevier, 2010), pp. 1249–50.

36. Myerson M, Soffer S. Lipoma as an etiology of tarsal tunnel syndrome: a report of two cases. *Foot Ankle Int.* 1989; 10(3):176–9.

37. Adam A, Dixon AK, Gillard JH, Schaefer-Prokop CM. *Grainger and Allison's Diagnostic Radiology: A Textbook of Medical Imaging, Vol. 2*, 6th edn. (Churchill-Livingstone-Elsevier, 2014), pp. 1135–6.

38. van der Heijden L, Gibbons CLM, Dijkstra PDS, et al. The management of diffuse-type giant cell tumour (pigmented villonodular synovitis) and giant cell tumour of tendon sheath (nodular tenosynovitis). *J Bone Joint Surg Br.* 2012; 94-B:882–8.

39. Gibbons CLMH, Khwaja HA, Cole AS, Cooke, PH, Athanasou NA. Giant-cell tumour of the tendon sheath in the foot and ankle. *J Bone Joint Surg Br.* 2002; 84-B:1000–3.

40. Bickels J, Isaakov J, Kollender Y, Meller I. Unacceptable complications following intra-articular injection of yttrium 90 in the ankle joint for diffure pigmented villonodular synovitis. *J Bone Joint Surg Am.* 2008; 90(2):326–8.

41. Wong K, Sallomi D, Janzen D, et al. Monoarticular synovial lesions: radiographic pictoral essay with pathologic illustration. *Clin Radiol.* 1999; 54:273–84.

42. Galat DD, Ackerman DB, Spoon D, Turner NS, Shives TC. Synovial chondromatosis of the foot and ankle. *Foot Ankle Int.* 2008; 29(3):312–17.

43. Kliman ME, Freiberg A. Ganglia of the foot and ankle. *Foot Ankle Int.* 1982; 3(1):45–6.

44. Carranza-Bencano A, Fernandez-Centeno M, Leal-Cerro A, et al. Xanthomas of the Achilles tendon: report of a bilateral case and review of the literature. *Foot Ankle Int.* 2005; 20(5):314–16.

45. Parker L, Singh D, Biz C. The dot-in-circle sign in Madura foot. *J Foot Ankle Surg.* 2009; 48(6):690–2.

46. Coughlin MJ, Mann RA, Saltzmann CL. *Surgery of the Foot and Ankle. Vol 1*, 8th edn. (Philadelphia: Mosby-Elsevier, 2007) p. 721.

47. Adam A, Dixon AK, Gillard JH, Schaefer-Prokop CM. *Grainger and Allison's Diagnostic Radiology: A Textbook of Medical Imaging, Vol. 2.* 6th edn. (Churchill-Livingstone-Elsevier 2014), pp. 1093–4.

48. Shawen SB, McHale KA, Temple HT. Correction of ankle valgus deformity secondary to multiple hereditary osteochondral exostoses with Ilizarov. *Foot Ankle Int.* 2000; 21(12):1019–22.

49. Adam A, Dixon AK, Gillard JH, Schaefer-Prokop CM. *Grainger and Allison's Diagnostic Radiology: A Textbook of Medical Imaging, Vol. 2.* 6th edn. (Churchill-Livingstone-Elsevier 2014), pp. 1098–9.

50. Brin YS, Lebel D, Yafe D, Melamed E, Nyska M. Treatment with CT guided radiofrequency thermal ablation for osteoid osteoma of the foot and ankle. A report of six cases. *J Bone Joint Surg Br.* 2008; 90-B(Suppl III):518.

51. Temple HT, Mizel MS, Murphey MD, Sweet DE. Osteoblastoma of the foot and ankle. *Foot Ankle Int.* 1998; 19(10):698–703.

52. Gajewski DA, Burnette JB, Murphey MD, Temple HT. Diferentiating clinical and radiographic features of enchondroma and secondary chondrosarcoma in the foot. *Foot Ankle Int.* 2006; 27(4):240–4.

53. Fin BR, Temple HT, Chiricosta FM, Mizel MS, Murphey MD. Chondroblastoma of the foot. *Foot Ankle Int.* 1997; 18(4):236–42.

54. Brant WE, Helms CA. *Fundamentals of Diagnostic Radiology*, 4th edn. (Philadelphia: Wolters Kluwer–Lippincott Williams and Wilkins, 2012) pp. 995–6.

55. Ricca RL, Kuklo TR, Shawen SB, Vick DJ, Schaefer RA. Periosteal chondroma of the cuboid presenting in a 7-year-old boy. *Foot Ankle Int.* 2000; 21(2):145–9.

56. Adam A, Dixon AK, Gillard JH, Schaefer-Prokop CM. *Grainger and Allison's Diagnostic Radiology: A Textbook of Medical Imaging, Vol. 2.* 6th edn. (Churchill-Livingstone-Elsevier 2014), pp. 1100–1.

57. Park I, Micic ID, Jeon I. A study of 23 unicameral bone cysts of the calcaneus: open chip allogogeneic bone graft versus percutaneous injection of bone powder with autogenous bone marrow. *Foot Ankle Int.* 2008; 29(2):164–70.

58. Chang CH, Stanton RP, Glutting J. Unicameral bone cysts treated by injection of bone marrow or methylprednisolone. *J Bone Joint Surg Br.* 2002; 84-B(3):407–12.

59. Garceau GJ, Gregory CF. Solitary unicameral bone cysts. *J Bone Joint Surg Am.* 1954; 36-A:267–80.

60. Greenspan A, Raiszadeh K, Riley GM, Matthews D. Intraosseous lipoma of the calcaneus. *Foot Ankle Int.* 1997; 18(1):53–6.

61. Casadei R, Ruggieri P, Moscata M, Ferraro A, Picci P. Aneurysmal bone cyst and giant cell tumour of the foot. *Foot Ankle Int.* 1996; 17(8):487–95.

62. Chowdhry M, Chandrasekar CR, Mohammed R, Grimer RJ.

Curettage of aneurysmal bone cysts of the feet. *Foot Ankle Int.* 2010; 31(2):131–5.

63. K, Perka C, Schmidt GR. Treatment of stages 2 and 3 giant cell tumour. *Arch Orthop Trauma Surg.* 2001; 121:83–8.

64. Becker WT, Dohle J, Bernd L, et al. Local recurrence of giant cell tumours of long bones after intralesional treatment with and without adjuvant therapy. *J Bone Joint Surg Am.* 2008; 90-A:1060–7.

Malignant Tumors of the Foot and Ankle

Jonathan S. Palmer, Panagiotis D. Gikas, Dishan Singh,
Timothy W. R. Briggs, and Paul O'Donnell

Introduction

Primary musculoskeletal malignancies are uncommon and represent approximately 1% of the cancer burden in adults and 10% in children[1-2]. Malignant tumors involving the foot and ankle are even less common and probably less than 5% of all malignancies of bone and soft tissues affect the foot[3]. Due to their low rates of occurrence the true burden of disease is difficult to establish. Unlike bone tumors elsewhere, malignant neoplasms affecting the foot are more likely to be primary than metastatic.

In the foot malignant tumors can arise from any of the tissues, including soft tissue, bone, nerves, and blood vessels. An understanding of the basic principles of the management of bone and soft tissue malignancies is critical for any orthopedic surgeon.

The clinical features of a malignant tumor arising in the foot and ankle may be similar to those of a benign tumor. Patients commonly present with pain and may attribute this to an antecedent traumatic episode, which can be misleading. Patients with sarcomas of the foot and ankle are often misdiagnosed and initially treated for benign pathologies. Early recognition of foot and ankle malignancies remains the biggest challenge in the management of these tumors. Sound knowledge is essential to ensure prompt recognition and appropriate management.

The following chapter looks in detail at the more common types of malignant tumors affecting the foot and ankle. The principles of management are discussed in general toward the end of the chapter.

Soft Tissue Sarcoma

Soft tissue sarcomas arise from extraskeletal tissues including fat, muscle, ligaments, synovium, and neurovascular structures. Soft tissue sarcomas are rare. The annual incidence is approximately two to three cases per 100 000 people, which accounts for less than

1% of adult and 8% of pediatric malignancies[4]. They are typically classified histologically according to their tissue of origin or as tumors of uncertain differentiation: it may be impossible to characterize the lesion (undifferentiated/unclassified sarcomas).

Soft tissue sarcomas are particularly rare in the foot and ankle. Most patients complain of a swelling, which may or may not be painful. A long history does not exclude the diagnosis. A careful history and examination are essential. Soft tissue swellings that are large, rapidly growing, deep to the fascia, and painful are more likely to be malignant[5].

There are over 50 subtypes of soft tissue sarcoma and cases involving the foot and ankle have been described for many of them, including synovial sarcoma, clear cell sarcoma, the condition previously described as malignant fibrous histiocytoma (now undifferentiated pleomorphic sarcoma), leiomyosarcoma, and fibrosarcoma[6]. However, in a review of 12 370 patients with soft tissue malignancies only 638 cases (5%) involved the foot and ankle[6]. Despite their infrequent occurrence, certain subtypes of soft tissue sarcoma seem to have a predilection for the foot and ankle. These are discussed below. The principles of management are discussed at the end of the chapter and can be applied to any malignant sarcoma involving the foot and ankle.

Synovial Sarcoma

Synovial sarcoma accounts for approximately 8 to 10% of all soft tissue sarcomas. Its peak incidence is in the third decade of life, with 30% arising in those aged under 20 years. Synovial sarcoma is slightly commoner in males and it is the commonest soft tissue sarcoma to arise in the foot and ankle, comprising 45 to 56% of all sarcomas in this region[7]. Typically the tumors arise in a periarticular position (Figure 18.1), although very rarely they occur within the joint. They are typically considered high-grade

(a) 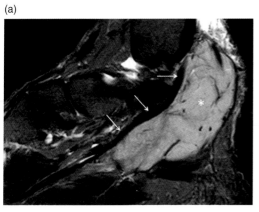 (b)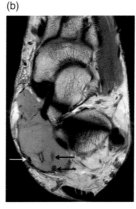

Figure 18.1 Synovial sarcoma in the left tarsal tunnel of a 42-year-old male. (**a**) Sagittal STIR MRI shows a large, homogeneous mass in the tarsal tunnel (*), inferior to the flexor digitorum longus tendon (arrows). (**b**) Axial PD MRI shows encasement of the posterior tibial artery (white arrow) and medial and lateral plantar nerves (black arrows). Below knee amputation was performed.

(a) 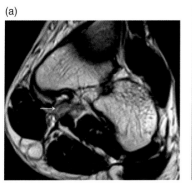 (b)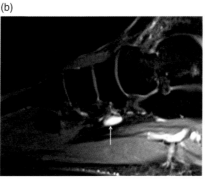

Figure 18.2 Synovial sarcoma in the plantar aspect of the left foot in a 21-year-old male. The mass had been present for 18 months with no significant growth and was thought to represent a benign synovial mass, possibly a ganglion – these relatively non-specific, non-aggressive clinical and imaging features are a significant pitfall in the management of this tumor. (**a**) Coronal T2 MRI and (**b**) sagittal T1 post-contrast MRI with fat saturation, showing a small, solid, enhancing mass (arrow) located dorsal to the knot of Henry.

tumors with characteristically invasive features and a tendency to metastasize.

The name synovial sarcoma is a misnomer as these tumors do not originate from cells within the synovium. The exact cell of origin is unknown and in the WHO classification of tumors they are included among sarcomas of uncertain differentiation, lacking a precise, normal tissue counterpart[1]. Three main subtypes of synovial sarcoma exist:

- biphasic – with epithelial and spindle cells in varying proportions
- monophasic – consisting of sheets of spindle cells only
- poorly differentiated – a more aggressive subtype with signs of necrosis, hemorrhage, and a high mitotic index.

Almost all synovial sarcomas demonstrate a reciprocal translocation t(X;18), which is not seen in other sarcomas. This fuses the SYT (SYnovial Tumor) gene from chromosome 18 with one of three SS (Synovial Sarcoma) genes (SSX 1, 2 and 4) from chromosome X.

The resultant fusion gene produces a protein which is thought to underlie synovial sarcoma pathogenesis by deregulating gene expression[8]. The SYT/SSX 1 fusion gene is more commonly associated with biphasic synovial sarcoma.

There are no clinical features or examination findings that distinguish synovial sarcoma from other soft tissue tumors. One review of 14 patients with synovial sarcoma of the foot and ankle found that pain, tenderness, edema, and an enlarging mass were the commonest symptoms[7]. However, frequently the mass behaves indolently and is present for considerable periods of time, sometimes years. Such non-specific features make prompt diagnosis a challenge. Indeed, the same study reported that six out of 14 patients had been initially diagnosed with benign pathologies including ganglion cyst, plantar fasciitis, and non-specific synovitis (Figure 18.2). Ten patients also gave a history of trauma prior to the onset of symptoms[7]. Initial conservative management led to delays in definitive diagnosis and management with a median duration of symptoms of 14 months prior to

311

presentation[7]. It is the commonest malignancy to be mistaken for a benign condition.

Synovial sarcoma is an aggressive tumor, which commonly metastasizes. As with other soft tissue sarcomas, negative prognostic factors include high grade, large tumor size, and metastases at the time of presentation. Hajdu et al. reviewed 126 cases and concluded that patients with tumors smaller than 5 cm had better five-year survival rates (79%) than those with tumors larger than 5 cm (33%)[9]. A large population-based study of 1268 patients with synovial sarcoma demonstrated that adults tend to have a worse outcome than children[10] with five-year survival rates estimated to be 83% for children and 62% for adults. The same study also showed more favorable outcomes for tumors involving the extremities. That said, of 14 cases involving the foot and ankle eight died of metastatic disease[7].

Undifferentiated Pleomorphic Sarcoma (or Malignant Fibrous Histiocytoma)

Undifferentiated pleomorphic sarcoma (UPS) may arise in both soft tissues and bone. They are relatively common and account for 20 to 30% of all soft tissue sarcomas. The peak prevalence is in the fifth decade of life and males are more affected than females (M:F, 1.5:1). Most patients present with a slowly enlarging, painless mass. These tumors commonly affect the extremities and 50% involve the lower limb[11]. Approximately 7% of malignant tumors affecting the foot are of this type[12].

Its true cell of origin is unknown and many feel that it represents the final common pathway of many different tumors, which become undifferentiated as they progress[13]. The WHO declassified malignant fibrous histiocytoma and renamed it as an undifferentiated pleomorphic sarcoma not otherwise specified, NOS[1]. Several subtypes have been described based on the predominant cellular features. These include storiform-pleomorphic, myxoid, giant cell, and angiomatoid. The storiform-pleomorphic subtype accounts for approximately 50 to 60% of these tumors and the remainder are usually of the myxoid type (25%)[11].

As with other soft tissue sarcomas, patients with larger and more deeply invested tumors tend to have a worse prognosis. Patients under 60 years of age with a small, low-grade myxoid type tumor typically have a better prognosis. Local recurrence is common and occurs in up to 50% of patients treated with radical, complete excision.

Clear Cell Sarcoma of Soft Tissue

Clear cell sarcoma of the soft tissue is a rare malignant tumor, which was first described by Enzinger in 1965[14]. Due to the presence of differentiated melanocytes this tumor has also been referred to as "malignant melanoma of soft parts"; however, it is recognized as being distinct from malignant melanoma.

The extremities are the principal site of involvement, with approximately 40% of these tumors arising in the foot and ankle[15]. It mainly affects young adults (mean 22 years)[16] but as it is so rare the exact incidence is unknown. They usually arise deep in the soft tissues and are commonly fixed to surrounding tendons or aponeuroses. Approximately 8% of soft tissue malignancies affecting the foot and ankle are clear cell sarcomas[6].

Patients usually present with a slow-growing mass, which is painful or tender in 50% of cases[15].

The prognosis is poor for patients with this tumor. Five-year survival rate has been estimated at 67%, which declines to 33% and 10% at 10 and 20 years respectively[17]. Patients succumb to widespread metastases, which can develop many years after complete surgical excision. Tumor size and necrosis are poor prognostic indicators[17].

Bone Tumors

Bone sarcomas involving the foot and ankle are rare. However, unlike elsewhere in the skeletal system, malignancies arising in this region are more likely to be primary tumors than metastases.

Patients rarely present with systemic symptoms[18] and the commonest complaint is pain. Often patients are initially treated for benign pathologies and delays in diagnosis are common.

Ewing's Sarcoma

The commonest primary malignant bone tumor to arise in the foot and ankle is Ewing's sarcoma. Out of a series of 8452 bone tumors only 54 were found to be malignant lesions arising in the foot[19]. Of these 54 cases 20 were Ewing's sarcomas (37%)[19].

Ewing's sarcoma typically occurs during childhood or adolescence, with the vast majority of cases

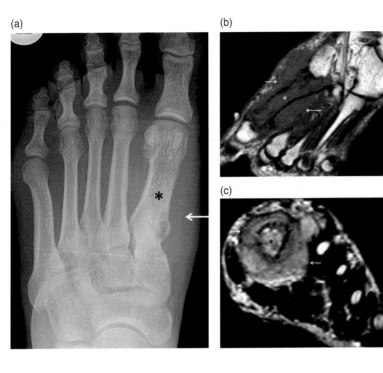

Figure 18.3 Ewing's sarcoma in the first metatarsal of a 25-year-old male. (**a**) Dorsoplantar radiograph showing permeative bone destruction (*) and extra-osseous mass (arrow). (**b**) T1-weighted coronal and (**c**) T2-weighted axial MRI showing infiltration of the first metatarsal (*) and surrounding mass (arrow).

arising before the age of 25. It can arise in any bone but is most frequently found in the diaphyses of the long bones of the lower limb, and flat bones such as the pelvis. It is the second most common primary malignant bone tumor to occur in children after osteosarcoma.

In a review of 16 patients with Ewing's sarcoma of the foot the mean age of the patients was 17 years (range 10–42)[18]. The tumor involved the metatarsals (Figure 18.3) or phalanges in 10 of the 16 patients, with the remainder arising in the calcaneus, navicular, and talus[18]. All the patients presented with pain and swelling in the foot, and fever was present in four cases[18]. As with other malignant tumors the diagnosis of Ewing's sarcoma in the foot is often delayed. The diagnosis took an average of 14 months, with many patients initially being treated for benign conditions[18]. Delays in diagnosis put patients at risk of developing advanced disease and in this case series 7 out of 16 patients had metastases at diagnosis[18].

Ewing's sarcoma shows variable neural differentiation and is morphologically similar and genetically identical to primitive neuroectodermal tumor (PNET). They are part of a spectrum of tumors collectively termed the Ewing's sarcoma family. The cell of origin for Ewing's sarcoma is not known but it is thought to arise from mesenchymal stem cells. It has a typical histological appearance consisting of small round cells that stain blue with hematoxylin and eosin (H&E).

In most cases, a genetic translocation occurs between the EWS gene on chromosome 22 and the FLI-1 gene on chromosome 11[20]. The resultant fusion protein regulates the expression of other genes leading to the development of the cancer.

Ewing's sarcoma is an aggressive tumor with poor survival. The five-year survival for patients with non-metastatic disease is 50 to 70%[21–22]. Positive prognostic indicators include non-pelvic tumors and younger age groups[22]. Survival is significantly reduced if metastases are present at the time of diagnosis (five-year survival 10–15%). In the case series mentioned above the overall five-year survival for tumors affecting the foot was 53%[18]. Those patients with metastases at presentation had an overall five-year survival of only 14%[18].

Osteosarcoma

Osteosarcoma is the commonest primary sarcoma of bone. It typically arises in patients in their second decade of life with a second peak occurring in the elderly population with preexisting Paget's disease. Approximately half of all osteosarcomas arise around the knee. Involvement of the foot is rare. Only 0.2 to 2% of all primary osteosarcomas occur in the foot[23].

The mean age of patients with osteosarcoma affecting the foot is estimated to be approximately 35 years[24]. This is over a decade older than expected for patients with osteosarcoma. The calcaneus is the most commonly affected bone and as in other tumors of the foot and ankle, pain is the most common presenting complaint[24]. Diagnosis is frequently delayed and has been reported to take up to two years[24]. Once again patients are frequently misdiagnosed with other conditions including osteoblastoma, chondroblastoma, osteomyelitis, and chondrosarcoma[25].

The exact cause of osteosarcoma is unknown. Patients who survive the inherited form of retinoblastoma are at an increased risk of developing osteosarcoma later in life as a result of a shared chromosomal abnormality involving the Rb1 gene on chromosome 13[26]. However, this genetic defect only accounts for a small number of osteosarcomas. Previous radiation therapy and preexisting conditions such as Paget's disease, hereditary multiple exostosis, and fibrous dysplasia are all linked to the development of osteosarcoma.

Various types of osteosarcoma have been described including intramedullary (conventional) osteosarcoma, parosteal osteosarcoma, and periosteal osteosarcoma. The microscopic appearance of intramedullary osteosarcoma varies according to the subtype:

- osteoblastic osteosarcoma: predominately osteoid/bony matrix
- chondroblastic osteosarcoma: predominately chondroid matrix
- fibroblastic osteosarcoma: predominately spindle cell matrix with little osteoid.

In a case series of 52 osteosarcomas[24] affecting the foot all were found to be intramedullary osteosarcomas with variations in subtype: osteoblastic osteosarcoma (46%), chondroblastic osteosarcoma (25%), fibroblastic osteosarcoma (29%). The tumor was high grade in over 80% of cases. Only one patient had an osteosarcoma arise from previously Pagetoid bone.

Osteosarcoma is an aggressive malignancy, which traditionally has had very poor outcomes. Advances in neo-adjuvant chemotherapy in conjunction with surgical resection have improved patient outcomes with overall five-year survival reaching 65%[27].

Outcomes for disease affecting the foot and ankle are hard to define as the published literature relies on case reports and case series. One series of 14 patients with osteosarcomas involving the foot reported 9 patients dying after a mean of 2½ years[24].

Chondrosarcoma

Chondrosarcomas are malignant cartilage-forming tumors that can arise in any bone but are commoner in the proximal femur, pelvis, and ribs. They tend to occur in older age groups (40–75 years). They are not commonly found in the foot and ankle, and most examples cited in the literature are case reports or case series. The Scottish Bone Tumour Registry reported that 3% of 403 chondrosarcomas arose in the bones of the foot with a mean age at presentation of 52 years (range 17–83)[28]. Chondrosarcomas arising in the foot are commoner in males (M:F, 9:2), compared to elsewhere in the body where the incidence is nearly equal[28].

Chondrosarcomas are described as either primary or secondary, based on whether the tumor has arisen de novo (primary) or from a preexisting benign lesion, such as an enchondroma (secondary). They are also described as central or peripheral. Central chondrosarcomas develop in the medullary cavity (Figure 18.4) and represent around 90% of chondrosarcomas, whereas peripheral tumors are rarer and tend to arise in the cartilage cap of a preexisting osteochondroma.

Microscopically chondrosarcomas vary according to grade with lower grade tumors showing immature chondrocytes and being calcified. Higher grade tumors have hyperchromatic malignant cells with areas of necrosis and degeneration.

At the time of writing, there is no unique chromosomal abnormality common to all chondrosarcomas. Patients with conditions that lead to the development of multiple enchondromas (such as Ollier's disease and Maffucci's syndrome) or osteochondromas (such as hereditary multiple exostoses or diaphyseal aclasis) are at increased risk of developing chondrosarcoma.

The grade of chondrosarcoma is the single most important predictor of outcome. Patients with higher grade tumors are more prone to local recurrence, metastases, and death. Tumors affecting the foot are most commonly grade 2 at the time of presentation [28]. Interestingly, some studies suggest that they have a

(a)

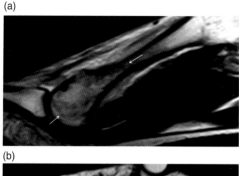

(b)

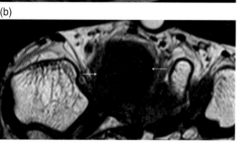

(c)

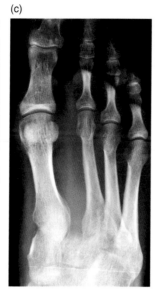

Figure 18.4 Grade 2 chondrosarcoma in a 37-year-old male, treated by second ray excision. (a) Sagittal T2 and (b) axial T1 MRI of the left foot show a chondral tumor in the distal second metatarsal (arrows). Extra-osseous tumor suggests aggressive disease rather than simple enchondroma, and biopsy confirmed grade 2 chondrosarcoma. (c) DP radiograph: the tumor was treated by ray excision.

greater tendency to metastasize when compared to similar lesions affecting the hand – of the 11 reported patients three had local recurrence and all died with metastatic spread[28]. The exact reason for this is unclear and more research is required to determine whether this reflects a more aggressive type of chondrosarcoma arising in the foot.

Investigations

If a malignant tumor of the foot or ankle is suspected a careful history and examination is essential and any areas of tenderness or swelling should be documented. Radiological investigations are required to help make the diagnosis and also to assist with staging, biopsy acquisition, and response to treatment.

Radiographs

Radiographs have a low yield for soft tissue sarcomas, although a soft tissue mass, calcification, and local bone destruction may be evident. Bone sarcomas may have more significant findings. Osteosarcomas of the foot and ankle show a mixture of lysis and sclerosis, and typically the margins of the tumor are poorly defined. Ewing's sarcoma may show typical features with a diffuse lytic lesion, cortical erosion (Figure 18.3) and periosteal reaction. Chondrosarcomas commonly show endosteal scalloping, cortical destruction, calcification, and bone expansion[28].

Pathological fractures may be present in any of the sarcomas affecting the foot.

Magnetic Resonance Imaging

MRI is valuable in the assessment of malignant tumors. It is not only accurate in detecting sarcomas but also assessing the extent of spread including invasion of bone, articular surfaces, local neurovascular structures (Figure 18.1), and the surrounding soft tissues. By demonstrating the extent of the malignant tumor, MRI often determines the type of amputation/resection required to achieve clear margins. The characteristic anatomical location of certain sarcomas in the foot may enable a specific diagnosis to be made, or at least help narrow down the differential diagnosis[29]. MRI is also used to evaluate response to treatment where patients have undergone preoperative chemo/radiotherapy.

Computed Tomography

CT can be helpful in assessing the local extent of a bone tumor, either benign or malignant, evaluating many of the radiographic features seen on plain films, but in greater detail. For example, the margin of the lesion with respect to host bone, the cortical response, the nature of the periosteal reaction, and presence and type of matrix mineralization can be helpful in tumor characterization. CT of the chest is reliable for detecting pulmonary metastases, which enables staging of disease.

Table 18.1 The Enneking staging system for musculoskeletal sarcoma[31]

Stage	Grade	Site
Ia	Low	Intracompartmental
Ib	Low	Extracompartmental
IIa	High	Intracompartmental
IIb	High	Extracompartmental
III	Any grade + local or distant metastases	Either intra- or extracompartmental

Radionuclide Bone Scan

Bone scans are used in primary bone sarcomas to assess distant skeletal metastases and are performed using radiolabeled ^{99m}technetium methylene diphosphonate. They are also useful in detecting skip lesions where there are non-contiguous foci of tumor, within the same bone or occasionally limb. In the foot and ankle such lesions would normally be detected by MRI scanning.

Biopsy

If a malignant tumor is suspected a biopsy should be carried out by either the operating surgeon or an experienced radiologist. This is best done at a specialist center where radiologists and surgeons can contribute to the decision making process as part of a multidisciplinary approach. Due to the paucity of soft tissues around the foot and ankle a needle biopsy is usually straightforward and sufficient to make the diagnosis. The biopsy should be taken in the line of any future surgical incision so that the tract can be excised at the time of definitive surgery. A poorly placed biopsy tract can potentially impair surgical options, leading to an otherwise avoidable amputation[30]. A biopsy will also determine tumor grade, thereby determining the need for systemic treatment.

Staging

There is no unique staging system for malignant tumors involving the foot and ankle. The Enneking staging system[31] is most commonly used to stage bone sarcomas (see Table 18.1) while soft tissue sarcomas are more likely to be staged using the American Joint Committee for Cancer Staging System[32]. The latter system has more grading levels than the Enneking system and documents lymph node spread as well as tumor size.

Treatment

The therapeutic goals in the management of foot and ankle malignancies include local tumor control, restoration of function, long-term survival, and quality of life. The cornerstone of treatment is surgical excision. As with all tumor surgery a multidisciplinary approach should be adopted and patients should be managed in a specialist center that regularly deals with musculoskeletal tumors.

Sarcomas of the foot and ankle have a low prevalence and should be managed on a case-by-case basis. There is insufficient published data to apply a one approach fits all policy. Adequate tumor excision with a wide margin is critical and should take precedence over function and cosmesis. Anatomically, the compartments of the foot are compact and resecting a malignant tumor with safe margins can be problematic[33]. Due to a lack of fascial boundaries and the thin cortices of the tarsal bones, some treat the hindfoot and midfoot as a single compartment[34], recommending trans-tibial (Figure 18.5) or Syme amputation for aggressive tumors involving the talus and calcaneum[28]. Below-knee amputation has also been recommended for all osteosarcomas involving the foot and ankle[35].

Well-localized soft tissue sarcomas can be treated with wide excision and radiotherapy; however, patients are at risk of pathological fractures and de novo sarcoma formation in the irradiated bone.

Neoadjuvant chemotherapy is often used in Ewing's sarcoma and osteosarcoma. Following surgical excision patients are continued on adjuvant chemotherapy based on the response to treatment seen on histological assessment of the excised tumor. The role of chemotherapy in soft tissue sarcomas of the extremity remains unclear.

Approximately, 20% of patients with sarcomas involving the distal lower extremity will have some form of amputation (Figures 18.4 and 18.5)[36]. Limb-sparing surgery should be considered if adequate margins are excised and a durable, functional, and pain free extremity can be achieved[37]. Distal tibial replacements offer a limb-sparing strategy for sarcomas in this region (Figure 18.6).

Metastatic Disease

Metastatic lesions within the foot and ankle occur infrequently. Most of the published literature relies on case reports and such scarcity makes it challenging

(a)

(c)

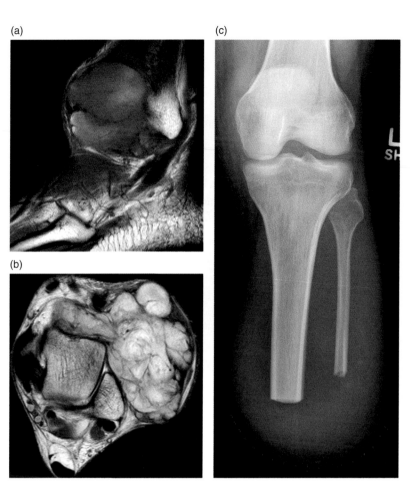

(b)

Figure 18.5 Extraskeletal myxoid chondrosarcoma in a 26-year-old male. (a) Sagittal T1 and (b) axial proton density MRI scan, showing a large mass anterolateral to the ankle, treated by below knee amputation (c).

for the general orthopedic surgeon to identify and diagnose these patients promptly. A study from the Mayo Institute involving 75 000 patients with primary malignancies found only ten patients with metastases to the foot and ankle.

The first case was described in 1920 and involved a metastatic deposit in a metatarsal from a prostate malignancy[38]. A review of 38 histologically confirmed metastases found the most frequent primary was in the genitourinary tract or colon, and that the tarsal bones were most frequently affected (50%)[39].

As this is such an uncommon presentation a high level of vigilance is required. Many patients are initially treated for benign conditions of the foot before the diagnosis is confirmed. The true prevalence of disease may be underestimated as people are not always investigated appropriately.

The presence of lesions within the foot tends to correlate with diffuse metastatic disease and a poor prognosis[40]. With this in mind, treatment goals have an emphasis on pain relief, with local radiotherapy being the most commonly described method for achieving this.

Summary

The commonest pitfall in the management of patients with foot and ankle malignancies is the incorrect diagnosis of a benign condition. Many orthopedic surgeons will never see a case of primary malignancy affecting the foot and ankle, whereas benign tumors affecting the foot and ankle are relatively common. Patients very rarely present with systemic symptoms consistent with a malignancy, and the commonest presenting complaint is one of pain. Some have suggested an MRI for all patients with soft tissue tumors around the foot and ankle measuring more than 2 cm[37]. If there is any doubt

(a)   (b)

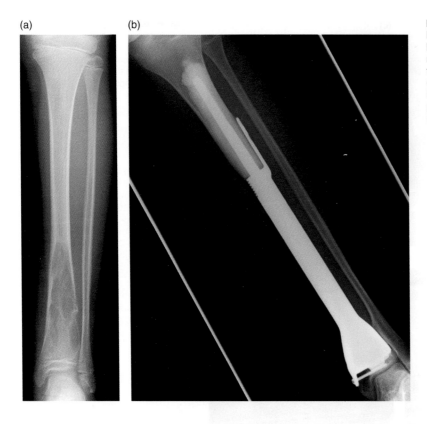

Figure 18.6 Osteosarcoma of the distal left tibia in a ten-year-old female, treated by distal tibial replacement. (**a**) AP radiograph shows a well-defined lytic tumor in the distal tibial diametaphysis (biopsy proven osteosarcoma). Cortical buckling laterally consistent with pathological fracture, stabilized in plaster. (**b**) Postoperative radiograph.

in the clinical diagnosis or there is a failure to respond to initial treatment then an MRI should be performed.

Despite the delays in diagnosis seen with malignancies of the foot and ankle the outcomes are not significantly worse than for similar tumors arising elsewhere. In fact, some authors have shown improved survival for patients with distal lower limb sarcomas, compared to similar tumors at more central anatomical sites[36]. This has led to the hypothesis that malignant tumors of the foot and ankle may have a different biological behavior when compared to sarcomas at other skeletal sites. Reasons for this are not understood and may include the relatively small tumor volume at presentation, limited blood supply, and the cooler temperatures found in tumors of the lower extremity[36].

Key Points

- Malignant tumors of the foot and ankle are rare and represent less than 5% of sarcomas affecting the musculoskeletal system.

- Clinical features of malignant tumors affecting the foot and ankle are similar to benign conditions.

- Approximately 50% of sarcomas affecting the foot and ankle are synovial sarcomas.

- The commonest bone sarcoma of the foot is Ewing's sarcoma.

- Patients with suspected malignant lesions of the foot and ankle should be managed in a specialist center with a multidisciplinary team.

- Surgical excision remains the mainstay of treatment for sarcomas and many patients will require an amputation in order to achieve clear surgical margins.

- The use of massive endoprosthesis offers a limb-sparing solution for cases where a tumor can be excised with an adequate margin and a functional, pain-free limb can be reconstructed.

- Despite advances in surgery and neoadjuvant treatment 23% of patients with primary extremity sarcoma eventually experience distant metastases.

References

1. Fletcher CDM, Bridge JA, Hogendoorn PCW, Mertens F. *World Health Organization Classification of Tumours of Soft Tissue and Bone*, 4th edn, (Lyon: IARC Press, 2013).

2. Miller RW, Young JL Jr, Novakovic B. Childhood cancer. *Cancer*.1995; 75(1 Suppl):395–405.

3. Papagelopoulos PJ, Mavrogenis AF, Badekas A, Sim FH. Foot malignancies: a multidisciplinary approach. *Foot Ankle Clin*. 2003; 8(4):751–63.

4. Weiss S, Goldblum J. General considerations. In Weiss S, Goldblum J, eds. *Enzinger and Weiss's Soft Tissue Tumors* (St Louis, Missouri: CV Mosby, 2001), pp. 1–19.

5. Datir A, James SL, Ali K, Lee J, Ahmad M, Saifuddin A. MRI of soft-tissue masses: the relationship between lesion size, depth, and diagnosis. *Clin Radiol*. 2008; 63(4):373–8.

6. Kransdorf MJ. Malignant soft-tissue tumors in a large referral population: distribution of diagnoses by age, sex, and location. *AJR Am J Roentgenol*. 1995; 164(1):129–34.

7. Scully SP, Temple HT, Harrelson JM. Synovial sarcoma of the foot and ankle. *Clin Orthop Relat Res*. 1999; (364):220–6.

8. Pollock, RE. ed. *Soft Tissue Sarcomas*. (American Cancer Society Atlas of Clinical Oncology, 2002).

9. Hajdu SI, Shiu MH, Fortner JG. Tendosynovial sarcoma. a clinicopathological study of 136 cases. *Cancer*. 1977; 39:1201–17.

10. Sultan I, Rodriguez-Galindo C, Saab R, Yasir S, Casanova M, Ferrari A. Comparing children and adults with synovial sarcoma in the Surveillance, Epidemiology, and End Results program, 1983 to 2005: an analysis of 1268 patients. *Cancer*. 2009; 115(15):3537–47.

11. Murphey MD, Gross TM, Rosenthal HG. From the archives of the AFIP. Musculoskeletal malignant fibrous histiocytoma: radiologic-pathologic correlation. *Radiographics*. 1994; 14(4):807–26.

12. Bakotic BW, Borkowski P. Primary soft-tissue neoplasms of the foot: the clinicopathologic features of 401 cases. *J Foot Ankle Surg*. 2001; 40(1):28–35.

13. Akerman M. Malignant fibrous histiocytoma: the commonest soft tissue sarcoma or a nonexistent entity? *Acta Orthop Scand Suppl*, 1997; 273:41–6.

14. Enzinger FM. Clear-cell sarcoma of tendons and aponeuorses. An analysis of 21 cases. *Cancer*. 1965; 18:1163–74.

15. Speleman R, Sciot F. Clear cell sarcoma of soft tissue. In *World Health Organization Classification of Tumours Pathology and Genetics of Tumours of Soft Tissue and Bone*, ed. C Fletcher, K Unni, F Mertens (Lyon: IARC Press, 2002), pp. 211–12.

16. Dim DC, Cooley LD, Miranda RN. Clear cell sarcoma of tendons and aponeuroses: a review. *Arch Pathol Lab Med*. 2007; 131(1):152–6.

17. Lucas DR, Nascimento AG, Sim FH. Clear cell sarcoma of soft tissues. Mayo Clinic experience with 35 cases. *Am J Surg Pathol*. 1992; 16(12):1197–204.

18. Adkins CD, Kitaoka HB, Seidl RK, Pritchard DJ. Ewing's sarcoma of the foot. *Clin Orthop Relat Res*. 1997; 343:173–82.

19. Dahlin DC, Unni KK. *Bone Tumors: General Aspects and Data on 8,542 Cases*, 4th edn. (Springfield, IL: Charles C Thomas, 1986).

20. Downing JR, Head DR, Parham DM, et al. Detection of the (11;22) (q24;q12) translocation of Ewing's sarcoma and peripheral neuroectodermal tumour by reverse transcription polymerase chain reaction. *Am J Pathol*. 1993; 143:1294–300.

21. Nesbit ME Jr., Gehan EA, Burgert EO Jr., et al. Multimodal therapy for the management of primary, nonmetastatic Ewing's sarcoma of bone: a long-term follow-up of the First Intergroup study. *J Clin Oncol*. 1990; 8(10):1664–74.

22. Burgert EO Jr., Nesbit ME, Garnsey LA, et al. Multimodal therapy for the management of nonpelvic, localized Ewing's sarcoma of bone: intergroup study IESS-II. *J Clin Oncol*. 1990; 8(9):1514–24.

23. Wu KK. Osteogenic sarcoma of the tarsal navicular bone. *J Foot Surg*. 1989; 28(4):363–9.

24. Choong PF, Qureshi AA, Sim FH, Unni KK. Osteosarcoma of the foot: a review of 52 patients at the Mayo Clinic. *Acta Orthop Scand*. 1999; 70(4):361–4.

25. Biscaglia R, Gasbarrini A, Böhling T, Bacchini P, Bertoni F, Picci P. Osteosarcoma of the bones of the foot: an easily misdiagnosed malignant tumor. *Mayo Clin Proc*. 1998; 73(9):842–7.

26. Hansen MF, Koufos A, Gallie BL, et al. Osteosarcoma and retinoblastoma: a shared chromosomal mechanism revealing recessive predisposition. *Proc Natl Acad Sci USA*. 1985; 82(18):6216–20.

27. Bielack SS, Kempf-Bielack B, Delling G, et al. Prognostic factors in high-grade osteosarcoma of the extremities or trunk: an analysis of 1,702 patients treated on neoadjuvant cooperative osteosarcoma study group protocols. *J Clin Oncol*. 2002; 20(3):776–90.

28. Patil S, de Silva MV, Crossan J, Reid R. Chondrosarcoma of the bones of the feet. *J Foot Ankle Surg*. 2003; 42(5):290–5.

29. Wetzel LH, Levine E. Soft-tissue tumors of the foot: value of MR imaging for specific diagnosis. *AJR Am J Roentgenol.* 1990; 155(5):1025–30.

30. Mankin HJ, Mankin CJ, Simon MA. The hazards of the biopsy, revisited. Members of the Musculoskeletal Tumor Society. *J Bone Joint Surg Am.* 1996; 78(5):656–63.

31. Enneking WF, Spanier SS, Goodman MA. A system for the surgical staging of musculoskeletal sarcoma. *Clin Orthop Relat Res.* 1980; 153:106–20.

32. American Joint Committee on Cancer. *AJCC Cancer Staging Manual,* 5th edn. (Philadelphia, PA: Lippincott, Williams & Wilkins, 1997) pp. 171–80.

33. Chou LB, Ho YY, Malawer MM. Tumors of the foot and ankle: experience with 153 cases. *Foot Ankle Int.* 2009; 30(9):836–41.

34. Enneking, WF. *Musculoskeletal Tumor Surgery.* (New York: Churchill Livingstone, 1983).

35. Ozdemir HM, Yildiz Y, Yilmaz C, Saglik Y. Tumors of the foot and ankle: analysis of 196 cases. *J Foot Ankle Surg.* 1997; 36(6):403–8.

36. Zeytoonjian T, Mankin HJ, Gebhardt MC, Hornicek FJ. Distal lower extremity sarcomas: frequency of occurrence and patient survival rate. *Foot Ankle Int.* 2004; 25(5):325–30.

37. DeGroot H 3rd. Approach to the management of soft tissue tumors of the foot and ankle. *Foot Ankle Spec.* 2008; 1(3):168–76.

38. Bloodgood JC. Bone tumors, benign and malignant: a brief summary of the salient features, based on a study of some 370 cases. *Am J Surg.* 1920; 34:229–37.

39. Zindrick MR, Young MP, Daley RJ, Light TR. Metastatic tumors of the foot: case report and literature review. *Clin Orthop Relat Res.* 1982; 170:219–25.

40. Billingsley KG, Lewis JJ, Leung DH, Casper ES, Woodruff JM, Brennan MF. Multifactorial analysis of the survival of patients with distant metastasis arising from primary extremity sarcoma. *Cancer.* 1999; 85(2):389–95.

Chapter 19

The Diabetic Foot

Cameron R. Barr and Lew C. Schon

Introduction

Management of the ever-increasing number of diabetic feet is an important issue for orthopedic foot and ankle surgeons. A thorough understanding of the pathophysiology and treatment options is necessary to provide optimal care for these patients. Within the multidisciplinary team, the orthopedic surgeon has a unique opportunity to play a critical role in the care of the diabetic patient.

Globally in 2013 an estimated 382 million people had diabetes. The International Diabetes Federation states that by 2035 this number will increase to 592 million[1]. Diabetes is more common in developed countries. The American Diabetes Association currently estimates that more than 10% of all Americans over the age of 20 have diabetes. This number steadily increases with age, and 26% of the population older than 65 years has diabetes[2]. Up to 25% of diabetic patients will be affected by foot disorders at some point in their life[3]. Foot ulcers are the most common medical complication causing diabetics to seek medical treatment. Each year in the United States over 65 000 non-traumatic lower limb amputations are performed in diabetics. Diabetes and its complications can and should be viewed as an epidemic, with the worldwide total yearly cost of the disease topping £360 billion ($465 billion)[1].

Pathogenesis

Diabetes is a metabolic disease with systemic manifestations involving the nervous, vascular, immune, and musculoskeletal systems. The etiology of diabetic foot problems is multifactorial. Sensory neuropathy is usually the underlying cause of ulceration and infection. Peripheral vascular disease is also common and hinders healing, but in itself rarely causes foot pathology[4]. If and when an infection does develop in the diabetic foot, the body's immune response is weakened and less effective.

Neuropathy

Diabetic neuropathy is described as a distal, symmetric polyneuropathy[5-6]. It is a length-dependent axonopathy involving both myelinated and unmyelinated nerves, with a predilection for the distal sensory and autonomic fibers, with relative sparing of motor fibers[7]. Metabolic, ischemic, and possibly even hormonal factors drive the nerve damage[5-8]. Although not fully understood the metabolic factors causing nerve damage include the intraneural accumulation of the end products of glycosylation and sorbitol, disruption of the hexosamine and protein kinase C pathways, and activation of the poly(ADP-ribose) polymerase pathway[9-11]. The common end pathway is the cellular build-up of reactive oxygen species, which cause metabolic neural damage.

The role of nerve ischemia in diabetic neuropathy is supported by the finding of thickened endoneural blood vessel walls in neuropathic patients[12]. It has also been shown that diabetic patients with advanced neuropathy have reduced oxygen tension in the peripheral nerves[13]. The impairment in antithrombotic mechanisms may also play a part in the pathogenesis, as there is a decreased level of thrombomodulin and tissue plasminogen activator in the peripheral nerve microvessels of diabetic patients[14]. It is probable that ischemic and metabolic factors work together in the development of peripheral neuropathy, but the exact interaction is not fully understood.

Risk factors for the development of diabetic neuropathy principally relate to the duration and severity of hyperglycemia[15]. More recent epidemiologic studies have focused on additional factors, which include hypertension, smoking, dyslipidaemia, and elevated body mass index[16-17].

Neuropathy alone does not cause diabetic foot pathology, it is the insensitivity combined with abnormal foot pressures that leads to ulceration and tissue breakdown. Brand showed in animal models that with low-level repetitive trauma to tissue, inflammation followed by necrosis will develop. With the inability to sense and respond to mechanical stresses, repetitive trauma from high pressure in the diabetic foot ultimately leads to tissue breakdown. Brand concluded that there are three factors that determine the probability of actual foot ulceration: the severity and location of sensory loss, the magnitude of the forces on the foot, and the walking distance it takes for repetitive stress to induce a state of inflammation[18]. Skin breakdown in diabetics frequently results from deformities from conditions that create bony prominences, such as the proximal phalangeal joints of claw toes, bony ridges from arthritic joints, malunited fracture fragments, or protuberances from Charcot neuroarthropathy. These prominences are vulnerable to pressure from the floor, shoes, or braces.

Dysfunction of the autonomic nervous system compounds the pathological process. With loss of skin temperature regulation, loss of perspiration, and arteriovenous shunting, the plantar skin becomes dry, thickened, and coarse. This leads to fissures and cracks[19]. The fissure leaves a breach in the integument with a vulnerability to infection, but the thickened callus and fissured tissues can also result in pressure areas and shear forces that can lead to deep ulceration.

Vascular

Peripheral vascular disease is four to six times more prevalent in the diabetic population[20]. In diabetics, the arterial calcification process is more diffuse than in those without the disease; it involves the entire circumference of the vessels[4,19]. Furthermore, occlusive disease is rapidly progressive, which prevents compensation with the opening of the collateral circulation. In diabetics the distribution of the vascular disease also differs with more distal vascular involvement. There is commonly popliteal trifurcation and tibioperoneal disease[21]. Interestingly the dorsalis pedis artery is frequently spared.

Studies on the microcirculation based on histology, arterial casting, and vascular resistance show that the changes in the small vessels of the foot are not occlusive[22]. Although patients with diabetes have a thickened capillary basement membrane, the lumen itself is not narrowed[23]. A pathological vascular process at the subarteriolar level that correlates to diabetic foot pathology has not been conclusively identified[4,23]. It is thought that peripheral vascular

disease hinders the healing of the diabetic foot, but alone is rarely the cause of foot pathology.

Immune Response

Diabetics are more susceptible to infections, largely due to their impaired immune response. Leukocyte chemotaxis and function are dramatically reduced[24]. Thus once neuropathic and vascular factors permit pathogens to enter and colonize the foot, the diabetic host is less efficient in combating the infection. With an environment of hyperglycemia, hypoxia, hypertonicity, edema, and an impaired immune response the environment is optimal for continued bacterial growth[19]. A hemoglobin A1c greater than 8% is independently associated with surgical site infection[25].

Evaluation

A thorough lower extremity physical examination is essential in the evaluation of a diabetic patient presenting with foot problems. Inspection of the affected limb alone can provide many important clues to the overall heath of the foot. This includes wear patterns on shoes, hair growth or lack thereof, erythema, edema, open wounds, and nail deformity.

The patients should be assessed in both static (seated and standing) and dynamic (walking and maneuvering) modes. The overall alignment of the foot, range of motion, and any bony prominences should be noted.

Neurologic Evaluation

Evaluation and quantification of sensory neuropathy are critical aspects in the examination of the diabetic foot. Although light touch, two-point discrimination, and proprioception are simple and rapid assessments of neuropathy, more quantitative measures are important for prognostic value. These include vibratory testing, nerve conduction studies, temperature testing, and monofilament testing[4]. By far the most commonly used is the Semmes–Weinstein monofilament (Figure 19.1). The monofilament consists of nylon filaments of varying thickness that are pressed onto the skin until they bend. The smallest monofilament that the patient can feel represents the threshold of sensation. Monofilament testing has been shown to have a higher reproducibility than vibration threshold perception[26]. It is frequently quoted that being able to feel a 5.07 monofilament, which is equivalent to a 10 g

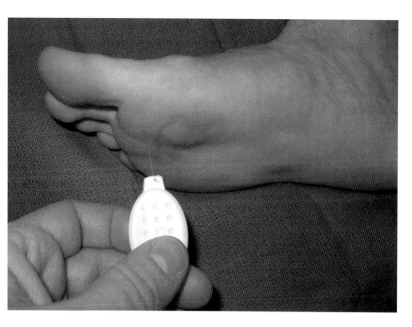

Figure 19.1 Sensory examination with 10 g Semmes–Weinstein monofilament.

force, is needed for protective sensation. It has been shown that failure to perceive such a monofilament is associated with an increased risk of foot ulceration and amputation[27]. Although the 5.07 monofilament is easy to use, economical, and widely accepted, nearly 10% of patients with sensation at this level still go on to develop ulceration and neuroarthropathy[19].

Vascular Evaluation

A vascular evaluation is necessary to inform treatment options. Beyond palpation of pulses and the timing of capillary refill, the most commonly used assessment of blood flow is with Doppler studies[4]. Doppler ultrasound can be used to measure arterial pressure. The ankle–brachial index (ABI) is the ratio of the systolic blood pressure measured at the ankle to the pressure in the arm. Wagner determined that an ABI of 0.45 was the minimum required for healing of diabetic foot lesions[28]. Although only a guideline, the prognostic value of an ABI can be strengthened with the addition of absolute toe pressures. The absolute toe pressure often quoted to achieve wound healing is 45 mmHg[19]. It is important to keep in mind, however, that pressure values can be falsely elevated in calcified vessels. In this setting, more pressure is required to compress the stiffened vessels. Thus an ABI of greater than 1.0 should raise the possibility of calcification[4]. The shape of the waveform is important and is normally bi- or triphasic. A monophasic waveform can indicate proximal disease.

Transcutaneous oxygen measurements are also used as a measure of vascularity and healing potential. Pinzur et al. found a direct correlation with healing of amputations and transcutaneous oxygen pressure $(TcPO_2)$[29]. When the $TcPO_2$ was greater than 30 mmHg over 90% of amputations healed, whereas when the $TcPO_2$ was less than 30 mmHg only 66% healed. The measurement has also been linked to the response to hyperbaric oxygen treatments[19].

If and when the patient is found to have vascular insufficiency, evaluation by a vascular surgeon or interventional radiologist is often warranted. An arteriogram can be used to localize specific points of occlusion and plan angioplasty or revascularization procedures. Coupled with local wound care and debridement, such procedures can often lead to limb salvage.

Imaging Overview

Imaging studies are critical in the evaluation of the diabetic foot and its complications. The most commonly used techniques include plain radiography, ultrasonography, MRI, and bone scintigraphy.

With its wide availability and low cost, radiographs remain the staple first-line imaging for the diabetic foot. They provide baseline information on joint changes, bone infection, soft tissue gas, and foreign bodies. Although they are less sensitive and specific for many diabetic complications than other imaging modalities, they are essential in evaluating the basic foot and ankle structure. Weightbearing radiographs of the foot and ankle should be obtained in all cases if possible.

Ultrasound is another widely available, non-invasive imaging modality, which is extensively used. It is helpful in the detection of inflammatory soft tissue changes, fluid collections, joint effusions, and foreign bodies. It can also be useful in guiding diagnostic aspiration.

MRI may be the most important modality for evaluation of the diabetic foot. Its strength lies in its ability to evaluate both soft tissue and bone, detecting bone marrow changes. MRI is useful for identifying soft tissue abscesses, particularly in swollen feet with cellulitis or Charcot neuroarthropathy. The imaging is multiplanar, which allows precise identification of the involved structures, and it is invaluable for directing surgical management. Nevertheless it is important to remember that the bone edema found in osteomyelitis and neuroarthropathy remains difficult to differentiate with MRI alone[30].

The most commonly used nuclear medicine techniques in the diabetic foot include three-phase bone scanning with technetium-99m (^{99m}Tc) and indium-111 (^{111}In) labeled white blood cell (WBC) scans[30]. Although less expensive than MRI, a ^{99m}Tc bone scan is highly non-specific and can remain positive for over a year following fracture or surgery[4]. Alone the ^{99m}Tc scan cannot easily differentiate osteomyelitis from neuroarthropathy. The addition of an extra scan at 24 hours, a four-phase bone scan, has not been found to help[31]. The ^{111}In white cell scan, in contrast, has a greater specificity for infection. Several studies have shown that by combining a ^{99m}Tc scan and ^{111}In white cell scan the sensitivity and specificity for differentiating infection from neuroarthropathy can be raised to over 90% and 80% respectively.

Clinical Problems and Treatment

Ulceration

Foot ulcers are the most common medical complication causing diabetics to seek medical attention. Fifteen percent of patients with diabetes will eventually develop an ulcer in their lifetime. Such ulcers have a tremendous impact on patients' quality of life. The majority require an ambulatory assist device or are unable to ambulate independently, and view their condition as significantly interfering with their

daily lives[32]. Ulceration is often the precursor to infection and osteomyelitis, and ulcers lead to over 65 000 amputations per annum in the United States alone[2].

Over 70% of ulcers occur in the forefoot, followed by the heel and midfoot[19]. Much work has been done to identify risk factors for the development of foot ulcers. The International Working Group on the Diabetic Foot[33] stratified over 200 diabetic patients into four risk groups: group 0 consisted of patients without neuropathy, group 1 consisted of patients with neuropathy but without deformity or peripheral vascular disease, group 2 consisted of patients with neuropathy and deformity or peripheral vascular disease, and group 3 consisted of patients with a history of foot ulceration or a lower extremity amputation. During a three-year follow-up period, ulceration occurred in 5%, 14%, 19%, and 56% of patients in groups 0, 1, 2, and 3, respectively. All the amputations occurred in groups 2 and 3. Additional risk factors include an abnormal tendo Achillis reflex, insensitivity to a 10 g monofilament, reduced pulses, increased age, and previous podiatric attendance. Factors associated with increased healing potential of ulcers include a serum albumin greater than 30 g/L and a total lymphocyte count of more than 1.5×10^9/L. The combination of sensory neuropathy and autonomic skin changes places soft tissue at high risk for breakdown. With continued pressure, usually over unprotected bony prominences, ulceration can develop.

Two commonly cited classification systems of diabetic ulcers are the Wagner classification[28] and the Brodsky depth–ischemia classification[34]. The Wagner classification, developed at Rancho Los Amigos Hospital, has historically served as a basis for evaluation. There are six grades, 0 to 5, based on depth of lesion and presence of gangrene (Table 19.1). There is an important divide in the system between the first four grades and the final two, with grades 4 and 5 being related to loss of vascularity, rather than depth of lesion.

The Brodsky depth–ischemia classification (Table 19.2) is a modification of the Wagner classification, with an alphanumeric system to separate the classification of the depth of the foot wound from the vascularity of the foot. The soft tissue is given a numbered depth (Grade 0–3). The perfusion of the foot is examined and given a letter (Grade A–D). This combination of soft tissue and vascularity assessment better helps guide prognosis and treatment

Table 19.1 Wagner classification for diabetic foot ulcers

Grade	Definition	Description
0	Foot at risk	Thick callus, no break in skin, prominent bony lesion
1	Superficial ulcer	Full thickness destruction of skin
2	Deep ulcer	Penetrates through skin, fat, tendons, and ligaments but not through bone. Includes penetration into a joint
3	Abscess and deep ulcer	Localized osteomyelitis or abscess
4	Limited gangrene	Limited necrosis in toes or forefoot
5	Extensive gangrene	Necrosis of complete foot with systemic effects

Table 19.2 Depth–ischemia classification for ulcers, developed by Wagner and modified by Brodsky

Grade	Description
Depth classification	
0	At-risk foot, no ulcer (Figure 19.2)
1	Superficial ulcer, not infected (Figure 19.3)
2	Deep ulceration exposing tendon or joint, with or without superficial infection (Figure 19. 4)
3	Extensive ulceration with exposed bone and deep infection (Figure 19.5)
Ischemia classification	
A	No ischemia
B	Ischemia without gangrene
C	Partial (forefoot) gangrene of the foot
D	Complete gangrene of the foot

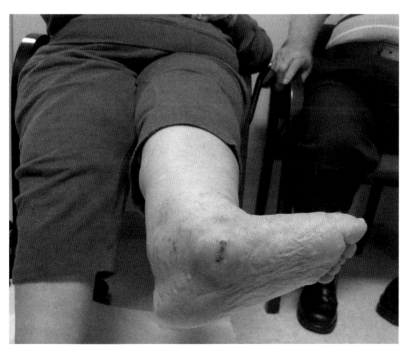

Figure 19.2 Grade 0 ulcer: foot at risk for ulceration, note the subcutaneous hemosiderin.

(Figures 19.2 to 19.5). Brodsky outlines a logical, stepwise approach for treating diabetic ulcers[34]. The surgeon first assesses the soft tissue wound using the numeric, depth component of the depth–ischemia classification system. This includes visual inspection and palpation of the wound with a probe to determine which, if any, underlying deep structures are exposed.

The typical grade 1 lesion, superficial ulceration with healthy granulation tissue, is treated as an outpatient, whereas the deeper grades usually require surgical care. Following this the ischemic component, A to D, of the depth–ischemia classification system is used to determine if there is adequate vascularity to allow healing. If palpable pulses are absent, vascular

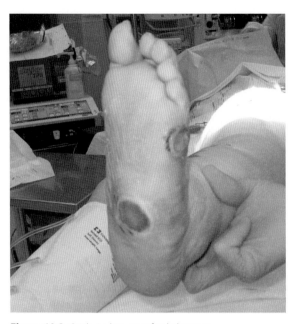

Figure 19.3 Grade 1 ulcer: superficial ulceration.

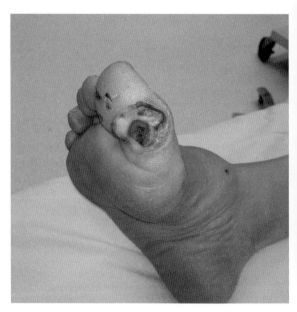

Figure 19.4 Grade 2 ulcer: deep ulceration.

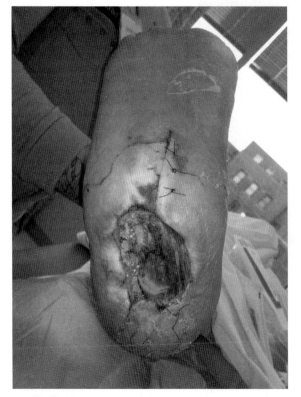

Figure 19.5 Grade 3 ulcer: extensive ulceration with exposed bone and deep infection.

studies are carried out. This is critical, as vascular reconstruction is often needed for wound healing. Finally, the ulcer is assessed for infection. If more than simple superficial colonization, the patient should be admitted to hospital for intravenous antibiotics. These ulcers often require surgical debridement to clear the ulcer bed of infected tissue. The ultimate goal of debridement is to achieve a wound with healthy granulation tissue with no infected or non-viable tissue.

Once the above steps have been taken, the ultimate treatment in ulcer care can be initiated – *pressure relief*. This comes in many forms, both non-operative and operative. Non-operative pressure relief includes footwear modification, total contact casts, and walking boots. Although the specific pressure-relieving device is chosen based on both provider and patient preference, a few points are worth mentioning here. Firstly, total contact casting, changed at two- to four-weekly intervals, remains the "gold standard" for most plantar sided ulcers, with an 85 to 90% healing rate of grade 1 and 2 ulcers[35-36]. These casts are not without problems. Guyton[37] found an overall complication rate of 30% per patient and 5% per cast. Although most of the complications were new abrasions or ulcers, which healed spontaneously, patients should be made aware of this before cast application. Prefabricated walking boots also reduce plantar foot pressure. The reduction in pressure is equal to, or can be greater than, that achieved by total contact casting[38-39]. The advantage of cost and ease of application must be weighed against the risk of patient non-compliance.

Sometimes pressure relief requires surgical intervention, with the creation of a plantigrade foot with no bony prominences. Sometimes this is simply achieved with tendo Achillis lengthening, to correct equinus and unload the forefoot, followed by total contact casting. This combination has been found to be very effective in the treatment of recurrent forefoot ulcers[40]. Other procedures are tailored to the specific ulcer and its location, but there are unifying surgical concepts[4]. The majority of procedures focus on resection of the bone causing the excessive pressure, as well as removal of non-viable and infected tissue. It is important that the incision for bone resection should be distinct from the ulcer. For example, with a plantar ulcer the incision for bone resection, or exostectomy, can be made on the medial or lateral border of the foot, and the ulcer is debrided directly. Once the underlying pressure has been relieved and the ulcer is clean and non-infected, the treatment returns to casting or shoe modification until healing is complete.

Infections

Foot infection is common in the diabetic patient, with foot infections accounting for the largest number of diabetes-related inpatient hospital days. They are often pivotal events leading to progressive clinical deterioration[41].

Diabetic foot infections are usually polymicrobial. Ge et al.[42] looked at the microbiological profiles of 825 infected diabetic foot ulcers and found an average of 2.4 organisms per ulcer. Gram-positive cocci (staphylococci, group B streptococci, enterococci), gram-negative rods (*Escherichia coli*, *Enterobacter*, *Proteus*, *Pseudomonas*), and anaerobes (*Bacteroides*, *Clostridium*) are commonly found together. Antibiotic-resistant organisms such as methicillin-resistant *Staphylococcus aureus* (MRSA) and vancomycin-resistant enterococcus and staphylococcus (VRSA) are now becoming more frequent and are associated with poorer outcomes in patients with diabetic foot infections[41].

A diabetic foot infection can present with a number of clinical scenarios, including cellulitis, abscesses, and osteomyelitis. A thorough examination of the foot is essential. The ability to probe to bone

through an ulcer alone has a positive predictive value of 89% for the presence of underlying osteomyelitis[43]. In addition to a white blood cell count with differential, laboratory studies should include an ESR, CRP, albumin, and prealbumin. It should be remembered that fewer than 50% of diabetic patients with infections have leukocytosis[3]. Deep cultures of soft tissue and bone are paramount in typing the microorganisms and their antibiotic sensitivity. Superficial swabs are notoriously inaccurate[4]. In imaging the foot MRI is most useful, as it allows the extent of bone and soft tissue involvement to be determined.

Treatment of diabetic foot infections is both non-operative and operative and often overlaps with the ulcer care discussed above. Most superficial infections are treated with a course of antibiotics. The choice and duration of antibiotic treatment depend on the severity of infection and the patient. Often broad-spectrum antibiotics are initiated, until specific microorganisms have been cultured, and antibiotic sensitivities determined.

Abscesses and osteomyelitis usually require surgical debridement. Despite the case series of Embril et al.[44], where 80% of cases of diabetic foot osteomyelitis went into remission with antibiotic treatment alone, the classic teaching remains that complete eradication of infection requires surgical intervention.

Forefoot osteomyelitis is usually treated with ablative surgery of the toes, including transection or disarticulation. Infection can travel along the flexor and extensor tendons, thus it is important to inspect the remaining proximal tissues, with this in mind, at the time of surgery. There is always a balance to be struck between removing all the involved tissue and retaining enough skin and subcutaneous tissue to allow primary closure of the wound.

Ulceration under prominent metatarsal heads is common, and leads to metatarsal osteomyelitis. Metatarsal head resection can be considered if the infection is localized to the head alone. Head resection is effective, although it is common for the adjacent metatarsal head to develop a transfer lesions and ulcerate, requiring an additional head resection. If head resection is not sufficient, partial or complete ray resection may be necessary. Multiple ray resections are a favorable option over transmetatarsal amputation as they allow for better postoperative shoe options, although a forefoot with three or fewer rays is prone to further ulceration as result of the high pressure under the remaining heads.

327

Midfoot osteomyelitis is commonly seen at the base of the fifth metatarsal in the varus hindfoot. Debridement is the standard treatment for this, but it is important to attempt to reattach the peroneus brevis to prevent worsening of the hindfoot varus. If reattachment is not possible, future triple, or even pantalar, arthrodesis may be necessary.

Hindfoot osteomyelitis is usually addressed through partial or total calcanectomies. This can be approached though a longitudinal, midline posterior and plantar incision. These procedures often require the use of negative-pressure dressings to assist with wound healing and carry a high failure rate. Revision to a below-knee amputation is sometimes required.

Nearly 50% of diabetic patients with foot infections eventually end up with an amputation[45]. A thorough discussion of amputations is beyond the scope of this review; however, a few important points are worth mentioning. Amputation should be viewed as a reconstructive procedure to regain energy-efficient ambulation. With advancements in surgery and prosthetics the outcomes for diabetic amputees have improved. Before any amputation a complete clinical evaluation should be undertaken including a vascular and nutritional assessment. A $TcPO_2$ level greater than 30 mmHg and a toe pressure greater than 45 mmHg are associated with a healing rate of approximately 90%[19]. A serum albumin greater than 30 g/L and a total lymphocyte count of more than 1.5×10^9/L is also associated with better wound healing[3]. Resection should be at, or above, the level of viable soft tissue and bone. There are numerous amputation levels, which include partial digital, digital, ray, transmetatarsal, Chopart (midtarsal), Syme, below the knee, and above the knee. The length of the residual limb is inversely proportional to the patient's energy expenditure during ambulation[3].

Charcot Neuroarthropathy

Charcot neuroarthropathy is a chronic and progressive disease following the loss of protective sensation. It is characterized by joint destruction and fragmentation and can result in significant foot deformity. The resulting deformity hinders shoe and brace use, and the bony malalignment may lead to ulceration and eventual infection. Diabetes is the leading cause of Charcot neuroarthropathy in the twenty-first

century, with the incidence in the diabetic population ranging from 1 to 37%[3]. The feet are the most common location for neuroarthropathy, and it is bilateral in approximately 30% of patients[4]. Interestingly, there does not appear to be a direct relationship between the severity of the diabetic neuropathy and neuroarthropathy, which is even seen in very mild type II diabetes.

There are two major theories that exist for the pathogenesis of Charcot neuroarthropathy. The first postulates underlying neurotraumatic destruction. It is thought that with loss of protective sensation, repetitive, mechanical micro-trauma in the insensate foot leads to joint destruction and collapse. The second is neurovascular destruction. It is postulated that autonomic dysfunction increases blood flow through arteriovenous shunting. The high blood flow leads to bone resorption, weakening, and eventually failure. In all probability the two theories play a combined role in the ultimate pathogenesis of the neuroarthropathy.

More recent studies suggest that inflammatory cytokines may have a role in the development of Charcot neuroarthropathy. It is proposed that an increase in the expression of cytokines, such as tumor necrosis factor and interleukin-1, stimulates osteoclast formation and bone resorption. Baumhauer et al.[46] confirmed an increase in both inflammatory markers and osteoclasts in pathologic specimens using immunologic staining.

Eichenholtz described the staging system of Charcot neuroarthropathy.

Stage I, the development phase, is characterized radiologically by osteopenia, fragmentation, and joint subluxation or dislocation. Clinically there is edema, warmth, and erythema. Osseous fragmentation and joint dislocation are seen on radiographs. Stage I usually lasts for two to six months.

Stage II, the coalescence phase, marks the initiation of the reparative process. Radiographs show coalescence of the fragments, sclerosis, and absorption of fine bone debris. Clinically there is decrease in erythema, temperature, and swelling.

Stage III is the reconstruction phase. Radiologically there is arthrosis and fibrous ankylosis, with the bone fragments becoming rounded. Clinically the foot cools and stabilizes, with or without deformity. Stage II and III usually last for a combined period of 18 to 24 months.

Brodsky classified Charcot neuroarthropathy into four anatomic regions of involvement[4]. Type 1

(a)

(b)

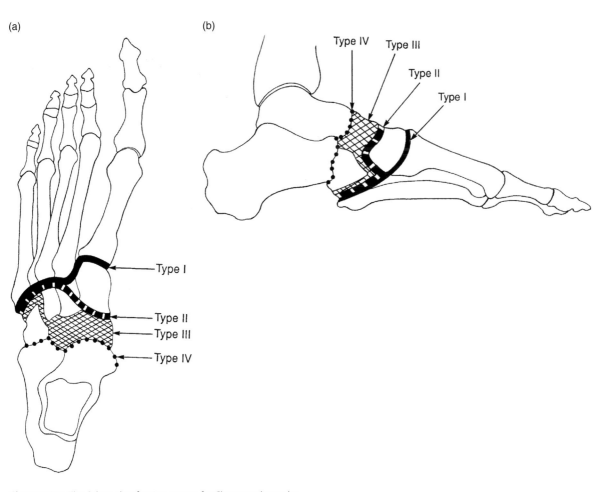

Type IV   Type III

Type II

Type I

Type I

Type II
Type III

Type IV

Figure 19.6 The Schon classification system for Charcot arthropathy.

(midfoot) involves the metatarsocuneiform and naviculocuneiform joints and is the most common presentation, accounting for 60% of cases. Type 2 (hindfoot) involves the subtalar, talonavicular, or calcaneocuboid joints. There are two subgroups of type 3. Type 3A (ankle) involves the tibiotalar joint. Type 3B (os calcis) is a small group in whom the tendo Achillis avulses the calcaneal tubercle, in the so called "parrot-beak." Over 90% of Charcot neuroarthropathy is of type 1 and 2.

The Schon classification reflects the anatomic location (I to IV), severity of the collapse (A to C), and radiographic severity (α and β)[47-48]. The classification has been found to be reliable and reproducible. It can be used for diagnosis, planning, treatment, and prognosis (Figures 19.6 to 19.10). Type I involves the metatarsocuneiform joints. A plantar prominence develops medially under either the first metatarsal base or the medial cuneiform. Most type I feet then abduct, with the collapse progressing plantar-laterally. Type II involves the naviculocuneiform joint and extends laterally to the fourth and fifth metatarsalcuboid joints. A lateral rocker bottom deformity typically develops under the subluxed cuboid. Type III involves the perinavicular region with fragmentation, fracture, or osteonecrosis of the navicular. There is shortening of the medial column with supination and adduction of the foot. These feet ulcerate under the fifth metatarsal tuberosity or the cuboid. Type IV involves the midtarsal joint. The navicular subluxes laterally on the talus, with abduction of the midfoot and the calcaneus moving into valgus. The calcaneal pitch decreases and a rocker bottom deformity develops at the calcaneocuboid joint. Type IV injuries

(a)

(b)

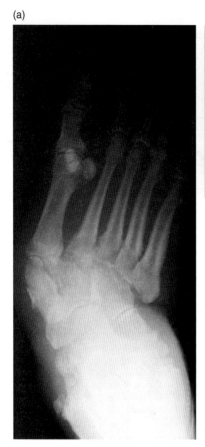

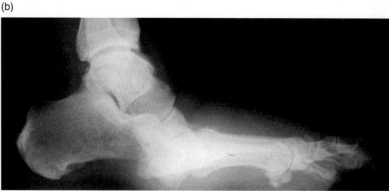

Figure 19.7 Schon type I: (a) AP and (b) lateral views.

ulcerate under the talar head, the navicular, and the plantar aspect of the distal calcaneus.

The clinical severity scale associated with the Schon stratifies feet at risk for ulceration and osteomyelitis (Figure 19.11). Stage A describes feet with a low arch, but the arch remains above the plane of the metatarsal heads and calcaneus. Stage B represents collapse of the arch to the level of the metatarsal heads and calcaneus. Stage C identifies an arch below the plane of the metatarsal heads and calcaneus, and carries a poor prognosis with a high risk of chronic ulcers and infection.

The radiographic severity is the final component. Alpha represents a better prognosis with less likelihood of requiring aggressive intervention. The following criteria must all be met for a foot to be classified as alpha:

1. AP talus–first metatarsal angle less than 35°
2. lateral talus–first metatarsal angle less than 30°

3. lateral calcaneal–fifth metatarsal angle greater than 0°
4. no dislocation – we think that patients in the beta category often benefit from realignment and fusion.

In the acute phase it can be difficult to differentiate between Charcot neuroarthropathy and infection. In the acute Charcot patient the involved foot is usually red, swollen, and warm. The systemic signs of fever, elevated white cell count, ESR, and CRP are not reliable in distinguishing between the two entities. A subtle diagnostic test that can be used is that the erythema associated with a Charcot foot improves with elevation, but that associated with infection does not. Furthermore, whereas patients with Charcot arthropathy may localize discomfort to the foot alone, patients with infection often appear and feel more systemically ill. When differentiation cannot be made clinically, a biopsy of the area in

(a)

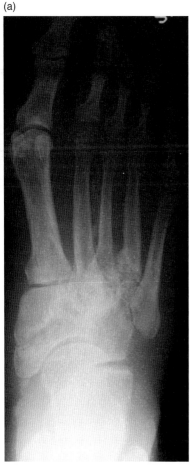

(b)

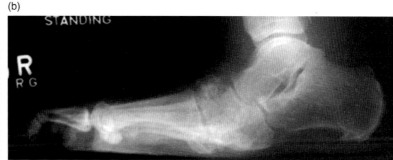

Figure 19.8 Schon type II: (**a**) AP and (**b**) lateral views.

question can help. It should also be borne in mind that infection is rare in the absence of a history of ulceration or previous surgery. In essence, if the skin has not been breached the implication is that the infection has arisen from hematogenous spread – a rare occurrence.

In contrast to acute Charcot neuroarthropathy, subacute and chronic cases present with disruption of the foot at a single or multiple joints. Patients may have a widened foot, bony prominences, and collapse of the foot with a rocker-bottom deformity.

Imaging the Charcot foot involves multiple modalities. Radiographs can be normal in the first days to weeks, often only revealing soft tissue swelling. Ultimately, however, the radiographs show joint destruction and bony fragmentation, followed by resorption and reconstruction as outlined above in the Eichenholtz staging system. MRI can also help to identify neuropathic fractures, as well as assisting in the differentiation of Charcot neuroarthropathy from some infections. Nevertheless, while MRI is useful in imaging abscesses, the MRI changes found in osteomyelitis and Charcot neuroarthropathy are often similar[30].

Nuclear scintigraphy, including the ^{99m}Tc bone scan and the ^{111}In labeled white blood cell scan, can help distinguish Charcot from osteomyelitis. Whereas a technetium bone scan alone may not differentiate the two pathologies, the addition of ^{111}In labeled white blood cell scan has been shown to aid in the diagnosis of osteomyelitis, having a sensitivity of 93% to 100% and a specificity of 80%[49].

The treatment goal for Charcot neuroarthropathy is to establish a plantigrade foot that is amenable to bracing or orthotic management and does not ulcerate or become infected. General guidelines have been

331

(a)

(b)

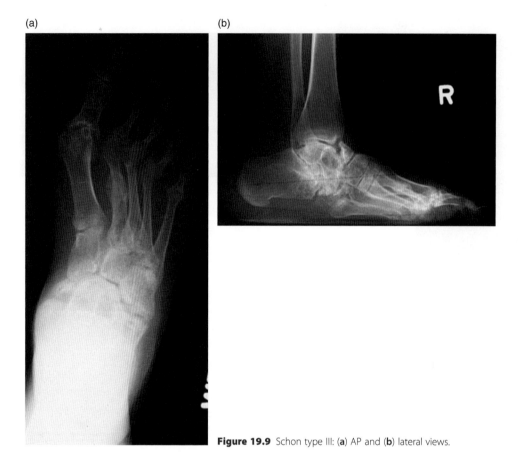

Figure 19.9 Schon type III: (**a**) AP and (**b**) lateral views.

developed based on the Eichenholtz and Schon deformity types (Table 19.3).

An Eichenholtz stage I Charcot foot is initially treated non-operatively, with rest, elevation, and a total contact cast. At first, the cast is changed on a weekly basis as the swelling reduces rapidly, and the cast becomes loose during the week. After a while the swelling becomes less marked and the interval between cast changes can be increased to several weeks. The patient is typically kept non-weightbearing during the treatment of stage I. Some providers use a prefabricated boot, as an alternative to a total contact cast, although bony deformity can make the fitting of the boot suboptimal[4,50]. When the inflammatory stage has settled with healing of the fragmentation on radiographs and return of a normal skin temperature, the patient is transitioned into a weightbearing removable orthosis. Typically, this consists of a molded total-contact polypropylene AFO or Charcot restraint orthotic walker (CROW).

Stage III allows final fitting with accommodative shoes and insoles.

Recently an immobilization treatment protocol, allowing early full weight bearing in the cast or brace, has been tried. This was in part recommended to try and reduce the incidence of contralateral limb fracture, which has been found to be as high as 72% in high-risk patients.[51] De Souza reported successful five-year follow-up management of Charcot neuroarthropathy in 33 of 34 patients using a weightbearing total contact cast.[52]

Surgical treatment is undertaken for infection, ulceration, and unstable or unbraceable deformity. Classically, surgery has been delayed until Eichenholtz stage III, as there is a high risk of complication in the earlier stages[3]. Surgical options are typically broken down into exostectomy and arthrodesis.

If an ulcer overlies an infected, or non-infected, bony prominence, where tarsal bones have shifted into non-anatomic positions following fracture or

(a)

(b)

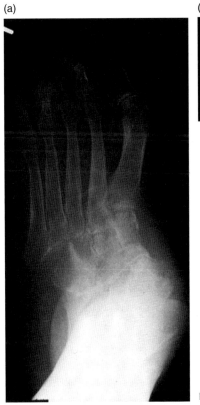

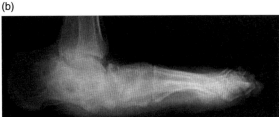

Figure 19.10 Schon type IV: (**a**) AP and (**b**) lateral views.

fragmentation[49], exostectomy is a simple and effective technique. Excision of the prominent bone is flat to the floor, and is usually undertaken through a lateral incision for the cuboid, a medial incision for the navicular or cuneiforms, and a plantar incision for a central bony mass. If there is an ulcer or infection, this is debrided. The cuboid is most often involved. Following exostectomy, bracing and antibiotics for infection are used. Brodsky and Rouse showed good results with a 90% limb salvage rate[53].

For more severe, unstable deformities arthrodesis may be indicated (Table 19.4, Figure 19.12). In these cases the arthrodesis is for salvage, creating a plantigrade foot, free from ulceration and infection[4]. Arthrodesis with internal fixation in the setting of Charcot neuroarthropathy is complex, often requiring osteotomies and a prolonged period of rigid immobilization with protected weight bearing for up to three months[49]. The surgery is frequently staged when infection is present, with initial debridement and exostectomy to heal the ulcer, and secondary reconstruction with arthrodesis. The rate of bony

union is between 36 and 100%, but even fibrous union has been shown to give acceptable clinical results[19,49].

External fixation can be used in high-risk patients, such as the obese, the immunocompromised, and those with a longstanding ulcer with osteomyelitic bone. Pinzur treated 26 consecutive patients with Charcot midfoot deformity and multiple comorbidities with a ring external fixator. At one-year follow-up, 92% of patients were ulcer and infection free and able to walk with custom orthoses[54]. Cooper had a 96% limb salvage rate at 22 months when treating 83 patients with Charcot arthropathy of the midfoot and hindfoot with external fixation[55].

Amputation rates in Charcot neuroarthropathy are close to 3%[49]. The decision to proceed with amputation is multifactorial and necessitates careful discussion between the patient and surgeon. In terms of burden to society, a recent analysis comparing single-stage limb reconstruction to amputation showed similar cost of care in the first year[56].

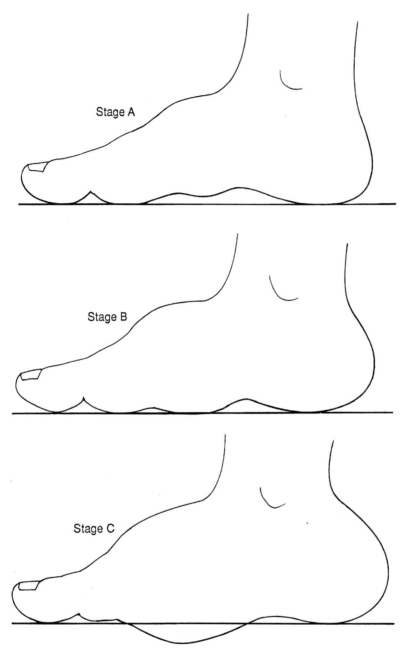

Figure 19.11 The Schon classification system clinical severity scale.

Stage A

Stage B

Stage C

Ankle Fractures

Ankle fractures in the diabetic population have significantly higher rates of in-hospital mortality, postoperative complications, length of stay, and non-routine discharges.[57] Infection, malunion, hardware failure, Charcot neuroarthropathy, and amputation are all increased in this patient population.

A review of 160 000 ankle fractures showed that nearly 6% had diabetes[57]. The diabetic patients had a higher rate of complications than the non-diabetics. Furthermore, those patients with complicated diabetes have significantly higher complication rates than those with uncomplicated diabetes. Wukich et al.[58] found that those with peripheral neuropathy,

Table 19.3 Treatment algorithm for Charcot foot based on Eichenholtz stage and Schon

Category	Management modalities
Eichenholtz I (any type, any stage)	Elevation, restricted weight bearing, cast or brace
Eichenholtz II (any type, any stage)	Walking cast, brace, custom-molded ankle–foot orthosis, restricted activities
Eichenholtz III Types I–IV (asymptomatic)	Extra-depth shoes, accommodative orthotic devices, occasionally custom-molded ankle–foot orthosis
Types I–IV (with persisting ulcer despite bracing, casts, or accommodative orthosis)	Exostectomy or corrective fusion (see Table 19.4)
Types I–IV (in the presence of osteomyelitis)	Excision of osteomyelitic bone, realignment of foot, external fixation

Table 19.4 Fusion techniques for Schon deformity types

Deformity type	
IA	Fuse involved TMTJ using screws or plantar plate
IB	Fuse involved metatarsocuneiform joints medially with plantar plate. If lateral fourth or fifth TMTJ collapses, fuse and apply lateral plantar plate
IC	Fuse entire TMTJ complex with plantar closing wedge osteotomy, apply medial and lateral plantar plates
IIA	Fuse naviculocuneiform joint with plantar plate or screws
IIB	Fuse naviculocuneiform joint and fourth and fifth TMTJ if collapsed with plantar lateral plate or screws
IIC	Fuse metatarsonaviculocuneiform joints and fourth and fifth TMTJ with plantar-based closing wedge osteotomy and medial and lateral plantar plates
IIIA	Fuse talonavicular and/or naviculocuneiform joints
IIIB	Fuse talonavicular and/or naviculocuneiform joints and fourth and fifth TMTJ with plantar plate if collapsed
IIIC	Fuse entire involved midtarsus medially and laterally with closing wedge osteotomy and medial and lateral plantar plates
IVA	Triple arthrodesis
IVB	Triple arthrodesis
IVC	Triple arthrodesis; may require plantar closing wedge osteotomy and medial and lateral plates

nephropathy, or peripheral artery disease had a 3.8 times higher rate of complications than those with uncomplicated diabetes.

The reason for the increased complication rates is multifactorial. In general both soft tissue and fracture healing are impaired. The combination of local ischemia and elevated blood glucose creates a poor environment for wound healing[59,60]. Under hypoxic conditions, fibroblast proliferation and migration is inhibited, impairing local collagen production[60]. In addition, hyperglycemia results in high levels of protein glycosylation, which hinders fibroblast and basement membrane function, and inflammatory cell receptors[59]. The final result is tenuous soft tissue healing.

The impaired fracture healing seen in diabetics is not fully understood. Most of our knowledge comes from studies in small animal models, which have shown that both the type of collagen and collagen content in the early stages of fracture healing are abnormal in the diabetic[61]. Other studies have shown a decrease in gene expression for the regulation of osteoblast differentiation and a decrease in local platelet-derived growth-factor levels, which leads to decreased cellular proliferation[62]. In the final analysis there is delayed ossification with a decrease in the mechanical strength of the fracture callus.

A diabetic patient with an ankle fracture needs careful evaluation. It is important to note any history of neuropathy, Charcot neuroarthropathy, peripheral artery disease, previous ulceration, and previous infections, as these all affect treatment and outcome.

Routine foot and ankle radiographs to assess fracture pattern and to evaluate for Charcot neuroarthropathy are obtained. The ultimate goal in both the diabetic and non-diabetic population is to create a stable, congruent joint, which allows continued function. This can be achieved either operatively or non-operatively. All fractures are initially reduced and splinted, being careful to preserve the soft tissue envelope.

Non-operative management is reserved for non-displaced, stable fractures, or for patients who cannot tolerate a surgical intervention as a result of medical comorbidities or peripheral vascular disease for example.

Non-operative treatment, as in the non-diabetic population, is with immobilization in a cast or boot.

It is important to recognize that the duration of immobilization and non-weightbearing will need to be increased in the diabetic patient, often by a factor of two to three times. Frequent follow-up is also necessary to monitor for loss of reduction. If this occurs reduction and fixation should be considered.

There is a number of small case series documenting the outcome of the non-operative treatment of diabetic ankle fractures. McCormack and Leith treated 26 ankle fractures in diabetic patients, of which seven were treated non-operatively in a cast.

(a) (b)

(c) (d)

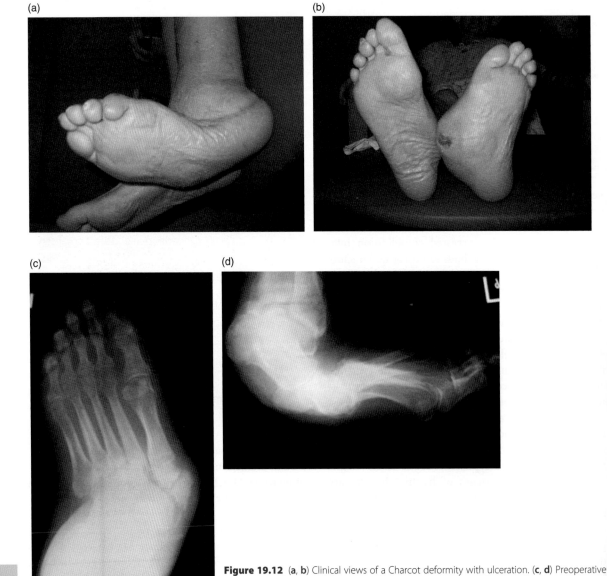

Figure 19.12 (**a**, **b**) Clinical views of a Charcot deformity with ulceration. (**c**, **d**) Preoperative radiographs of type IIC deformity. (**e**, **f**) Postoperative radiographs show fixation with a plantar plate and oblique screws. (**g**, **h**) Clinical views postoperatively.

(e)

(f)

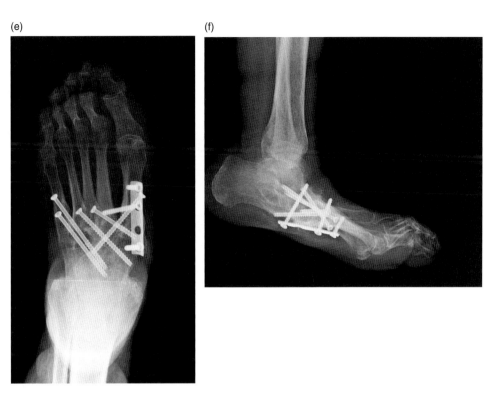

(g)

(h)

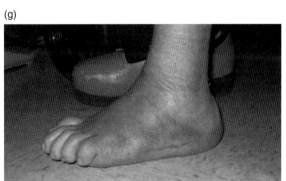

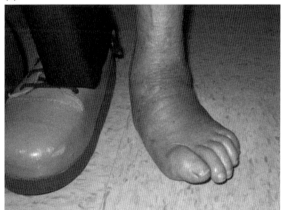

Figure 19.12 (*cont.*)

Five of the seven developed an asymptomatic malunion and the other two healed uneventfully. The incidence of significant complications in diabetic patients was 42.3%, compared to 0% in non-diabetic patients. The authors suggest that even displaced fractures can be treated non-operatively in the low-demand diabetic patient, although they did not comment on either fracture severity or the functional level of the patients with eventual malunion[63]. On the other hand

Schon and Marks reported their results of 28 neuropathic ankle fractures of which 13 were displaced and 15 were non-displaced. All were treated non-operatively with three to nine months of immobilization. Although all non-displaced fractures healed without infection or Charcot arthropathy, all displaced fractures went on to non-union or malunion[64].

Thus we recommend surgical treatment for displaced and unstable ankle fractures with an incongruent joint. General principles should be followed, including allowing the soft tissues to settle before surgery, and rigid fixation. Prolonged postoperative immobilization, of two to three times that for routine ankle fractures, is recommended. Strict non-weightbearing should be used for at least eight weeks followed by protected weight bearing for another eight to twelve weeks.

The surgical construct should be chosen based on the degree of peripheral neuropathy and the bone density. Those patients with mild neuropathy and non-osteoporotic bone may do well with standard small-fragment instrumentation using an interfragmentary compression screw and a neutralization plate. It is important, however, to handle the soft tissues and bone carefully. Periosteal stripping should be minimized. Full thickness skin flaps and wide skin bridges when using two incisions are optimal.

In those patients with peripheral neuropathy or poor bone quality a more rigid construct is necessary to prevent loss of reduction. Several surgical techniques have been proposed in this regard. Increasing the biomechanical strength of the fixation has been shown to minimize postoperative complications[64–68]. Koval et al. used retrograde 1.6 mm K-wires across the reduced fibular fracture to improve screw purchase prior to lateral plate fixation. Biomechanical testing showed 81% greater resistance to bending and twice the resistance to motion during torsional testing. Of 19 patients treated with this technique, all went on to union without loss of reduction[67].

Schon and Marks[64] have advocated multiple tetracortical fibula-to-tibia screws through a one-third tubular plate in the proximal fibular fragment (Figure 19.13). This construct has been shown to be significantly stiffer in resisting axial and external rotation loads compared to intramedullary K-wire augmentation of the fixation[65]. Perry et al. had good results in six failed neuropathic ankle fractures using a 4.5 mm dynamic compression plate and screws in this manner[68].

In unstable ankle fractures or fracture–dislocations, Jani et al. recommended supplementing standard fracture fixation with transarticular fixation. In 15 diabetic patients with neuropathy, large Steinmann pins were passed retrograde in a transcalcaneal route across the ankle and subtalar joints. After prolonged immobilization with implant removal at 12 to 16 weeks, 13 of the 15 patients had a stable ankle, which allowed weightbearing activity. Nevertheless, there was a 25% complication rate, including four cases

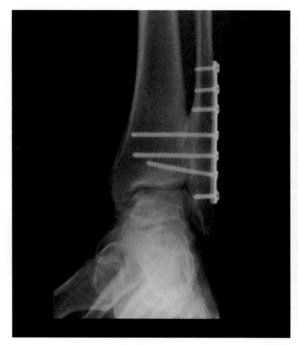

Figure 19.13 Tri-cortical fixation for an ankle fracture in a diabetic patient.

of post-traumatic arthritis and three cases of retained intramedullary implants[66].

Locking plate technology may also be beneficial in diabetic ankle fracture fixation. It should reduce the localized failure and loosening of individual screws in the osteoporotic bone often seen in diabetics. Minimally invasive surgical techniques should also be considered in the treatment of diabetic ankle fractures with tenuous soft tissue envelopes. Retrograde insertion of a lateral plate through a small incision over the distal fibula followed by percutaneous screw insertion can be used. External fixation, either alone or in conjunction with limited internal fixation, is also gaining in popularity.

Overall the outcome of surgical treatment for diabetic ankle fractures is significantly worse than for non-diabetic ankle fractures. Egol et al. evaluated predictors of outcome in operatively treated ankle fractures and found that the absence of diabetes alone was predictive of improved functional recovery[69]. At one-year follow-up, 92% of non-diabetic patients regained more than 90% of their baseline function. Only 71% of diabetic patients achieved the same. SooHoo et al. looked at over 50 000 ankle fractures treated surgically and clearly found an increased complication rate in the diabetic population[70]. The rates of infection in patients with and without complicated diabetes were 7.7% and 1.4%, respectively. There was also a significant increase in the rate of amputation among patients with complicated diabetes (3.9%) relative to the overall patient population (0.2%).

Key Points

- Up to 25% of diabetic patients will be affected by foot disorders at some point during their life.
- Each year in the United States alone, over 65 000 non-traumatic lower limb amputations are performed in the diabetic population.

Ulceration

- The combination of sensory neuropathy and abnormal skin pressure from bony prominences leads to ulceration and infection.
- Perception of a 10 g/ 5.07 Semmes–Weinstein monofilament is needed for protective sensation.
- Total contact casting is the gold standard for mechanical relief of plantar ulcerations.
- Most diabetic foot infections are polymicrobial.
- Treatment is largely determined by the Wagner or Brodsky grade.
- HBA1c greater than 8% is independently associated with surgical site infection.

Charcot Neuroarthropathy

- Charcot neuroarthropathy is a chronic and progressive joint disease following loss of protective sensation.
- An acute Charcot foot can be confused with infection.
- The treatment goal for Charcot arthropathy is to establish a plantigrade foot that is amenable to bracing or orthotic treatment, while avoiding ulceration and infection.
- Surgical treatment is undertaken for infection, ulceration, and unstable or unbraceable deformity.
- Surgical options are typically broken down into exostectomy and arthrodesis.
- Amputation is not uncommon in the setting of Charcot arthropathy and failed surgery, with annual rates close to 3%.

Ankle Fractures

- Unstable ankle fractures may be best treated with augmented internal fixation.
- The immobilization time should be doubled or tripled.
- Ankle fractures in the diabetic population are at increased risk for complications.

References

1. International Diabetes Federation. The global burden. www.idf.org/ diabetesatlas/global-burden. Accessed June 27, 2014.

2. American Diabetes Association. National diabetes fact sheet. www.diabetes.org/diabetes-basics/statistics. Accessed June 27, 2014.

3. Philbin TM. The diabetic foot. In *Orthopaedic Knowledge Update: Foot and Ankle*, 4th ed. (Rosemont: American Academy of Orthopaedic Surgeons, 2008), pp. 273–330.

4. Brodsky JW. The diabetic foot. In Coughlin MJ, Mann RA, Saltzman CL eds. *Surgery of the Foot and Ankle*, 8th edn. (St. Louis: Mosby-Year Book Inc, 2007), pp. 1281–368.

5. Callaghan BC, Cheng HT, Stables CL, Smith AL, Feldman EL. Diabetic neuropathy: clinical manifestations and current treatments. *Lancet Neurol.* 2012; 11:521–34.

6. Dyck PJ, Kratz KM, Karnes JL, et al. The prevalence by staged severity of various types of diabetic neuropathy, retinopathy, and nephropathy in a population-based cohort: the Rochester Diabetic Neuropathy Study. *Neurology.* 1993; 43:817–24.

7. Malik RA. The pathology of human diabetic neuropathy. *Diabetes.* 1997; 46(Suppl 2): S50–S53.

8. Edwards JL, Vincent AM, Cheng HT, Feldman EL. Diabetic neuropathy: mechanisms to management. *Pharmacol Ther.* 2008; 120:1–34.

9. Das Evcimen N, King GL. The role of protein kinase C activation and the vascular complications of diabetes. *Pharmacol Res.* 2007; 55:498–510.

10. Oates PJ. Aldose reductase, still a compelling target for diabetic neuropathy. *Curr Drug Targets.* 2008; 9:14–36.

11. Sugimoto K, Yasujima M, Yagihashi S. Role of advanced glycation end products in diabetic neuropathy. *Curr Pharm Des.* 2008; 14:953–61.

12. Fagerberg SE. Diabetic neuropathy: a clinical and histological study on the significance of vascular affections. *Acta Med Scand Suppl.* 1959; 345:1–97.

13. Newrick PG, Wilson AJ, Jakubowski J, Boulton AJ, Ward JD. Sural nerve oxygen tension in diabetes. *Br Med J* (Clin Res Ed). 1986; 293:1053–4.

14. Hafer-Macko CE, Ivey FM, Sorkin JD, Macko RF. Microvascular tissue plasminogen activator is reduced in diabetic neuropathy. *Neurology.* 2007; 69:268–74.

15. Genuth S. Insights from the Diabetes Control and Complications Trial/Epidemiology of Diabetes Interventions and Complications Study on the use of intensive glycemic treatment to reduce the risk of complications of type 1 diabetes. *Endocr Pract.* 2006; 12(Suppl 1):34–41.

16. Dyck PJ, Davies JL, Wilson DM, Service FJ, Melton LJ, O'Brien PC. Risk factors for severity of diabetic polyneuropathy: intensive longitudinal assessment of the Rochester Diabetic Neuropathy Study cohort. *Diabetes Care.* 1999; 22:1479–86.

17. Tesfaye S, Chaturvedi N, Eaton SE, et al. Vascular risk factors and diabetic neuropathy. *N Engl J Med.* 2005; 352:341–50.

18. Brand PW. Tenderizing the foot. *Foot Ankle Int.* 2003; 24:457–61.

19. Laughlin RT, Calhoun JH, Mader JT. The diabetic foot. *JAAOS.* 1995; 3:218–25.

20. Barker WF. Peripheral vascular disease in diabetes: diagnosis and managment. *Med Clin North Am.* 1971; 55:1044–55.

21. Arora S, LoGerfo FW. Lower extremity macrovascular disease in diabetes. *J Am Podiatr Med Assoc.* 1997; 87:327–31.

22. Conrad MC. Large and small artery occlusion in diabetics and nondiabetics with severe vascular disease. *Circulation.* 1967; 36:83–91.

23. Arora S, LoGerfo FW. Lower extremity macrovascular disease in diabetes. *J Am Podiatr Med Assoc.* 1997; 87:327–31.

24. Delamaire M, Maugendre D, Moreno M, Le Goff MC, Allannic H, Genetet B. Impaired leucocyte functions in diabetic patients. *Diabet Med.* 1997; 14:29–34.

25. Wukich DK, Crim BE, Frykberg RG, Rosario BL. Neuropathy and poorly controlled diabetes increase the rate of surgical site infection after foot and ankle surgery. *J Bone Joint Surg Am.* 2014; 96:832–9.

26. McCabe CJ, Stevenson RC, Dolan AM. Evaluation of a diabetic foot screening and protection programme. *Diabet Med.* 1998; 15:80–4.

27. Tan LS. The clinical use of the 10g monofilament and its limitations: a review. *Diabetes Res Clin Pract.* 2010; 90:1–7.

28. Wagner FW. A classification and treatment program for diabetic, neuropathic and dysvascular foot problem. *Instr Course Lect.* 1979; 28:143–65.

29. Pinzur MS, Sage R, Stuck R, Ketner L, Osterman H. Transcutaneous oxygen as a predictor of wound healing in amputations of the foot and ankle. *Foot Ankle.* 1992; 13:271–2.

30. Tomas MB, Patel M, Marwin SE, Palestro CJ. The diabetic foot. *Br J Radiol.* 2000; 73:443–50.

31. Sanverdi SE, Ergen BF, Oznur A. Current challenges in imaging of the diabetic foot. *Diabet Foot Ankle.* 2012; 3:10.3402/dfa.v3i0.18754 [doi].

32. Evans AR, Pinzur MS. Health-related quality of life of patients with diabetes and foot ulcers. *Foot Ankle Int.* 2005; 26:32–7.

33. Peters EJ, Lavery LA. Effectiveness of the diabetic foot risk classification system of the International Working Group on the Diabetic Foot. *Diabetes Care.* 2001; 24:1442–7.

34. Brodsky JW. Outpatient diagnosis and care of the diabetic foot. *Instr Course Lect.* 1993; 42:121–39.

35. Frigg A, Pagenstert G, Schafer D, Valderrabano V, Hintermann B. Recurrence and prevention of diabetic foot ulcers after total contact casting. *Foot Ankle Int.* 2007; 28:64–9.

36. Nabuurs-Franssen MH, Sleegers R, Huijberts MS, et al. Total contact casting of the diabetic foot in daily practice: a prospective follow-up study. *Diabetes Care.* 2005; 28:243–7.

37. Guyton GP. An analysis of iatrogenic complications from the total contact cast. *Foot Ankle Int.* 2005; 26:903–7.

38. Baumhauer JF, Wervey R, McWilliams J, Harris GF, Shereff MJ. A comparison study of plantar foot pressure in a standardized shoe, total contact cast, and prefabricated pneumatic walking brace. *Foot Ankle Int.* 1997; 18:26–33.

39. Pollo FE, Brodsky JW, Crenshaw SJ, Kirksey C. Plantar pressures in fiberglass total contact casts vs. a new diabetic walking boot. *Foot Ankle Int.* 2003; 24:45–9.

40. Lewis J, Lipp A. Pressure-relieving interventions for treating diabetic foot ulcers. *Cochrane Database Syst Rev.* 2013; 1:CD002302.

41. Lipsky BA, Berendt AR, Deery HG, et al. Diagnosis and treatment of diabetic foot infections. *Plast Reconstr Surg.* 2006; 117:212S–238S.

42. Ge Y, MacDonald D, Hait H, Lipsky B, Zasloff M, Holroyd K. Microbiological profile of infected diabetic foot ulcers. *Diabet Med.* 2002; 19:1032–4.

43. Grayson ML, Gibbons GW, Balogh K, Levin E, Karchmer AW. Probing to bone in infected pedal ulcers. A clinical sign of underlying osteomyelitis in diabetic patients. *JAMA.* 1995; 273:721–3.

44. Embil JM, Rose G, Trepman E, et al. Oral antimicrobial therapy

for diabetic foot osteomyelitis. *Foot Ankle Int.* 2006; 27:771–9.

45. Eneroth M, Apelqvist J, Stenstrom A. Clinical characteristics and outcome in 223 diabetic patients with deep foot infections. *Foot Ankle Int.* 1997; 18:716–22.

46. Baumhauer JF, O'Keefe RJ, Schon LC, Pinzur MS. Cytokine-induced osteoclastic bone resorption in charcot arthropathy: an immunohistochemical study. *Foot Ankle Int.* 2006; 27:797–800.

47. Schon LC, Easley ME, Weinfeld SB. Charcot neuroarthropathy of the foot and ankle. *Clin Orthop.* 1998; 349:116–31.

48. Schon LC, Easley ME, Cohen I, Lam PWC, Badekas A, Anderson CD. The acquired midtarsus deformity classification system: interobserver reliability and intraobserver reproducibility. *Foot Ankle Int.* 2002; 23:30–6.

49. van der Ven A, Chapman CB, Bowker JH. Charcot neuroarthropathy of the foot and ankle. *J Am Acad Orthop Surg.* 2009; 17:562–71.

50. Pinzur MS, Shields N, Trepman E, Dawson P, Evans A. Current practice patterns in the treatment of Charcot foot. *Foot Ankle Int.* 2000; 21:916–20.

51. Clohisy DR, Thompson RC Jr. Fractures associated with neuropathic arthropathy in adults who have juvenile-onset diabetes. *J Bone Joint Surg Am.* 1988; 70:1192–200.

52. de Souza LJ. Charcot arthropathy and immobilization in a weight-bearing total contact cast. *J Bone Joint Surg Am.* 2008; 90:754–9.

53. Brodsky JW, Rouse AM. Exostectomy for symptomatic bony prominences in diabetic Charcot feet. *Clin Orthop.* 1993; 296:21–6.

54. Pinzur MS. Neutral ring fixation for high-risk nonplantigrade Charcot midfoot deformity. *Foot Ankle Int.* 2007; 28:961–6.

55. Cooper PS. Application of external fixators for management of Charcot deformities of the foot and ankle. *Foot Ankle Clin.* 2002; 7:207–54.

56. Gil J, Schiff AP, Pinzur MS. Cost comparison: limb salvage versus amputation in diabetic patients with charcot foot. *Foot Ankle Int.* 2013; 34:1097–9.

57. Ganesh SP, Pietrobon R, Cecilio WA, Pan D, Lightdale N, Nunley JA. The impact of diabetes on patient outcomes after ankle fracture. *J Bone Joint Surg Am.* 2005; 87:1712–18.

58. Wukich DK, Joseph A, Ryan M, Ramirez C, Irrgang JJ. Outcomes of ankle fractures in patients with uncomplicated versus complicated diabetes. *Foot Ankle Int.* 2011; 32:120–30.

59. Chaudhary SB, Liporace FA, Gandhi A, Donley BG, Pinzur MS, Lin SS. Complications of ankle fracture in patients with diabetes. *J Am Acad Orthop Surg.* 2008; 16:159–70.

60. Hunt TK, Linsey M, Sonne M, Jawetz E. Oxygen tension and wound infection. *Surg Forum.* 1972; 23:47–9.

61. Topping RE, Bolander ME, Balian G. Type X collagen in fracture callus and the effects of experimental diabetes. *Clin Orthop Relat Res.* 1994; 220–8.

62. Lu H, Kraut D, Gerstenfeld LC, Graves DT. Diabetes interferes with bone formation by affecting the expression of transcription factors that regulate osteoblast differentiation. *Endocrinology.* 2003; 144:346–52.

63. McCormack RG, Leith JM. Ankle fractures in diabetics.

Complications of surgical management. *J Bone Joint Surg Br.* 1998; 80:689–92.

64. Schon LC, Marks RM. The management of neuroarthropathic fracture-dislocations in the diabetic patient. *Orthop Clin North Am.* 1995; 26:375–92.

65. Dunn WR, Easley ME, Parks BG, Trnka H-J, Schon LC. An augmented fixation method for distal fibular fractures in elderly patients: a biomechanical evaluation. *Foot Ankle Int.* 2004; 25:128–31.

66. Jani MM, Ricci WM, Borrelli J, Jr., Barrett SE, Johnson JE. A protocol for treatment of unstable ankle fractures using transarticular fixation in patients with diabetes mellitus and loss of protective sensibility. *Foot Ankle Int.* 2003; 24:838–44.

67. Koval KJ, Petraco DM, Kummer FJ, Bharam S. A new technique for complex fibula fracture fixation in the elderly: a clinical and biomechanical evaluation. *J Orthop Trauma.* 1997; 11:28–33.

68. Perry MD, Taranow WS, Manoli A, Carr JB. Salvage of failed neuropathic ankle fractures: use of large-fragment fibular plating and multiple syndesmotic screws. *J Surg Orthop Adv.* 2005; 14:85–91.

69. Egol KA, Tejwani NC, Walsh MG, Capla EL, Koval KJ. Predictors of short-term functional outcome following ankle fracture surgery. *J Bone Joint Surg Am.* 2006; 88:974–9.

70. Soohoo NF, Krenek L, Eagan MJ, Gurbani B, Ko CY, Zingmond DS. Complication rates following open reduction and internal fixation of ankle fractures. *J Bone Joint Surg Am.* 2009; 91:1042–9.

Introduction

The pediatric foot presents a wide spectrum of normal and developmental variants, from congenital abnormalities in otherwise healthy individuals, to complex problems resulting from a generalized developmental abnormality or a broader syndrome. Generally speaking, patients who have a stable, plantigrade foot should initially be treated with a course of non-operative management. Conversely, patients with deformities that create pain or difficulty with ambulation are more often managed with surgical intervention.

Normal Variation

The "normal" shape of the pediatric foot is, at best, a moving target. Normal arch height is not well defined, although in infancy the foot is normally flat, with the arch gradually rising over the first five years or so. The shape and posture of the foot does not necessarily indicate which pathologies will occur in it. Differentiating a normal variant from a pathological foot is based upon an assessment of the complete picture, including the foot position, the patient's symptoms, physical examination, and radiographic findings.

Accessory ossicles are a common radiographic finding. In fact, more than 20% of children have an accessory bone on radiographic imaging[1]. These are generally an incidental finding and most are of limited or no clinical significance. The os trigonum and os naviculare will be discussed in further detail as they do cause occasional symptoms.

Os Trigonum

The medial and lateral posterior processes of the talus appear between eight and 11 years of age and then join to the talus in the subsequent year. The posterolateral process forms the lateral border of the groove

for the flexor hallucis longus (FHL) as it courses behind the ankle[2]. In approximately 13% of patients the posterolateral process remains unfused as the os trigonum (Figure 20.1).

Injury to the os trigonum typically occurs in patients who perform activities that require maximal plantar flexion, such as ballerinas who dance en pointe. However, a single traumatic event involving extreme plantar flexion of the ankle can injure the os trigonum. The patient presents with posterior ankle pain. On physical examination, forced ankle plantar flexion reproduces the pain, which must be distinguished from FHL tenosynovitis, which is also frequently seen in ballet dancers. Careful examination can often identify FHL tenosynovitis, which typically causes tenderness in the posteromedial ankle on deep palpation over the FHL tendon when the hallux is put through a range of motion. However, in the acute setting it may be difficult to distinguish between the diagnoses on examination alone.

Radiographs will show the os trigonum. A true os can be distinguished from a fracture of the posterior process by its smooth, well-corticated margin. A fracture has a rough, irregular border. If the diagnosis is unclear a CT or MRI scan can be utilized to further evaluate the posterior ankle. CT is useful for distinguishing an os from a fracture.

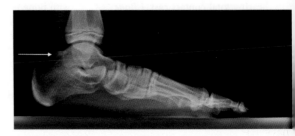

Figure 20.1 Lateral radiograph demonstrating an os trigonum.

MRI will demonstrate an increased signal if the os is injured, as well as in the case of tenosynovitis of the FHL tendon.

Treatment of a painful os trigonum starts with a period of immobilization with a cast or walking boot. If the pain persists despite immobilization, excision of the os using either an open or arthroscopic approach is appropriate.

Accessory Navicular

The presence of an accessory navicular has an autosomal dominant inheritance pattern with incomplete penetrance[4]. The reported prevalence is near 10%[2], thus an accessory navicular is often an incidental finding, although it can become symptomatic. An accessory navicular may be classified as type I in which an ossicle exists in the substance of the posterior tibial tendon, type II in which there is a distinct synchondrosis between the main body of the navicular and the accessory bone, and type III in which there is a "cornuate navicular" or enlarged medial process of the navicular.[3]

Despite clinical experience often associating a painful accessory navicular with pes planovalgus, a study evaluating the relationship of the accessory navicular to the development of a pediatric flat foot showed that the accessory ossicle does not contribute to the development of a flat foot[6]. The histology of a painful accessory navicular has shown microfracture through the cartilaginous synchondrosis, acute and chronic inflammation, and cellular proliferation indicating attempted repair[5].

The child with a symptomatic accessory navicular presents with pain over the medial tuberosity at, or near, the insertion of the tibialis posterior tendon. The pain may be especially prominent over the plantar medial aspect of the navicular tuberosity, not just over the medial edge. The pain may be increased with pressure from tight-fitting shoes.

X-rays can be used to classify the type of accessory navicular. An external oblique radiograph (Figure 20.2), the opposite of the usual internal oblique, best visualizes the synchondrosis or bony ossicle. Important to surgical planning is that it is primarily plantar and proximal to the navicular tuberosity on the lateral radiograph.

The initial treatment of a symptomatic accessory navicular is with padding or stretching of the shoe over the bony prominence, and the avoidance of tight

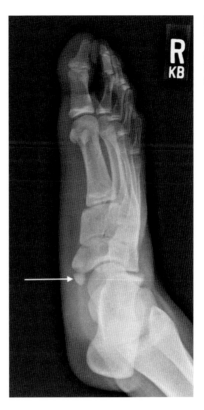

Figure 20.2
External oblique radiograph demonstrating type II accessory navicular.

shoes. If there is an associated planovalgus deformity, an orthosis with a medial heel wedge, to induce varus, and an arch support may help. However, the arch support may press directly on the bony prominence of the navicular, unless specifically designed with a padded flange to protect the prominence. If orthoses fail a period of immobilization in a short-leg walking cast or a walking boot is tried.

If non-operative treatment fails, surgical management involves excision of both the painful ossicle and prominent medial navicular tuberosity. The ossicle is carefully dissected from the surrounding tendon, the prominent navicular tuberosity is removed with a micro-saw, and the tendon is reconstructed for maximal functional outcome. The redundant tendon is advanced and maximally tightened into the navicular and surrounding soft tissues, with the foot held in inversion, in order to maximize tibialis posterior function. Similar to the classic Kidner procedure, the tendon must be advanced to prevent iatrogenic dysfunction and weakness of the tibialis posterior muscle, although there has been disagreement about this in the literature[7].

343

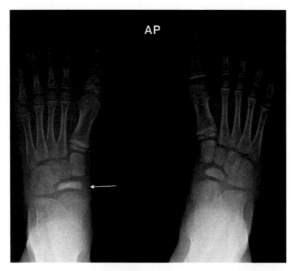

Figure 20.3 Anteroposterior radiograph demonstrating normal navicular (right) and the flattened, sclerotic navicular typical of Köhler's disease (left, with arrow).

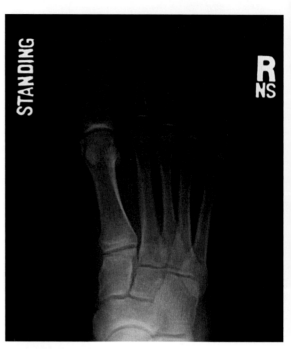

Figure 20.4 Radiograph demonstrating the typical findings of Freiberg's infraction of the third metatarsal head.

Osteochondroses

Sever's Disease

Sever's disease is believed to be an overuse injury of the calcaneal apophysis. The usual presentation is in an active child who participates in running and jumping activities. Generally, the child will complain of pain over the posterior or plantar aspect of the heel, aggravated by activity. The heel is tender to palpation. Treatment is universally non-operative and the disease process is self-limited, although not necessarily quick to resolve. Treatment consists of heel wedges to elevate the heel and reduce the tension in the plantar fascia and the tendo Achillis (TA) through the growth plate. Stretching of the TA is helpful but it can be difficult to get the child to participate in this on a regular basis. Forced rest with cast immobilization for four to eight weeks may assist recalcitrant cases. The disease will eventually resolve when the apophysis closes.

Köhler's Disease

Köhler's disease is an osteochondrosis of the navicular, of unknown cause. There are two predominant theories as to its etiology:

1. The location of the navicular coupled with the fact that it ossifies relatively late makes it susceptible to mechanical compression injury.

2. Periodic compression of the navicular leads to AVN.

Köhler's disease most commonly presents in children around the age of five and is more common in boys than girls. Few patients give a history of specific trauma relating to the onset. They usually complain of pain, tenderness, and swelling in the midfoot. Radiographs demonstrate a flattened, sclerotic navicular (Figure 20.3).

Treatment is non-operative because the symptoms and radiographic changes spontaneously resolve over 18 months to three years. Restricted weight bearing and the use of walking casts, or boots, are prescribed according to the patient's pain.[2]

Freiberg's Infraction

Freiberg's disease is an osteochondrosis of the metatarsal head, most commonly of the second metatarsal, although it also occurs in the third. The cause is poorly understood but it is believed to be a result of AVN. It usually occurs in adolescents after 13 years of age and is more common in girls than boys.

The patients usually complain of pain underneath the metatarsal head. Radiographs show subchondral lucency and collapse of the metatarsal head (Figure 20.4).

Initial non-operative treatment is with a hard-soled shoe, boot, or cast. A metatarsal pad can also be used to help offload pressure from the metatarsal head. If the pain persists, surgical intervention may be warranted.

Several surgical options exist for the treatment of Freiberg's disease. The affected area is predominantly on the dorsal aspect of the metatarsal head and the plantar condyles are relatively spared. A dorsal closing wedge osteotomy will rotate the better preserved plantar cartilage into the area of articulation with the phalanx. Alternatively, if the dorsal cartilage is in satisfactory condition, the collapsed segment of the metatarsal head is curetted and the resulting defect filled with cancellous autograft to buttress the subchondral bone and cartilage joint surface. In the latter case metatarsal shortening, for example with a Weil osteotomy, may be attempted in an effort to decrease the joint pressure. Finally, in select cases, metatarsal head allograft or metatarsal head resection may be attempted[9].

Congenital Deformity

Congenital Talipes Equinovarus (Clubfoot)

Clubfoot is a common congenital deformity found in one to two of every 1000 live births. It is more frequent in males. While clubfoot tends to occur in multiple members of the same family, it does not follow typical genetic inheritance patterns. The majority of congenital talipes equinovarus (CTEV) cases are idiopathic, although it may result from an underlying neuromuscular condition or syndrome. Thus a patient with CTEV, particularly if it is rigid, should be evaluated for neuromuscular disease, including arthrogryposis, diastrophic dwarfism, Möbius syndrome, Streeter's dysplasia, spinal dysraphism, and fetal alcohol syndrome.

The congenital idiopathic clubfoot is diagnosed clinically. Patients have a consistent and predictable pattern of deformity, comprised of cavus, forefoot adductus, hindfoot varus, and equinus (Figure 20.5). Furthermore, there is dysplasia of the talar neck, which consistently deviates in a medial and plantar direction. The navicular is subluxed medially and there is internal rotation of the calcaneus.

Several etiologies have been proposed for the idiopathic clubfoot. These include a primary germ plasm defect, soft tissue abnormalities with a "retractive

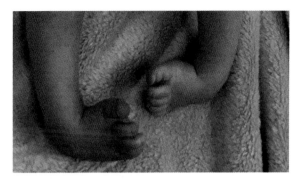

Figure 20.5 A child with bilateral clubfoot deformity.

fibroblastic response," and developmental arrest of the foot. None of these theories fully explains all of the features of CTEV encountered in practice, and for this reason it is believed that the etiology is multifactorial[2].

The initial treatment of the idiopathic clubfoot has alternated between operative and non-operative. At the current time there is a consensus for early non-operative treatment[13–15]. By contrast, the neuromuscular clubfoot is typically rigid, and resistant to non-operative correction.

The Ponseti method is based upon weekly changes of a long-leg cast, with gradual correction by manipulation of each component of the deformity. The acronym "CAVE" describes the order of correction and also conveniently defines the clinical deformity. It stands for Cavus, Adductus, Varus, and Equinus. Correction is usually achieved with the use of five or six casts. Nevertheless, aggressive attempts to manipulate and cast a rigid equinus deformity can result in dorsiflexion through the midfoot and the creation of a rocker bottom foot. Thus TA tenotomy is required in over 85% of patients in order to achieve adequate correction of the equinus. The tenotomy is delayed until satisfactory correction of all other components of the deformity have been achieved.

After the completion of cast treatment, the patient is placed into a foot abduction orthosis, the Denis–Brown bar and shoes, to maintain correction. The brace holds the feet in 70° of external rotation and 5 to 10° of dorsiflexion. It is used all the time for three to four months and thereafter during sleep for a period of two to four years. Compliance with use of the brace is important in achieving a successful outcome. Fifteen to 20% of patients treated successfully with the Ponseti method require subsequent lateral transfer of the anterior tibial tendon to correct dynamic forefoot supination during swing phase. At a mean follow-up of 34 years, 78% of 71 idiopathic congenital clubfeet, in 45 patients, treated with the Ponseti method had good or excellent outcomes, even though 30 of the 71 required later anterior tibial tendon transfer[14].

An alternative non-surgical treatment is with the French physiotherapy, or "functional" method. This has proven to be equally effective[16]. The functional method requires daily manipulation of the foot for two months. The foot is strapped with non-adhesive strapping in between manipulation sessions. After approximately two months the manipulation is reduced to three times per week for up to six months. Nighttime splinting is used for two to three years thereafter. This method of treatment is not as popular as the Ponseti method as it requires daily treatment, with considerable parental training and participation.

A prospective comparison of these two non-surgical treatment methods included 267 feet in 176 patients treated with the Ponseti method and 119 feet in 80 patients treated with the functional method. Initial correction was similar for the two groups with 94% correction in the Ponseti group and 95% in the functional group. In the Ponseti group, 37% of feet relapsed and two-thirds of these required surgical intervention. Twenty-nine percent of the feet in the functional group relapsed, and all of these required surgical intervention. Good results were obtained in 72% of the feet treated with the Ponseti method and 67% of the French physiotherapy method. The study concluded that while a trend demonstrating better results with the Ponseti method was identified, it was not significant. The authors further noted that parents chose the Ponseti method twice as often as the functional method[17].

Idiopathic clubfeet that are resistant to non-surgical treatment and neuromuscular clubfeet require surgical treatment at about one year of age, once the child is able to walk. There are multiple surgical variations, but all consist of a series of soft tissue releases to correct the foot position. The calcaneofibular ligament, posterior talofibular ligament, and superficial deltoid ligament are released, the TA and medial tendons (PTT, FDL, and FHL) are lengthened, and the tibiotalar, subtalar, and talonavicular capsules are released[18].

Long-term complications following clubfoot surgery usually can be considered as either the result of undercorrection, or recurrence, on the one hand, and overcorrection on the other. Dorsal subluxation of the navicular, valgus overcorrection, a dorsiflexed first metatarsal, or dorsal bunion, and ankle pain and stiffness are all recognized complications, which may require further surgical intervention[21].

Congenital Vertical Talus

A congenital vertical talus is defined by a severely plantar flexed talus with dorsal dislocation of the navicular. The fixed hindfoot equinus produces a rocker-bottom deformity of the foot with a tight TA. The underlying etiology of the vertical talus is unknown but the deformity is often associated with neuromuscular conditions such as myelomeningocele, arthrogryposis, prune-belly syndrome, spinal muscular atrophy, neurofibromatosis, congenital dislocation of the hip, Tasmussen's syndrome, and trisomy 13–15 and 18.

On examination there is a rocker-bottom deformity of the foot, the talar head is prominent in the plantar-medial foot, and the heel is in equinovalgus, with a dorsiflexed and abducted forefoot. The lateral x-ray shows a severely plantar flexed talus, with the longitudinal axis of the talus lying almost parallel to that of the tibia. The calcaneus lies in equinus. As the navicular does not ossify until three years of age, its dorsally dislocated position is not seen. Its position must be inferred from the dorsally dislocated position of the midfoot and forefoot. If a congenital vertical talus is suspected a forced plantar flexion radiograph is taken. If a line drawn along the longitudinal axis of the talus passes plantar to the midfoot and first metatarsal, this indicates that the navicular and midfoot dislocation is fixed, confirming the diagnosis (Figure 20.6). If the line passes through the first metatarsal, there is a congenital *oblique* as opposed to *vertical* talus. Thus while both an oblique and vertical talus have a similar clinical appearance, with a rocker-bottom deformity, the difference between the two is that the midfoot is reducible with an oblique talus.

Recent studies have demonstrated considerable success with manipulation and serial casting to correct the deformity in both the idiopathic and rigid vertical talus associated with neuromuscular or genetic disease[22-23]. The technique involves weekly serial casting with gradual deformity correction, similar to the management of a clubfoot deformity. As in the

(a)

(b)

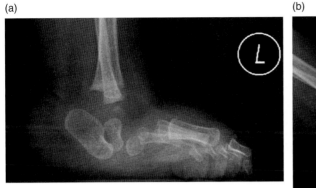
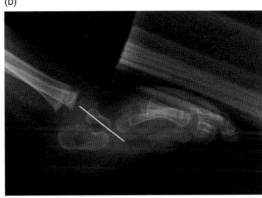

Figure 20.6 (a) A lateral radiograph showing a congenital vertical talus. (b) Forced plantar flexion radiograph demonstrating persistent dorsal midfoot subluxation on the plantar flexed talus, confirming the diagnosis of congenital vertical, as opposed to oblique, talus.

treatment of a clubfoot, all components of the deformity are corrected by manipulation and casting, except the equinus. With a dorsal force imparted on the plantar-medial aspect of the talar head, the midfoot and forefoot are manipulated into a plantar flexion and inversion, in order to gradually reduce the navicular onto the plantar flexed talus. After several casts, talonavicular reduction is confirmed radiographically. If the talar–first metatarsal angle in maximal forced plantar flexion is less than 30°, talonavicular stabilization in a reduced position is held with a percutaneous Kirschner wire, with or without a small talonavicular arthrotomy to confirm anatomic alignment of the joint. The TA can then be released percutaneously to correct the equinus deformity. The final cast and wire are left in place for approximately four weeks at which point the wire is removed and bracing is instituted to prevent recurrence.

If serial casting fails, presentation is delayed, or if the deformity is rigid and irreducible, surgery is performed at around one year of age. The surgery consists of:

1. reduction of the navicular onto the talus by releasing the capsular structures and the tibialis anterior tendon
2. lengthening of the long toe extensors and peroneal tendons
3. reduction of the cuboid onto the calcaneus through release of the bifurcate ligament and capsular structures
4. transfer of the tibialis anterior tendon to the neck of the talus

5. temporary pin fixation of the talonavicular joint to maintain alignment.

This is followed by six to twelve weeks in a cast. In older children, excision of the navicular and a Grice extra-articular talocalcaneal arthrodesis may be necessary.

Neglected deformities are challenging. It is usually not possible to correct the foot with joint-sparing surgery in the older child with a symptomatic foot. A corrective triple arthrodesis with soft tissue releases is usually necessary.

Calcaneovalgus Foot

A calcaneovalgus foot in a newborn occurs as a result of intra-uterine molding. The foot will be in extreme dorsiflexion with eversion of the hindfoot and abduction of the forefoot. The calcaneovalgus foot is passively correctable and is treated with stretching and observation.

Flexible Flat Foot (Pes Planovalgus)

It is important to distinguish between a *flexible* and *rigid* flat foot. A flexible flat foot will have normal or excessive mobility of the subtalar joint. When the child is non-weightbearing the arch should reconstitute. In a flexible flat foot when the patient moves up onto tip-toes the heel should move into varus. A rigid flat foot does not correct.

In infancy the foot is normally flat. The arch gradually constitutes over the first five years or so, although in 15 to 20% of children the flat foot persists into adulthood. Flexible flat foot is a common cause

347

(a)   (b)

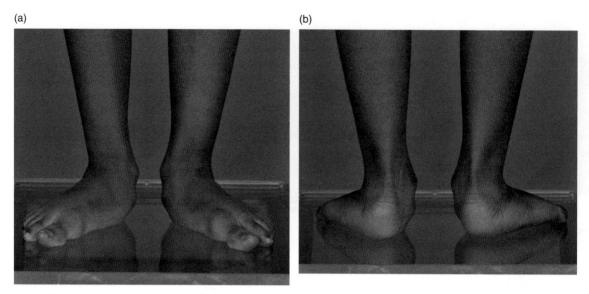

Figure 20.7 (**a**) A child with bilateral congenital pes planovalgus. (**b**) Note the severe heel valgus and abduction of the forefoot – the "too-many-toes" sign.

for parental concern, although the child is rarely symptomatic. It is almost always bilateral and there is often a family history. It is associated with rotational abnormalities of the lower extremities and may be associated with ligamentous laxity. Typically the medial arch is flat, with a valgus hindfoot and an abducted forefoot (Figure 20.7).

A rigid flat foot is uncommon, is often intermittently painful, and is pathological. A rigid flat foot is usually caused by a tarsal coalition or a vertical talus. These conditions are discussed elsewhere in this chapter.

The typical flexible flat foot is also associated with TA tightness. As the calcaneus externally rotates beneath the talus, it assumes a valgus posture and the calcaneal pitch flattens. This allows the TA to shorten. A vicious cycle is established: as the vector of the TA's pull moves lateral to the midline, it pulls the hindfoot further into valgus, further shortening the TA, and so on. The position of the forefoot should be evaluated with the hindfoot held in subtalar neutral. In more severe flat foot deformities, the forefoot will rotate into supination as the heel valgus is corrected. This is important in surgical planning to help determine the need for a plantar flexion osteotomy of the medial column to help correct the forefoot supination and varus.

Standing radiographs allow quantification of the degree of deformity. The lateral radiograph shows Meary's angle, which is the angle created between the longitudinal axis of the talus and that of the first metatarsal (normal 0°). Talonavicular coverage is evaluated on the AP view of the foot. This is useful both in evaluating the amount of deformity and planning surgery to correct the deformity (Figure 20.8). It is important to check the radiographs for causes of a rigid, or pathological, flat foot deformity such as an accessory navicular, congenital vertical talus, and tarsal coalition. If in doubt, CT or MRI scanning may be necessary.

The majority of patients are asymptomatic and no treatment is required. The treating surgeon should explain the condition and reassure the parents. Importantly, there is no evidence that orthoses correct foot shape in the long term, and thus orthotic treatment is used for symptomatic relief only as needed. It is best achieved with a molded, cushioning insole, without rigid components.

Initially over-the-counter orthoses with a varus heel wedge and arch support can be tried. Customized orthoses, while potentially more effective in correcting the static foot position, are expensive as the child grows and replacement becomes necessary. Stretching of the TA may help when the child is old enough to understand the treatment and can be taught to comply with the exercise regime. A UCBL (University of California Biomechanics Laboratory) orthosis can be considered. This is a custom device made from

(a)

(b)

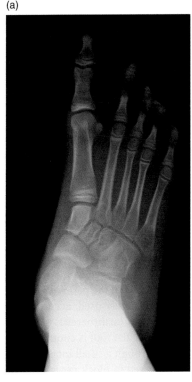

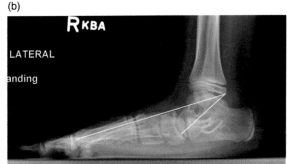

Figure 20.8 (a) Anteroposterior radiograph demonstrating uncovering of the talar head by the navicular and abduction. (b) Lateral radiograph, note Meary's angle between the lines.

rigid plastic, which has a deep molded heel cup to hold the hindfoot, an arch support to control the midfoot, and a lateral wall to control the lateral border of the foot. While a UCBL can provide passive correction of the deformity, it can be quite uncomfortable, especially at older ages, as the foot becomes less flexible.

Surgical correction may be considered in severely symptomatic cases (Figure 20.9). There are three components to the correction.

Firstly, an Evan's type lateral column lengthening osteotomy is performed. This is done just proximal to the calcaneocuboid joint, passing between the anterior and middle calcaneal facets of the subtalar joint. The insertion of a bone wedge into the osteotomy rotates the midfoot and forefoot around the talar head to correct the abduction deformity. Avoiding overcorrection is important, as it can result in lateral column overload. It is also important to ensure that the graft lies lower than the floor of the sinus tarsi, to avoid painful subtalar impingement. Intraoperatively, the calcaneocuboid joint must be radiographically

evaluated to prevent dorsal subluxation of the distal calcaneal segment.

Secondly, it is necessary to decide whether to correct forefoot supination. This decision is made intraoperatively, after the calcaneal lengthening has been performed. If the forefoot is more than 15° supinated and the foot lacks the flexibility to correct this, a plantar flexion opening wedge osteotomy through the medial cuneiform (Cotton osteotomy) is performed. The osteotomy is performed through a dorsal approach. The anterior tibial tendon is identified and protected. A guide pin is inserted from dorsal to plantar in the central portion of the cuneiform. There is a tendency to aim the guide pin perpendicular to the "floor," which causes the guide pin to lie distally in the plantar aspect of the cuneiform. Thus it is important to aim the guide pin directly perpendicular, or slightly proximal, relative to the dorsal surface of the cuneiform. The position of the guide pin is checked fluoroscopically and then an oscillating saw is used to make a dorsal to plantar cut in the cuneiform. The cut is gently levered open with an

Thirdly, the patient will also require lengthening of the TA or gastrocnemius. Tendo Achillis lengthening, especially if undertaken percutaneously, can lead to overlengthening. Thus we prefer gastrocnemius lengthening. In a modified Strayer-type procedure, a medial incision is made just distal to the muscle belly of the gastrocnemius, avoiding the sural nerve. The two borders of the tendon are visualized, and the tendon of the gastrocnemius is then divided in its entirety, sharply from medial to lateral. Alternatively, the release may be achieved by incising the anterior fascia of the gastrocnemius more proximally, at the level of the muscle belly. This is indicated in less severe deformity, and produces more controlled lengthening and, ultimately, less weakening of the gastrocnemius.

Additional soft tissue procedures, such as shortening of the posterior tibial tendon and spring ligament complex, lengthening of the peroneus brevis, and arthroereisis, are occasionally used, according to surgical preference. Use of an arthroereisis screw in the treatment of the pediatric flat foot is controversial. It is an implant inserted through a small incision over the sinus tarsi and is designed to block excessive subtalar pronation. It has been shown to improve the radiographic parameters in correction of the pediatric flat foot. Its mechanism of action is not fully understood. It has a blocking effect on the rotational motion of the subtalar joint and may also change the tension of the interosseous ligaments, stabilizing the subtalar joint. Arthroereisis screws have numerous complications including migration, subtalar pain, permanent subtalar stiffness, subtalar arthritis, and implant removal. Acceptable satisfaction rates have been reported[8]; however, many do not use the technique.

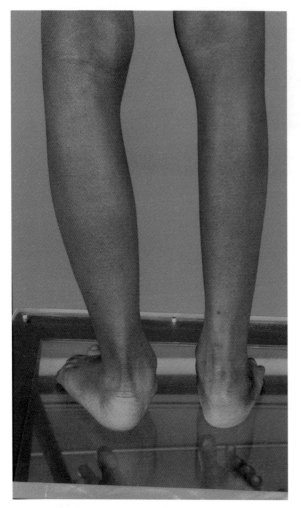

Figure 20.9 Postoperative clinical photo: notice the correction in hindfoot position and forefoot abduction on the right, compared to the uncorrected left, side.

osteotome and a wedge of cortico-cancellous graft is used to hold open the cuneiform, usually by 6 to 8 mm. As with the calcaneal osteotomy, the use of internal fixation is left to the surgeon's discretion, and is based on the stability of the graft.

An alternative to the dorsal opening wedge osteotomy is a medial cuneiform plantar-based closing wedge osteotomy. This is performed through a medial approach, which can also be used, if desired, to imbricate the medial talonavicular joint and the posterior tibial tendon. Resection of a plantar-based wedge of the medial cuneiform plantarflexes the first ray. Fixation in the form of a percutaneous Kirschner wire or a staple is required[24].

Metatarsus Adductus

Metatarsus adductus is adduction or varus of the forefoot on the midfoot. It is a spectrum from a mild flexible deformity to a severe fixed deformity. It is thought to be caused by intra-uterine compression, and is associated with torticollis and developmental dislocation of the hip. The incidence is difficult to quantify as mild deformities are often ignored, but is estimated at 1 in a 1000 live births[10].

Metatarsus adductus is classically characterized by several features, described by Kite. These are:

1. active medial deviation of the foot
2. high arch

3. concave medial foot border
4. fixed forefoot adductus with the hindfoot in neutral
5. a bean-shaped sole of the foot.[11]

It is not uncommon for children with metatarsus adductus to also have a component of internal tibial torsion, which contributes to their intoed appearance.

Radiographs typically show adduction, or varus, of the metatarsals at the TMTJ, with valgus of the hindfoot.

- Mild flexible metatarsus adductus, which spontaneously corrects with peroneal contraction, is treated with reassurance, as it will spontaneously correct. Parents may be shown how to gently stretch the foot and stimulate it to actively correct.

- Moderate metatarsus adductus is defined as that which can be passively corrected by the examiner but does not correct actively. It is usually treated with passive stretching. Children younger than six months may also be treated with a period of corrective casting. There is debate about whether treatment is actually required since most of these moderate deformities will resolve naturally by two years of age.

- Rigid uncorrectable metatarsus adductus, which cannot be passively corrected, should be treated with stretching and cast application. The problem is largely cosmetic, but difficulties fitting shoes and occasional discomfort with activity, which persist following non-operative treatment, are reasonable indications for surgery. Patients younger than six months can be treated surgically with release of the abductor hallucis and first TMTJ capsulotomy. When the child is older, persistent metatarsus adductus can be treated surgically with multiple valgus osteotomies of the metatarsal bases. Alternatively a closing wedge osteotomy of the cuboid, with transposition of the wedge into the medial cuneiform, as an opening wedge, can be used.

Skewfoot

Skewfoot is a curious condition in which there is adduction of the forefoot, lateral navicular subluxation, and hindfoot valgus producing a serpentine or Z-shaped deformity. Skewfoot is rare and there is little written about the condition. The AP radiograph of the foot will demonstrate adductus of the forefoot with relative external rotation of the midfoot and lateral talonavicular uncoverage producing the hindfoot valgus. Asymptomatic patients do not need active treatment. If the patient is symptomatic, they usually present with pain in the arch as a result of the hindfoot valgus, as well as lateral column pain from the forefoot adductus. If non-surgical treatment fails, calcaneal osteotomy to correct hindfoot valgus, correction of forefoot adductus, and TA lengthening or gastrocnemius recession can be undertaken[12].

Tarsal Coalition

Tarsal coalitions result from a failure of embryonic mesenchymal segmentation and lead to an abnormal connection between two or more tarsal bones. Calcaneonavicular or talocalcaneal coalitions are the commonest. Tarsal coalition is thought to be an autosomal dominant condition with an incidence in the general population of less than 1%. They are bilateral in 50 to 60% of cases.[19]

Coalitions can be fibrous, cartilaginous, osseous, or any combination thereof. Fully ossified coalitions are the minority and referred to as complete; most coalitions are made up of a mixture of tissues. Coalitions are not just abnormal connections between tarsal bones but, often, in particular with talocalcaneal coalitions, reflect abnormal joint morphology.

A calcaneonavicular coalition is an abnormal connection between the anterior process of the calcaneus and the lateral tuberosity of the navicular. Talocalcaneal coalitions are a failure of formation of a portion of the subtalar joint. The middle facet of the subtalar joint is most commonly involved, but the coalition can involve the anterior facet and the distal portion of the posterior facet. The majority of both talocalcaneal and calcaneonavicular coalitions are a combination of abnormal bony morphology and fibrous tissue. In some cases there is a complete bony bridge. Extensive coalitions are associated with the development of a ball-and-socket ankle.

Historically, a patient presenting with a rigid valgus hindfoot deformity, peroneal muscle spasm, and pain has been diagnosed as suffering with a "peroneal spastic flat foot." Tarsal coalitions are the primary cause of the peroneal spastic flat foot, but as peroneal spastic flat foot is not a pathological diagnosis that determines treatment, the term has fallen into disuse. Tarsal coalitions typically present in childhood

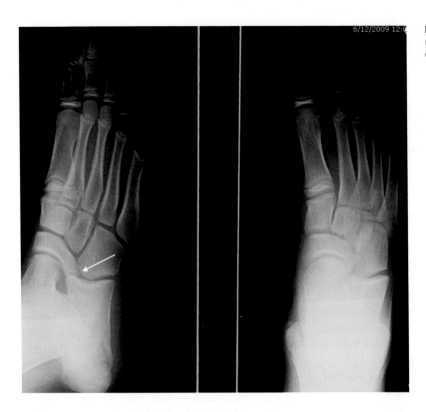

Figure 20.10 Oblique and AP radiographs demonstrating calcaneonavicular coalition.

or early to mid-adolescence, although some are diagnosed in adulthood. Often the parent, or child, gives a history of a minor sprain that has not resolved. Some patients report recurrent ankle sprains as a result of the restriction of subtalar motion. Children with talocalcaneal coalitions tend to present with pain located in the sinus tarsi, along the medial aspect of the subtalar joint near the middle facet, or in the arch of the foot. Patients with calcaneonavicular coalitions have pain in the sinus tarsi, near the anterior process of the calcaneus and the coalition itself.

Physical examination usually reveals a valgus hindfoot position with restricted movement of the subtalar and midtarsal joints. Great care must be exercised to lock the ankle in ankle maximum dorsiflexion, as compensatory tibiotalar laxity may obscure the loss of inversion–eversion. Passive manipulation of the subtalar joint is often met with resistance as a result of peroneal spasm. The heel also does not correct into a varus position when the patient rises on to tip-toe.

Radiographically the oblique view of the foot is the best for identifying a calcaneonavicular coalition, with a bar projecting from the anterior process of the calcaneus, connecting it to the lateral process

of the navicular (Figure 20.10). The coalition is often described on the lateral view as showing an "anteater sign," as the elongated anterior process of the calcaneus is said to resemble an anteater's nose.

A talocalcaneal coalition is best seen on the lateral x-ray. The view across the subtalar joint is obscured both by the coalition and the valgus position of the subtalar joint. Classically there is a C-sign, which is common but not pathognomonic. If a line is drawn around the curve of the talar dome and extended along the posteroinferior portion of the sustentaculum tali in the normal individual there will be a gap behind the sustentaculum tali; if a coalition is present the line is continuous without a break (Figure 20.11). The axial view of the heel is also useful in the evaluation of a talocalcaneal coalition, as the middle facet angles abnormally plantarward and a bony bridge between the talus and calcaneus may be visualized.

It is not uncommon for a talar beak to form on the dorsal aspect of the talar neck in the presence of a coalition. It is believed that this beak forms either as a result of the abnormal ankle motion or alternatively as a result of the impingement of the navicular on the talus, as a result of abnormal transverse tarsal joint motion.

If a coalition is suspected on examination or x-ray, a CT or MRI scan is obtained. The scan helps quantify the size of a talocalcaneal coalition, better images the joint morphology, and excludes a second coalition existing in the same foot (Figure 20.12). While MRI may be useful in evaluating fibrous or cartilaginous coalitions, CT is preferred as it is more useful in surgical planning because it shows the bone contour and morphology.

Treatment usually begins with a period of non-surgical management. In the acute case where an injury has brought on the pain, a four- to six-week period of immobilization in a short-leg cast or boot is tried. If the presentation is with chronic pain, an attempt at treatment with a UCBL orthosis to reduce the stresses of hindfoot movement on the foot is made.

If non-operative management fails, surgical treatment may be considered. Surgical treatment of a calcaneonavicular coalition is excision through a dorsolateral incision. The key to the procedure is complete removal of the coalition, avoiding the tendency to perform a triangular resection leaving too much bone on the medial-plantar aspect. Once the coalition has been excised, the EDB muscle belly is mobilized from its bed in the sinus tarsi and interposed as a soft tissue spacer in the void left by the coalition. The cut surfaces of the bone are sealed with bone wax. Postoperatively, the patient is immobilized for two to four weeks, after which therapy commences in an attempt to regain subtalar motion.

Talocalcaneal coalitions can either be treated by excision or with subtalar arthrodesis. Some base the choice of procedure upon the size of the coalition, while others base the decision on the activity level of the patient, opting for excision in a younger patient with a large coalition to attempt to preserve motion. However, a substantial number of patients suffer with persistent pain after excision, as the underlying subtalar joint is not normal. These patients require a second procedure – a subtalar arthrodesis.

Excision of a talocalcaneal coalition can be performed through a medial approach, centered just plantar to the sustentaculum tali. The FHL and FDL are identified, released from their sheaths, and retracted plantarward. The coalition is identified and complete excision undertaken using a burr, saw, or osteotome. Excision of the coalition is in part confirmed when the subtalar is seen to move. The exposed bone, following excision, may be covered with bone wax or transposed fat to try and prevent

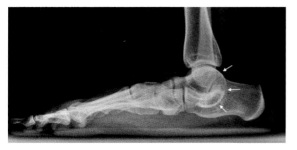

Figure 20.11 Lateral radiograph demonstrating talonavicular coalition: note the "C-sign."

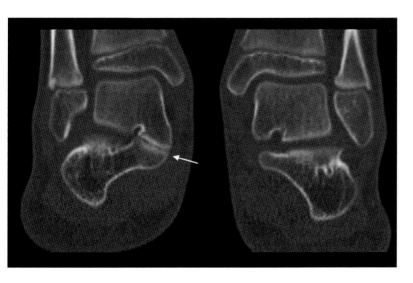

Figure 20.12 CT scan demonstrating a normal middle facet, and a coalition involving all of the middle facet.

reformation of the coalition. This medial approach has the advantage of directly identifying the neurovascular bundle, but the disadvantage that there is difficulty in localizing the plane of the coalition, which is often oblique, creating a risk of damaging the adjacent articular surface. An alternative is resection from the lateral side, through a sinus tarsi approach, which allows the joint to be visualized and protected. The coalition is removed piecemeal with curettes, identifying the coalition's posterior and anterior margins, and working forward or backward. Distraction with a lamina spreader is very helpful. It is worth considering concomitant correction of an associated planovalgus deformity at the time of coalition resection. This can be achieved with a calcaneal lengthening osteotomy and gastrocnemius recession. Good short- to mid-term results have been reported with combined excision and correction[25].

Subtalar arthrodesis can be performed through either a medial approach, a lateral approach, or a combination of the two. It is important to correct any deformity of the hindfoot at the same time, because an in situ fusion can result in persistent pain attributable to abnormal loading in weight bearing. Deformity correction usually requires excision of the coalition prior to the arthrodesis.

Neurologic Deformity

The Cavus Foot

Cavus foot deformity in a child has an underlying neurological cause in approximately two-thirds of patients. A pediatric neurological opinion should be considered if the cause of the deformity is not obvious, and is mandatory if the deformity is unilateral. The conditions most often associated with bilateral pes cavus include hereditary sensorimotor neuropathies (HMSN)[26] or "Charcot–Marie–Tooth" (CMT), cerebral palsy, polio, Friedreich's ataxia, and myelomeningocele. The unilateral cavus foot is relatively rare and warrants an MRI of the spine to assess for an intraspinal anomaly such as a syrinx, Chiari malformation, or diastematomyelia. MRI of the brain and spinal cord, EMG, and nerve-conduction studies, as well as genetic testing, to differentiate between the various subtypes of the HMSNs, can be useful.

Cavus in itself is usually benign and causes few symptoms; its importance is when it is associated with varus. The cause of the cavovarus foot posture is muscular imbalance. The intrinsic foot musculature, the tibialis anterior and the peroneus brevis, are relatively weak, which allows the peroneus longus and tibialis posterior to dominate the weaker muscles resulting in the classic deformity of a high arched foot with a varus hindfoot. The weakness of the tibialis anterior forces the long toe extensors to be recruited as ankle dorsiflexors. The increased pull of the long toe extensors produces a reciprocal tightness of the toe flexors. Coupled with the weakened intrinsic muscles, claw toe deformities develop with extension of the MTPJs and flexion of the PIP and DIP joints.

Patients present in two ways, either with concern about the shape of the foot or as a result of lateral ankle pain and instability. The cavovarus position of the foot results in overload of the lateral column and a tendency to sustain inversion injuries of ankle. Older patients will often describe a long history of recurrent ankle sprains. Lateral column overload is common and there may be a callus, or even a painful ulcer, under the lateral aspect of the fifth metatarsal base. Pain may also present as a result of tightness of the plantar fascia, which is almost universal in patients with pes cavovarus.

Physical examination is performed with the patient both standing and seated. While standing, note the static position of the foot (Figure 20.13), with hindfoot varus seen from behind or with the "peek-a-boo" heel sign seen from the front. The patient will have a high arch and often forefoot adduction. In the case of CMT, the patient may have significant atrophy of lateral and anterior compartments of the leg, often referred to as "stork legs." In CMT heel walking is difficult because of weakness of the extensors.

With the patient seated, careful neurological examination and recording of the strength of the different muscle groups should be made; sensory deficits may be present in patients with CMT. The correctability of the deformity is evaluated by holding the ankle in a neutral position while passively inverting and everting the subtalar joint. If, in the seated or prone position, the heel can be shown to correct into valgus, the deformity is not fixed, and joint-sparing surgery is appropriate. If the heel varus is rigid, then arthrodesis of the hindfoot is indicated. We find this easier than undertaking a Coleman block test. If a patient stands with a varus heel, but the heel can be corrected into valgus when non-weightbearing, this implies that the heel varus is forefoot-driven by a plantar flexed first ray.[20]

(a)

(b)

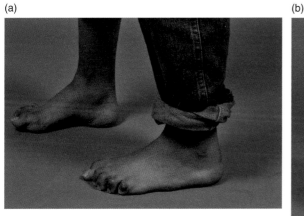
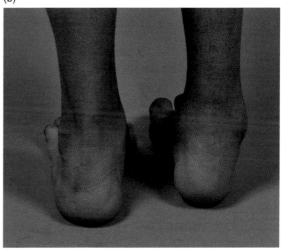

Figure 20.13 A patient with cavovarus foot deformity: note the high arch, clawed toes, and heel varus.

Radiographs of the ankle may show varus malalignment on the mortise view and a posteriorly displaced fibula on the lateral. On the standing lateral view the calcaneal pitch is frequently increased with a reciprocal decrease in the talar declination angle. The midfoot has a "stacked" appearance, with the navicular and cuneiforms appearing higher than the cuboid, and the forefoot is rotated such that the metatarsals have less overlap than usual (Figure 20.14).

Radiographs are crucial for determining the apex of the deformity. This guides the surgeon in the choice of which procedures will be necessary to correct the deformity. The location of the apex in the sagittal plane is used to determine whether the deformity is an anterior (midfoot) or posterior (hindfoot) cavus. Additionally, a plan for correction in the coronal plane is needed, as the forefoot is pronated to compensate for hindfoot varus. Understanding the 3D nature of the cavus deformity is essential in planning correction of this multiplanar deformity.

Painful cavus feet are generally treated surgically. Conservative management with bracing such as an AFO may help temporarily; insoles are often unsuccessful because it is difficult to create a sufficiently high arch in the material for contact with the plantar foot.

The commonest indication for surgical intervention is pain as a result of lateral column overload, lateral ankle instability as a result of varus instability, and occasionally lateral ulceration. Generally, a

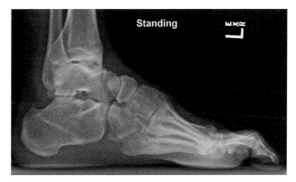

Figure 20.14 Lateral radiograph of a cavovarus foot.

combination of bony and soft tissue procedures will be necessary to correct the deformity. Posterior tibial tendon lengthening or transfer through the interosseous membrane to the lateral cuneiform removes a deforming force and, in the case of the transfer, converts it to an ankle dorsiflexor. Procedures commonly included in a flexible cavus foot reconstruction include plantar fascia release, peroneus longus to brevis transfer, posterior tibial tendon lengthening or transfer, lateralizing calcaneal osteotomy, and dorsiflexion osteotomy of the medial forefoot – usually of the first ray. It is critical to remind many HMSN/CMT patients that if they have a foot drop, correction of the deformity will not necessarily render them brace free, as posterior tibial tendon transfer functions largely as a tenodesis, and tends to stretch over time.

355

Toe Deformities

Hallux Valgus

Cases of juvenile hallux valgus are often familial, bilateral, and 88% occur in girls. Most cases occur in patients with no underlying disorder, although juvenile hallux valgus is seen in cerebral palsy or in association with soft tissue disorders such as Ehlers–Danlos or Marfan's syndrome. As with the adult deformity, juvenile hallux valgus is associated metatarsus primus varus, with an intermetatarsal angle of greater than or equal to 10°. As the proximal phalanx deviates into valgus, the adductor hallucis acts as a deforming force pulling the proximal phalanx and sesamoid complex laterally, while the abductor hallucis rotates plantarward into a non-functional position. Without the dorsal buttress of the metatarsal head, the sesamoids are then free to translate and rotate with resulting pronation of the hallux. Lateral bowstringing of the EHL and FHL then tends to accentuate the deformity as they shorten.

Pediatric patients with hallux valgus seek treatment either for pain over the medial eminence or for cosmesis and difficulty fitting into shoes. Pain is usually exacerbated by the pressure of shoes.

Weightbearing x-rays are routine. The hallux valgus angle and intermetatarsal angle are measured, as is the DMAA, as juvenile bunions tend to have an increased DMAA. This has three implications. Firstly, the bunion is congruent, and therefore not correctable by a procedure that rotates the phalanx around the metatarsal. Secondly, the average juvenile hallux valgus is more severe than the average adult hallux valgus. Thirdly, there are high rates of recurrence and of incomplete correction due to the difficulty of realigning the articular surface.

Non-operative treatment includes shoe modification with the use of a wide toe box. Toe spacers, bunion pads, and bunion splints may also be tried, but it should be explained to the patient that none of these will alter the long-term foot shape.

Most surgeons recommend avoiding surgical intervention until after first metatarsal physeal closure due to a high recurrence rate in the growing child, and concern for a growth arrest[27]. In planning surgery it is important to recognize that the distal metatarsal joint surface faces laterally and use an osteotomy that realigns the DMAA. One option is an osteotomy that corrects first metatarsal varus by translation and, at the same time, allows varus rotation of the metatarsal head to correct the DMAA. A Scarf osteotomy or biplanar distal chevron osteotomy, excising a wedge to allow medial rotation of the head, is widely used. Another option is a double osteotomy with a proximal osteotomy to correct the first metatarsal varus, and a distal osteotomy to realign the DMAA. One study reported a lateral hemiepiphyseodesis of the first metatarsal, but this is not widely practiced[28].

Polydactyly

Polydactyly is the most common congenital toe deformity with an incidence of 1.7 per 1000 live births. There is a strong genetic component with a positive family history in 30% of cases and bilateral involvement approximately 50% of the time. It occurs more commonly in black children and males are involved slightly more than females.

Postaxial polydactyly (duplication of the fifth toe) is most common, occurring 80% of the time as opposed to preaxial polydactyly (duplication of the hallux). Polydactyly is divided into type A, which is a well-formed digit, and type B, which is a rudimentary digit. Treatment is by surgical excision of the duplicated toe at near one year of age.

Syndactyly

Simple syndactyly is congenital webbing of the toes involving the soft tissue structures only. Syndactyly is usually "incomplete" with the webbing including only part of the webspace, although it can be "complete." The webbing is typically a cosmetic problem and surgery is usually not indicated. Complex syndactyly with bony fusion of adjacent toes is seen in patients with Apert's syndrome.

Curly Toe

Curly toes are common, usually affecting the third or fourth toes. The toe is flexed and medially deviated at the PIPJ. The toe supinates and comes to lie beneath the adjacent normal toe. The cause is a congenital tightness of the flexor digitorum longus and brevis. Curly toes are frequently bilateral and there is often a family history with a pattern of autosomal dominant inheritance. Initial treatment is with observation as about one-fourth will resolve without intervention. Persistent deformity at age six, accompanied by pain,

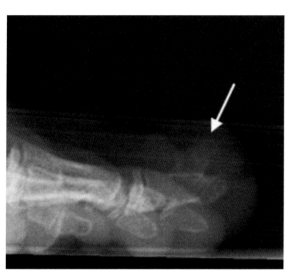

Figure 20.15 A lateral radiograph of subungual exostosis.

is an indication for surgery. The pain is usually from dorsal irritation by shoes on the normal digit, which is raised by the underlapping of the curly toe. While flexor-to-extensor tendon transfer has been described with satisfactory results, a simple flexor tenotomy will almost always correct the deformity and is the authors' preferred surgical approach.

Subungual Exostosis

Subungual exostosis is a benign condition in which an osteochondroma grows on the dorsomedial surface of the distal phalanx of the hallux, just beneath the nail.

It typically presents during the second decade of life, and is more common in females. Pain and toenail deformity are presenting symptoms. The lesion is firm and palpable beneath the nail and often displaces, or erodes through, the nail plate. The mass can be seen on x-ray (Figure 20.15). Surgical excision is generally curative, but usually requires repair or reconstruction of the nail bed. Most cases have resolution of symptoms but some permanent deformity of the hallux nail.

Key Points

- Congenital idiopathic clubfoot is usually treated with the non-surgical Ponseti method.
- "CAVE" describes the order of correction with the Ponseti method. Tendo Achillis tenotomy is required in over 85% of patients.
- In infancy the foot is normally flat, and the arch gradually constitutes, although in 15 to 20% the flat foot persists into adulthood.
- The flexible flat foot rarely requires surgery. Orthoses do not alter the long-term shape of the foot.
- The rigid flat foot is uncommon, and usually due to a talocalcaneal or calcaneonavicular coalition.
- Approximately two-thirds of cavovarus feet have an underlying neurological cause.
- Juvenile hallux valgus is more severe, and more recalcitrant to correction, than in adults. Surgery has a significant recurrence rate.

References

1. Coskun N, Yuksel M, Cevener M, et al. Incidence of accessory ossicles and sesamoid bone in the feet: a radiographic study of the Turkish subjects. *Surg Radiol Anat.* 2009; 31(1):19–24.

2. Herring JA. Disorders of the foot. In *Tachdjian's Pediatric Orthopaedics*, 4th edn. (Philadelphia, PA: Saunders Elsevier, 2008).

3. Sella EJ, Lawson JP, Ogden JA. The accessory navicular synchondrosis. *Clin Orthop Rel Res.* 1986; 209:280–5.

4. Kiter E, Erduran M, Günal I. Inheritance of the accessory navicular bone. *Arch Orthop Trauma Surg.* 2000; 120(10):582–3.

5. Grogan DP, Gasser SI, Ogden JA. The painful accessory navicular: a clinical and histopathological study. *Foot Ankle.* 1989; 10(3):164–9.

6. Sullivan JA, Miller WA. The relationship of the accessory navicuar to the development of the flat foot. *Clin Orthop Rel Res.* 1979; 144:233–7.

7. Cha SM, Shin HD, Kim KC, Lee JK. Simple excision vs the Kidner procedure for type 2 accessory navicular associated with flatfoot in a pediatric population. *Foot Ankle Int.* 2013; 34(2):167–72.

8. Metcalfe SA, Bowling FL, Reeves ND. Subtalar joint arthroereisis in the management of pediatric flexible flatfoot: a critical review of the literature. *Foot Ankle Int.* 2011; 32(12):1127–39.

9. Ajis A, Seybold JD, Myerson MS. Osteochondral distal metatarsal allograft reconstruction: a case series and surgical technique. *Foot Ankle Int.* 2013; 24(8):1158–67.

10. Wynne-Davies R. Family studies and the cause of congenital

clubfoot, talipes equinovarus, talipes calcaneovalgus and metatarsus varus. *J Bone Joint Surg Br.* 1964; 46(3):445–63.

11. Kite JH. Congenital metatarsus varus. *J Bone Joint Surg Am.* 1967; 49:388–97.

12. Mosca VS. Flexible flatfoot and skewfoot. An instructional course lecture. *J Bone Joint Surg Am.* 1995; 77(12):1937–45.

13. Kite J. *The Clubfoot* (New York: Grune & Stratton, 1964).

14. Cooper DM, Dietz FR. Treatment of idiopathic clubfoot. A thirty-year follow-up note. *J Bone Joint Surg Am.* 1995; 77:1477–89.

15. Ponset IV. *Congenital Clubfoot: Fundamentals of Treatment* (Oxford: Oxford University Press, 1966).

16. Bensahel H, Guillaume A, Czukonyi Z, Desgrippes Y. Results of physical therapy for idiopathic clubfoot: a long-term follow-up study. *J Pediatr Orthop.* 1990; 10(2):189–92.

17. Richards BS, Faulks S, Rathjen KE, Karol LA, Johnston CE, Jones SA. A comparison of two nonoperative methods of idiopathic clubfoot correction: the Ponseti method and the French functional (physiotherapy) method. *J Bone Joint Surg Am.* 2008; 90(111):2313–21.

18. Turco VJ. Surgical correction of the resistant club foot. One-stage posteromedial release with internal fixation: a preliminary report. *J Bone Joint Surg Am.* 1971; 53(3):477–97.

19. Kulik SA, Clanton TO. Tarsal coalition. *Foot Ankle Int.* 1996; 17:286.

20. Coleman SS, Chesnut WJ. A simple test for hindfoot flexibility in the cavovarus foot. *Clin Orthop Relat Res.* 1997; 123:60–2.

21. Zide JR, Myerson M. The overcorrected clubfoot in the adult: evaluation and management – topical review. *Foot Ankle Int.* 2013; 34:1312–18.

22. Dobbs MB, Purcell DB, Nunley R, Morcuende JA. Early results of a new method of treatment for idiopathic congenital vertical talus. *J Bone Joint Surg Am.* 2006; 88(6):1192–200.

23. Chalayon O, Adams A, Dobbs MB. Minimally invasive approach for the treatment of non-isolated congenital vertical talus. *J Bone Joint Surg Am.* 2012; 6(94):e73.

24. Mosca VS. Flexible flatfoot in children and adolescents. *J Child Orthop.* 2010; 4(2):107–21.

25. Mosca VS, Bevan WP. Talocalcaneal tarsal coalitions and the calcaneal lengthening osteotomy: the role of deformity correction. *J Bone Joint Surg Am.* 2012; 94(17):1584–94.

26. Saporta AS, Sottile SL, Miller LJ, Feely SM, Siskind CE, Shy ME. Charcot–Marie–Tooth disease subtypes and genetic testing strategies. *Ann Neurol.* 2011; 69(1):22–33.

27. Coughlin MJ. Juvenile hallux valgus: etiology and treatment. *Foot Ankle Int.* 1995; 16(11):682–97.

28. Davids JR, McBrayer D, Blackhurst DW. Juvenile hallux valgus deformity: surgical management by lateral hemiepiphyseodesis of the great toe metatarsal. *J Pediatr Orthop.* 2007; 27(7):826–30.

Chapter 21

Fractures and Dislocations of the Ankle

Daniel Thuillier and Bruce Sangeorzan

Introduction

The "ankle" is composed of the tibiotalar and the distal tibiofibular joints, which work in combination with the rest of the structures of the lower leg to allow standing and walking. The term "ankle fracture" is used to describe the very common malleolar fracture patterns and these are described in the first part of this chapter. Impaction injuries into the weightbearing surface of the tibial plafond are usually termed "pilon" fractures. Pilon fractures need special consideration, and are described separately in the second part of this chapter.

The importance of the tibiotalar joint is in allowing successful force transmission from the foot, via the talus, to the distal tibia during standing and walking. In order to do this the talus needs to maintain its position underneath the distal tibia and to move freely from plantar flexion to dorsiflexion. This ankle movement relies on the complex interactions between the bony structures of the distal tibia and fibula and the surrounding ligaments, tendons, muscles, and nerves. Treatment aims to restore ankle bony and soft tissue anatomy.

Pathogenesis: Etiology, Epidemiology, and Pathophysiology

The incidence of ankle fractures in the United States is 187/100 000 adults per annum[1] or 4.2 per 1000 Medicare enrollees.[2] The incidence of ankle fractures seems to be increasing, this is unsurprising as age and BMI are two of the most significant risk factors for fracture. History of previous ankle fracture is also a risk factor[3–4]. The highest incidence of ankle fractures occurs in older women aged 75 to 84 years[3,5]. In contrast below the age of 50 ankle fractures are commoner in men than women.

Ankle fractures result most commonly from acute trauma, either during sport, or during a fall while running, jumping, or descending stairs or a ladder. The position of the foot during injury, as well as the direction of the force causes different fracture patterns. Understanding the anatomy of the fracture is key to understanding their pathophysiology and planning their treatment.

Anatomy and Biomechanics

Bony Anatomy

The distal tibia and distal fibula form a mortise (Figure 21.1), within which the talar dome sits. The term mortise is taken from the woodworking mortise and tenon joint, where a joint is formed between a recess (the mortise) and a corresponding projection (tenon), which mates with it. The ankle mortise is maintained by both bony and ligamentous structures.

Medial Structures: Medial Malleolus and Deltoid Ligament

The medial flare of the distal tibia forms the medial malleolus. In its normal position it helps prevent the talus from translating medially. The deltoid ligament stabilizes the medial ankle, and is composed of superficial and deep components. The superficial deltoid ligament fans out from the medial malleolus to attach to the talus, calcaneus, and navicular, and prevents eversion of the hindfoot. The thick deep deltoid ligament runs from the medial malleolus to the medial talus and is crucial in preventing abduction of the talus. Running directly posterior to the medial malleolus are the tendons of tibialis posterior, flexor digitorum longus (FDL), and flexor hallucis longus (FHL), from medial to lateral. The posterior tibial artery and nerve are described as lying between the FHL and FDL tendons. The posterior aspect of the medial malleolus usually has a groove for the posterior tibial tendon (PTT). The saphenous nerve and

(a)

(b)

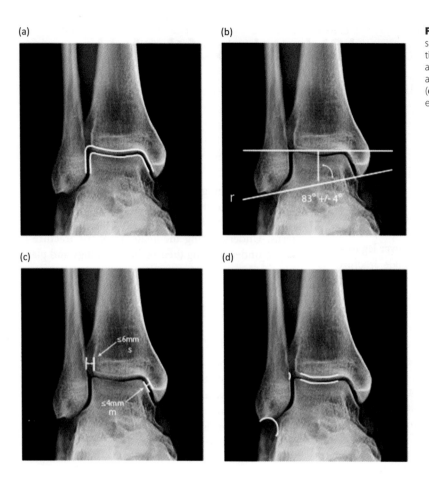

(c)

(d)

Figure 21.1 (a) Outline of the mortise showing equal joint space. (b) Shows the tibial plafond and axis of rotation (r) of the ankle. (c) The medial clear space (m) and the syndesmotic space (s). (d) Demonstrates the marks for establishing normal fibular length.

vein run superficially over the medial malleolus in the subcutaneous fat.

Midline Structures: Talar Dome, Plafond, and Posterior Malleolus

The tibial plafond sits at approximately 87° to the mechanical axis of the tibia. It is covered with articular cartilage and articulates directly with the talar dome. It has a small sagittal ridge dividing it into a wider lateral and smaller medial part.

The talar dome closely matches the curvature of the distal tibial plafond. It is bi-lobed with the sagittal prominence of the tibial plafond sitting within the groove. This fit is crucial as studies have shown that translating the talus 1 mm may increase joint pressures by as much as 40%[6–7], predisposing the ankle to post-traumatic arthritis. The slightly larger radius of the lateral portion of the talar dome results in dorsiflexion causing the foot to externally rotate slightly. Additionally the talar dome is wider anteriorly than it

is posteriorly, thus the talus has a more stable fit within the mortise when the ankle is dorsiflexed. The distal fibula accommodates the differential width, by rotating slightly as the talus dorsiflexes, and the wider portion moves into the mortise.

The posterior malleolus is part of the weightbearing articular surface and injury to it does affect ankle joint function. It has also been postulated that the posterior malleolus helps to prevent posterior translation of the talus[8], although there is contradictory evidence on this. Early research in cadavers demonstrated that resection of up to 40% of the posterior malleolus, leaving the lateral structures intact, resulted in little to no translation with posteriorly directed forces[9–10]. On the other hand, it has been shown in cadavers that with an axially directed force and resection of 25% of the plafond there is increased posterior talar translation[11].

The posterior malleolus is also the attachment point for the posterior inferior talofibular ligament (PITFL). With combined fractures of the posterior malleolus and the fibula the PITFL often remains intact. As a result reduction of the fibula and posterior malleolus is linked. The regions of the tibia that attach to the PITFL and the anterior inferior tibiofibular ligament (AITFL) posteriorly are eponymously named, with the PITFL being attached to the Volkmann fragment (posterolateral) and AITFL to the Chaput fragment (anterolateral).

Lateral Structures: Lateral Malleolus and Syndesmosis

The distal fibula articulates with the distal tibia as well as the lateral aspect of the talus. It sits slightly posteriorly in the crescent-shaped incisura of the distal tibia. The fibula rotates slightly in ankle dorsiflexion to accommodate the wider anterior aspect of the talar dome. The syndesmotic ligaments hold the fibula in place. There are four main ligaments, which help to maintain this relationship – the interosseous membrane (IOM), AITFL, PITFL and the inferior transverse ligament (ITL) (Figure 21.2). These ligaments help resist external rotation of the fibula by the talus and with the deltoid ligament also resist lateral translation.

The more superficial ligaments are also important in maintaining ankle function. The anterior talofibular ligament (ATFL) runs from the distal fibula to the talar neck. It helps prevent anterior translation of the ankle in slight plantar flexion and is the most commonly injured ligament in ankle sprains. The calcaneofibular ligament (CFL) runs from the distal tibia to the calcaneus, deep to the peroneal tendons. It primarily resists ankle inversion.

Just posterior to the lateral malleolus run the peroneal tendons in their tendon sheath. They are kept in place by the strong peroneal retinaculum. The superficial peroneal nerve pierces the peroneal fascia approximately 10 to 12 cm from the distal tip of the lateral malleolus and then courses superficially and anteriorly to cross the tibiotalar joint in front of the fibula, adjacent to the peroneus tertius – the nerve is at risk in lateral approaches to the fibula.

Presentation

History

Patients usually present with a history of trauma, although neuropathic patients may present simply with swelling or deformity. It should not to be forgotten that neuropathic patients also present with pain.

The history should include the time of injury and the nature of the trauma, including if possible the exact mechanism and position of the foot. It is important to specify the location of pain both in the foot and ankle, as well as generally.

It is particularly important to record comorbidities such as peripheral vascular disease and

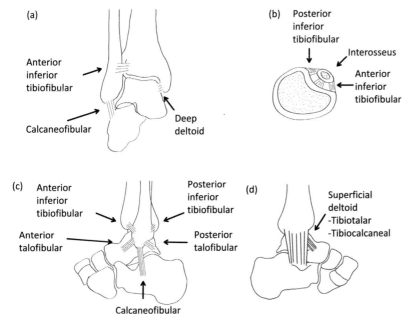

Figure 21.2 Ligaments of the ankle. (**a**) Anterior ankle. (**b**) Axial view showing components of the syndesmosis. (**c**) Lateral ankle ligaments. (**d**) Medial ankle ligaments.

361

diabetes[12–14]. Lifestyle factors including smoking, occupation, and recreational activities should also be noted.

Physical Examination

The physical examination in all trauma patients should start with the "ABC" of airway, breathing, and circulation, with systemic stabilization if necessary. Local examination of the foot and ankle should be prompt and can often be undertaken as the patient is being stabilized. In particular signs of vascular or skin compromise as well as gross deformity should be noted. Swelling, evidence of previous trauma, and surgical scars should be recorded. The bony prominences of the foot and ankle are palpated, including the medial and lateral malleoli, the base of the fifth metatarsal, navicular tuberosity, calcaneus, and proximal fibula.

Vascular examination is important in all cases. Vascular injuries acutely require urgent treatment, whereas, chronically, peripheral vascular disease will impact upon surgical treatment. The vascular examination should include palpating both the dorsalis pedis and posterior tibial pulses and noting capillary refill. If the pulses are not palpable, Doppler ultrasound should be used to record their presence.

Neurological examination should include testing skin sensation in the distribution of the superficial peroneal, deep peroneal, saphenous, sural, and tibial nerves. Additionally great toe dorsiflexion (deep peroneal) and plantar flexion (tibial nerve) should be assessed[15]. There is debate about the management of nerve injuries, with some advocating urgent repair and others recommending observation, even if the nerve injury is complete[16–17]. Damage to the tibial nerve is an important factor in determining limb viability, nevertheless good results are seen with tibial nerve injury[18], thus absence of the tibial nerve is not, in itself, an indication for amputation.

Compartment Syndrome

Compartment syndrome of the leg or foot can complicate ankle trauma, although it is commoner after tibial shaft fracture. Compartment syndrome should always be considered in patients who have pain disproportionate to their injury, or neurological abnormality. If there is any clinical suspicion of a compartment syndrome then compartment pressures should be measured.

Imaging

The indications for radiographs in ankle trauma have been widely studied to try and eliminate unnecessary radiographs. The Ottawa ankle rules advocate obtaining radiographs for anyone who has tenderness who cannot bear weight, has medial tenderness over the posterior edge of the medial malleolus or navicular, or lateral tenderness over the posterior edge of the fibula and base of the fifth metatarsal. Special care should be taken in intoxicated or obtunded patients, those with peripheral neuropathy, or with swelling that prevents direct palpation of bony prominences.

Radiographs

Standard imaging includes three views of the ankle. Some authors have looked at limiting the study to two views, a lateral and mortise, but this approach has been shown to miss as many as 18% of fractures[19]. Physical examination for tenderness should help guide further imaging of the tibia, knee, and foot. Additionally, any patient whose ankle radiographs show evidence of a syndesmosis injury, without a fibular fracture, should have full-length tibial and fibular films, to exclude a proximal fibula fracture.

The fracture pattern, integrity of the ligamentous structures, and the weightbearing surfaces should be noted on the radiographs. Normal radiographic relationships are shown in Figure 21.1. In general the mortise view should show equal ankle joint space laterally, superiorly, and medially.

As radiographs for trauma are usually not obtained weight bearing, they may fail to show ligament injury. This most commonly occurs in Weber B, supination external rotation type II fractures where it is unclear whether the deltoid ligament is disrupted, or not. In those patients stress imaging may be helpful[20]. The timing and technique remains controversial. Some have advocated gravity stress views, where the patient's foot is placed with the lateral malleolus toward the ground and a mortise radiograph is taken[21–22]. A manual stress test where the physician forcibly dorsiflexes and externally rotates the hindfoot while obtaining a mortise radiograph has also been described[23]. Still others have advocated weightbearing radiographs as a true measure of physiologic stress. The timing of these radiographs (emergency room vs. first clinic visit) is up to the surgeon, and to some degree the ability of the patient to tolerate them.

Advanced Imaging

Complex imaging such as CT or MRI scans is generally not required for the evaluation of malleolar fractures. CT scans are helpful if there is concern about impaction of the tibial plafond, the morphology of a fracture extending into the plafond is unclear, or if there is uncertainty as to the fracture configuration. MRI scanning can be helpful in the evaluation of soft tissue structures, but is rarely indicated in the setting of an acute ankle fracture, as the soft tissue edema makes interpretation difficult, and clinical decision making is not helped.

Classification

Lauge–Hansen Classification

This classification scheme (Figure 21.3) was developed as a result of cadaver research. The foot was placed into a specified position and a force applied. The resulting fracture patterns were divided into two part descriptive names, with the first part being the position of the foot (supination or pronation) and the second the direction of the force (external rotation, abduction, or adduction). Increasing severity was designated by numbers. This combination creates characteristic fracture patterns of the malleoli.

Supination adduction. The lateral structures fail first (fibula or calcaneofibular ligament) and the talus is then driven up into the talar dome.

Fibular fracture pattern: transverse, usually below the tibiotalar joint

Medial malleolar pattern: vertical, often with impaction of the medial plafond.

Supination external rotation. This is the commonest pattern following a twisting injury where the failure line moves rotationally around the ankle, starting laterally and moving posteriorly to the medial side. The structures are injured in the following order:

1. anterior talofibular ligament
2. lateral malleolus
3. posterior inferior tibiofibular ligament or posterior malleolus
4. deltoid ligament or medial malleolus.

The fibular fracture pattern is short oblique at the level of the tibiotalar joint. The medial malleolus is an oblique avulsion at the shoulder of the plafond.

Pronation abduction. This fracture pattern starts medially with disruption of either the deltoid or medial malleolus. It then moves laterally through the syndesmosis and eventually the fibula fracture with a bending motion.

Fibular fracture pattern: transverse, comminuted fracture at the level of the joint

Medial malleolar fracture pattern: transverse avulsion fracture, often distal to the plafond.

Pronation external rotation. A twisting mechanism, which starts medially with disruption of the medial malleolus or deltoid ligament, and then extends through the syndesmosis eventually leading to fibular fracture.

Fibular fracture pattern: a short spiral oblique fracture proximal to tibial plafond

Medial malleolar fracture pattern: transverse avulsion fracture, often distal to the plafond.

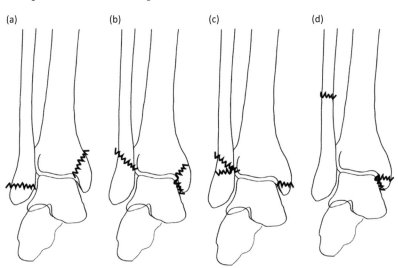

Figure 21.3 Lauge–Hansen classification of ankle fractures. (**a**) Supination adduction; (**b**) supination external rotation; (**c**) pronation abduction; (**d**) pronation external rotation.

363

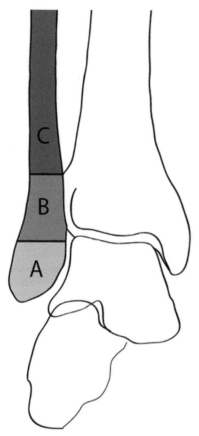

Figure 21.4 Weber ankle fracture classification. The fibular fracture is designated A, B, or C, according to the level of the fracture.

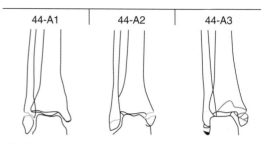

44-A   infrasyndesmotic lesion
44-A1 isolated
44-A2 with fractured medial malleolus
43-A3 with posteromedial fracture

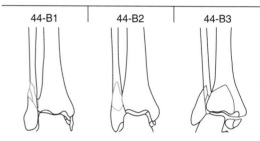

44-B   transsyndesmotic fibular fracture
44-B1 isolated
44-B2 with medial lesion
44-B3 with medial lesion and Volkmann's fracture

Weber/AO Classification

The Weber classification system (Figure 21.4) is broken down into three different fracture types based solely on the location of the fibular fracture.

A: Distal to the plafond
B: At the level of the plafond
C: Proximal to the plafond.

The AO classification (Figure 21.5) is based upon the Weber classification, but adds subclassifications to account for additional injuries to the medial and posterior malleoli.

Treatment

The overall aim in treating ankle fractures is to restore a stable, congruent ankle joint. This anatomy is restored, while the soft tissue injury is minimized.

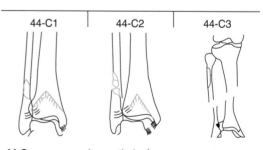

44-C   suprasyndesmotic lesion
44-C1 fibular diaphyseal fracture, simple
44-C2 fibular diaphyseal fracture, multifragmentary
44-C3 proximal fibular lesion

Figure 21.5 AO classification of ankle fractures. (Source: *AO Surgery*, copyright by AO Foundation, Switzerland)

Initial Treatment

Initial treatment includes reduction and temporary stabilization. Reduction decompresses the soft tissues and provisionally restores alignment. This can usually be achieved closed. Even if future surgical intervention is planned, a poor reduction should not be tolerated. *If proper reduction cannot be obtained in the emergency room or clinic then the patient should promptly be taken to the operating room for an open reduction.* After reduction, the patient should be placed in a well-molded and padded splint to hold the reduction. Post-reduction films should be obtained to confirm the position.

Bosworth fractures are rare fractures where the proximal aspect of the distal fibula is trapped posterior to the distal tibia (Figure 21.6). They need to be recognized as closed reduction will not be possible, and may even cause further harm. Bosworth fractures should be treated with early open reduction and internal fixation.

Vascular Compromise

If signs of vascular compromise are present the ankle should be promptly reduced in the emergency department. If this does not restore blood supply to the foot, or if a vascular injury is readily apparent, for example with visible pulsatile bleeding, a vascular opinion should be obtained immediately. If vascular repair is necessary a temporary external fixator is applied before undertaking the vascular repair, in order to restore stability and protect the repair. External fixation is usually advocated, as it is generally faster to apply and minimizes the ischemic time. External can then be revised to internal fixation, once the vascular supply has been stabilized.

Open Fractures

Patients with open ankle fractures should receive immediate intravenous antibiotics in the emergency department followed by timely surgical debridement in the operating room. The recommended antibiotics in our institution are:

- all open fractures: second-generation cephalosporin
- larger (>10 cm) or grossly contaminated wounds: second-generation cephalosporin and an aminoglycoside
- farmyard wounds: second-generation cephalosporin and penicillin.

Historically, a six- to eight-hour window post-injury for surgical debridement has been regarded as the gold standard. Recent data has called this into question, showing equivalent results with debridement at up to 24 hrs[24]. This study also demonstrated that early admission to a definitive trauma center appears to have a significant benefit in reducing the rate of infection. It is possible that early resuscitation

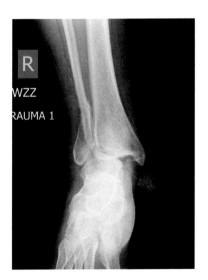
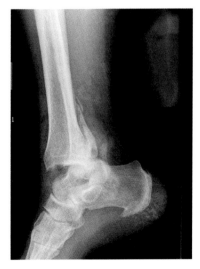

Figure 21.6 Bosworth fracture. Note the position of the fibula behind the distal tibia, this makes closed reduction very difficult.

365

and antibiotic administration may play a role in this[24].

Whenever possible, definitive surgical fixation of the fracture should be undertaken at the time of the surgical debridement. However, it is important that the overlying skin can be closed without tension over the hardware. This is often possible for small, simple wounds, but if there is a large wound that cannot be closed, then the fracture site should be thoroughly debrided and external fixation applied. The external fixation needs to be placed well away from the zone of injury and clear of possible future incisions. The external can then be changed to internal fixation at the time of definitive soft tissue coverage, if the soft tissues allow.

If additional soft tissue coverage is needed, such as a local or free flap, this should only be undertaken once all necrotic tissue has been debrided. This debridement may require multiple trips to the operating room, to allow proper assessment of soft tissues. Nevertheless, coverage should be undertaken as early as possible, although the timing of definitive soft tissue coverage has not been shown to be a factor in the later development of infection[24].

Definitive Treatment

The goal is to obtain a stable, congruent joint with normal movement. This is achieved with anatomic reduction, stable fixation, and the early institution of joint range of motion[25]. *The key is to anatomically reduce the talus and restore the components of the mortise to maintain that position.*

The components include:

- restoration of fibular length and rotation
- reduction of the syndesmosis
- reduction of the medial malleolus
- reduction of the posterior malleolus
- reduction of any step off, gapping, or impaction of the tibial plafond.

If these components can be achieved by non-operative means then no surgical intervention is needed. If they cannot, then surgical treatment should be considered. As with all surgical treatment the benefits should outweigh the risks. Factors such as age, medical comorbidities, especially peripheral vascular disease and diabetes, occupation, cigarette smoking, recreational activities, and ability to comply with postoperative protocols need to be considered and

discussed with the patient before finally confirming the treatment plan.

Specific Considerations for Operative Treatment
Weber A

Distal fractures of the fibula are the result of supination/adduction tension forces. The fractures are often very distal and fixation can only be achieved using either a tension band wire, or a tension band plate and screws.

Any associated medial malleolar fracture is the result of impaction of the talus through the shoulder of the tibial plafond. The medial tibial joint surface is also often impacted as well, and this needs disimpaction before fixation. The fracture is opened and the subchondral bone is elevated. The resultant bone defect is filled with autograft or allograft. The medial malleolar fracture is usually vertical and should be fixed either with horizontal lag screws or a buttress plate and lag screws. Remember that the lag screws should be placed perpendicular to the fracture line. It is important to check that the screws do not penetrate the joint.

Weber B

In treating Weber B fibular fractures the emphasis is on the restoration of fibular length and rotation (Figure 21.7). There is often a long oblique fracture pattern, which lends itself to lag screw fixation with either one or two screws. A lateral or posterolateral neutralization plate is then used to stabilize the construct. If there is fibular comminution, then a bridging plate should be used. The medial malleolar fracture is also fixed.

After the malleolar fractures have been fixed, an on-table stress radiograph should be obtained to assess integrity of the syndesmosis. Approximately 39% of Weber B fractures will be associated with a syndesmosis injury[26]. If the syndesmosis is incompetent, it should be stabilized. There are many described methods and to date no method has proven more effective than any other. Our preferred method is either one or two 3.5 mm screws placed parallel to the tibiotalar joint, with the most distal approximately 1 cm above the joint at the level of the physeal scar. This screw is placed from posterolateral through the fibula to the anteromedial tibia, through three cortices. When placing the screws one must take care to

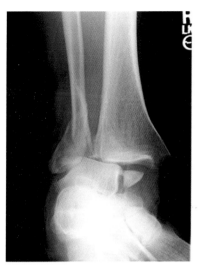
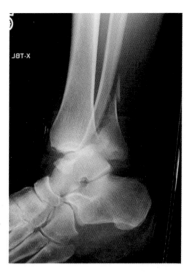
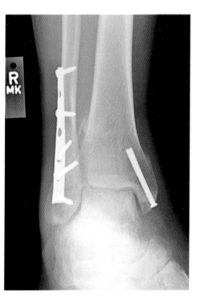
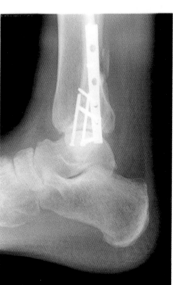

Figure 21.7 Weber B fibular fracture with a medial malleolar fracture. A posterolateral fibular plate captures the oblique fracture with posterior to anterior lag screws. Intraoperative stress testing demonstrated the syndesmosis to be intact.

reduce the fibula into the incisura. Good intraoperative imaging is important (Figure 21.8).

A posterior malleolar fracture is often present. It is known as a Volkmann fragment and contains the tibial attachment of the PITFL. If present the Volkmann fragment must be reduced, although primary reduction of the fibula is often necessary to achieve this, as the two structures are linked by the PITFL. An added benefit of fixation of the Volkmann's fragment is that it may also stabilize the syndesmosis, by refunctioning the PITFL.

As the posterior malleolus is covered with weightbearing articular cartilage, we would recommend fixing all but the smallest posterior malleolar fractures. Fixation usually takes the form of lag screws or a posterolateral buttress plate. If posterior malleolar fixation is required the surgical approach is posterolateral, and therefore the incision for the fibula is posterolateral, to allow both structures to be accessed.

The medial malleolar fracture is usually oblique at the level of the shoulder of the plafond. This can usually be fixed using two 4.0 mm partially threaded lag screws, at least 40 mm in length to ensure compression.

367

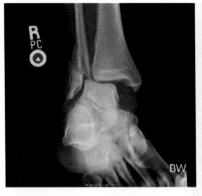
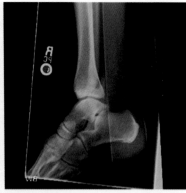

Figure 21.8 Distal fibular fracture with deltoid ligament disruption. The distal fibula was fixed using lag screws and a lateral neutralization plate. A locking plate was chosen because the patient was diabetic. Intraoperative stress testing revealed a diastasis. Syndesmosis screws were added.

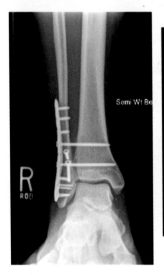
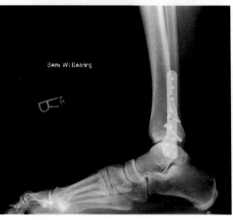

Weber C

High fibular fractures are almost always associated with a syndesmosis injury, as the fracture pattern starts medially and moves up through the syndesmosis, rupturing the interosseous ligament (Figure 21.9). With disruption of the syndesmosis surgical fixation is almost always indicated. For very high fibula fractures, also known as *Maisonneuve fractures*, reduction of the fracture itself is not always needed *as long as the fibular length and rotation are maintained*. As the interosseous membrane is disrupted, fixation of the syndesmosis is required, usually with two screws. The same principles of accurate reduction of the fibula in the incisura apply.

As with Weber B fractures a Volkmann fragment may be present, and it should be reduced and held with a single lag screw if small, or if it extends proximally a buttress plate.

The medial malleolar fracture is usually a small horizontal fracture at the level of the plafond, which can be fixed using two lag screws or a tension band wire.

Postoperative Protocol

In general, young active patients, in whom there is little concern for fracture healing, benefit from early range of motion and weight bearing. Our usual postoperative protocol is splintage for two weeks. The splint is then removed and replaced with a controlled ankle motion (CAM) walker. The patient is kept non-weightbearing. At six weeks radiographs are obtained and progressive weight bearing is initiated, starting at 50% and increasing 25% every two weeks, as tolerated. Neuropathic patients, or patients with peripheral vascular disease, should have their ankle protected for an extended period of time.

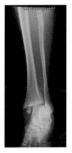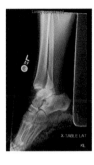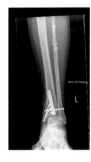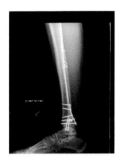

Figure 21.9 A trimalleolar fracture with high Weber C fibular fracture. The high fibular fracture has been fixed to re-establish length and rotation of the fibula. The large posterior malleolar fragment has been fixed using a buttress plate. The syndesmosis is disrupted therefore a syndesmosis screw has been added.

No standard protocol for syndesmosis fixation exists. We typically follow the same protocol as for patients without syndesmosis fixation. The patients are told that their screws are likely to break and if they are symptomatic from a broken screw, or having difficulties with dorsiflexion, then the screws are removed at six to nine months. We do not advocate routine screw removal as it requires an additional surgery with possible complications.

Outcomes

With accurate reduction approximately 80% of patients will achieve good to excellent long-term results[27]. Bhandari et al. showed that at two years, ankle fracture patients achieved scores similar to the normal population in six of eight domains in the SF 36. Unsurprisingly, perhaps, it was patients' physical function and physical role scores that remained significantly lower. In this series smoking, lower education, and presence of a medial malleolar fracture were predictive of poorer outcomes[28]. In other long-term studies, fractures involving the medial malleolus (Figure 21.10) have shown poorer outcomes with bimalleolar fractures having only 52% excellent results at 13 years' follow-up[1]. Fractures with a posterior malleolar component have also shown poorer long-term outcomes. With the posterior and medial malleolar fracture variants, the poorer long-term results may be a result of injury to the articular cartilage predisposing toward post-traumatic arthritis[29].

Pilon Fractures

Introduction

Destot first used the term "pilon," which comes from the French word for pestle, as in pestle and mortar, in 1911 to describe fractures of the distal flare of the tibial metaphysis. Pilon fractures are impaction fractures of the tibial plafond, extending into the tibial metaphysis. There is often comminution of the tibial plafond with direct injury of the articular surface and chondrocytes, in addition to the soft tissue injury. Soft tissue compromise and post-traumatic arthritis remain major concerns in the treatment of pilon fractures. They are challenging fractures to treat.

Pathogenesis, Etiology, and At-Risk Patients

Pilon fractures are the result of an axially directed force pushing the talus through the tibial plafond. The position of the foot at the time of impact is thought to direct the force and dictate the fracture pattern. With a dorsiflexed foot the plafond fracture is primarily anterior. When the foot is plantar flexed the primary fracture is posterior and central impaction occurs with a neutral foot position. As the distal tibia fails, the fibula will often fracture, resulting in the foot moving into valgus. Alternatively if the fibula remains intact, the foot moves into varus. The comminution of the plafond can be severe, but there are usually identifiable fragments: the Volkmann fragment attached to the PITFL, and Chaput fragment attached to the AITFL and the medial malleolus. The size and pattern of the fragments vary.

The high-energy axial loading force, which causes the pilon fracture, is most often the result of falls from a height or motor vehicle accidents. They are relatively rare injuries representing only 10% of lower extremity injuries[30]. The highest incidence of pilon fractures is in men aged 35 to 40 years[30]. The incidence appears to be increasing in developed countries. This is thought to be the result of seatbelts and airbags, as more drivers are surviving motor vehicle accidents, with lower extremities that remain unprotected[31].

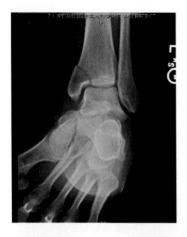
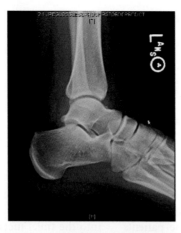
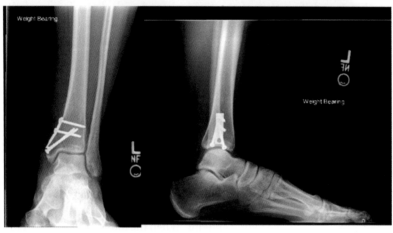

Figure 21.10 This isolated medial malleolar fracture is large, resulting from impaction of the talus. A buttress plate/lag screw construct has been used to achieve fixation.

Presentation, History, and Examination

The evaluation of the patient is similar to that for simpler ankle fractures. Special attention should be paid to the skin. Even in closed injuries there may be areas of skin that are at risk, and fracture blisters or abrasions are often present. These need to be noted in planning surgical incisions.

Imaging

Radiographs

The standard three views of the ankle should be obtained in addition to an AP and lateral of the full tibia. Sometimes when there is severe comminution traction views, in an external fixator, may be helpful.

Advanced Imaging

Understanding the fracture pattern is crucial in accurate surgical planning. This is best achieved with a CT

scan. The scan can be obtained in the emergency room, although if temporary external fixation is used, scanning after application of the fixator is recommended, as it is easier to interpret. MRI scans are rarely helpful.

Classification

Classification schemes for pilon fractures are not universally accepted. The AO classification is the most widely used.

AO Classification

Fractures of the distal tibia, as with most joints in the AO system, are separated into A, B, and C representing extra-articular, partially articular, and fully articular. Each group is then further subdivided into 1, 2, or 3 based upon the amount and degree of comminution. Pilon fractures generally fall into the B and C types (Figure 21.11).

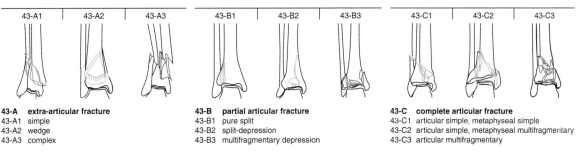

| 43-A1 | 43-A2 | 43-A3 | 43-B1 | 43-B2 | 43-B3 | 43-C1 | 43-C2 | 43-C3 |

43-A extra-articular fracture
43-A1 simple
43-A2 wedge
43-A3 complex

43-B partial articular fracture
43-B1 pure split
43-B2 split-depression
43-B3 multifragmentary depression

43-C complete articular fracture
43-C1 articular simple, metaphyseal simple
43-C2 articular simple, metaphyseal multifragmentary
43-C3 articular multifragmentary

Figure 21.11 AO classification of pilon fractures. (Source: *AO Surgery*, copyright by AO Foundation, Switzerland)

Initial Treatment

The acute treatment of pilon fractures tends to be more complex than the treatment of malleolar fractures, as a result of the more extensive soft tissue injury. Open fractures and vascular injuries require urgent treatment.

Reduction and splinting have a limited role, except in non- or minimally displaced fractures and in the severely debilitated patients with very limited functional goals. The majority of these fractures will require surgical treatment. Prior to the adoption of internal fixation, treatment of pilon fractures using traction and casting had dismal results with high rates of malunion, non-union, and arthritis.

The adoption of modern internal fixation techniques has greatly improved the results of these injuries[32], nevertheless complication rates remain high with an up to 37% rate of either deep infection or wound complications[33]. This is as a result of the high energy of the injury and the paucity of the soft tissue envelope surrounding the distal tibia – there is little in the way of muscular cover. Early internal fixation in this setting is prone to wound breakdown and subsequent infection. Osteomyelitis can be devastating in this setting, often resulting in amputation. Thus to try and minimize the surgical trauma to the compromised soft tissue envelope external fixation, with or without limited internal fixation, was adopted, by some, as definitive treatment for pilon fractures[26]. Despite good reported results and the avoidance of the soft tissue complications with external and minimal internal fixation, deep infection, pin-site problems, malreduction and non-union rates have remained unsatisfactorily high[34]. This has led to a staged approach of initial external fixation and later definitive open reduction and internal fixation[35–37].

This staged treatment involves initial reduction, held by external fixation, performed in the first 24 hours. This restores length and will relieve pressure on the soft tissues. Restoring length is crucial as this can be very difficult to regain once healing begins. When the external fixator is placed, it should be placed with the pins well outside both the zone of injury and possible future incision. The fibula may be internally fixed acutely, at the same time[36]. This allows accurate reduction of the fibula, restoring length and rotation, and giving a marker as to the level of the tibial plafond. At times soft tissue swelling can be so pronounced that closing the skin over the lateral wound may not be possible, in these cases the fibula fixation should not be attempted.

Fracture blisters filled with blood or serous fluid are often present. There are no data as to the best way to treat these. Some surgeons prefer to aspirate them sterilely in the operating room, others prefer to cover them with a petroleum dressing and allow them to decompress on their own.

Definitive Fixation

In treating pilon fractures the aim is to restore stability and congruence to the joint, so that it can move and load physiologically. As with simple ankle fractures the aim of surgery is anatomic reduction, stable fixation, and the commencement of early joint range of motion exercises[25]. Despite this post-traumatic arthritis may occur, even with anatomic reduction, as a result of primary cartilage injury at the time of injury. However, anatomic reduction will result in the best functioning ankle for the longest period of time and help prevent post-traumatic arthritis[38]. It will also make later salvage surgery, such as ankle fusion, easier. Internal or external fixation or a combination of both may be needed to achieve this. No matter

371

whether internal or external fixation is employed the steps of reconstruction are:

1. restoration of length
2. reconstruction of the articular surface
3. bone grafting any defects
4. attaching the articular surface/metaphysis to the tibial diaphysis.

External Fixation or Hybrid

We recommend using a delta frame construction with two high 5 mm tibial Schanz half-pins, a calcaneal transfixion pin, and a midfoot pin to prevent equinus. Length can usually be judged from the reduction of the fibula. With external fixation ligamentotaxis helps reduce the fragments of the tibial plafond and metaphysis. Additional pins can be added to reduce and stabilize larger fragments. Limited bone graft and internal fixation are also, on occasions, added through minimal incisions.

The advantage of external fixation is that surgical incisions to insert hardware are not required, thus eliminating complications from surgical wounds, excluding pin-site infections, which are common. There are disadvantages, however; in particular external fixation does not allow early joint range of motion exercises. Indeed if the fixation crosses the subtalar joint unaffected joints can also become stiff. Consequently we recommend using external fixation only for those patients where soft tissue compromise and wound healing is a major concern (Figure 21.12), or as a temporary measure to aid soft tissue recovery, while awaiting definitive surgery.

Internal Fixation

Internal fixation remains the best and most consistent method for achieving an anatomic reduction and accurately restoring the articular surface. Good preoperative planning is essential and it is important to recognize the fracture patterns and fragments and their extension into the metaphysis, to optimize the choice of surgical approach and fixation (Figures 21.13 and 21.14).

Approaches to the Ankle

A number of factors should be taken into consideration when planning the approach/es.

- The fracture patterns and proposed fixation dictate the surgical approach.

- The skin most at risk overlies the anteromedial tibia.
- If fracture blisters or other lesions, which may heal in a timely fashion, are present, it may be better to let these heal, rather than choose an alternative incision.
- Historically the minimum skin bridge width has been 7 cm[39]. More recently this has been questioned and skin bridges as small as 5 cm have been successfully used with modern staged techniques[40].
- All incisions should be made using minimal dissection, raising full thickness skin flaps.

Direct Lateral Approach

Description: direct lateral, in line with the fibula

Access: fibula for fibular fracture

Structures at risk: superficial peroneal nerve proximally, sural nerve distally

Problems: difficulty accessing the tibia, especially access to the posterior plafond.

Anterolateral

Description: straight incision centered at the ankle parallel to the interosseous membrane proximally and the fourth metatarsal distally

Access: entire anterior tibial plafond

Structures at risk: superficial peroneal nerve

Problems: medial tibial shoulder difficult to access. A separate incision may be needed for access to the medial malleolus.

Anteromedial

Description: start just medial to the tibial crest and follow the tibialis anterior curving medially across the joint to just distal to the medial malleolus

Access: medial joint and medial malleolus for traditional incision, extendable to the entire anterior joint surface

Structures at risk: deep peroneal nerve and artery, saphenous nerve

Problems: extensive dissection of the anteromedial tibial face, which may put the skin at risk.

Posteromedial

Description: incision just medial to the tendo Achillis and deep through the FHL sheath

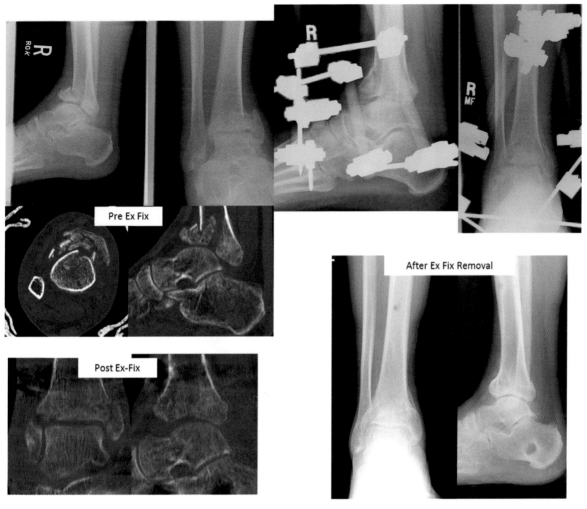

Figure 21.12 Isolated tibial plafond injury with substantial comminution. As a result of the severity of the soft tissue injury this patient was treated definitively in an external fixator. The fracture healed, all be it with an imperfect reduction.

Access: the entire posterior and medial tibia

At risk: tibial artery and nerve

Problems: difficulty accessing the posterolateral tibia

Posterolateral

Description: a longitudinal incision along the posterior edge of the fibula

Access: fibula and posterior malleolus/plafond

At risk: superficial peroneal nerve proximally

Problems: high historical rate of wound problems[41]; inability to access posteromedial tibia.

Stage 1 Restoration of Length

In a staged approach, the length should have been restored and held acutely with the external fixator and fibular fixation. Slight adjustments may need to be made. If length has not been restored acutely, a universal distractor can be used to help restore it. The proximal Schanz pin is placed parallel to the normal anatomic plafond and the distal pin is placed into the talar neck or the calcaneus. If the fibula is fractured and has not been fixed acutely, then it should be fixed first using either a direct lateral or posterolateral approach (Figure 21.13).

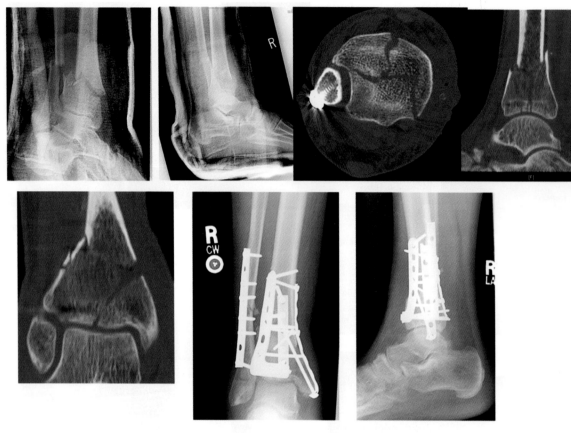

Figure 21.13 This pilon fracture shows the typical Volkmann, Chaput, and medial malleolar fragments on the CT scan (AO type C). This patient had a staged approach, with early external and fibular fixation, followed by CT scanning. The tibia was then fixed using a posterolateral approach for the posterior malleolar buttress plate. An anteromedial incision was used for the anterior plate as well as the medial malleolar plate, stabilizing both the medial and lateral columns.

Stage 2 Articular Restoration

In stage 2 the articular surface is restored. This can be difficult if the joint surface is very comminuted. Ligamentotaxis from the restoration of length may approximately reduce some fragments. The Volkmann and the Chaput fragments, with their relatively constant position and attachment to the distal fibula, can be a good starting point from which to reconstruct the articular surface of the distal tibia. Additionally the talar dome may provide a good template for the tibial plafond. Once the pieces are reconstructed they can be held provisionally using Kirschner wires (Figure 21.13).

Definitive fixation using screws or mini-fragment plates can then be undertaken. Larger fragments can sometimes be captured through a standard medial or anterolateral plate.

Stage 3 Bone Grafting of Defects

As a result of the axial forces that cause pilon fractures, metaphyseal impaction is often present. As a result, after restoring the articular surface, voids may be present in the metaphysis. Whenever possible these should be filled with autograft. The iliac crest remains the gold standard and has the highest number of viable stem cells; however, the proximal tibial metaphysis at Gerdy's tubercle is another good option with less

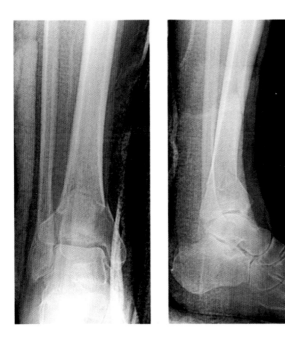
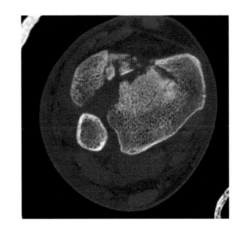
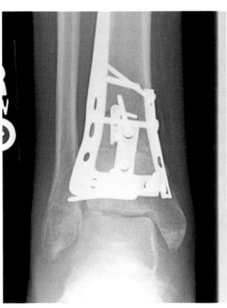
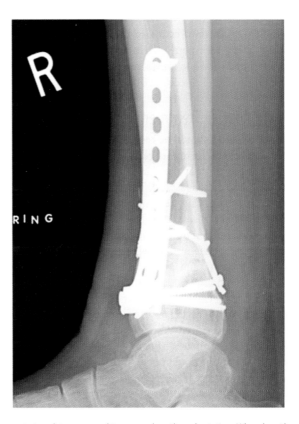

Figure 21.14 A pilon fracture without a fibular fracture. In this case a posterior plate was used to secure length and rotation. When length and rotation have been re-established the anterior comminution is easier to reduce and fix.

postoperative morbidity. If autograft is not possible then allograft or structural bone substitutes, such as calcium phosphate, may be used. Whenever possible grafting should be undertaken at the time of definitive fixation as it will help to provide structural support.

Stage 4   Fixation of the Metaphysis to the Diaphysis

The type of fixation needed will again depend largely on the fracture pattern. In general one needs to ensure that both the medial and lateral columns are supported, to prevent varus or valgus malunion, and ensure that the joint is perpendicular to the mechanical axis of the tibia. This can be performed using a variety of plate and screw techniques. Traditionally a clover-shaped plate was placed medially on the tibia with additional screws or small plates as needed.

Newer pre-contoured plates offer a lower profile fit than traditional plates, and this may reduce later impingement on the soft tissues. Pre-contoured plates are available for the medial, anterior, and anterolateral portions of the tibia. Additionally, newer plates often have options for both locking and non-locking screws. Locking screws offer better angular stability, which may be helpful in highly comminuted fractures or in osteoporotic bone. Non-locking screws can allow reduction and compression of the fracture fragments using a lag technique. Thus hybrid fixation with locking and non-locking screws through the same plate is now often used (see Figures 21.13 and 21.14).

Postoperative Treatment

The soft tissues should be respected and handled with care at all times during surgery. Special care should be taken to ensure that the skin is closed with minimal tension in a layered fashion. The deep layers are closed with absorbable sutures and the skin with non-absorbable sutures such as nylon. Tension-relieving stitches, such as a modified Allgower–Donati, or vertical mattress are useful. The leg should then be placed in a bulky dressing and a posterior plaster slab with a stirrup to hold the ankle in neutral. The patient should keep the leg elevated for the next one to two weeks.

Range of motion exercises of the ankle and subtalar joints are commenced as soon as the wounds heal and the soft tissues allow – usually at one to two weeks. Range of motion should not be initiated at the expense of wound healing. At this point the patient's splint and sutures can be removed and they are placed into a CAM walker to allow range of motion exercises. The patient is kept non-weightbearing until there is evidence of bone healing, which is usually at six to twelve weeks.

Outcome

There are many factors that influence the outcomes of pilon fractures. Many of these are a result of the injury itself. Open fractures, fractures with soft tissue compromise, bone loss, and more severe fracture patterns (AO C3) have been shown to have worse outcomes regardless of treatment[42–43]. This is probably as a result of the energy imparted to the articular cartilage at the time of injury and the potential for infection or soft tissue compromise. Other factors including misalignment, instability, and incongruence of the tibial plafond have been shown to be associated with a poorer outcome. These factors may be helped by surgical intervention. Unfortunately articular cartilage incongruity following fixation has also been shown to predict a poorer outcome[38].

The commonest immediate complication of surgery is wound problems, with a traditional incidence as high as 37%[33]. Using a modern, staged technique the incidence can be reduced to 0 to 17%[36]. Infection and chronic osteomyelitis remain a problem, especially after open injuries.

The commonest late complication is post-traumatic arthritis. The true rate is very difficult to determine as it requires long-term follow up, but the rate is quoted as being between 13 and 54%[38]. The severity of the fracture and joint incongruity are thought to contribute. Malunion and non-union are also predictors of failure, and they have been shown to be commoner when using external fixation as the definitive fixation technique[34].

Even utilizing modern techniques, Pollak et al. demonstrated that at three years patients with pilon fractures remained significantly disabled compared to age-matched controls, with 33% reporting significant stiffness, 33% reporting ongoing pain, and only 57% of people returning to work[30].

Key Points
Ankle Fractures
- The Lauge–Hansen classification scheme is based on foot position and the direction of the force.
- Bosworth fractures are a rare fracture pattern, where the distal fibula is trapped behind the distal tibia, and require open reduction.
- Shifting of the talus by 1 mm can cause a 40% increase in tibiotalar forces.
- Preoperative stress imaging tests the integrity of the deep deltoid ligament.
- Intraoperative stress imaging tests the integrity of the syndesmosis.
- Syndesmosis injuries are almost always seen with Weber C fractures, and in 30% of Weber B fractures.

- The PITFL usually remains attached to the posterior malleolar fragment.
- Medial and posterior malleolar fractures have worse long-term outcomes.
- Malreduction of the fibula or the medial malleolus may lead to subtle instability, an alteration of joint forces, and post-traumatic arthritis.

Pilon Fractures

- The constant fragments in a pilon fracture tend to be the Chaput fragment (AITFL), the Volkmann fragment (PITFL), and the medial malleolus.
- A modern staged surgical technique involves primary initial external fixation +/– ORIF of the fibula to restore length.
- Once the soft tissue injury allows, secondary internal fixation is undertaken.
- This staged approach has resulted in a reduced rate of wound complications, in comparison to acute ORIF.

- Failure of fixation of the medial column can lead to a varus malunion or deformity.
- The anteromedial skin is traditionally at risk following a pilon fracture.
- The posterolateral approach has been reported as having the highest rate of wound complication.
- More severe fracture patterns (AO C3) have worse outcomes than less severe fracture patterns (AO B, C1, C2), in all probability as a result of damage to the articular cartilage at the time of the injury.
- Articular incongruity, joint instability, malalignment, and injury severity are associated with increased rates of post-traumatic arthritis.
- The most common short-term complication is wound problems (0–37%) and the most common long-term problem is post-traumatic arthritis (13–54%).
- Three years after a pilon fracture at least a third of patients remain significantly disabled compared to their healthy, age-matched counterparts.

References

1. Day GA, Swanson CE, Hulcombe BG. Operative treatment of ankle fractures: a minimum ten-year follow-up. *Foot Ankle Int.* 2001; 22(2):102–6.

2. Lauge N. Fractures of the ankle; analytic historic survey as the basis of new experimental, roentgenologic and clinical investigations. *Arch Surg.* 1948; 56(3):259–317.

3. Daly PJ, Fitzgerald RH Jr., Melton LJ, Ilstrup DM. Epidemiology of ankle fractures in Rochester, Minnesota. *Acta Orthop Scand.* 1987; 58(5):539–44.

4. Valtola A, Honkanen R, Kröger H, Tuppurainen M, Saarikoski S, Alhava E. Lifestyle and other factors predict ankle fractures in perimenopausal women: a population-based prospective cohort study. *Bone.* 2002; 30(1):238–42.

5. Court-Brown CM, McBirnie J, Wilson G. Adult ankle fractures: an increasing problem? *Acta Orthop Scand.* 1998; 69(1):43–7.

6. Ramsey PL, Hamilton W. Changes in tibiotalar area of contact caused by lateral talar shift. *J Bone Joint Surg Am.* 1976; 58(3):356–7.

7. Lloyd J, Elsayed S, Hariharan K, Tanaka H. Revisiting the concept of talar shift in ankle fractures. *Foot Ankle Int.* 2006; 27(10):793–6.

8. Harper MC. Posterior instability of the talus: an anatomic evaluation. *Foot Ankle.* 1989; 10(1):36–9.

9. Raasch WG, Larkin JJ, Draganich LF. Assessment of the posterior malleolus as a restraint to posterior subluxation of the ankle. *J Bone Joint Surg Am.* 1992; 74(8):1201–6.

10. Herscovici D Jr., Sanders RW, Infante A, DiPasquale T. Bohler incision: an extensile anterolateral approach to the foot and ankle. *J Orthop Trauma.* 2000; 14(6):429–32.

11. Scheidt KB, Stiehl JB, Skrade DA, Barnhardt T. Posterior malleolar ankle fractures: an in vitro biomechanical analysis of stability in the loaded and unloaded states. *J Orthop Trauma.* 1992; 6(1):96–101.

12. Liu J, Ludwig T, Ebraheim NA. Effect of the blood HbA1c level on surgical treatment outcomes of diabetics with ankle fractures. *Orthop Surg.* 2013; 5(3):203–8.

13. Nasell H, Ottosson C, Törnqvist H, Lindé J, Ponzer S. The impact of smoking on complications after operatively treated ankle fractures – a follow-up study of 906 patients. *J Orthop Trauma.* 2011; 25(12):748–55.

14. Ovaska MT, Mäkinen TJ, Madanat R, et al. Risk factors for deep surgical site infection following operative treatment of ankle fractures. *J Bone Joint Surg Am.* 2013; 95(4):348–53.

15. Mohler LR, Hanel DP. Closed fractures complicated by peripheral nerve injury. *J Am Acad Orthop Surg.* 2006; 14(1):32–7.

16. Seddon HJ. A review of work on peripheral nerve injuries in Great Britain during World War II.

J Nerv Ment Dis. 1948; 108(2):160–8.

17. Sedel L. The surgical management of nerve lesions in the lower limbs. Clinical evaluation, surgical technique and results. *Int Orthop.* 1985; 9(3):159–70.

18. MacKenzie EJ, Bosse MJ. Factors influencing outcome following limb-threatening lower limb trauma: lessons learned from the Lower Extremity Assessment Project (LEAP). *J Am Acad Orthop Surg.* 2006; 14(10 Spec No.):S205-10.

19. Vangsness CT Jr., Carter V, Hunt T, Kerr R, Newton E. Radiographic diagnosis of ankle fractures: are three views necessary? *Foot Ankle Int.* 1994; 15(4):172–4.

20. McConnell T, Creevy W, Tornetta, 3rd P. Stress examination of supination external rotation-type fibular fractures. *J Bone Joint Surg Am.* 2004; 86-A(10):2171–8.

21. Michelson JD, Varner KE, Checcone M. Diagnosing deltoid injury in ankle fractures: the gravity stress view. *Clin Orthop Relat Res.* 2001; 387:178–82.

22. van den Bekerom MP, Mutsaerts EL, van Dijk CN. Evaluation of the integrity of the deltoid ligament in supination external rotation ankle fractures: a systematic review of the literature. *Arch Orthop Trauma Surg.* 2009; 129(2):227–35.

23. Gill JB, Risko T, Raducan V, Grimes JS, Schutt RC Jr. Comparison of manual and gravity stress radiographs for the evaluation of supination–external rotation fibular fractures. *J Bone Joint Surg Am*, 2007; 89(5):994–9.

24. Pollak AN, Jones AL, Castillo RC, Bosse MJ, MacKenzie EJ, LEAP Study Group. The relationship between time to surgical debridement and incidence of infection after open high-energy lower extremity trauma. *J Bone Joint Surg Am.* 2010; 92(1):7–15.

25. Mehta S, Gardner MJ, Barei DP, Benirschke SK, Nork SE. Reduction strategies through the anterolateral exposure for fixation of type B and C pilon fractures. *J Orthop Trauma.* 2011; 25(2):116–22.

26. Tornetta P 3rd, Weiner L, Bergman M, et al. Pilon fractures: treatment with combined internal and external fixation. *J Orthop Trauma.* 1993; 7(6):489–96.

27. Stufkens SA, van den Bekerom MP, Kerkhoffs GM, Hintermann B, van Dijk CN. Long-term outcome after 1822 operatively treated ankle fractures: a systematic review of the literature. *Injury.* 2011; 42(2):119–27.

28. Bhandari M, Sprague S, Beate H, et al. Health-related quality of life following operative treatment of unstable ankle fractures: a prospective observational study. *J Orthop Trauma.* 2004; 18(6):338–45.

29. De Vries JS, Wijgman AJ, Sierevelt IN, Schaap GR. Long-term results of ankle fractures with a posterior malleolar fragment. *J Foot Ankle Surg.* 2005; 44(3):211–17.

30. Pollak AN, McCarthy ML, Bess RS, Agel J, Swiontkowski MF. Outcomes after treatment of high-energy tibial plafond fractures. *J Bone Joint Surg Am.* 2003; 85-A(10):1893–900.

31. Burgess AR, Dischinger PC, O'Quinn TD, Schmidhauser CB. Lower extremity injuries in drivers of airbag-equipped automobiles: clinical and crash reconstruction correlations. *J Trauma.* 1995; 38(4):509–16.

32. Rüedi T. Fractures of the lower end of the tibia into the ankle-joint. *Injury.* 1969; 1:92–9.

33. Ovadia DN, Beals RK. Fractures of the tibial plafond. *J Bone Joint Surg Am.* 1986; 68(4):543–51.

34. Anglen JO. Early outcome of hybrid external fixation for fracture of the distal tibia. *J Orthop Trauma.* 1999; 13(2):92–7.

35. Blauth M, Bastian L, Krettek C, Knop C, Evans S. Surgical options for the treatment of severe tibial pilon fractures: a study of three techniques. *J Orthop Trauma.* 2001; 15(3):153–60.

36. Sirkin M, Sanders R, DiPasquale T, Herscovici D Jr. A staged protocol for soft tissue management in the treatment of complex pilon fractures. *J Orthop Trauma.* 1999; 13(2):78–84.

37. Watson JT, Moed BR, Karges DE, Cramer KE. Pilon fractures. Treatment protocol based on severity of soft tissue injury. *Clin Orthop Relat Res.* 2000; 375:78–90.

38. Anderson DD, Van Hofwegen C, Marsh JL, Brown TD. Is elevated contact stress predictive of post-traumatic osteoarthritis for imprecisely reduced tibial plafond fractures? *J Orthop Res.* 2011; 29(1):33–9.

39. Thordarson DB. Complications after treatment of tibial pilon fractures: prevention and management strategies. *J Am Acad Orthop Surg.* 2000; 8(4):253–65.

40. Howard JL, Agel J, Barei DP, Benirschke SK, Nork SE. A prospective study evaluating incision placement and wound healing for tibial plafond fractures. *J Orthop Trauma.* 2008; 22(5):299–306.

41. Bhattacharyya T, Crichlow R, Gobezie R, Kim E, Vrahas MS. Complications associated with the posterolateral approach for pilon fractures. *J Orthop Trauma.* 2006; 20(2):104–7.

42. Barbieri R, Schenk R, Koval K, Aurori K, Aurori B. Hybrid external fixation in the treatment of tibial plafond fractures. *Clin Orthop Relat Res.* 1996; 332:16–22.

43. Weber M, Burmeister H, Flueckiger G, Krause FG. The use of weightbearing radiographs to assess the stability of supination-external rotation fractures of the ankle. *Arch Orthop Trauma Surg.* 2010; 130(5):693–8.

Fractures and Dislocations of the Hindfoot and Midfoot

Mark B. Davies and Chris M. Blundell

Introduction

Fractures and dislocations of the foot come in a wide spectrum of patterns, which depend upon the position of the foot at the time of injury and the degree and direction of force applied. Low-energy injuries of the hind- and midfoot are common after torsional injury. The findings in low-energy injuries can be subtle and radiographic changes may be easily missed. They often result in soft tissue injuries or avulsion fractures seen on the dorsal aspect of the talus and navicular and also on the lateral aspect of the cuboid. Calcaneal fractures are most frequently seen in falls from a height.

High-energy injuries, such as those following road traffic accidents, can lead to much more complex foot trauma associated with poorer outcomes and significant long-term disability. This is especially true when these injuries are associated with a breach in the soft tissue envelope, major visceral injuries, or injuries to the axial and appendicular skeleton. Associated injuries take priority and should be managed in a multidisciplinary manner according to Advanced Trauma Life Support principles.

General Principles of Managing Hindfoot and Midfoot Injuries

In most open injuries the soft tissue break occurs on the dorsum of the foot, as the skin is thin and the bones are superficial. In open injuries soft tissue stabilization is the primary goal. Open injuries through the skin of the sole of the foot are often the result of higher energy injuries, such as crush, blast, penetrating trauma, or falls from a height. Early reduction of fractures and dislocations is recommended especially with compromised skin and neurovascular structures (Figure 22.1). In the presence of open wounds, thorough wound toilet followed by temporary external fixation and selective internal fixation is warranted (Table 22.1).

Imaging in Hindfoot and Midfoot Trauma

Plain radiographs are the baseline for imaging foot injuries, but in the emergency setting standard views are often compromised or inadequate. In most complex cases CT scanning is used to define fracture lines, and to plan the surgical approach, a strategy for reduction, and method of fixation. MRI offers little in the

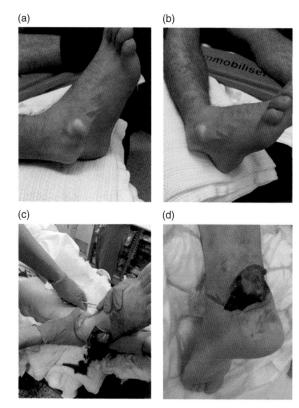

Figure 22.1 (**a**, **b**) Closed medial peritalar dislocation. Note the blanching to the skin from the prominent dislocated head of the talus with tenting of the peroneus tertius tendon. (**c**) Open medial peritalar dislocation. (**d**) Open extra-articular fracture of the posterior calcaneal tubercle.

Table 22.1 Principles in the treatment of mid- and hindfoot trauma

- Advanced Trauma Life Support principles
- Normal clotting parameters, serum lactate, and core temperature govern damage-limitation surgery
- Photograph, wash, and dress wounds
- Reduce dislocations
- Relieve threatened skin
- Apply splintage/make safe in an external fixator
- CT scan to assess fracture configuration
- Plan definitive fixation with/without soft tissue management

Table 22.2 Talus fractures

- Injuries are often associated with multiply injured patients and so may be missed
- Hawkins classification is of value in prognosis
- Increasing grade leads to higher rate of avascular necrosis and worsening outcomes
- Fractures are best visualized with CT, which then guides the approach
- Surgical approaches should respect the vascularity of the talus
- Stable fixation of anatomical reduction secures the best outcome
- Consider the use of titanium implants to permit MRI investigation of talus vascularity
- Salvage options are complex and carry poor outcomes overall

management of acute trauma, although it is useful in assessing the vascularity of the talus in the recovery period. As a consequence some prefer to use titanium fixation, rather than stainless steel, to allow later MRI scanning, minimizing the artifact from metal scatter.

Surgical Anatomy of the Hindfoot and Midfoot

Bony Anatomy

The hindfoot consists of the talus and the calcaneus. The talus acts as a passive, intercalated segment between the leg, the calcaneus, and the midfoot. Together they create a mobile unit that provides stability in all phases of gait, transmits the forces for propulsion, allows the foot to adapt to variable ground surfaces, and supplies proprioceptive feedback regarding foot position.

The bones of the midfoot are the navicular, cuboid, and the three cuneiforms. The midtarsal joint, which is also known as Chopart's joint, comprises the calcaneocuboid and the talonavicular joints, with the latter contributing the majority of midfoot motion. The midfoot is unlocked and permits significant accommodative foot motion through the midtarsal joint in stance phase, but it locks and forms a stable locked lever in the propulsive phase of the gait cycle. Preservation of midfoot function by accurate anatomical reconstruction after injury leads to better functional outcomes. As the midtarsal joint is a functional entity any navicular or cuboid fracture cannot be considered in isolation. The principles for treating talus fractures are outlined in Table 22.2.

It is helpful to consider the foot as two functional columns: a medial column including the talus,

navicular, and the three cuneiform bones with the three medial metatarsals, and a lateral column, which includes the calcaneus, cuboid, and the lateral two metatarsals (Figure 22.2). The medial column provides a stable arch, which transmits the forces of propulsion, while the lateral column acts as a shock absorber permitting adaptation of foot position to the terrain.

The relative lengths of the two columns vary with foot morphology. A planovalgus foot results from relative lengthening of the medial column, or shortening of the lateral column. The converse can be considered to be true in a cavovarus foot. In a traumatized foot a column may be acutely shortened – if this is left untreated, the foot will be deformed. Thus in the traumatized foot careful analysis of the CT scans and consideration of column length is important in reconstruction. In principle, each column should have its length and alignment re-established, to restore the hindfoot–forefoot relationship. This may necessitate bridge fixation across mobile joints such as the talonavicular, calcaneocuboid, and the fourth and fifth TMTJs. This can be achieved with internal, external, or a combination of both fixation methods. Any joints that are spanned need to be mobilized as soon as the fractures have healed by removing the spanning fixation.

In the authors' experience, primary arthrodeses are technically challenging in the acute setting. Cases to be considered for primary arthrodesis are often the highest energy injuries with most comminution, such that compression across these crushed joints risks shortening the column. Thus the authors prefer to

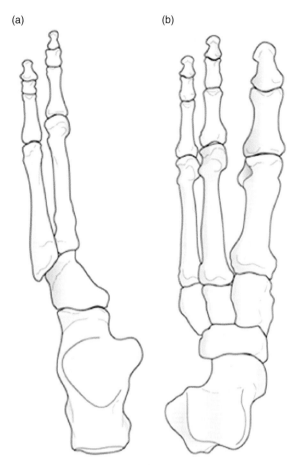

(a)   (b)

Figure 22.2 (a) The lateral and (b) the medial columns of the foot.

restore the foot shape and perform secondary arthrodeses, as salvage procedures.

Vascular Anatomy

The arterial supply to the foot is through the posterior tibial, dorsalis pedis, and peroneal arteries. There is a generous blood supply to the long bones of the foot and those tarsal bones providing tendon origins or insertions. However, the talus and the navicular have tenuous blood supplies, which has implications for surgical treatment and the outcome of injury.

Sixty percent of the surface of the talus is covered in articular cartilage. The remaining 40% is occupied by joint capsular reflections and ligament insertions. There are no tendon origins or insertions. The vascular supply to the talus comes from anastomoses between the anterior and posterior tibial arteries and the peroneal artery[1]. The talar body is supplied from the anastomoses inferiorly in the tarsal canal, superiorly from the dorsalis pedis artery, and medially through branches within the deep deltoid ligament. In talar neck fractures the vascularity of the talus can be damaged, not only from the injury itself, but also from the surgical approach used to treat the injury. Magnetic resonance angiography has quantified the relative contributions of the major vessels to the talus as 47% from the posterior tibial artery, 36% from the anterior tibial artery, and 17% from the peroneal artery[2].

The vascular supply to the navicular is also from both the dorsalis pedis and the posterior tibial arteries, as well as an indirect supply through the tendon attachment of the tibialis posterior onto the tubercle. The arterial supply is radial in nature leaving the central area of the navicular prone to avascular change. The blood supply to the cuboid and cuneiforms is less tenuous and infarction of these bones following trauma is uncommon.

Lastly, the microvascular supply to the soft tissue envelope of the posterior and lateral aspects of the hindfoot needs to be appreciated. Terminal branches of the posterior peroneal artery supply the angiosomes of the skin flap raised in an extended lateral approach to the hindfoot to afford access to the calcaneus in open fracture fixation[3].

Fractures of the Calcaneus

The calcaneus is the most frequently injured bone in the tarsus. Many injuries are severe with almost 20% of calcaneal fractures breaching or compromising the skin. Nevertheless some injuries are minor affecting the inferior aspect of the posterior tubercle after minor falls. These fractures may simply require symptomatic relief.

As well as providing a lever arm for propulsion in gait, the calcaneus is a significant part of the longitudinal arch of the foot. It provides a cradle for the talus superiorly with three articulating facets, the largest of which is the posterior facet. These allow accommodation in walking on uneven surfaces and are instrumental in the locking and unlocking of the midtarsal joint during the gait cycle. However, apart from the posterior tubercle and some trabecular condensations, the calcaneus has very thin cortices. This means that it is prone to injury in falls from a height.

Extra-Articular Fractures of the Calcaneus

Excluding open injuries as a consequence of a direct blow to the heel, any activity that results in a strong

381

(a)

(b)

(c)

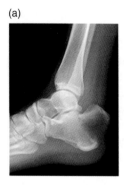 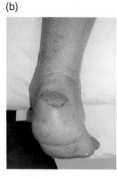 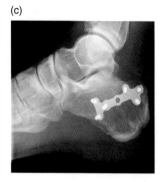

Figure 22.3 Closed tongue-type extra-articular fracture of the calcaneus with threatened overlying skin. It was treated with emergency open reduction and locked plate fixation through a lateral approach.

contraction of the gastrocnemius–soleus complex can result in an avulsion fracture at its insertion on the calcaneus. This is particularly true in osteopenic bone and in neuropathic patients, who are usually diabetic. With the lack of significant soft tissue cover, the single most important consideration is whether the skin overlying an avulsion fracture is compromised (Figure 22.3). Skin compromise occurs in 20% of these fractures[4]. Any threatened skin requires urgent treatment in the form of fracture reduction and fixation to reduce the risk of soft tissue loss and the requirement for free tissue transfers and even transtibial amputation[4]. The authors' preferred method of fixation is through a lateral approach and to apply a locked plate across the fracture, as attempts to use lag screw fixation require surgical incisions close to the compromised soft tissue envelope. In those fractures with minimal displacement and no soft tissue compromise, management in a walking cast may be possible. It is rare to have to fix these fractures in the diabetic patient.

Fractures of the Anterior Process of the Calcaneus

Broadly, these fractures fall into two distinct groups and account for 15% of all calcaneal fractures[5]. Firstly, the anterior process of the calcaneus is prone to injury as part of a high-energy disruption of the midtarsal joint, and the cuboid compresses the anterior process[6]. In these cases, the principles of restoration of the lateral column of the foot need to be applied. This is discussed later in the chapter.

Secondly, and more commonly, fractures of the anterior process are avulsion injuries induced by the midfoot being forced into an adducted and plantar flexed position. In this injury tension across the bifurcate ligament avulses the anterior process.

A high index of suspicion is required for these injuries with careful palpation over the sinus tarsi and lateral to the extensor digitorum brevis muscle belly, and scrutiny of plain radiographs. Often the oblique and lateral views are the most helpful, but if doubt persists a CT scan is indicated. Anterior process fractures are frequently misdiagnosed as ankle sprains[5].

In small, minimally displaced fracture fragments, a compressive bandage or a weightbearing cast or boot will allow symptoms to settle. Up to 25% of patients take a year to become pain free[7]. In some symptomatic cases with larger fracture fragments and in the event of progression to symptomatic nonunion, surgery to excise the fragment may be necessary[7]. Outcomes in those fractures that are missed or go on to non-union are often poor with persistent pain irrespective of the late treatment instituted.

Intra-Articular Fractures of the Body of the Calcaneus

Seventy-five percent of calcaneal fractures are intraarticular, with 90% resulting from a fall from a height[8]. The majority of injuries occur in males between the ages of 30 and 60 years. Ten percent of calcaneal fractures are associated with spinal column injuries and a similar figure are bilateral. The dense talus acts as a hammer to the posterior facet of the subtalar joint, creating a primary fracture line that splits the calcaneus into an anteromedial fragment containing the sustentaculum tali and a posterolateral fragment incorporating the lateral portion of the posterior facet. Essex-Lopresti described a secondary fracture line. This could be of two types, a joint depression or a tongue type[9]. The joint depression splits the posterior facet of the subtalar joint into two, creating joint incongruity. Radiologically this leads to a flattened Bohler's angle. Bohler's angle is the angle formed by the intersection of a line drawn from the tip of the anterior process to the posterior aspect of the posterior facet with the line from the latter to the tip of the posterior tubercle. This angle normally measures 20 to 40°. When Bohler's angle is flattened this implies that there is posterior facet depression and loss of calcaneal height. This angle is important, as a reduced Bohler's angle is associated with a poor outcome[10]. Almost two-thirds of fractures extend into the calcaneocuboid joint.

The overall effect of significant calcaneal injury is usually loss of calcaneal height and an increase in calcaneal width. This can lead to impingement between the lateral calcaneal wall and the tip of the fibula, with the peroneal tendons painfully trapped between the two. The enveloping soft tissues around the calcaneus are also injured. Open fractures are not uncommon and plantar wounds, in particular, have a worse prognosis than medial or lateral wounds. Injury to the heel fat pad can lead to chronic pain.

Several classification systems have been suggested to aid in the management of these fractures. No single classification has achieved universal acceptance[9,11–12]. Although it does not include the calcaneocuboid joint, the most familiar classification was described by Sanders[12] and uses axial CT views of the posterior facet to assess the number of longitudinal fracture lines of the posterior facet of the subtalar joint, grading them in increasing severity from type 1 to 4:

- Type 1 is undisplaced (<2 mm)
- Type 2 has one intra-articular fracture line
- Type 3 has two intra-articular fracture lines
- Type 4 has three or more intra-articular fracture lines.

The position of the fracture lines (Figure 22.4) is used to note the position of the fracture line on the posterior facet (for example 2b, or 3ab).

The treatment of intra-articular calcaneal fractures can be non-surgical, with analgesia, splintage, and physiotherapy, or surgical, with open reduction and internal fixation (Figure 22.5). Factors governing the outcomes following these injuries can be divided into patient related, fracture related, and surgeon related. Patients who smoke, are over the age of 50, have significant comorbidities, who are manual workers, or are involved with litigation seem to have a poorer outcome[10]. Fracture-related issues associated with a poorer outcome are those associated with the energy of the injury namely: open fractures, bilateral fractures,

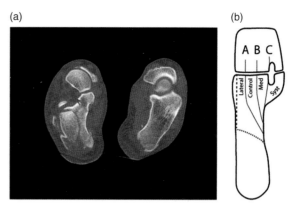

Figure 22.4 (a) Axial CT scans of both calcanei. On the left foot, the scans show a Sanders 3bc fracture of the posterior facet. Note the fracture of the inferomedial aspect of the right posterior tubercle. (b) Line diagram of the axial cut through the posterior facet demonstrating the fracture line configuration for the Sanders classification[12].

polytrauma, a Bohler's angle of less than 0° and Sanders type 4 fractures. Intuitively, the quality of articular reduction should correlate with the surgical outcome.

There remains clinical uncertainty as to the optimal management for adults with a displaced intra-articular calcaneal fracture, as there is insufficient high-quality evidence to establish whether operative or non-operative treatment is better. Two large randomized controlled trials comparing surgical and non-surgical treatment have been reported. In Canada, a trial showed no conclusive proof that open reduction and internal fixation achieved better results than non-operative treatment[10]. Further subgroup analysis suggested that the results of operative treatment were marginally better in young women, non-manual employees, non-smokers, and those who were not pursuing compensation. With the numerous confounding variables that apply to these fractures, a pragmatic prospective randomized controlled study was required. This led to the inception and completion of the UK Heel Fracture Trial. The results from this study show that after excluding those fractures "with gross deformity," the remaining cases with more than 2 mm displacement of the posterior facet, treated with an extended lateral approach, demonstrate no improvement in outcome when comparing internal fixation with non-operative treatment[13]. Of course this does not take into account that it is easier to perform a subtalar fusion for post-traumatic arthrosis of the posterior facet in a reconstructed calcaneum, as opposed to a severely malunited one.

(a)

(b)

(c)

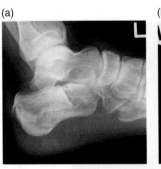
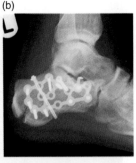
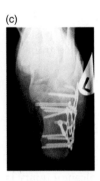

Figure 22.5 (**a**) Lateral radiograph showing an intra-articular fracture of the calcaneus with depression of the posterior facet. (**b**) Lateral and (**c**) axial radiographs of the calcaneus following open reduction and internal fixation.

(a)

(b)

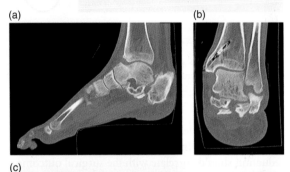

(c)

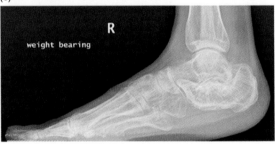

Figure 22.6 (**a**) CT image of a malunion of an intra-articular fracture of the calcaneus demonstrating a dorsiflexion deformity of the talus leading to restricted ankle dorsiflexion. (**b**) Note the subfibular impingement of the lateral calcaneal wall. (**c**) Lateral plain radiograph of a malunion of the calcaneus showing the loss of heel height.

The rationale for surgical treatment of Sanders type 2 and 3 fractures has been directed at open fractures, those with subfibular impingement, and those cases where a malunion would lead to a dorsiflexed talus and subsequent restricted ankle dorsiflexion (Figure 22.6). Other criteria for fixation include greater than 3 mm displacement of the posterior facet or varus malalignment of the posterior tubercle. In may ways the most important factor is Sanders group's demonstration that a subtalar fusion following initial open reduction and internal fixation (ORIF) of a calcaneal fracture has a better outcome than subtalar arthrodesis of a malunited fracture, which was not reduced acutely[14]. Open reduction and internal fixation is best performed through an extended lateral approach, once the soft tissue envelope shows signs of wrinkling. Reconstruction of the calcaneus aims to reduce the posterior facet of the subtalar joint, the calcaneocuboid joint, Bohler's angle, and any varus or valgus malalignment. With wound complications being a concern, minimally invasive techniques have been tried with some low-grade evidence that they are an effective alternative in less severe, Sanders type 2 fractures[15–16].

Fractures of the Talus

In a seminal paper in 1952, Coltart reviewed the records of the British Royal Air Force personnel treated for fractures of the talus[17]. This series of 228 cases represented 1% of all fractures and dislocations within this population. About a quarter of these were classified as "chip and avulsion fractures" with the remaining three-quarters described as "serious" injuries. Seventy percent of these serious injuries were high-energy injuries secondary to flying accidents. It still remains true that talar fractures should be considered as low- or high-energy injuries.

Low-Energy Fractures of the Talus
Avulsion Fractures

In minor inversion or eversion injuries of the ankle, the talus is prone to injury[18]. Although excluded from the Ottawa rules[19], avulsion fractures from the neck of the talus occur (Figure 22.7a). These injuries occasionally need immobilization and physiotherapy, but usually recover completely. It should be noted that an avulsion of this sort may be the radiographic marker of a midtarsal dislocation. In midtarsal injuries there will be more swelling and there may also be bony avulsions from the lateral column.

Acute Osteochondral Fractures of the Talar Dome

Torsional forces to the ankle can subject the shoulders of the talar body to shearing of the articular surface and osteochondral fractures. Such damage may occur in up to 6.5% of all ankle sprains[20]. Plain radiographs may appear normal, especially if there is minimal subchondral bone involvement. In the very swollen ankle following injury, further imaging with CT or MRI may be selected to reveal the diagnosis. Acute diagnosis and treatment of the larger fragments is recommended because internal fixation or fragment excision permit early rehabilitation and a good outcome[21] (Figure 22.7b,c,d).

High-Energy Fractures of the Talus

Included in this group of injuries are dislocations involving the talus and fractures of the lateral process, talar head, talar neck, and talar body.

High-energy injuries involving the talus are rarely isolated and, as stated above, life-threatening injuries should be prioritized. Talar extrusions and fractures of the talar neck and body are frequently open, requiring urgent treatment. After initial debridement, internal fixation may be safely delayed in cases of heavy contamination or if the fracture pattern is too technically challenging for the available surgical team[22]. Most Level I trauma center surgeons acknowledge that, after wound toilet and adequate reduction, definitive fixation can wait more than eight hours. Nearly half felt that a delay of 24 hours or more in fixation was acceptable management. The quality of treatment was considered more important than the speed of treatment[23].

Monitoring Post-Injury Progress and Hawkins Sign

In 1970, Hawkins observed a subchondral radiolucent band within the talar dome on plain radiographs[24]. It is best appreciated on the AP radiograph, but can also be detected on the lateral. If present, this sign appears between six and nine weeks post injury[25] with the lucency thought to represent hyperemia from a metabolically active, vascularized talar dome (Figure 22.8). The lucent line does not have to span the whole width of the talar dome in order to be deemed present. Tezval et al.[25] found the presence of this sign to be a reliable prognostic indicator that avascular necrosis will not develop at a later stage. However, conversely

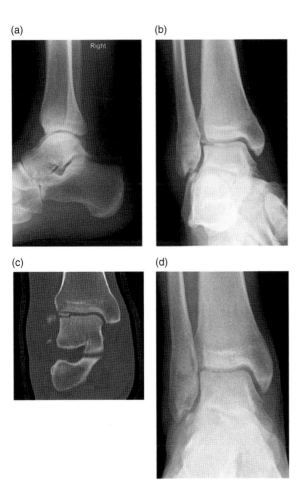

Figure 22.7 (**a**) Lateral plain radiograph demonstrating avulsion of the capsule from the neck of the talus following an ankle inversion injury. (**b**) Plain radiograph and (**c**) CT of an acute osteochondral fracture of the lateral talar dome. The fracture fragment has inverted. (**d**) Six months post open reduction and internal fixation of the fracture with bioabsorbable pins.

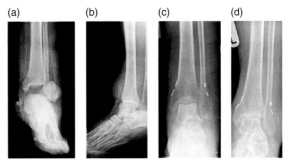

Figure 22.8 (**a**, **b**) Closed extrusion of the talus. (**c**) Six weeks after open reduction of the talus with Tightrope® (Arthrex) stabilization of the syndesmosis. Note the very sclerotic appearance of the talar dome. (**d**) Three months post injury. Note Hawkins' sign suggesting re-vascularization of the talus.

the absence of a Hawkins sign does not dictate that the talus is avascular.

Dislocations of the Hindfoot

Dislocations of the talus are rare high-energy injuries ranging from subtalar dislocation, through total talar dislocation, to complete open talar extrusion. Subtalar, or peritalar, dislocation usually occurs in a road traffic accident or in athletes who land awkwardly. Medial or lateral subtalar dislocation is defined by where the calcaneus lies relative to the talus. Approximately 10% of these injuries are open, but even in closed injuries, the soft tissue envelope may be compromised necessitating urgent reduction (Figure 22.1). Closed reduction is usually successful but if there are interposed soft tissue structures, for example the tibialis posterior tendon, or there is an associated interlocked impacted fracture of the talar head or the navicular, then open reduction may be necessary. Following successful reduction, immobilization in a cast is recommended. The authors' preferred choice is a removable walking cast, to permit early physiotherapy to avoid joint stiffness. Avascular necrosis of the talus is uncommon following subtalar dislocations, as the talus remains reduced within the ankle mortise, preserving its blood supply.

In total dislocations of the talus, the talus is most commonly extruded anterolaterally (Figure 22.8). More often than not, these injuries are open but even in closed injuries, the skin and soft tissues are invariably threatened. These injuries therefore require urgent reduction. An extruded talus should be retrieved and reimplanted, despite being avascular. This allows more options for delayed reconstruction[26].

Lateral Process Fractures

Lateral talar process fractures account for approximately 25% of all talar fractures. They are frequently high-energy injuries and result from an everted or externally rotated foot being forced into dorsiflexion – a mechanism of injury typically associated with snowboarding[27]. There is commonly an associated dislocation of the ankle or subtalar joint (Figure 22.9). In those injuries where there is no concurrent dislocation, the radiographic findings can be subtle, and the fracture is easily missed. Although Broden's views, with the leg internally rotated 45° and the x-ray beam tilted 10 to 40° to the head, increase the likelihood of making this diagnosis, a CT scan more accurately assesses the fracture.

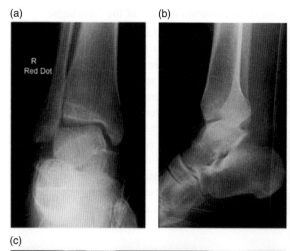
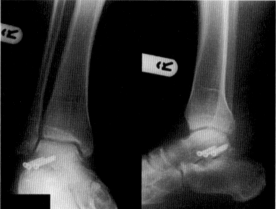

Figure 22.9 (a, b) Plain radiographs of a lateral process fracture with subluxation of both the ankle and subtalar joints. (c) Postoperative radiographs showing reduction and fracture fixation.

Lateral talar process fractures were also classified by Hawkins[24]:

Type I – simple two-part fracture

Type II – comminuted fracture

Type III – chip fracture of the anteroinferior lateral process.

Type I and type III fractures can be managed in a non-weightbearing cast, if they are undisplaced. In those lateral process fractures associated with a dislocation, the injury is frequently irreducible, necessitating open reduction. A lateral subtalar approach affords excellent access[27]. In order to confer stability and to lessen the risk of non-union, internal fixation of the process is recommended in fractures displaced by more than 2 mm (Figure 22.9)[28]. In comminuted fractures where the fragments measure less than 1 cm, the fragments should be excised.

Fractures of the Talar Neck

These fractures are usually high-energy injuries, which are associated with polytrauma, where dorsiflexion in conjunction with supination of the foot results in a fracture of the talar neck. A small number of fractures occur as a result of a heavy object falling onto the dorsum of the foot. Approximately 20% of these fractures are open with many of the remainder having compromised skin and soft tissues[24,29]. Nearly a quarter of these fractures are associated with a medial malleolar fracture[24].

Hawkins initially devised a classification with three discrete groups of increasing severity[24]. A fourth group was later added by Canale and Kelly (Figure 22.10), which represents the most severe fracture dislocation of the head of the talus from the talonavicular joint[29]. The Hawkins–Canale classification system is useful as it reflects injury severity, which helps when counseling the patient about prognosis and functional recovery. Vascular damage occurs with greater displacement, and when it does occur the vessels within the tarsal canal are principally affected.

Type I fractures are undisplaced with a vertical fracture line through the neck extending onto the inferior aspect of the talus between the middle and posterior subtalar facets.

In type II fractures, there is associated dislocation or subluxation of the subtalar joint. The primary fracture line is vertical and sometimes extends into the posterior facet. The dorsiflexion force applied to the talar neck is often associated with rotation and, although in most instances the talar body fragment dislocates posteriorly, the body fragment can also dislocate either medially or laterally.

In type III fractures, the vertical fracture line involves the posterior facet (Figure 22.11). The body fragment dislocates from the ankle mortise and the subtalar joint, either to adopt a rotated position within the mortise or occasionally to twist on the intact fibers of the deep deltoid ligament, and comes to lie posterior to the posterior malleolus and medial to the tendo Achillis.

Type IV fractures are rare, and only small case series are reported[29-30]. A vertical neck fracture is associated with extrusion of the body and, in addition, the talar head dislocates from the talonavicular joint. This group of fractures had a universally poor outcome in Canale and Kelly's series, although better results have been reported in other series[30].

The principles for treating talus fractures are outlined in Table 22.3.

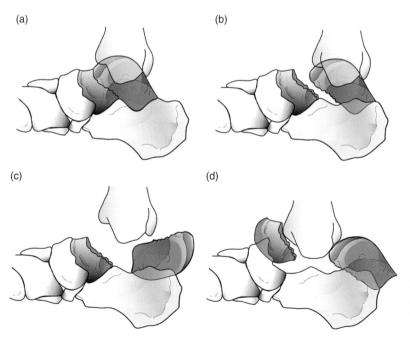

Figure 22.10 Combined classification of fractures of the neck of the talus according to Hawkins[24] and Canale and Kelly[29]. (**a**) type I; (**b**) type II; (**c**) type III; and (**d**) type IV.

Table 22.3 Principles in treating talus fractures

- Make correct diagnosis early
- Maintain appropriate lateral and medial column length
- Maintain appropriate relationship between the forefoot and the hindfoot
- Preserve talonavicular joint function
- Preserve the fourth and fifth tarsometatarsal joints
- Use stable fixation to maintain anatomic reductions or primary arthrodeses
- Allow adequate time for bone and soft tissue healing

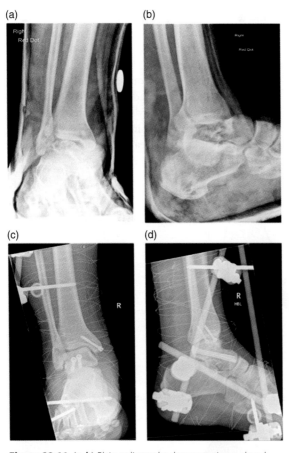

(a)　　　　　(b)

(c)　　　　　(d)

Figure 22.11 (**a**, **b**) Plain radiographs demonstrating a closed Hawkins type III fracture of the neck of the talus. (**c**, **d**) Postoperative images demonstrating a medial malleolar osteotomy and two lagged screws inserted percutaneously from a posterolateral approach. Note the postoperative immobilization in a monolateral external fixator to permit easy management of the soft tissue envelope.

Initial Management

Closed reduction under suitable relaxation and analgesia is necessary in all fracture dislocations where the soft tissue envelope is compromised. Multiple attempts may further damage the soft tissues. If closed reduction fails open reduction is mandatory.

Surgical Approaches for Talar Neck Fractures

The single most important factor determining surgical approach is the fracture pattern. Care must be taken not to shorten the talus when there is comminution, and as comminution of the medial wall is commoner, an anteromedial approach is often necessary. In many instances, judging the quality of the reduction necessitates a combined anteromedial and anterolateral approach, although an Ollier approach is an alternative[31–33]. Vascular studies confirm these approaches are safe although a previously unidentified medial branch to the talar neck is at risk with the anteromedial approach[2].

It should also be borne in mind that, as primary open reduction and internal fixation is indicated in all open fractures[32], the traumatic wounds are an important determinant of the surgical approach. In the authors' experience, using the same technique as in pilon fracture fixation[34], where the incision is placed directly over the displaced fracture line, avoids further periosteal stripping with disruption of the remaining blood supply to the fracture fragments and permits accurate reduction of the most displaced and comminuted elements of both talar and navicular fractures.

In the anterolateral approach, there is an area bare of arterial supply on the lateral talar neck, which permits safe surgical access without compromising the branches from the anterior tibial or the artery of the tarsal canal. It is important to avoid unnecessary dissection, either plantar or dorsal, on the talar neck to preserve the anastomotic vessels[2].

Medial malleolar osteotomy is less damaging, and therefore preferable to a wide soft tissue dissection when restoring medial talar neck length[2]. Lateral malleolar osteotomy, similarly, does not compromise the talar blood supply[2]. Medial malleolar osteotomies are more likely to be required than lateral malleolar osteotomies in order to aid reduction of type III talar neck fractures and in fractures involving the talar body[35] (Figures 22.12 and 22.13). It may also be possible to use a malleolar fracture to access the talus (Figure 22.14).

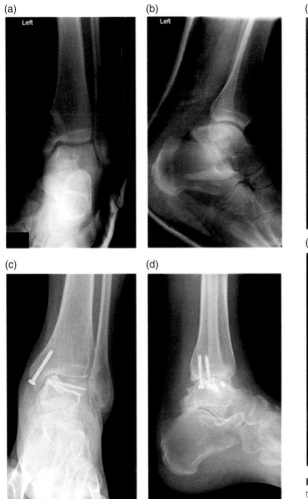

Figure 22.12 (**a, b**) Shear fracture of the body of the talus with subluxation of the subtalar joint. (**c, d**) Postoperative views following open reduction and internal fixation through a medial malleolar osteotomy.

Percutaneous fixation can be also be employed. From the posterolateral aspect of the ankle, screws are passed from the posterior aspect of the talus into the anteromedial aspect of the talar head (Figure 22.11). Inserting the screws close to the tendo Achillis helps avoid neurovascular injury.

Choice of Fixation Method
Studies have shown no difference in the strength of fixation when comparing screws passed from anterior to posterior, posterior to anterior, and a fixed angle blade plate, in a bone model of a talar neck fracture with dorsomedial comminution[36]. Spanning external

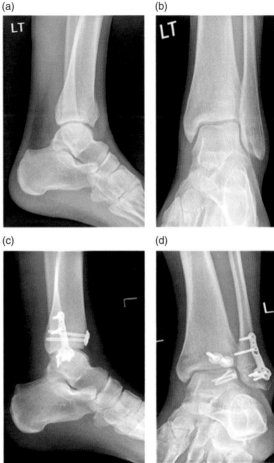

Figure 22.13 (**a, b**) Fracture of the lateral aspect of the body of the talus associated with a fracture of the tibial plafond. (**c, d**) Postoperative views following ORIF of both fractures. The talar fracture was approached through a lateral malleolar osteotomy.

or fine wire fixation has a role in acting as a splint postoperatively, as it allows the soft tissues to be monitored (Figure 22.11). It may also have a role in definitive treatment.

Outcome
Malunion, Arthrosis, and Non-Union
Historical non-operative fracture management led to almost 50% of patients having poor results, secondary to osteoarthrosis as a result of malunion[29]. As little as 3° of malunion of a talar neck fracture results in a significant reduction in subtalar motion and the development of arthrosis[37]. In those patients who do not have a malunion or arthrosis, functional outcomes are generally good[38]. However, even in those

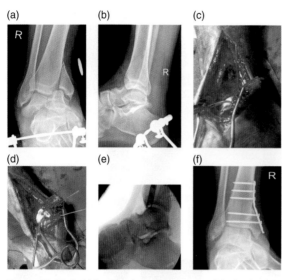

Figure 22.14 (**a**, **b**) Sagittal plane shear fracture of the body of the talus associated with a vertical shear fracture of the medial malleolus. (**c**, **d**) Intraoperative photographs showing temporary K-wire fixation of a shear fracture of the talus, accessed through a medial malleolar fracture. (**e**, **f**) Postoperative views of the talus, secured with bioabsorbable pins, and anti-glide plate fixation of the medial malleolus.

it is difficult to gauge whether the 85 to 90% AVN rate represents reality, especially as modern management techniques have shown only a 38% incidence of AVN[33].

Malunion, comminution of the talar neck, and open fracture are significantly associated with AVN[29,41]. Interestingly there was no correlation between the timing of fixation and the development of AVN[33]. Post-traumatic arthrosis developed in 54% of cases, in the ankle, subtalar, or both joints[33].

Infection is most commonly seen following open injury. Nevertheless it can occur as a result of surgery and careful soft tissue handling is essential. Superficial wound problems may be treated with antibiotics in conjunction with negative pressure dressings. Once deep infection is established the bone must be thoroughly debrided, which, in effect, involves resection of part of the talus. This may precipitate hindfoot arthrodesis, using a staged approach with impregnated bone cement to fill bone cavities and temporary or definitive external fixation. Close liaison with microbiologists, to guide antibiotic therapy, and plastic surgeons, to ensure wound coverage, is helpful.

patients treated with ORIF, malunion has been noted in one-third of cases[38] often as a result of overzealous lagging of medial fragments. Poor outcomes are also seen as a result of hardware failure, non-union, and talar dome collapse. Residual steps in the articular surface after reduction are likely to progress to arthrosis[30].

Screws placed anteriorly in the medial talus in a posterolateral direction are thought to increase the risk of malreduction by dorsiflexing the talar neck, as the screws cannot be accurately placed perpendicular to the fracture line[39]. Non-union is rare in type I and II fractures[24]. After internal fixation of isolated talar neck fractures almost 90% unite[30].

Avascular Necrosis

Early series of type I talar neck fractures treated in a cast had an AVN rate of 0 to 13%[24,29], although in one of the series, an undiagnosed, concomitant talar dome fracture may have skewed the figure[29]. In type II injuries treated using a variety of techniques from cast to ORIF, the AVN rate rose to between 42 and 50%[24,29]. Historically type III fractures have been treated with many methods including closed reduction, ORIF, primary talectomy, and talectomy with a Blair fusion[24,29,40]. With such a variety of techniques

Fractures of the Body of the Talus

Differentiation between a fracture of the talar body and a neck fracture can be difficult. Some have even proposed that any fracture extending into the posterior facet of the subtalar joint is classified as a body fracture[42]. Despite this shear forces can leave primary fracture lines in the coronal, sagittal, or horizontal planes[35] (Figure 22.15). Body fractures are typically high energy and sustained in road traffic accidents or falls from a height. In almost a third of cases they are open[43–44]. The range of Injury Severity Scores associated with these injuries is from 9 to 50, with a mean of 15, thus these patients are often polytrauma victims[44].

Body fractures occur from hyperdorsiflexion of the foot in conjunction with axial loading. This imparts a shear force through the talar body. They are frequently associated with either a talar neck or tibial plafond fracture[30].

Talar body fractures were classified by Boyd and Knight in 1942[45]. They described "minor" and "major" fracture patterns dependent upon the energy of the injury. They were then subdivided into "simple" and "comminuted," with these subdivided into "undisplaced" and "displaced." In undisplaced fractures cast immobilization was recommended, recognizing that a proportion would subsequently

(a)

(b)

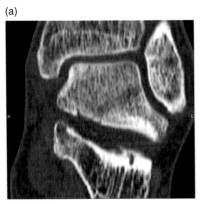
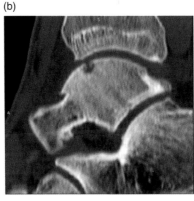

Figure 22.15 CT scan images demonstrating a healed shear fracture of the body of the talus together with cystic degeneration within the ankle. The fracture was not diagnosed until 12 months post injury.

require fusion, of either the ankle or subtalar joints. With simple displaced fractures, ORIF was recommended. If there are extruded fragments devoid of blood supply primary fusion may be needed. In comminuted displaced fractures primary talectomy and tibiocalcaneal fusion was the treatment of choice in 1942. The Orthopaedic Trauma Association classification[46] also divides these injuries into non-comminuted and comminuted fractures, and relates these factors to involvement of the ankle and subtalar joints. These classifications fail to provide a comprehensive description of all fracture types.

We recommend investigation with a CT scan in suspected talar body fractures in order to better define the fracture planes and ascertain the degree of displacement, as this is under-recognized on plain radiographs

In fractures with less than 2 mm of displacement, treatment in a below-knee, non-weightbearing cast for four to eight weeks is an accepted treatment with good outcomes[45,47]. These minimally displaced fractures can occasionally be missed and diagnosed as an ankle sprain (Figure 22.15). Displaced fractures tend to require surgical treatment with ORIF[43–44]. Surgical approaches are governed by a similar rationale to talar neck fractures: namely fracture pattern, the degree of comminution, and surgeon preference. Occasionally fractures of the posterior part of the talar body require exposure through a posterolateral or posteromedial approach with the patient in a prone position[48]. In very comminuted body fractures, internal fixation may not be possible and some authors advocate delayed primary tibiocalcaneal fusion[49–50].

The prognosis for displaced body fractures is uniformly poor. Body fractures only have a 29% satisfactory outcome, compared to 64% of neck fractures[47]. One reason for this is that AVN is commoner after talar body than neck fractures[35], as a result of disruption of the anastomotic vessels within the tarsal canal. With coronal shear fractures, the blood supply is jeopardized if the fracture lines disrupt the vascular supply from the deltoid ligament, which renders the posterior body at risk of AVN. The worst outcome is seen in horizontal shear fractures as the superior part of the talar dome is supplied by end arterioles. The presence of AVN may become evident by collapse of the talar body (Figure 22.16). Avascular necrosis is even commoner in open fractures[44].

In the early postoperative period, superficial wound infection and wound dehiscence are not infrequent. Any resultant deep infection can be difficult to eradicate. Staged resection of the dead, infected bone and subsequent fusion can be undertaken. In some instances trans-tibial amputation may be the only solution.

Post-traumatic ankle and subtalar arthrosis is common after talar body fractures. This is secondary to the cartilage damage at the time of injury, collapse of the talar dome, and malunion, which has effects on hindfoot biomechanics (Figure 22.16c,d). Malunion is relatively common because of the technical difficulty of reducing these complex fracture fragments through the constraints of the surgical exposures. Non-union is relatively uncommon[35].

Fractures of the Head of the Talus

Approximately 10% of talar fractures involve the talar head. These fractures are rarely isolated, and are usually seen in combination with fractures of the talar neck or talar body, or disruption of Chopart's joint. The mechanism of injury is a high-energy force

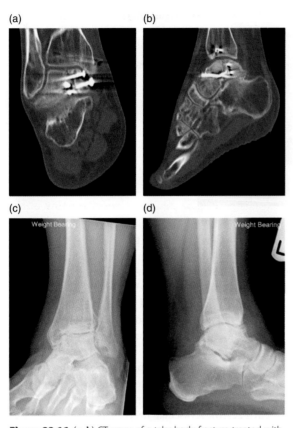

(a)   (b)

(c)   (d)

Figure 22.16 (**a**, **b**) CT scans of a talar body fracture treated with internal fixation through a medial malleolar osteotomy, demonstrating a non-union with backing out of the metalwork and collapse of the fracture fragments. (**c**, **d**) Arthrosis of the ankle joint following a talar body fracture.

applied vertically through the sustentaculum tali or anterior process of the calcaneum crushing the talar head, or a shear force applied through axial loading of the navicular. Talar head fractures are frequently associated with subtalar or lateral column injuries[51].

Stable injuries can be managed in a weightbearing cast with regular radiographs to check for fracture fragment displacement. Unstable injuries are treated with ORIF through an anteromedial approach. Care should be taken to restore the relative length of the medial and lateral columns and reduce the subtalar joint.

The accurate reduction of talar head fragmentation from crushing injury can be challenging. Therefore malreduction is not uncommon, leading to altered hindfoot biomechanics and subsequent arthrosis. In addition, AVN occurs in up to 10% of cases.

Fractures of the Posterior Process of the Talus

The posterior process of the talus is comprised of two tubercles between which is a groove containing the tendon of the flexor hallucis longus. Both tubercles can be injured in athletic individuals, often presenting late with persistent posterior ankle pain following injury. In pronation injuries, the medial tubercle can avulse[52]. Either in sudden or in repeated extremes of plantar flexion, the lateral tubercle can fracture, from impaction on the posterior tibial plafond. Lateral tubercle fractures are eponymously known as Shepherd's fractures[53]. The fracture may be visible on plain radiographs, but CT can differentiate the acute injury from a well-corticated os trigonum.

A period of cast immobilization appears to be effective in acute cases. Patients presenting with chronic posterior ankle pain and swelling, with restricted plantar flexion and signs of posterior impingement, are best treated by surgical excision – either open or arthroscopically[54].

Salvage for Talus Fractures

The principles of salvage surgery for talar fracture are similar to the salvage of calcaneal fracture, except that the calcaneus is more amenable to corrective osteotomy for malunion. Some authors have suggested that very comminuted fractures of the talus are managed with a talectomy, but pain on weight bearing and instability have consigned this to history[17,24,29].

The outcome following excision of the body of the talus with a Blair tibiocalcaneal fusion seems to be slightly more acceptable than excision arthroplasty[29,40]. Nevertheless if the talar body becomes avascular and collapses, total talectomy with tibiocalcaneal arthrodesis is the only option. Non-union rates are high and functional outcomes with a short and stiff limb are poor, irrespective of the fixation technique used – intramedullary nail, locking plate, or circular frame.

Treatment of symptomatic non-union requires great care in view of the poor blood supply, but restoring the shape of the talus in conjunction with bone graft and rigid fixation can be attempted. If, however, the non-union is as a result of talar collapse secondary to AVN then the necrotic bone should be resected and the affected joints arthrodesed. This may require ankle, subtalar, or tibiotalocalcaneal fusion[49–50]. Rarely a pantalar arthrodesis, which includes the midtarsal joint, is required.

Traditionally, triple fusion is a good salvage for malunion[29]. Treatment should be as for a non-union, with restoration of the talar shape, with or without bone grafting, and rigid internal fixation. Ideally the malunion should be taken down as close to the original fracture as possible to minimize a second hit to the blood supply. In practice this can be difficult and may involve malleolar osteotomy and removal of preexisting hardware. Malunion surgery poses a significant reconstructive challenge, as there is a risk of turning a malunion into non-union; for this reason care must be exercised when taking on these cases.

Fractures and Dislocations of the Navicular

Navicular fractures may be traumatic or stress. Stress fractures of the navicular tend to occur in athletes involved in sports that require explosive propulsion, such that repetitive forces along the longitudinal axis of the second metatarsal drive the metatarsal base into the medial cuneiform, which in turn drives into the central portion of the navicular[55]. It has been postulated that a long second metatarsal, or a short first metatarsal, predisposes to navicular fractures.

Bone scintigraphy and MRI are both useful for establishing the diagnosis, but CT demonstrates whether the fracture is fresh or there is an established non-union. This helps determine treatment[56]. In the presence of a fresh fracture, cast immobilization and a period without weight bearing is the treatment of choice. In an established non-union, with sclerosis and cysts, open reduction and internal fixation with freshening of the fracture edges and bone grafting is undertaken.

Dorsal avulsion fractures, sustained as part of an ankle sprain, are common[19,57]. With torsional foot injuries avulsion of the navicular tuberosity, where the tibialis posterior tendon inserts, are characteristic[55,57]. Partial avulsions can often be treated in a cast. Complete avulsions are usually treated with ORIF.

Isolated injuries of the navicular are uncommon, indeed it has been stated that it is not possible to have an isolated dislocation of the navicular without injury to the lateral column[58]. The medial column is a fundamentally stable bony construct with the navicular as the keystone; very powerful interosseous and plantar ligament complexes support it. Thus large amounts of energy are required to fracture the navicular and almost two-thirds of such fractures involve surrounding structures within the mid- or hindfoot[59].

Sixty percent of these injuries occur in the third to fifth decades of life[57]. In almost half the diagnosis is missed[18] with resulting long-term disability and compromised foot function[18,60]. Almost 75% of these injuries occur in road traffic accidents and a large proportion of the remainder occur in falls from a height[61]. Almost a third are open[62].

A high index of suspicion is required to exclude concurrent injuries to the lateral column, the hindfoot, and the TMTJ. CT scanning is the best way of fully defining these injuries. Careful scrutiny of the images for avulsed ligamentous attachments helps to determine the full extent of the injury. Poorly treated disruptions of the midtarsal and TMTJs are associated with long-term arthrosis[61]. It should be stressed that simply treating the navicular injury will not optimize recovery, it is important to restore the length of the medial and lateral columns and the longitudinal arch[61].

Initial attempts to classify navicular body fractures pre-date the era of CT scanning and were hindered by the lack of 3D imaging[18]. Nonetheless, it was appreciated that longitudinal forces applied to the forefoot tend to generate a shear fracture through the navicular. This tends to create three distinct types of body fracture, which were described by Sangeorzan[62]. In type I fractures there is a transverse fracture in the coronal plane associated with a displaced dorsal fragment that is less than half of the navicular when viewed in the sagittal plane. Type II fractures are commonest, with a primary fracture line passing from the dorsolateral aspect of the navicular to the plantar-medial cortex (Figure 22.17). Type III fractures are typified by central and lateral comminution, often with preservation of a large medial fragment. Type III fractures were most commonly associated with lateral column disruption.

Historically treatment mainly consisted of either open or closed reduction and cast immobilization[18], open reduction and K-wire fixation, or primary naviculo-cuneiform or triple fusion[57]. These are deemed suboptimal by modern standards[62]. Current treatment is with open reduction and stable internal fixation, in order to minimize long-term disability[61–63].

Open reduction can be achieved through a combination of dorsomedial and dorsolateral approaches, taking care to minimize stripping of the periosteum

393

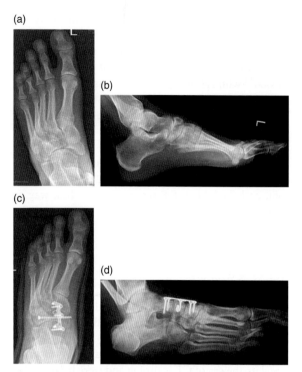

(a)

(b)

(c)

(d)

Figure 22.17 (**a**, **b**) Plain radiographs demonstrating a type II fracture of the body of the navicular. There is some associated crushing of the cuboid. (**c**, **d**) Postoperative views following open reduction with lagged screw fixation of the sagittal fracture line and locked bridge plate fixation to maintain the medial column length.

from the fracture fragments. Intraoperative distraction[55] or external fixation can aid fracture reduction[63]. Subsequent internal fixation with interfragmentary lag screws and neutralization plates aims to achieve rigid, stable fixation with preservation of the length of the medial column. The use of locking or non-locking plates and whether to span the joints of the medial column remain controversial[59,64–65]. In some, medial column length may be definitively maintained by external fixation[63]. Any metalwork used to span joints in the medial column should be removed after three months to avoid hardware failure[65].

There are a number of sequelae to high-energy injuries of the navicular. Avascular necrosis has been reported in isolated navicular dislocation[66], but the incidence in navicular body fractures ranges from zero to 30% in complex midfoot trauma[59,62,64]. Historically, fractures of the body of the navicular have had poor outcomes with a significant proportion of patients requiring salvage arthrodeses, mainly for post-traumatic arthrosis[18]. The Sangeorzan

classification appears to be a reliable predictor of outcome for navicular body fractures[62]. Clinical outcomes are most favorable in type I fractures with the poorest results in type III injuries. The best results were achieved when at least 60% of the articular surface of the talonavicular joint was accurately reconstructed. More recent series of navicular body fractures treated with reduction and internal fixation demonstrate that approximately 17% develop post-traumatic arthrosis. Nevertheless whether it is arthrosis secondary to articular surface damage or foot deformity causing the poor outcomes remains unclear.

In summary, the patient has the best chance of a positive outcome if an accurate, early diagnosis is made together with accurate restoration of column length using stable fixation methods.

Fractures of the Cuboid

The cuboid is integral to the lateral column of the foot. It has articulations with the calcaneus, the lateral cuneiform, the bases of the fourth and fifth metatarsals, and, on occasions, with the navicular. The most frequent fractures involving the cuboid are avulsions of its many ligamentous attachments[67], with displaced fractures solely involving the cuboid being rare. In adults solitary injuries to this bone probably only occur as stress fractures, with the literature regarding high-energy injuries solely to the cuboid being confined to isolated case reports[68].

As with the navicular, the cuboid is often injured in association with its surrounding structures. In the classic "nutcracker" fracture, the cuboid is crushed when an abduction force is applied to the forefoot, when the hindfoot is everted. This causes subluxation of the talonavicular joint and "cracking" of the cuboid between the anterior process of the calcaneus and the fourth and fifth metatarsals[69]. There is often medial column failure with either avulsion of the navicular tuberosity or a tear of the tibialis posterior tendon[55]. Alternatively, the cuboid can be fractured by longitudinally applied forces through the lateral two rays or by a direct crushing blow[55]. Associated injuries within the lateral column include anterior process fractures of the calcaneus and dislocation or disruption of the fourth and fifth TMTJs.

Patients present with a swollen foot, inability to bear weight, tenderness over the cuboid, and, on occasions, tenderness of the medial column. A high

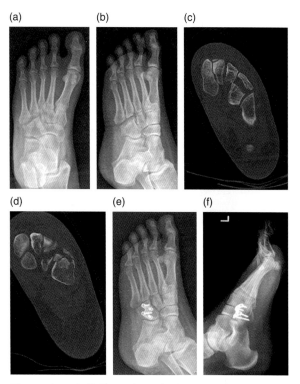

(a) (b) (c)

(d) (e) (f)

Figure 22.18 (**a, b**) Plain radiographs demonstrating a split-depression fracture of the cuboid following a forced forefoot abduction injury. (**c, d**) CT scans aid in the operative planning and show the extent of the injury. (**e, f**) Postoperative radiographs showing reduction and locked plate fixation of the cuboid fracture.

index of suspicion of injuries to both columns, together with good quality imaging, aid the diagnosis. Plain radiographs to include an oblique view are a basic requisite, but CT scans provide excellent imaging of any joint depression or loss of cuboid length[70] (Figure 22.18). MRI is useful to diagnose stress fractures.

Cuboid fractures may be most simply classified as undisplaced or displaced. The displacement may involve only the articular surface, or it may result in cuboid, and consequent lateral column, shortening. Lateral column shortening is often associated with medial column disruption.

Undisplaced cuboid fractures can be managed in a cast until comfort permits weight bearing. In injuries to the cuboid, where there is loss of cuboid length, treatment should be directed at restoration of length, as postoperative shortening of the lateral column is poorly tolerated[60,62–63,70]. Reduction of any depressed intra-articular fragments is recommended as persistent incongruity of joint surfaces ultimately leads to

post-traumatic arthrosis[63]. Use of intraoperative external fixation spanning the lateral column aids reduction. Through a longitudinal incision, along the line from the tip of the fibula to the axis of the fourth metatarsal, a trapdoor of the lateral wall of the fractured cuboid can be elevated to allow reduction of the displaced articular surface. Iliac crest grafting together with plating can then be used to maintain length and reduction. Nevertheless, if maintaining reduction is difficult then a spanning external fixator or locking plate may be used to hold length (Figure 22.19).

Cuneiform Fractures

The three cuneiforms are keystones within the rigid transverse arch of the foot and provide a stable medial column for the transmission of propulsive forces during gait. They are not prone to isolated injuries but are regularly involved in injuries to the tarso-metatarsal complex, as torsional injury causes small flake fractures from ligament avulsions. Although these small avulsed fragments seem trivial on a CT scan, they can indicate significant instability, which may require treatment.

The cuneiforms are not particularly vulnerable to injury when longitudinal forces are applied to the medial three rays, the energy preferentially disrupts the intercuneiform ligaments or fractures the navicular. On rare occasions isolated injuries of the cuneiforms are the result of a direct blow to the dorsum of the midfoot. The medial cuneiform is most frequently injured[55], and is plantarly dislocated[71]. Dorsal dislocations of the cuneiforms can occur with axial loading and forced plantar flexion, but are rare. As in all midfoot injuries, a high index of suspicion and early imaging with CT scans is helpful. Undisplaced injuries may be managed in a cast but displaced fractures and dislocations should be treated with stable anatomical fixation. This may mean bridging comminuted fractures with locking plates or consideration of primary arthrodesis[55,71]. Dislocations of the cuneiform bones with minimal or no trauma may be seen in neuropathic patients, where they represent early Charcot neuroarthropathy.

Fractures and Dislocations of the Hindfoot and Midfoot in Childhood

Fractures of the talus are rare in childhood, particularly under the age of ten years[72–73], with the

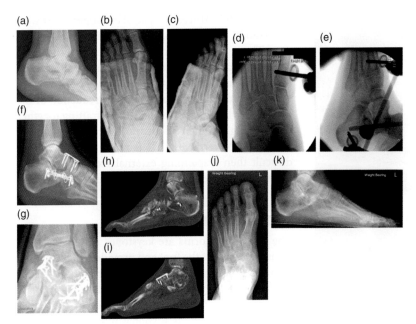

Figure 22.19 (**a**, **b**, **c**) Plain radiographs demonstrating a peritalar dislocation. (**d**, **e**) Emergency reduction with temporizing external fixation. The intraoperative fluoroscopy shows a crush fracture of the anterior process of the calcaneus. (**f**, **g**) Locked bridge fixation across the midtarsal joints to maintain the length of both columns of the foot. (**h**, **i**) CT scans show the reduction of the talonavicular and subtalar joints. (**j**, **k**) Final weightbearing images of the foot following removal of metalwork.

literature limited to small case series. In the teenage years, the incidence increases marginally, with the mechanism of injury and treatment similar to that of adulthood[73–74]. From these small case series, it appears that there may be a risk of AVN of up to 25% following talar neck fractures[73]. Fractures of the navicular and cuboid are extremely uncommon in childhood and are seldom covered in textbooks.

Key Points

Calcaneal Fractures

- 15% of fractures are of the anterior process – diagnosis may be difficult.
- 75% of fractures of the calcaneum are intra-articular involving the posterior facet of the subtalar joint.
- There is debate as to the benefits of fixation of displaced intra-articular fractures.
- Secondary subtalar fusion following intra-articular fractures is more successful if the heel shape has been restored by primary fixation.

Talar Neck Fractures

- High-energy injuries with 25% open fractures.
- Fracture configuration is the most important factor determining the surgical approach.

- Malunion is poorly tolerated – consider ORIF with any displacement.
- Avascular necrosis is associated with open fracture and comminution, but *not* time to surgery.

Lateral Process of Talus Fractures

- Lateral process of talus fractures are 25% of talar fractures.
- Associated with subtalar dislocation.
- Non-displaced fractures are treated in a cast.
- Displace excise if fragment <1 cm; fix if >1 cm.

Talar Body Fractures

- Defined by the presence of a primary fracture line through the posterior facet (cf talar neck fracture).
- ORIF if >2 mm displacement.
- Poor prognosis – only 24% satisfactory outcome.

Navicular Fractures

- Isolated fractures rare – CT for associated lateral column and tarsometatarsal injury.
- Sangeorzan classification is recommended.
- Surgical priority is the restoration of medial and lateral column lengths with stable fixation.

References

1. Mulfinger GE, Trueta J. The blood supply of the talus. *J Bone Joint Surg.* 1970; 52B:160–7.

2. Prasarn ML, Miller AN, Dyke JP, et al. Arterial anatomy of the talus: a cadaver and gadolinium-enhanced MRI study. *Foot Ankle Int.* 2010; 31(11):987–93.

3. Freeman BC, Duff S, Allen PE, et al. The extended lateral approach to the hindfoot: anatomical basis and surgical implications. *J Bone Joint Surg.* 1998; 80B:139–42.

4. Gardner MJ, Nork SE, Barei DP, et al. Secondary soft tissue compromise in tongue-type calcaneus fractures. *J Orthop Trauma.* 2008; 22:439–45.

5. Judd DB, Kim DH. Foot fractures frequently misdiagnosed as ankle sprains. *Am Fam Phys.* 2002; 66(5)785–95.

6. Jahss MH, Kay BS. An anatomic study of the anterior superior process of the os calcis and its clinical application. *Foot Ankle.* 1983; 3:268–81.

7. Degan TJ, Morrey BF, Braun DP. Surgical excision for anterior process fractures of the calcaneus. *J Bone Joint Surg.* 1982; 64A:519–24.

8. Tennent TD, Calder PR, Salisbury RD, et al. The operative management of displaced intra-articular fractures of the calcaneum: a two-centre study using a defined protocol. *Injury.* 2001; 32(6):491–6.

9. Essex-Lopresti P. The mechanism, reduction technique and results in fractures of the os calcis. *Br J Surg.* 1952; 39:395–419.

10. Buckley R, Tough S, McCormack R, et al. Operative compared with non-operative treatment of displaced intra-articular calcaneal fractures. *J Bone Joint Surg.* 2002; 84A:1733–44.

11. Eastwood DM, Gregg PJ, Atkins RM. Intra-articular fractures of the calcaneum. Part I. Pathological anatomy and classification. *J Bone Joint Surg.* 1993; 75B:183–8.

12. Sanders R, Fortin P, DiPasquale T, et al. Operative treatment of 120 displaced intra-articular fractures of the calcaneus. *Clin Orth.* 1993; 290:87–95.

13. Griffin D, Parsons N, Shaw E, et al. Operative versus non-operative treatment for closed, displaced, intra-articular fractures of the calcaneus: randomised controlled trial. *BMJ.* 2014; 24:349.

14. Radnay CS, Clare MP, Sanders R. Subtalar fusion after displaced intra-articular calcaneal fractures: does initial operative treatment matter? *J Bone Joint Surg.* 2009; 91A:541–6.

15. Rammelt S, Amlang M, Barthel S, et al. Percutaneous treatment of less severe intraarticular calcaneal fractures. *Clin Orthop Relat Res.* 2010; 468:983–90.

16. Schepers T, Vogels LM, Schipper IB, et al. Percutaneous reduction and fixation of intra-articular calcaneal fractures. *Oper Orthop Traumatol.* 2008; 20(2):168–75.

17. Coltart WD. Aviator's astragalus. *J Bone Joint Surg.* 1952; 34B:545–66.

18. Main BJ, Jowett RL. Injuries of the midtarsal joint. *J Bone Joint Surg.* 1975; 57B:89–97.

19. Stiell IG, Greenberg GH, McKnight RD, et al. A study to develop clinical decision rules for the use of radiography in acute ankle injuries. *Ann Emerg Med.* 1992; 21(4):384–90.

20. Bosien WR, Staples OS, Russell SW. Residual disability following acute ankle sprains. *J Bone Joint Surg.* 1955; 37A:1237–43.

21. Verhagen RA, Struijs PA, Bossuyt PM, et al. Systematic review of treatment strategies for osteochondral defects of the talar dome. *Foot Ankle Clin.* 2003; 8:233–42.

22. Marsh J, Saltzman C, Iverson M, et al. Major open trauma of the talus. *J Orthop Trauma.* 1995; 9:371–6.

23. Patel R, Van Bergeyk A, Pinney S. Are displaced talar neck fractures surgical emergencies? *Foot Ankle Int.* 2005; 26(5):378–81.

24. Hawkins LG. Fractures of the neck of the talus. *J Bone Joint Surg.* 1970; 52A:991–1002.

25. Tezval M, Dumont C, Klaus M. Prognostic reliability of the Hawkins sign in fractures of the talus. *J Orthop Trauma.* 2007; 21(8):538–43.

26. Smith CS, Nork SE, Sangeorzan BJ. The extruded talus: results of re-implantation. *J Bone Joint Surg.* 2006; 88A:2418–24.

27. Valderrabano V, Perren T, Ryf C, et al. Snowboarder's talus fracture: treatment outcome of 20 cases after 3.5 years. *Am J Sports Med.* 2005; 33(6):871–80.

28. Ahmad J, Raikin SM. Current concepts review: talar fractures. *Foot Ankle Int.* 2006; 27(6):475–82.

29. Canale ST, Kelly FB. Fractures of the neck of talus. Long-term evaluation of seventy-one cases. *J Bone Joint Surg.* 1978; 60A:143–56.

30. Lindvall E, Haidukewych G, DiPascuale T, et al. Open reduction and stable fixation of isolated, displaced talar neck and body fractures. *J Bone Joint Surg.* 2004; 86A:2229–34.

31. Rammelt S, Zwipp H. Talar neck and body fractures. *Injury.* 2009; 40:120–35.

32. Sanders R, Pappas J, Mast J, et al. The salvage of open grade IIIB ankle and talus fractures. *J Orthop Trauma.* 1992; 6:201–8.

33. Vallier HA, Nork SE, Barei DP, et al. Talar neck fractures: results

and outcomes. *J Bone Joint Surg.* 2004; 86A:1616–24.

34. McCann PA, Jackson M, Mitchell ST, et al. Complications of definitive open reduction and internal fixation of pilon fractures of the distal tibia. *Int Orthop.* 2011; 35(3):413–18.

35. Thordarson DB. Talar body fractures. *Orthop Clin N Am.* 2001; 32(1):65–77.

36. Attiah M, Sanders DW, Valdivia G, et al. Comminuted talar neck fractures: a mechanical comparison of fixation techniques. *J Orthop Trauma.* 2007; 21(1):47–51.

37. Daniels TR, Smith JW, Ross TI. Varus malalignment of the talar neck: its effect on the position of the foot and on subtalar motion. *J Bone Joint Surg.* 1996; 78A:1559–67.

38. Sanders DW, Busam M, Hattwick E, et al. Functional outcomes following displaced talar neck fractures. *J Orthop Trauma.* 2004; 18:265–70.

39. Swanson TV, Bray TJ, Holmes GB. Fractures of the talar neck. A mechanical study of fixation. *J Bone Joint Surg.* 1992; 74A:544–51.

40. Blair HC. Comminuted fracture and fracture-dislocations of the body of the astragalus: operative treatment. *Am J Surg.* 1943; 59:3.

41. Santavirta S, Seitsalo S, Kiviluoto O, et al. Fractures of the talus. *J Trauma.* 1984; 24:986–9.

42. Inokuchi S, Ogawa K, Usami N. Classification of fractures of the talus: clear differentiation between neck and body fractures. *Foot Ankle Int.* 1996; 20:595–605.

43. Ebraheim NA, Patil V, Owens C, et al. Clinical outcome of fractures of the talar body. *Int Orthop.* 2008; 32:773–7.

44. Vallier HA, Nork SE, Benirschke SK, et al. Surgical treatment of talar body fractures. *J Bone Joint Surg.* 2003; 85A:1716–24.

45. Boyd HB, Knight RA. Fractures of the astragalus. *South Med J.* 1942; 35:160–7.

46. Orthopaedic Trauma Association Committee for Coding and Classification. Fracture and dislocation compendium. *J Orthop Trauma.* 2007; 21(Supplement 10):89–94.

47. Mindell ER, Cisek EE, Kartalian G, et al. Late results of injuries of the talus: analysis of forty cases. *J Bone Joint Surg.* 1963; 45A:221–45.

48. Carmont MR, Davies MB. Buttress plate stabilisation of posterior malleolar ankle fractures: a familiar technique through an unfamiliar approach. *Curr Orthop.* 2008; 22(5):359–64.

49. Papa JA, Myerson MS. Pantalar and tibiotalocalcaneal arthrodesis for post-traumatic osteoarthrosis of the ankle and hindfoot. *J Bone Joint Surg.* 1992; 74A:1042–9.

50. Russotti GM, Johnson KA, Cass JR. Tibiotalocalcaneal arthrodesis for arthritis and deformity of the hind part of the foot. *J Bone Joint Surg.* 1988; 70A:1304–7.

51. Pennal GE. Fractures of the talus. *Clin Orthop.* 1963; 30:53–63.

52. Cedell CA. Rupture of the posterior talotibial ligament with the avulsion of a bone fragment from the talus. *Acta Orthop Scand.* 1974; 45:454–61.

53. Shepherd FJ. A hitherto undescribed fracture of the astragalus. *J Anat Physiol.* 1882; 17:82–3.

54. Davies MB. The os trigonum syndrome. *Foot.* 2004; 14(3):119–23.

55. Pinney SJ, Sangeorzan BJ. Fractures of the tarsal bones. *Orthop Clin N Am.* 2001; 32:21–33.

56. Oddy MJ, Davies MB. Stress fractures of the navicular. *Op Tech Sports Med.* 2009; 17(2)115–18.

57. Eichenholtz SN, Levine DB. Fractures of the tarsal navicular

bone. *Clin Orth Rel Res.* 1964; 34:142–57.

58. Dhillon MS, Nagi ON. Total dislocations of the navicular: are they ever isolated injuries? *J Bone Joint Surg.* 1999; 81B:881–5.

59. Evans J, Beingessner DM, Agel J, et al. Minifragment plate fixation of high-energy navicular body fractures. *Foot Ankle Int.* 2011; 32(5):485–92.

60. Dewar FP, Evans DC. Occult fracture-dislocation of the midtarsal joint. *J Bone Joint Surg.* 1968; 50B:386–8.

61. Richter M, Wippermann B, Krettek C, et al. Fractures and fracture dislocations of the midfoot: occurrence, causes and long-term results. *Foot Ankle Int.* 2001; 22(5):392–8.

62. Sangeorzan BJ, Benirschke SK, Mosca V, et al. Displaced intra-articular fractures of the tarsal navicular. *J Bone Joint Surg.* 1989; 71A:1504–10.

63. Swords MP, Schramski M, Switzer K, et al. Chopart fractures and dislocations. *Foot Ankle Clin N Am.* 2008; 13:679–93.

64. Cronier P, Frin JM, Steiger V, et al. Internal fixation of complex fractures of the tarsal navicular with locking plates. A report of 10 cases. *Orthop Traumatol Surg Res.* 2013; 99S:S241–S249.

65. Schildhauer TA, Nork SE, Sangeorzan BJ. Temporary bridge plating of the medial column in severe midfoot injuries. *J Orthop Trauma.* 2003; 17(7):513–20.

66. Pathria MN, Rosenstein A, Bjorkengren AG, et al. Isolated dislocation of the tarsal navicular: a case report. *Foot Ankle.* 1988; 9:146–9.

67. Sangeorzan BJ, Swiontkowski MF. Displaced fractures of the cuboid. *J Bone Joint Surg.* 1990; 72B:376–8.

68. Drummond DS, Hastings DE. Total dislocation of the cuboid bone: report of a case. *J Bone Joint Surg.* 1969; 51B:716–18.

69. Hermel BM, Gershon-Cohen J. The nutcracker fracture of the cuboid by indirect violence. *Radiology*. 1953; 60:850–4.

70. Weber M, Locher S. Reconstruction of the cuboid in compression fractures: short to midterm results in 12 patients. *Foot Ankle Int*. 2002; 23(11):1008–13.

71. Saxby TS, Sharp RJ, Rosenfeld PF. Plantar fracture-dislocation of the intermediate cuneiform: case report. *Foot Ankle Int*. 2006; 27(9):742–5.

72. Kenwright J, Taylor RG. Major injuries of the talus. *J Bone Joint Surg*. 1970; 52B:36–48.

73. Letts RM, Gibeault D. Fractures of the neck of the talus in children. *Foot Ankle*. 1980; 1:74–7.

74. Spak L. Fractures of the talus in children. *Acta Chir Scand*. 1954; 107:553–66.

Chapter 23

Fractures and Dislocations of the Forefoot

Timothy A. Coughlin and Ben J. Ollivere

Introduction

Forefoot trauma ranges in severity from the seemingly trivial "turf toe" to significant fracture dislocations of the tarsal bones and complex multicolumn injuries. Both ends of the spectrum provide their own unique challenges in treatment and diagnosis, but the main challenge is knowing when to operate and how to optimize the outcome. Even the most insignificant appearing fracture can result in significant long-term disability.

High-energy forefoot and midfoot trauma is a significant cause of long-term morbidity. The lifelong impact of a poorly functioning forefoot should not be underestimated. These patients often present with open injuries with soft tissue loss, and associated muscle and tendon damage. Patients presenting with ankle, pilon, and tibial plateau fractures should all be carefully examined and investigated to ensure that they do not have associated mid- and forefoot fractures. Long periods of non-weightbearing are often necessary, which coupled with the associated soft tissue damage results in a poorly functioning, stiff foot.

Lower energy trauma presents its own difficulties, with isolated Lisfranc and cuneiform fractures often being misdiagnosed in the Accident and Emergency department as sprains. Careful investigation of all persistently swollen midfeet following trauma is essential to reach the correct diagnosis early and improve the long-term outcome.

There is an increasing burden of fragility fractures in the elderly who present with complex metatarsal base fractures on a background of poorly controlled diabetes or osteoporosis. These patients present their own challenges with a "less is more" approach often being appropriate. Judicious use of internal fixation can, however, prevent long-term deformity and ulceration, and so should be considered in selected cases. In many ways older fragility fractures present a more difficult decision-making process than the high-energy fractures seen in younger patients. It is clearly in the patient's interest to have treatment decisions made by a senior foot and ankle or trauma surgeon.

The main principles of treatment in the forefoot include restoration of the stability of the medial column, allowing soft tissue healing, and ensuring that the foot continues to function as a stable tripod without loss of length or overload of the lesser rays. A stepwise approach to reconstruction with medial bridge plating of the first ray to maintain length, and reconstruction of the lesser rays, is usually appropriate. In many cases, metalwork should be removed after a suitable interval. Management of expectations can be difficult and treatment should be undertaken bearing in mind that a proportion of patients will require secondary fusion surgery. In summary, reconstruction of complex forefoot fractures is among the most challenging surgery.

Pathogenesis

The three parts of the foot have very different functions. The hindfoot is used for propulsion, deceleration, and as a shock absorber. The midfoot controls the relationship between the hindfoot and the forefoot. Fixing the midfoot and forefoot is key in locking the metatarsals to provide a sound platform through the third rocker to toe-off. The locked forefoot provides a platform for standing and a lever for push-off. During gait, load is distributed unevenly with the first metatarsal bearing one-third of the body's weight and the second to the fifth sharing the other two-thirds. The metatarsal heads and the toes are in contact with the floor for around 75% of the stance phase. A supple and functioning forefoot is required to maintain stability with the assistance of the windlass mechanism, allowing function of the major muscles and tendons crossing the ankle and ensuring the body's weight is correctly distributed under the metatarsal heads to prevent transfer metatarsalgia.

Lisfranc Injuries

The Lisfranc "joint" is usually used eponymously to mean the tarsometatarsal joint, although Lisfranc injuries often involve the tarsometatarsal, intermetatarsal, and intertarsal joints. The central stabilizing structure is the Y-shaped Lisfranc ligament, which runs from the medial cuneiform to the base of the second metatarsal; the ligament stabilizes the second metatarsal and is central to maintenance of the mid-foot arch. The second metatarsal is the keystone of the transverse arch, and thus rupture of the Lisfranc ligament tends to be the key to Lisfranc injuries. Although initially described as a specific injury, Lisfranc injuries are now taken to refer to any injury defunctioning the Lisfranc joint. These injuries are usually caused by axial loading or indirect rotational forces through the Lisfranc joint in a plantar flexed foot. The plantar directed "V" shape of the second metatarsal makes it susceptible to dorsal dislocation. This family of injuries can also be caused by direct crush injuries when a heavy load lands on the foot, usually resulting in a plantarly displaced fracture.

First Metatarsal Fractures

The first ray is relatively rigid, providing a stable lever arm around which the windlass mechanism functions during the third rocker of gait. Shortening of as little as 7 mm from malunion of a first metatarsal fracture can lead to transfer of load to the lateral side of the foot. This can often result in pain, with transfer lesions of the lesser rays.

The first metatarsal is wider, shorter, and stronger than the lesser metatarsals. As a result of its relative size and strength, when fractures do occur in the first metatarsal they are often resultant on a high-energy injury, with more comminution and a higher incidence of being open.

Fifth Metatarsal Fractures

Injuries to the fifth metatarsal are common, comprising 25% of all metatarsal fractures. They are a significant burden for surgeons and patients alike, with a surprising number of unsatisfactory results and dissatisfied patients. The three common fractures of the base of the fifth metatarsal all occur by different mechanisms.

1. Avulsion fractures are caused by the pull of peroneus brevis and are classically seen in dancers.

Affecting the proximal 1.5 cm of the fifth metatarsal these injuries do not place the blood supply at risk.
2. Jones' fractures are more distal and are caused by inversion injuries. They involve the intermetatarsal facet between the fourth and fifth metatarsals, usually 1.5 to 3 cm from the styloid process.
3. Stress fractures are the least common fracture and are seen in the diaphysis, distal to Jones' fractures.

The fifth metatarsal has a relatively poor blood supply and therefore all three types of fracture risk non-union[1]. The diaphyseal blood supply primarily comes from a single vessel entering the diaphysis at the junction of the proximal and middle thirds. Secondary arteries supply the tuberosity and base. This leaves a relatively avascular area in zone 2, where Jones' fractures occur, and accounts for the high rates of non-union with these fractures. The only level 1 evidence available shows a non-union rate of 33% for those treated in cast, falling to 6% for those who have open reduction and internal fixation[2].

Second to Fourth Metatarsal Fractures

Acute fractures of the middle metatarsals are rarely isolated and often occur as a result of a high-energy injury, usually either as an extension of a Lisfranc injury, or as a result of the metatarsal bases being forced plantarward. Stress fractures are usually isolated and found in the second and third metatarsals, which are relatively fixed in comparison to the first, fourth, and fifth rays. In stress fractures low bone mineral density is a risk factor for occurrence and also an independent risk factor for non-union.

Together the metatarsal heads form a curved cascade when looked at from above (Lelièvre's parabola). In the horizontal plane the plantar aspect of the second to the fourth metatarsal heads should all be on the same level. The first metatarsal head lies higher than the other four as the sesamoids are the weightbearing point.

Hallux Fractures and Dislocations

Intra-articular "corner" fractures of the proximal phalanx usually occur with a "stubbed toe" when the great toe is caught while walking barefoot or in sandals. Diaphyseal injuries are usually the result of direct trauma such as kicking a wall, and very high-energy axial loads can result in a pilon type fracture of the base of the toe. Patients commonly present late after the simpler great toe fractures.

Sesamoid Fractures

The two sesamoid bones of the hallux, which lie within the tendon of flexor hallucis brevis, and fibers of the abductor hallucis and adductor hallucis, also attach, respectively, to the tibial and fibular sesamoids. The two sesamoids are connected to each other by the intersesamoidal ligament. As a result of the lever arm of the first metatarsal head the sesamoids bear up to three times the body weight in the normal gait cycle, with the tibial sesamoid bearing a greater proportion of this due to its size and position.

The sesamoids are commonly injured during sport, usually as a result of either a direct axial loading force resulting in a comminuted fracture, or forced hyperextension of the first MTPJ. Stress fractures are seen three times more commonly than acute fractures, often in long-distance runners. The risk of a sesamoid fracture is increased by cavus deformity of the foot and hallux valgus deformity of the great toe.

Misdiagnosis is common, as bipartite or multipartite sesamoids are present in 20%[3] of the population as a result of the ossification centers failing to fuse. A bipartite or multipartite sesamoid is only bilateral in 25% of patients and so unilaterality is *not* a useful sign for assessing a fracture. To compound matters, when a bipartite sesamoid is fractured, it often does so through the fibrocartilagenous junctional zone making detection very difficult. It should therefore be more accurately termed a "diastasis" injury. Diagnosis may be aided by either MRI scanning or more traditionally bone scanning with areas of high signal or tracer uptake indicative of fracture.

Turf Toe

The term "turf toe" was coined in 1976 to describe a plantar capsulo-ligamentous injury of the hallux MTPJ[4]. The condition commonly affects athletes and ballet dancers, and is caused by hyperdorsiflexion of the first MTPJ, usually with an axial load applied with the foot in fixed equinus (such as when a ballerina attempts to land "en pointe"). This results in tearing of the plantar plate and the surrounding structures. Injuries have become commoner in sports people as the use of hard synthetic sports surfaces and soft-soled shoes has become commoner. Astroturf has a higher coefficient of friction than

living grass and loses some of its shock absorbency over time. This results in the forefoot being "fixed" to the playing surface, making hyperdorsiflexion injury more likely.

Turf toe is associated with significant morbidity with as many as 50% of athletes complaining of persisting symptoms five years following injury[5]. Once torn, unrestricted motion of the proximal phalanx causes significant compression of the dorsal articular surface of the metatarsal head. Turf toe may be associated with a sesamoid fracture.

Phalangeal Dislocations and Fractures

Fractures of the lesser toe phalanges are seen four times as frequently as those of the hallux[6]. Fractures of the proximal phalanx and dislocations of the proximal interphalangeal joint are usually sustained when barefoot, as the toe can easily catch and be forced into abduction. Distal phalangeal fractures are usually caused by a direct crushing injury or an axial loading force (a "stubbed" toe). Great care must be made not to miss a nailbed injury or open fracture as these injuries need thorough washout and repair of the nail bed.

Classification

There are many classification systems that have been proposed over the years for the various injuries of the forefoot – far too many to be considered in their entirety in this chapter. Many are just descriptive, but some guide treatment or deepen understanding of the pathophysiology and are worth consideration.

Lisfranc Injuries

Sprains of the Lisfranc joint are relatively common and have been classified by the grade of injury to the Lisfranc ligament[7]. Differentiation of the grades is aided by weightbearing AP films, to demonstrate instability.

- Grade 1: Pain at the site of the Lisfranc ligament with minimal swelling and no instability.
- Grade 2: Pain and swelling with associated laxity, but no instability. Diastasis present between the first and second metatarsals, but no collapse of the medial arch.
- Grade 3: Complete ligamentous disruption with diastasis and loss of the longitudinal arch.

Grade 3 injuries are usually a fracture dislocation, which can also be classified as below.

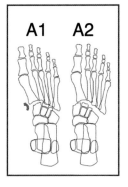 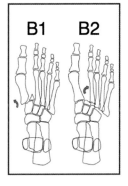 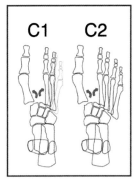

Figure 23.1 Myerson classification of Lisfranc injuries.

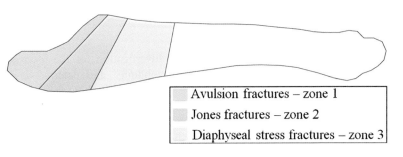

Figure 23.2 Dameron–Lawrence–Botte zonal classification of fractures of the base of fifth metatarsal.

Avulsion fractures – zone 1

Jones fractures – zone 2

Diaphyseal stress fractures – zone 3

Complete injuries of the Lisfranc joint, with ligament rupture and defunctioning of the base of the second metatarsal, were originally classified by Quénu and Küss in 1909[8], a classification that was subsequently modified in 1982 by Hardcastle[9] and finally updated in 1986 by Myerson[10]. The Myerson classification is in common use as it guides treatment and also indicates prognosis (Figure 23.1).

A: Homolateral

    A1: total incongruity medial displacement

    A2: total incongruity lateral displacement.

B: Isolated

    B1: partial incongruity medial displacement

    B2: partial incongruity lateral displacement.

C: Divergent

    C1: partial divergent displacement

    C2: total divergent displacement.

It is important to bear in mind that in the normal foot radiograph:

- The lateral border of the medial cuneiform should align with the lateral aspect of the first metatarsal.
- The medial aspect of the second metatarsal should align with the medial cortex of the middle cuneiform.
- The medial aspect of the third metatarsal should align with the medial edge of the lateral cuneiform.
- The medial aspect of the fourth metatarsal should align with the medial edge of the cuboid.

Fractures of the Base of the Fifth Metatarsal

Fractures of the base of the fifth metatarsal are most commonly classified using the Dameron–Lawrence–Botte zonal classification[11–12]. The classification (Figure 23.2) divides injuries into three zones: avulsion fractures of the tubercle (zone 1); Jones' fractures at the metadiaphyseal junction (zone 2); and diaphyseal stress fractures (zone 3). While this classification is useful, in that it does predict the likelihood of fracture union, it does suffer from the problem that in vivo many injuries cross more than one zone.

Jones' fractures and stress fractures within 1.5 cm of the tuberosity are also subclassified by the Torg classification[13]:

Type I: Acute fracture with sharp margins and no widening

Type II: Delayed union with some periosteal reaction, widened fracture site and intramedullary sclerosis

Type III: Non-union with intramedullary sclerosis.

Presentation

Clinical assessment can be difficult at the time of initial examination. A number of different forefoot injuries present with a painful, swollen, and contused foot. Initial evaluation of the patient should include a careful history including the mechanism and position of the foot at the time of injury. At least three radiographic views (AP, lateral, and oblique) of the foot should be obtained.

There is a surprisingly high incidence of vascular compromise and compartment syndrome associated with metatarsal fractures and careful examination of the vascularity of the foot, and in particular the toes distal to the fracture, should be undertaken. Any significant swelling with pain out of proportion to the injury and pain on passive motion of the toes should alert the clinician to the possibility of compartment syndrome. Although there is no universal agreement on the precise indications for fasciotomy in the foot, establishing the diagnosis is important. The presence, or absence, of pulses should always be documented.

All patients should be assessed for diabetes mellitus and, in particular, the presence of a peripheral neuropathy. This is easily assessed with a Semmes–Weinstein 10 gram monofilament. In those patients with diabetes, management should be as part of a multidisciplinary team, as tight control of the blood glucose will help optimize outcome. Patients who smoke tobacco should be advised to cease usage, as it is associated with higher overall complication rates, not just non-union.

Patients presenting with severe open injuries should be managed in a multidisciplinary team, with plastic and, if required, vascular surgical input. A staged approach to skeletal and soft tissue reconstruction is used. While clean grade I and II injuries can always be treated in a planned manner, severe grade III injuries, or those with contamination, should be treated as an emergency. Careful documentation of the neurovascular status, in particular plantar sensation, and operative findings at the initial debridement should be used to guide subsequent decision making. Limb salvage is not always the best option, but for the majority of isolated severe open foot fractures it should be the goal.

In many of the less severe fractures and soft tissue injuries of the forefoot diagnosis can be difficult. It is worth maintaining a high level of clinical suspicion and if doubt persists then a CT scan should be arranged to rule out fractures or dislocations. Patients presenting with severe swelling should be admitted for elevation and treatment with a pneumatic foot pump. Outcomes are generally better if prolonged periods of immobilization can be avoided.

Investigations

The majority of forefoot injuries can be adequately imaged with standard series x-rays, nevertheless specialist radiological views and more complex imaging modalities are frequently helpful.

X-Ray

X-ray is the standard investigation for the forefoot with anteroposterior, oblique, and lateral views (Figure 23.3). These will adequately show most injuries. Acutely radiographs are normally taken with the patient non-weightbearing as a result of pain or for fear of causing further damage. Nevertheless significantly more information, particularly in defining Lisfranc instability and collapse, can be garnered from weightbearing films and stress views. It is essential to correlate radiological and clinical findings. X-rays are often normal in stress fractures from two to six weeks of symptom onset, though they usually progress to show either the stress fracture itself or evidence of healing.

Special Views

Weightbearing Views. AP and lateral x-rays with the patient weight bearing can be useful to show displacement of the Lisfranc joint where there has been complete ligament rupture. This is often missed on standard non-weightbearing films. Where there remains any doubt weightbearing films of the uninjured side may be useful.

Stress Views of the Lisfranc Joint. Stress views can be used to ascertain the extent of the injury if this remains unclear after weightbearing x-rays. They are rarely performed in the emergency department in the acute setting, as to do so would usually require an anesthetic and interpretation can be difficult. They can, however, be very informative at the start of an operation if for no other reason than to document the degree of instability. The widespread availability of preoperative CT and MRI scanning has rendered these views obsolete in many centers.

Sesamoid Views. When assessing the sesamoids two sets of views are useful:

- The medial oblique view, to assess the tibial sesamoid, and the lateral oblique view, to assess the fibular sesamoid, show each sesamoid in a near AP or PA view (depending on technique) and clear the metatarsal head from the projection. The two views are taken with the foot in the AP position and the x-ray beam directed 15° cephalad with the MTPJ extended to 50°.

- Axial views, with the hallux held dorsiflexed, and a radiograph taken along the longitudinal axis of the sole of the foot to profile the two sesamoids, can also be helpful.

Contralateral x-rays should not be used for interpretation due to the significant variation in bipartite and multipartite sesamoids between sides.

CT Scan

A CT scan is commonly used to assess the extent of injury, especially of the Lisfranc joint. The complex overlapping geometry of the forefoot and midfoot can be clearly viewed with cross-sectional imaging and 3D reconstructions assisting in the assessment of the metatarsal arcade and other fracture patterns. CT is particularly useful in assessing the degree of plantar comminution, which may not be appreciated on plain radiographs. The use of volume rendered images (Figure 23.4) is particularly helpful in understanding fracture patterns, and hence in surgical planning. When assessing fractures using 3D-rendered views there is a risk of missing fractures, or oversimplification of fracture configurations, as these are inherently lower resolution images and should be carefully compared to plain slices.

MRI Scan

An MRI scan can aid in the diagnosis of metatarsal stress fractures, as x-rays can remain normal for up to six weeks. MRI may also show a stress *reaction* within

(a)   (b)

(c)

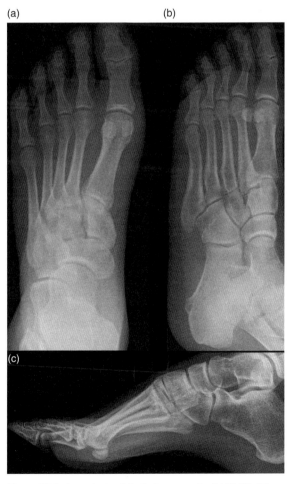

Figure 23.3 A standard radiological trauma series. (**a**) AP, (**b**) oblique, and (**c**) lateral. If the series can be obtained weight bearing this is ideal.

(a)   (b)

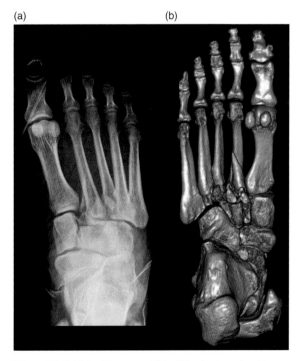

Figure 23.4 (**a**) An AP x-ray and (**b**) a 3D volume-rendered image of the same injury looking at the plantar aspect. While some comminution can be appreciated on the AP x-ray the comminution of the bases of the second to fourth metatarsals can be fully appreciated on the CT scan.

the metatarsal, showing low signal on the T1 and high signal intensity on T2 and STIR sequences, but with *no* evidence of extension into the cortices. A stress reaction should be treated in the same way as a stress fracture. The diagnosis of a stress reaction is never made on x-ray.

Sesamoid fractures can also be diagnosed on MRI, and the technique is particularly useful in identifying those patients with a diastasis injury of a bipartite or multipartite sesamoid. It may also reveal avascular necrosis of the sesamoid[14].

Bone Scan

To a large extent the use of technetium and other bone-scanning methods has been replaced by the wider accessibility and lower cost of MRI. They are occasionally used in the diagnosis of sesamoid fractures[15]. Bone scanning suffers the same problems in identifying metatarsal stress fractures and sesamoid fractures, with high sensitivity but poor specificity.

Treatment

When taken as a whole, injuries to the forefoot are most commonly managed non-operatively. Extreme care should be taken in patient selection, with some injury patterns requiring early, aggressive treatment in order to effect an optimal outcome. Non-operative management strategies will be considered in the first instance.

Non-Operative Management

Lisfranc Injuries

There is some controversy in the literature as to whether these injuries can be treated non-operatively at all. One approach, which is often quoted, is that injuries that show less than 2 mm of diastasis between the first and second metatarsal can be considered for non-operative treatment, although some report successful conservative management with up to 5 mm of displacement[16]. The majority of displaced injuries are treated operatively in most centers; however, there is a large number of undisplaced and base of metatarsal fractures that with appropriate follow-up can be successfully treated non-operatively.

If non-operative management is to be considered the patient should be placed into a non-weightbearing cast for a minimum of six to eight weeks, followed by a weightbearing cast for a further eight weeks.

Patients should be carefully followed with x-rays during this time period, as displacement can occur as swelling subsides. In the acute stages the taking of a weightbearing film is often not possible as a result of pain. However, many use a weightbearing film at two weeks to dynamically load the ligament. Displacement on the weightbearing radiographs is taken as an indication to revert to operative management. Patients often benefit from physiotherapy after removal of the plaster. The ongoing swelling may necessitate the wearing of supportive, accommodative shoes for many months after the injury.

Fractures of the Hallux

Fractures of the first metatarsal require accurate reduction, avoiding shortening or dorsiflexion, and operative intervention is often appropriate. When fractures are undisplaced a trial of conservative management is appropriate. This can be achieved with spica strapping, a short plantar splint, or a heel weightbearing shoe. There is a single study suggesting that pain scores were significantly lower in patients treated with a splint, as opposed to a spica[17].

Sesamoid Fractures

Sesamoiditis is a term used to describe pain arising from the sesamoid. It is not an inflammatory condition but, in most cases, is the result of a fracture. Brodsky et al. histologically examined 32 sesamoids excised at surgery for sesamoiditis[18]. A non-united fracture was demonstrated in 28. Two patients had diastases of a bipartite sesamoid, and two exhibited degenerate loss of cartilage. No patient had primary avascular necrosis. There was evidence of avascular necrosis secondary to fracture in nine patients. Of the fractures 16 were stress fractures, and in 12 the onset was related to a specific traumatic event.

Acute fractures of the sesamoids are seen in combination with dislocations of the MTPJ, or with a diagnosis of turf toe. The tibial sesamoid is more commonly fractured than the fibular sesamoid due to its size and position beneath the first metatarsal head. The non-operative management of sesamoid stress fractures is controversial, with multiple papers indicating that non-union frequently persists despite prolonged immobilization, the use of in-shoe orthoses, and non-weightbearing. Brodsky et al. in 2000[18] reported excellent and good results in all patients following sesamoid excision and reconstruction of the flexor hallucis brevis tendon. Acceptable results have also been reported with simple bone grafting without fixation in 90% of individuals[19] rising to 100% with the addition of percutaneous fixation[20]. Non-operative management of acute fractures is with forefoot immobilization for six to eight weeks where the fracture is undisplaced or with displacement of up to 5 mm[21].

Turf Toe

Turf toe can be a potent cause of morbidity in the elite athlete and should be taken seriously. The optimal assessment of a turf toe injury is with MRI scanning using a powerful magnet and a surface coil, reported by an experienced foot and ankle radiologist. Only then can a proper diagnosis be made and appropriate management instituted. The presence of ligament, bone, and cartilage injury as well as the integrity of the plantar plate will determine whether these injuries are managed operatively or non-operatively.

The management of MTPJ sprains is largely non-operative and the timing of return to activity is related to the grade of sprain. Management aims are to limit dorsiflexion until symptoms have settled.

Grade 1 injuries, where the plantar plate is only sprained, can be effected with bulky buddy strapping to the second toe for a period of one to two weeks followed by a gradual return to activity as symptoms allow.

Grade 2 injuries, where the plantar plate is partially torn, may be treated with buddy strapping or a short leg cast for one to two weeks, depending on the severity of symptoms, with return to activity as symptoms allow over a period of weeks.

Grade 3 injuries with a complete tear usually require short leg casting for one to two weeks and restricted activities, until pain-free active dorsiflexion has returned, which may take up to six weeks. On rare occasions, surgical repair of the avulsed plantar plate is necessary for persisting instability. This can be undertaken using a suture anchor or drill hole through the metatarsal.

First Metatarsophalangeal Joint Dislocation

Dislocation of the hallucal MTPJ is rare. Dorsal dislocations are classified on the radiographic appearance of the sesamoids. They were classified by Jahss.

- Type I: The plantar plate ruptures at its proximal attachment to the metatarsal neck. The sesamoids remain attached to the proximal phalanx. Consequently the plantar capsule interposes and blocks reduction. This necessitates open reduction through a dorsal approach.
- Type IIa: The inter-sesamoid ligament ruptures, but closed reduction is usually possible.
- Type IIb: There is transverse fracture of the sesamoids, and closed reduction is usually possible.

These are rare injuries, and each is treated on its individual merit. Repair of the plantar plate is advisable if open surgery is undertaken.

Lesser Metatarsal Fractures

In one study of patients with minimally displaced metatarsal fractures where tubular elastic bandages were compared with cast immobilization, there was no statistically significant difference in union rates between the two methods. The median pain score at one week favored bandage over plaster cast, but by four weeks there was no significant difference between the two treatments in the patients' pain[22].

The management of displaced fractures of the central metatarsals can be problematic. Mild displacement in the medial/lateral plane are well tolerated, but when the metatarsal head displaces into flexion or extension, or if the metatarsal is significantly shortened, this leads to transfer metatarsalgia in over a third of patients. If the displacement is dorsal, the adjacent metatarsals will develop calluses and transfer pain, and if plantarward, the affected metatarsal head may develop a callus under it and be painful.

The majority of metatarsal stress fractures can be treated with rest alone and do not necessarily need immobilization. Where a causative factor is involved, such as an increase in exercise, this should be stopped for a period of four to eight weeks[23]. If walking itself causes pain then crutches and partial weight bearing may be used for a period. Once pain has subsided activities can be *gradually* reintroduced, although if this is done too rapidly symptoms are likely to recur. If symptoms are neglected then a stress fracture can progress to a frank metatarsal fracture.

Fractures of the Base of the Fifth Metatarsal

The majority of fractures of the base of the fifth metatarsal can be treated non-operatively, with the success of treatment dependent on the location of the fracture.

- Zone 1 fractures can usually be treated with a compressive soft dressing and walking boot or cast. Non-union is uncommon and, when it does occur, it is usually an asymptomatic fibrous non-union.
- Zone 2 (Jones' fracture) have a higher non-union rate than zone 1 injuries, the non-union rate is quoted as being as high as 33%. There is a high incidence of failure after cast treatment of acute Jones' fractures, although cast-treated Torg type 1 fractures have reported union rates of up to 93%. Early intramedullary screw fixation, especially in Torg II and III fractures, results in quicker times to union and return to sports when compared with cast treatment[2]. It remains the first-line treatment in the majority of patients.
- Zone 3 acute fractures have a high refracture rate. The low-demand patient can be managed in a non-weightbearing cast for a period of six to eight weeks. If union has not been achieved in this timeframe operative management should be considered. The more active patients, and those with non-union, are more usually treated with intramedullary screw fixation.

Dislocations or Fractures of the Metatarsophalangeal Joints

The initial management of MTPJ joint dislocations, provided they are closed, is reduction under local anesthetic or a regional block. Reduction can be tricky, particularly if the sesamoids are entrapped in the joint, but in general exaggeration of the deformity and longitudinal traction will usually effect reduction. The joint should then be tested for stability throughout the arc of motion; instability is usually due to collateral ligament injury. An incongruous post-reduction film usually indicates disruption and interposition of the plantar plate, which will require operative treatment. Successful reductions should be maintained with neighbor strapping to the longest neighboring toe.

Lesser Phalangeal Fractures/Dislocations

Fractures of the lesser toe phalanges can nearly always be treated non-operatively, unless the fracture is open or significantly displaced. Similarly dislocations, provided they are closed, can be reduced and then treated

conservatively. In both cases strapping to the longest neighboring uninjured phalanx should be performed, with a strip of gauze between the clean toes and "silk" tape.

Surgical

Compartment Syndrome of the Foot

There are commonly considered to be four compartments in the foot, although some studies have described up to nine. Hematoma and interstitial edema cause a rise in pressure, which ultimately results in myoneural necrosis. Pain out of proportion to the injury and pain on a passive toe stretch may indicate the diagnosis, but the presence of the foot fractures themselves will make these painful, potentially clouding clinical assessment. Compartment pressure can be measured if there is uncertainty in the diagnosis.

The four compartments are medial, lateral, central, and interosseous.

Medial

This compartment contains the abductor hallucis and flexor hallucis brevis. The medial and plantar border is the plantar aponeurosis, laterally the intermuscular septum, and dorsally the first metatarsal. For compartment pressure measurement the needle is inserted at the base of the first metatarsal, into the bulk of the abductor hallucis.

Lateral

This contains the abductor digiti quinti minimi, fifth toe flexor digitorum brevis, and opponens digiti quinti minimi. The dorsal border is the fifth metatarsal, the plantar aponeurosis plantar and laterally, and the intermuscular septum medially. For compartment pressures insert the needle at the midpoint of the fifth metatarsal, 1 cm medial and plantar.

Central

This contains the flexor digitorum brevis, lumbricals, quadratus plantae, and adductor hallucis. The plantar aponeurosis is again the plantar border, the intermuscular septum medially and laterally, and the osseo-fascial tarsometatarsal structures dorsally. For compartment pressure again insert the needle at the base of the fifth metatarsal but go medial and plantar *through* the abductor hallucis.

Interosseous

The interosseous compartment contains the seven interossei, each is bordered by the interosseous fascia and the metatarsals. To measure the compartment pressure insert the needle through the second, third, and fourth web spaces until it punctures the extensor fascia.

Approach. Two approaches are described; a single medial incision or two dorsal incisions. The medial approach is considered the approach of choice. Start your incision 2.5 cm (one inch) distal to the medial malleolus and extend it to the proximal first metatarsal. Identify and protect the neurovascular bundle and incise and retract the fascia. The medial compartment can then be incised longitudinally. The lateral, central, and interosseous compartments are released by blunt dissection, retracting the flexor digitorum brevis to access the lateral compartment.

Two dorsal incisions can be used when the intention is to perform metatarsal fixation in addition to fasciotomy. For this approach center one incision over the second and one over the fourth metatarsal, trying to maintain as large a skin bridge as possible. The interosseous compartments can be directly released and blunt dissection used to access the central, medial, and lateral compartments.

There is significant controversy over the use of compartment decompression in the foot. The indications for decompression are controversial with experts failing to agree. The trauma associated with decompression, combined with the often-delayed diagnosis, leaves many patients better off treated conservatively, and *not* decompressed, rather than undergoing extensive surgery, with the risks of infection and wound-healing problems.

Nevertheless in patients with mangled forefeet or significant Lisfranc injuries, who require urgent surgery in any case, a compartment decompression is likely to improve the outcome. Surgical incisions should be sited to allow decompression. Postoperatively a VAC dressing reduces comorbidity and helps minimize the need for plastic surgical reconstruction.

Lisfranc Injuries

There are two windows for surgical intervention with Lisfranc injuries: in the first 24 hours, or around seven to ten days post injury, once the swelling has subsided. There are a number of surgical strategies for the treatment of Lisfranc injuries. The least invasive is closed reduction and percutaneous K-wire fixation. Although still practiced, K-wire fixation alone rarely achieves the stability required to obtain the best results. Accurate reduction can also be difficult to obtain closed, and so a low threshold should be used for open reduction and internal fixation.

Approach. Two dorsal incisions can be used to access the whole of the tarsometatarsal articulation. The dorsomedial incision is made between the extensor hallucis longus and brevis tendons, giving access to the first and second TMTJs. The dorsolateral incision is along the fourth metatarsal. The skin bridge should be full thickness and not be undermined. It should be kept as wide as possible to reduce the risk of necrosis. Care should be taken to preserve the dorsalis pedis artery and deep peroneal nerve, which can easily be damaged in the medial incision. In high-energy injuries it is not uncommon for the dorsalis pedis to be ruptured in any case, as a result of the trauma.

Fixation. The first, second, and third TMTJs are key to stability and should be rigidly stabilized with transarticular screws or bridging plates (Figure 23.5). Each surgeon will have their own preference as to whether to use plates or screws, although either is acceptable. Screws are transarticular and cause further damage to the joint surface, whereas plates can be bulky and are technically more difficult to implant. We usually commence fixation with either a medial plate or position screw from the first metatarsal to the medial cuneiform. This helps buttress accurate reduction of the lesser rays. The second metatarsal should be fixed to both the medial cuneiform, usually with a medial to lateral position screw, which replicates the ruptured Lisfranc ligament, and also longitudinally to the intermediate cuneiform. This can be achieved with either an axial screw or dorsal plate. Often this will be all that is required to maintain reduction but if there is any persisting subluxation of the third, fourth, or fifth TMTJs then these can also be held with either screws, for the third, or percutaneous K-wire fixation, for the fourth and fifth rays.

The patient should remain non-weightbearing for a period. Removal of hardware is controversial. Some advocate removal of the metalwork before the commencement of weight bearing and physiotherapy; others recommend delaying removal for at least four to six months. Some leave asymptomatic hardware, fearing redisplacement more than broken screws and plates. A sensible approach is to start weight bearing as appropriate, usually at six weeks with a supportive

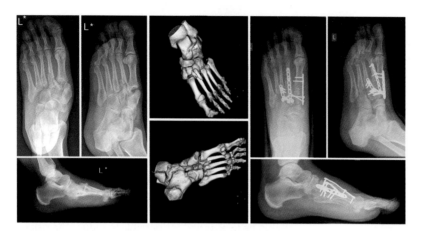

Figure 23.5 A Lisfranc injury showing fixation with screws and dorsal plates.

boot, but to leave the metalwork until the fracture and ligaments have healed, usually at four to six months. In doing this one has to accept there may be some metalwork breakage and irritation of the dorsal extensor tendons in the short term. There is some evidence that fusion of the second TMTJ may give superior results, and a single randomized controlled trial[24] suggests this may give superior functional results. However, in the absence of a conclusive study and given the technical difficulty of acute fusion, a pragmatic approach should be taken. In the presence of significant intra-articular damage a fusion may be preferable.

First Metatarsal Fractures

Surgical intervention for first metatarsal fractures depends on the pattern and energy of the injury. Significant displacement, particularly with shortening and dorsiflexion, and intra-articular fractures are indications for operative reduction and internal fixation.

Approach. There are two approaches to the first metatarsal. The dorsal approach can be used to fix diaphyseal fractures and allows good access for plate fixation. The skin incision is made dorsally in line with the first ray from the medial cuneiform to the dorsolateral proximal phalanx. Care must be taken to avoid the dorsalis pedis and cutaneous branches of the deep peroneal nerve. The metatarsal is accessed between the tendons of the extensor hallucis longus and brevis. A medial approach may also be used if the fracture involves the phalanges of the hallux.

Fixation. Simple long spiral fractures can be fixed using two or more out-of-plane 2.4 or 2.7 mm lag screws. If the spiral segment is too short to accommodate two screws a neutralization plate must be used, but this runs the risk of adhesions and reduced tendon gliding. Fractures of the first metatarsal are often high energy and therefore comminuted. In comminuted fractures bridge plating is usually the option of choice, with the aim of restoring length and alignment to refunction the windlass mechanism and the sesamoid mechanism (Figure 23.6).

Postoperatively a period of immobilization in a short leg cast is appropriate. Patients can then be transferred to a walking boot if suitable fixation has been achieved. In general, bridge plating requires a longer period of immobilization.

Lesser Metatarsal Fractures

Fractures of the bases of the lesser metatarsals should raise the strong suspicion that the patient has sustained an injury to the Lisfranc joint. If the Lisfranc ligament is intact minimal displacement of the proximal metatarsals is tolerated well. Comminuted intra-articular fractures of the TMTJ are usually part of a Lisfranc injury, but if isolated injuries may be treated best with primary arthrodesis to prevent painful post-traumatic arthritis. The second and third TMTJs move little and arthrodesis is well tolerated.

Diaphyseal and distal fractures are often isolated injuries. A dorsal approach along the fractured metatarsal is used for diaphyseal and subcapital fractures, provided the overlying soft tissues are not significantly contused. The main indication for open reduction and internal fixation is displacement that is going to compromise the metatarsal parabola and lead to later metatarsalgia. The majority of patients with complete displacement and no overlap of the

(a)

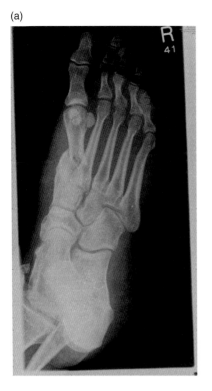

(b)

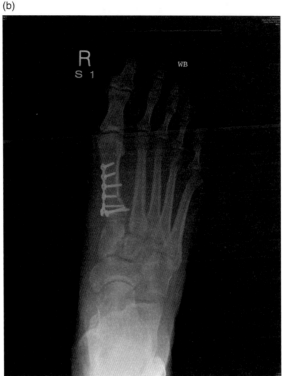

(c)

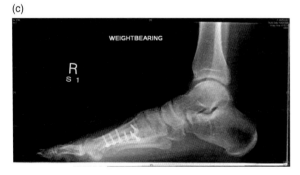

Figure 23.6 A fractured first metatarsal fixed with a plate inserted through a plantar-medial incision.

metatarsal fracture ends are going to have sufficient deformity to risk this, and they therefore merit consideration of reduction and internal fixation. Fixation is obtained with lag screws, a small plate, or a combination of both. Axial K-wires or TENS nails can be tricky to site but avoid further damage to the soft tissue envelope.

Fractures of the Base of the Fifth Metatarsal

The commonest reason for surgical intervention at the base of the fifth metatarsal is non-union of a

Jones' fracture. However, acute operative intervention may be considered in the active patient, and in particular high-level athletes, to reduce the risk of non-union and shorten the time to return to sport. Most non-unions can be addressed with a percutaneous lag screw fixation.

Approach. In many cases a percutaneous technique is often used; alternatively a lateral approach can be used to access the base of the fifth metatarsal. The skin is incised starting at the base of the fifth metatarsal extending as far distally as needed. The incision should be made at the junction of the dorsal

411

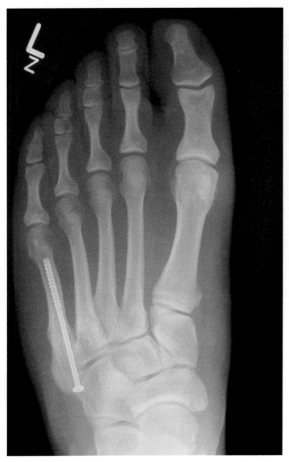

Figure 23.7 A fifth metatarsal zone 3 stress fracture internally fixed with a percutaneously inserted 5.0 mm screw.

and plantar skin, which is usually readily identifiable. Small branches of the sural nerve cross the surgical field and should be preserved. The abductor digiti quinti minimi muscle belly is divided to expose the underlying metatarsal.

Fixation. There are two common methods of fixation. In the majority, intramedullary screw fixation is used (Figure 23.7). The screw must be large enough, in any case greater than 4.5 mm, to gain purchase within the canal. It is not uncommon to need a 6.5 mm screw for the larger individual. For those patients with type 1 fractures a small fragment lag screw or a tension band wire can be used. Alternatively the fragment may be excised, and the peroneus brevis reattached with an anchor.

Initial immobilization is with a below-knee cast, which may be changed to a walking boot at the

two-week wound check. After this the patient can be allowed to weight bear as pain allows, although immobilization should not be removed for six weeks or until x-rays indicate evidence of union.

Fractures and Dislocations of the Hallux

Displaced intra-articular fractures involving the MTPJ, such as corner fractures, should be treated with open reduction and internal fixation if the fragment is large enough to be fixed. As a rule of thumb, fragments forming greater than 30% of the joint surface are suitable for fixation. Fractures of the proximal phalanx should be fixed when there is a significant rotational deformity or angulation. All open fractures of the hallux should be opened, debrided, and if appropriate stabilized.

Approach. The commonest approach used to access the hallux is the medial approach. This approach is extensile, giving access to the shaft of the first metatarsal and phalanges, as well as allowing access to the tibial sesamoid. There are three main structures at risk: the dorsomedial nerve, which is usually a terminal continuation of the superficial peroneal nerve; the medial plantar digital neurovascular bundle; and the plantar metaphyseal artery, which supplies the head of the first metatarsal. The plantar metaphyseal artery runs in the fatty soft tissues just proximal to the plantar capsular insertion into the first metatarsal head. Therefore the skin incision should be centered at the midpoint of the medial aspect of the metatarsal head and extend in the midline to the distal phalanx. To access the MTPJ the capsule must be opened and at the end of the procedure soundly repaired. When more proximal access to the metatarsal diaphysis is needed the approach is extended along metatarsal shaft, above the border of the abductor hallucis, which is retracted inferiorly.

Fixation. Corner fractures, when they require fixation, can be challenging, as the fragment is often small and reduction of the articular surface may be difficult. Fixation is usually effected with a 2.0 or 2.4 mm lag screw, applying cautious compression so as not to fracture the smaller fragment.

Shear fractures of the proximal phalanx should be reduced with pointed reduction forceps and then temporarily transfixed with a K-wire to maintain the reduction while definitive fixation is achieved. With open fractures K-wire transfixion is often an excellent treatment option.

Turf Toe

While the majority of turf toes are successfully treated non-operatively there are some instances where surgical management is preferable. There is little consensus in the literature as to the precise indications for surgery, but those cited include loss of push-off strength, significant instability, clawing, migration of the proximal sesamoid fragment, or diastasis of a bipartite sesamoid. Operative intervention is via an L-shaped medioplantar approach. The plantar plate, FHL, and sesamoids should all be assessed for injury and direct or suture anchor repair of the plantar structures undertaken. Early range of motion is important postoperatively to reduce the risk of arthrofibrosis of the sesamoids, and consequent hallux rigidus.

Dislocations or Fractures of the Lesser Phalanges

Dislocation of the lesser ray MTPJs is much more commonly chronic than acute, being secondary to hallux valgus or an inflammatory arthropathy, for example. There is usually no convincing history of trauma. These injuries will be irreducible in the casualty department, and the forefoot as a whole should be addressed.

Interphalangeal joint injuries are much commoner, and are usually traumatic. They can usually be reduced closed, and are treated with neighbor strapping. Occasionally a percutaneous axial K-wire fixation is required.

The occasional patients present late with recurrent or missed dislocation of the interphalangeal joint, usually of the fifth toe. This is best treated with a primary interphalangeal joint fusion secured with a longitudinal K-wire, or similar device.

Pitfalls

Missed Lisfranc Injuries

A significant proportion of Lisfranc injuries are missed. Late presentation with persisting symptoms makes reconstruction difficult, emphasizing the importance of early diagnosis. Significant foot trauma with gross swelling of the foot and plantar ecchymosis is an unstable Lisfranc injury, even with normal x-rays, until proven otherwise. A weightbearing radiograph, if pain allows, or a CT scan may help. Controversy exists as to when late is "too late" for open reduction and internal fixation, a problem that is frequently encountered in foot and ankle specialist practice. Certainly after six months the outcome is compromised, and TMTJ fusion is recommended.

Non-Operative Management of Lisfranc Injuries

Great caution should be taken if non-operative management is instituted. The risk of persisting incompetence of the Lisfranc ligament should not be underestimated. Weightbearing views should be used to assess the initial injury, looking for diastasis of the first and second metatarsals on the AP view and a talometatarsal angle of 0° on the lateral view. If the patient is unable to comply fluoroscopic stress views under general anesthetic may be helpful. It is important to follow the conservatively managed patient with regular weightbearing radiographs in the early stages, and if displacement occurs operative treatment should be pursued. Once the period of immobilization is complete, further weightbearing views should be obtained if symptoms persist to check for evidence of persisting incompetence.

Missed Open Phalangeal Fractures

While often seen as a trivial injury requiring little or no management great care must be made not miss an open fracture. The two key signs are bleeding from the eponychium or a laceration proximal to the nail bed. Prompt diagnosis and treatment with antibiotics is indicated, with delayed diagnosis or treatment potentially leading to osteomyelitis[25] and prolonged treatment.

Sesamoid Fractures

When there is an underlying deformity that precipitates a sesamoid fracture consideration must be given to treating this as well as the sesamoid fracture. The two deformities associated with increased risk are hallux valgus and cavus deformity. If this is not considered, particularly in the presence of a sesamoid stress fracture or non-union, the risk of treatment failure is high[26–27].

Key Points

Lisfranc

- Patients often present late through misdiagnosis or late presentation.

413

- Many patients with a persistently painful and swollen midfoot following trauma should have a Lisfranc injury considered and excluded.
- Base of metatarsal fractures are often a sign of Lisfranc disruption, even when the tarsometatarsal joint looks congruous.
- Initial investigation is with weightbearing x-rays or stress views. When these are not possible CT is mandated.
- When a conservative management course is followed, a weightbearing x-ray must be taken demonstrating that the midfoot is stable under load.
- In the acute case there is a role both for open reduction and internal fixation, and primary TMTJ fusion.

Fifth Ray

- Classification can be useful for determining risk of non-union. Fractures commonly cross the category zones and so rigid application of treatment rules should be avoided.
- Fractures in zone 2 have a non-union rate of 33% and so primary surgical intervention should be discussed with the patient.
- Zone 3 fractures have a high rate of re-fracture and where this occurs fixation should be considered.

- When using intramedullary screw fixation the screw used must be >4.5 mm in diameter; a 6.5 mm screw may be required in a larger patient.

Turf Toe

- Incidence is increasing due to the rise of synthetic sports surfaces.
- It causes long-term morbidity in 50% of athletes five years following injury.
- Commonly associated with a fracture or diastasis injury to the sesamoids.
- The majority of cases are treated non-operatively.

Sesamoid

- Bipartite sesamoids are only bilateral in 25%, thus imaging the uninjured side is of limited significance.
- Imaging is difficult and usually MRI or bone scans are required, the latter suffering from poor specificity.
- The majority of cases are fractures – either stress or acute.
- Treatment with sesamoidectomy gives good results, as does fixation +/– bone grafting.

References

1. Hetsroni I, Nyska M, Ben-Sira D, et al. Analysis of foot structure in athletes sustaining proximal fifth metatarsal stress fracture. *Foot Ankle Int.* 2010; 31(3):203–11.

2. Mologne TS, Lundeen JM, Clapper MF, O'Brien TJ. Early screw fixation versus casting in the treatment of acute Jones fractures. *Am J Sports Med.* 2005; 33(7):970–5.

3. Vranes R. Hallux sesamoids: a divided issue. *J Am Podiatry Assoc.* 1976; 66:687.

4. Bowers KD Jr, Martin RB. Turf-toe: a shoe-surface related football injury. *Med Sci Sports.* 1976; 8(2):81–3.

5. Clanton TO, Seifert S. Injuries to the metatarsophalangeal joint in athletes. *Foot Ankle.* 1986; 7:162–76.

6. Schnaue-Constantouris EM, Birrer RB, Grisafi PJ, Dellacorte MP. Digital foot trauma: emergency diagnosis and treatment. *J Emerg Med.* 2002; 22:163–70.

7. Burroughs K, Reimer C, Fields K. Lisfranc injury of the foot: a commonly missed diagnosis. *Am Fam Physician.* 1998; 58:118–24.

8. Quenu E, Küss G. Etude sur les luxations du metatarse (luxations metatarsotarsiennes) du diastasis entre le 1er et le 2e metatarsien. *Rev Chir.* 1909; 39:1093–134.

9. Hardcastle PH, Reschauer R, Kutscha-Lissberg E, Schoffmann W. Injuries to the tarsometatarsal joint. Incidence, classification and treatment. *J Bone Joint Surg Br.* 1982; 64(3):349–56.

10. Myerson MS, Fisher RT, Burgess AR, Kenzora JE. Fracture dislocations of the tarsometatarsal joints: end results correlated with pathology and treatment. *Foot Ankle.* 1986; 6(5):225–42.

11. Dameron TB Jr. Fractures of the proximal fifth metatarsal: selecting the best treatment option. *J Am Orthop Surg.* 1995; 3:110–14.

12. Lawrence ST, Botte MJ. Jones' fractures and related fractures of the proximal fifth metatarsal. *Foot Ankle* 1993; 14:358–65.

13. Lehman RC, Torg JS, Pavlov H, DeLee JC. Fractures of the base of the fifth metatarsal distal to the tuberosity: a review. *Foot Ankle.* 1987; 7(4):245–52.

14. Zanetti M, Weishaupt D. MR imaging of the forefoot: Morton neuroma and differential

diagnosis. *Semin Musculoskelet Radiol.* 2005; 9(3):175–86.

15. Chisin D, Peyser A, Milgram C. Bone scintigraphy in the assessment of hallucal sesamoids. *Foot Ankle Int.* 1995; 16:291–4.

16. Shapiro MS, Wascher DC, Finerman GA. Rupture of Lisfranc's ligament in athletes. *Am J Sports Med.* 1994; 22(5):687–91.

17. Maitra AK. Treatment of fractures of the hallux with a simple splint. *Injury.* 1987; 18(5):344–6.

18. Brodsky JW, Robinson AHN, Krause JO, Watkins D. Excision and flexor hallucis brevis reconstruction for the painful sesamoid fractures and non-unions: surgical technique, clinical results and histo-pathological findings. *J Bone Joint Surg Br.* 2000; 82:217.

19. Anderson RB, McBryde AM Jr. Autogenous bone grafting of hallux sesamoid nonunions. *Foot Ankle Int.* 1997; 18(5):293–6.

20. Blundell CM, Nicholson P, Blackney MW. Percutaneous screw fixation for fractures of the sesamoid bones of the hallux. *J Bone Joint Surg Br.* 2002; 84B:1138–41.

21. Rodeo SA, Warren RF, O'Brien SJ, Pavlov H, Barnes R, Hanks GA. Diastasis of bipartite sesamoids of the first metatarsophalangeal joint. *Foot Ankle Int.* 1993; 14:425–34.

22. Zenios M, Kim WY, Sampath J, Muddu BN. Functional treatment of acute metatarsal fractures: a prospective randomised comparison of management in a cast versus elasticated support bandage. *Injury.* 2005; 36(7):832–5.

23. Brukner P, Khan K. *Clinical Sports Medicine*, 2nd edn. (New York, NY: McGraw-Hill, 2001), p. 596.

24. Ly TV, Coetzee JC. Treatment of primarily ligamentous Lisfranc joint injuries: primary arthrodesis compared with open reduction and internal fixation. A prospective, randomized study. *J Bone Joint Surg Am.* 2006; 88(3):514–20.

25. Kensinger DR, Guille JT, Horn BD, Herman MJ. The stubbed great toe: importance of early recognition and treatment of open fractures of the distal phalanx. *J Pediatr Orthop.* 2001; 21(1):31–4.

26. Pagenstert GI, Valderrabano V, Hintermann B. Medial sesamoid nonunion combined with hallux valgus in athletes. *Foot Ankle Int.* 2006; 27:135–40.

27. Van Hal ME, Keene JS, Lange TA, Clancy WG Jr. Stress fractures of the great toe sesamoids. *Am J Sports Med.* 1982; 10:122–8.

Index